Clinical Manual Emergency Pediatrics

Sixth Edition

Clinical Manual of Emergency Pediatrics

Sixth Edition

Edited by

Jeffrey C. Gershel
Professor of Clinical Pediatrics, Albert Einstein College of Medicine, NYC Health + Hospitals Jacobi, Bronx, NY, USA

Ellen F. Crain
Professor Emerita of Pediatrics and Emergency Medicine, Albert Einstein College of Medicine, Bronx, NY, USA

Associate Editor

Sandra J. Cunningham
Associate Professor of Clinical Pediatrics and Clinical Emergency Medicine, Albert Einstein College of Medicine, NYC Health + Hospitals Jacobi, Bronx, NY, USA

Assistant Editor

James A. Meltzer
Assistant Professor of Pediatrics, Albert Einstein College of Medicine, NYC Health + Hospitals Jacobi, Bronx, NY, USA

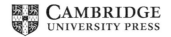

CAMBRIDGE
UNIVERSITY PRESS

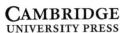

CAMBRIDGE
UNIVERSITY PRESS

University Printing House, Cambridge CB2 8BS, United Kingdom

One Liberty Plaza, 20th Floor, New York, NY 10006, USA

477 Williamstown Road, Port Melbourne, VIC 3207, Australia

314–321, 3rd Floor, Plot 3, Splendor Forum, Jasola District Centre, New Delhi – 110025, India

79 Anson Road, #06–04/06, Singapore 079906

Cambridge University Press is part of the University of Cambridge.

It furthers the University's mission by disseminating knowledge in the pursuit of
education, learning and research at the highest international levels of excellence.

www.cambridge.org
Information on this title: www.cambridge.org/9781316648636
DOI: 10.1017/9781108183109

Sixth edition © Cambridge University Press 2018

This book was previously published by Appleton-Century-Crofts and McGraw-Hill Companies, Inc.
First edition 1986, Appleton-Century-Crofts
Second edition 1992, McGraw-Hill Companies, Inc.
Third edition 1997, McGraw-Hill Companies, Inc.
Fourth edition 2003, McGraw-Hill Companies, Inc.
Fifth edition published by Cambridge University Press 2010
This Sixth edition published by Cambridge University Press 2018

A catalogue record for this publication is available from the British Library

Library of Congress Cataloguing in Publication data
Names: Crain, Ellen F., editor. | Gershel, Jeffrey C., editor. | Cunningham, Sandra J., editor. |
Meltzer, James, editor.
Title: Clinical manual of emergency pediatrics / edited by Ellen F. Crain, Jeffrey C. Gershel ; associate editor,
Sandra J. Cunningham ; assistant editor, James Meltzer.
Description: Sixth edition. | Cambridge, United Kingdom ; New York : Cambridge University Press, 2018. |
Includes bibliographical references and index.
Identifiers: LCCN 2018019470 | ISBN 9781316648636 (paperback)
Subjects: | MESH: Emergencies | Child | Infant | Emergency Medicine – methods |
Pediatrics – methods | Handbooks
Classification: LCC RJ370 | NLM WS 39 | DDC 618.92/0025–dc23
LC record available at https://lccn.loc.gov/2018019470

ISBN 978-1-316-64863-6 Paperback

Contents

Contributors

Robert Acosta, MD
Assistant Professor of Pediatrics
Albert Einstein College of Medicine
NYC Health + Hospitals Jacobi
Bronx, New York

Elizabeth Alderman, MD
Professor of Clinical Pediatrics
Children's Hospital at Montefiore
Albert Einstein College of Medicine
Bronx, New York

Tamar G. Baer, MD
Fellow
Division of Pediatric Endocrinology,
Diabetes and Metabolism
Columbia University Medical Center
New York, New York

Dan Barlev, MD
Associate Professor of Radiology
State University of New York at Stony
Brook
Winthrop University Hospital
Mineola, New York

Stephen M. Blumberg, MD
Assistant Professor of Pediatrics
Albert Einstein College of Medicine
NYC Health + Hospitals Jacobi
Bronx, New York

Haamid Chamdawala, MD, MPH
Fellow in Pediatric Emergency Medicine
Albert Einstein College of Medicine
NYC Health + Hospitals Jacobi
Bronx, New York

Katherine J. Chou, MD
Associate Professor of Clinical Pediatrics
and Clinical Emergency Medicine
Albert Einstein College of Medicine
NYC Health + Hospitals Jacobi
Bronx, New York

Anthony J. Ciorciari, MD
Associate Professor of Emergency
Medicine
Albert Einstein College of Medicine
NYC Health + Hospitals Jacobi
Bronx, New York

Keri A. Cohn, MD, MPH, DTM&H
Assistant Professor of Clinical
Pediatrics
The Children's Hospital of Philadelphia
Perelman School of Medicine at the
University of Pennsylvania
Philadelphia, Pennsylvania

Ellen F. Crain, MD, PhD
Professor Emerita of Pediatrics and
Emergency Medicine
Albert Einstein College of Medicine
Bronx, New York

Sandra J. Cunningham, MD
Associate Professor of
Pediatrics and Clinical Emergency
Medicine
Albert Einstein College of Medicine
NYC Health + Hospitals Jacobi
Bronx, New York

Michele Fagan, MD
Assistant Professor of Clinical
Pediatrics
Albert Einstein College of Medicine
The Children's Hospital at Montefiore
Bronx, New York

Kristine Fortin, MD, MPH
Assistant Professor of Clinical
Pediatrics
The Children's Hospital of
Philadelphia
Perelman School of Medicine at the
University of Pennsylvania
Philadelphia, Pennsylvania

Jeffrey C. Gershel, MD
Professor of Pediatrics
Albert Einstein College of Medicine
NYC Health + Hospitals Jacobi
Bronx, New York

Michael H. Gewitz, MD
Professor of Pediatrics
Maria Fareri Children's Hospital at WMC
Health
New York Medical College
Valhalla, New York

Beatrice Goilav, MD
Associate Professor of Pediatrics
Albert Einstein College of Medicine
The Children's Hospital at Montefiore
Bronx, New York

Waseem Hafeez, MBBS
Associate Professor of Pediatrics
Albert Einstein College of Medicine
The Children's Hospital at Montefiore
Bronx, New York

Dominic Hollman, MD
Clinical Assistant Professor of Pediatrics
Division of Adolescent Medicine
Lucile Packard Children's Hospital
Stanford University School of Medicine
Palo Alto, California

Joyce Hui-Yuen, MD, MS
Assistant Professor of Pediatrics
Hofstra-Northwell School of Medicine
Cohen Children's Medical Center
Lake Success, New York

Stephanie Jennings, MD
Clinical Assistant Professor of Pediatrics
Cleveland Clinic Lerner College of Medicine
Cleveland, Ohio

Olga Jimenez, MD
Assistant Professor of Pediatrics
Albert Einstein College of Medicine
NYC Health + Hospitals Jacobi
Bronx, New York

Daran Kaufman, MD
Assistant Professor of
Pediatrics
Albert Einstein College of Medicine
NYC Health + Hospitals Jacobi
Bronx, New York

Sari Kay, MD
Clinical Fellow
Pediatric Gastroenterology and
Nutrition
New York Presbyterian Hospital/Weill
Cornell Medicine
New York, New York

Jeffrey Keller, MD, FACS
Director of Pediatric Otolaryngology
The Mount Sinai Health System at
CareMount Medical Group
Mount Kisco, New York

Robert M. Kennedy, MD
Professor of Pediatrics
Washington University School of
Medicine
St. Louis Children's Hospital
St. Louis, Missouri

Sergey Kunkov, MD, MS
Associate Professor of Pediatrics
Stony Brook University School of
Medicine
Stony Brook Children's Hospital
Stony Brook, New York

Carolyn Lederman, MD
Assistant Clinical Professor
Columbia University
Edward. S. Harkness Eye Institute of
New York Presbyterian Hospital
New York, New York

Martin Lederman, MD
Associate Clinical Professor
Columbia University
Edward. S. Harkness Eye Institute of
New York Presbyterian Hospital
New York, New York

Shannon Liang, MD
Assistant Clinical Professor of Pediatric
Neurology
UC Davis School of Medicine
UC Davis Children's Hospital
Sacramento, California

C. Anthoney Lim, MD
Assistant Professor of Emergency Medicine
Icahn School of Medicine at Mount Sinai
New York, New York

Frank A. Maffei, MD
Associate Professor of Pediatrics
Temple University School of Medicine
Janet Weis Children's Hospital at
Geisinger
Danville, Pennsylvania

Theresa Maldonado, MD
Assistant Professor of Clinical Pediatrics
Albert Einstein College of Medicine
The Children's Hospital at Montefiore
Bronx, New York

Soe Mar, MD
Associate Professor in Neurology and
Pediatrics
Washington University School of Medicine
St. Louis, Missouri

Morri Markowitz, MD
Professor of Pediatrics
Albert Einstein College of Medicine
Children's Hospital at Montefiore
Bronx, New York

Alexandra D. McCollum, MD
Larchmont Pediatrics
CHLA Health Network Affiliate
Los Angeles, California

James A. Meltzer, MD
Assistant Professor of Pediatrics
Albert Einstein College of Medicine
NYC Health + Hospitals Jacobi
Bronx, New York

Scott Miller, MD
Assistant Professor of Pediatrics
Albert Einstein College of Medicine
NYC Health + Hospitals Jacobi
Bronx, New York

Stephanie Morris, MD
Instructor of Neurology
Washington University School of Medicine
St. Louis, Missouri

Vincent Nguyen, MD
Assistant Professor of Emergency Medicine
Albert Einstein College of Medicine
NYC Health + Hospitals Jacobi
Bronx, New York

Kirsten Roberts, MD
Assistant Professor of Pediatrics
Albert Einstein College of Medicine
NYC Health + Hospitals Jacobi
Bronx, New York

Daniel Rogers, MD
Associate Professor of Pediatrics
Geisinger Commonwealth School of
Medicine
Janet Weis Children's Hospital at Geisinger
Danville, Pennsylvania

Noé Romo
Assistant Professor of Pediatrics
Albert Einstein College of Medicine
NYC Health + Hospitals Jacobi
Bronx, New York

Michael E. Russo, MD
Fellow in Pediatric Infectious Diseases
The Children's Hospital of
Philadelphia
Philadelphia, Pennsylvania

Joshua M. Sherman, MD
Assistant Professor of Pediatrics
USC/Keck School of Medicine
Children's Hospital Los Angeles
Los Angeles, California

David P. Sole, DO
Clinical Assistant Professor of Emergency
Medicine
Temple University School of
Medicine at Geisinger
Philadelphia, Pennsylvania

Loretta Sonnier, MD
Assistant Professor
Department of Psychiatry and Behavioral
Sciences
Division of Forensic Psychiatry
Tulane University School of
Medicine
New Orleans, Louisiana

Aviva Sopher MD, MS
Assistant Professor of Pediatrics
Department of Pediatrics
Division of Endocrinology, Diabetes and
Metabolism
Columbia University Medical Center
New York, New York

Michelle Tobin, MD
Clinical Assistant Professor
Department of Pediatrics
Stony Brook Children's Hospital
Stony Brook, New York

Carmelle Tsai, MD
Fellow in Emergency Medicine
The Children's Hospital of Philadelphia
Philadelphia, Pennsylvania

Alexandra M. Vinograd, MD, MSHP, DTM&H
Assistant Professor of Clinical Pediatrics
The Children's Hospital of Philadelphia
Perelman School of Medicine at the
University of Pennsylvania
Philadelphia, Pennsylvania

Joshua Vova, MD
Adjunct Assistant Professor
Director of Rehabilitation
Children's Healthcare of Atlanta
Adjunct Assistant Professor
Morehouse School of Medicine
Atlanta, Georgia

Irfan Warsy, MD
Assistant Professor of Pediatrics
Maria Fareri Children's Hospital at WMC
Health
New York Medical College
Valhalla, New York

Mark Weinblatt, MD
Professor of Clinical Pediatrics
Stony Brook University School of Medicine
NYU Winthrop Hospital
Mineola, New York

Farhad Yeroshalmi, DMD
Clinical Associate Professor of Dentistry
Albert Einstein College of Medicine
NYC Health + Hospitals Jacobi
Bronx, New York

Preface

In this sixth edition of the *Clinical Manual of Emergency Pediatrics*, we have endeavored to remain true to our original intention: to provide a dependable, comprehensive, portable handbook that offers concise advice regarding the approach to the majority of conditions seen in a pediatric emergency department. For each topic, we have included essential points and priorities for diagnosis, management, and follow-up care, as well as indications for hospitalization and a bibliography to guide further reading.

There has been a significant paradigm shift in the care of sick and injured children. Many patients now receive acute care in primary care offices and free-standing urgicenters, which may lack the full range of resources that are available in the emergency department setting. Ill children are hospitalized less often, and they tend to be discharged back to their primary care providers sooner than ever before. In addition, increasing numbers of chronically ill and medically fragile children are receiving care in ambulatory sites. As a result of these changing practices, physicians working in non-emergency settings, such as private offices and clinics, may be faced with potential, or real, pediatric emergencies. Now, more than ever, these caregivers, as well as emergency physicians, can benefit from a practical handbook which provides a summary of the myriad acute conditions that may be encountered, along with a clear guide as to how to differentiate among them.

Since the publication of the first edition of this manual, online and portable resources have become readily available. However, many are not geared to pediatric conditions or presentations. It is our observation that there is a lack of detail, particularly when discussing differential diagnoses. Our hope is that this manual, which gathers the necessary facts and management recommendations in a user-friendly, easily accessible format, will facilitate decision-making and safe care.

In the sixth edition, we have maintained the book's unique features while making many changes that increase its utility. Because the scope of childhood illnesses and injuries seen in acute care settings is constantly increasing, we have revised and updated every chapter. We have added new sections on anti-NMDA receptor encephalitis, bedside ultrasound, commercial sexual exploitation of children, fever of unknown origin, newer "designer" drugs of abuse, ovarian emergencies, the returned traveler, and the "ouchless" emergency department. The endocrinology, gastroenterology, infectious diseases, ingestions, and neurology sections have been completely revised and updated.

A word of caution is in order. Although a manual for emergency care can be very useful, it may tempt physicians, particularly those still in training, to look for automatic solutions. It is not our intent that this text be used as a protocol book. We urge students and house staff to not use this manual as a substitute for their own critical thinking and sensitivity when caring for children and their families.

We owe special thanks to our associate editor, Sandra J. Cunningham, and assistant editor, James A. Meltzer, for their contributions and diligent editing. Their careful attention to detail has greatly improved the quality of the book, and helped to ensure that our recommendations were updated and evidence-based. Although the content of this sixth edition reflects the hard work of all the contributors and section editors, the final manuscript reflects our approach to any given illness or problem, and we are responsible for the book's content.

By what they have taught us and by their example, we are especially grateful to the pediatric emergency department nurses, attendings, and nurse practitioners at NYC Health + Hospitals Jacobi. We have become better teachers and caregivers by observing them and their interactions with patients and families.

We are particularly indebted to the Pediatric house staff, the Emergency Medicine house staff, and the Pediatric Emergency Medicine fellows at NYC Health + Hospitals Jacobi, as well as the medical students of the Albert Einstein College of Medicine. We have had the privilege of teaching and learning from all of them over the years. Their thoughtful questions provided the impetus for this manual.

This book is dedicated to the memory of Dr. Lewis M. Fraad, our beloved mentor, whose name has been memorialized in the name of our department, Lewis M. Fraad Department of Pediatrics at NYC Health + Hospitals Jacobi. Day in and day out he set an example for all of us by combining intellectual rigor with a deep respect for children and their families. He will always be with us when we are at our best.

Pediatric Emergency Management Code Card

Waseem Hafeez
Albert Einstein College of Medicine, The Children's Hospital at Montefiore

Anaphylaxis

Epinephrine: (1:1000) 0.01 mL/kg (max. 0.5 mL): IM thigh q 15 min × 3

H1: Diphenhydramine 1–2 mg/kg slow IV/IM (max. 50 mg)

H2: Famotidine 0.25 mg/kg IV (max. 20 mg)

Methylprednisolone: 2 mg/kg IV (max. <12 yr: 60 mg; ≥12 yr: 125 mg)

Bronchospasm: see Status Asthmaticus

Hypotension: Epinephrine infusion 0.1–1 mcg/kg/min)

Stridor: see Croup

Antibiotics (First Dose)

Ampicillin 100 mg/kg, Clindamycin 10 mg/kg, Gentamicin 2.5 mg/kg

Unasyn 50 mg/kg, Vancomycin 15 mg/kg, Zosyn 100 mg/kg of piperacillin

Cefoxitin 40 mg/kg, Ceftriaxone/Cefepime/Cefazolin/Cefotaxime 50 mg/kg

Asthma (Status Asthmaticus)

Albuterol neb: <20 kg, 2.5 mg; ≥20 kg, 5 mg

Albuterol continuous: 0.5 mg/kg/h

Albuterol MDI: 4–8 puffs (90 mcg/puff) q20 min

Ipratropium neb: <12 yr: 250 mcg; ≥12 yr: 500 mcg q20 min × 3 with albuterol ✓

Prednisone 1–2 mg/kg/day (max. 60 mg) PO, then 1–2 mg/kg/day

Methylprednisolone: 1–2 mg/kg (max. 125 mg) PO/IV/IM

Dexamethasone: 0.6 mg/kg (max. 10 mg) PO/IV/IM once

Magnesium sulfate: 40 mg/kg (max. 3 g) IV over 20 min (in 50 mL NS)

Epinephrine (1:1000): 0.01 mL/kg (max. 0.3 mL) SQ q 15 min × 3

Terbutaline 0.01 mg/kg IV load over 5 min then 0.2–10 mcg/kg/min

HFNC (with FiO_2 to keep O_2 sat >92%): <6 mo: 4–8 L/min; ≥ 6 mo: 6–10 L/min

BiPAP: IPAP = 8–10 cm H_2O/EPAP = 4–5 cm H_2O

Adrenal Crisis

Hydrocortisone stress dose: <3 yr: 25 mg; 3–12 yr: 50 mg; ≥12 yr: 100 mg

Burns

Parkland Formula for second and third-degree burn surface area:
NS/LR: 4 mL/kg/day × % BSA burn (half first 8 h, half over next 16 h)
Add maintenance fluids; do not add K^+ for first 48 h; < 20 kg add D_5

Diabetic Ketoacidosis

Deficit: NS/RL 10 mL/kg IV bolus over 1 h, may repeat × 1
Then NS or 0.45 NS with K^+ (½ KAcetate + ½ KPO_4) at 1½ maintenance
K^+: <3: add 60 mEq/L; 4–5: add 40 mEq/L; 5–6: add 20 mEq/L; >6: none
Add maintenance IVF over 24 h: use D_5 W if glucose <250–300 mg/dL
After 1 h: start IV regular insulin at 0.1 unit/kg/h
(if <5 yr or glucose >800 mg/dL: use 0.05 unit/kg/h)

Hypoglycemia

Glucose: <5 yr: 5 mL/kg D_{10} W; ≥5 yr: 2 mL/kg D_{25} W
Glucose infusion: D_5–$D_{12.5}$ at 6–8 mg/kg/min
Glucagon (IV/IM/SC q 20 min): <20 kg: 0.5 mg; ≥20 kg: 1 mg

Hypocalcemia

Ca Cl (10%): 0.2 mL/kg via central IV over 5–10 min (max. 1 g)
Ca gluconate (10%): 0.6 mL/kg (60 mg/kg) IV over 5–10 min (max. 3 g)

Hyperkalemia

Regular insulin 1 unit/5 g glucose plus 0.5–1 g/kg glucose
Albuterol neb <20 kg: 2.5 mg; ≥20 kg: 5 mg q 20 min × 2
Ca gluconate (10%) 0.6 mL/kg
K^+: 6–7 mEq/L: furosemide 1 mg/kg IV (max. 40 mg)
Kayexalate (no sorbitol): 1 g/kg (max. 50 g) PR

Hypertensive Emergency/Urgency

Hydralazine: 0.1–0.2 mg/kg (max. 20 mg) IV bolus q 4h
Isradipine: 0.05–0.1 mg/kg PO (max. 5 mg)
Labetalol: 0.25–1 mg/kg (max. 20 mg) IV over 2 min q 10 min
Labetalol infusion: 0.4–1 mg/kg/h (max. 3 mg/kg/h)
Nicardipine infusion: 0.5–2 mcg/kg/min

Increased Intracranial Pressure

Keep head in midline and elevate head of bed to 30°
Maintain euvolemia: NS at two-thirds maintenance

Mannitol: 0.5–1 g/kg (max. 25 g) IV over 20–30 min

Maintain pCO_2 30–35 mmHg; pO_2 80–100; pH 7.3–7.5

Rapid-Sequence Intubation (IV)

Premedicate (if indicated): atropine 0.02 mg/kg (max. 0.4 mg)

Sedation: etomidate 0.1–0.3 mg/kg (not in septic shock) or midazolam 0.1 mg/kg (max. 5 mg)

Asthma: ketamine 1–2 mg/kg or etomidate 0.1–0.3 mg/kg

Head injury/increased ICP: etomidate 0.1–0.3 mg/kg

Shock: None or ketamine 1 mg/kg or fentanyl 1 mcg/kg

Paralysis: rocuronium 1–1.2 mg/kg or vecuronium 0.1 mg/kg (max10 mg) or succinylcholine

(with atropine) infant 2–3 mg/kg; child/adolescent 1–1.5 mg/kg (max. 150 mg)

Status Epilepticus

Lorazepam: 0.1 mg/kg (max. 2–4 mg) slow IV, can repeat in once in 5 min

No IV: Diazepam 0.2–0.5 mg/kg PR (max. 20 mg); midazolam 0.2 mg/kg IM (max. 10 mg)

Fosphenytoin 20 mg PE/kg IV/IO over 10–15 min (max. 1.5 g PE)

Phenobarbital 15 mg/kg IV (max. 1 g) over 15–20 min (first-line for infants < 2 mo)

Valproate 30–40 mg/kg (max. 3 g) IV over 60 min

Levetiracetam 30–60 mg/kg IV load (max. 4.5 g)

Sedation and Analgesia

Dexmedetomidine 2 mcg /kg IV over 10 min

Etomidate: 0.15–0.2 mg/kg (max. 20 mg)

Fentanyl: 1–5 mcg /kg IV (max. 100 mcg); 1.5 mcg/kg intranasal (max. 60 mcg)

Hydromorphone: 0.015 mg/kg (max. 2 mg) IM/IV/SC

Ketamine: 1.5 mg/kg IV; 3–4 mg/kg IM (max. 75–150 mg)

Ketorolac 0.5 mg/kg (max. 30 mg) IM/IV

Midazolam: 0.1 mg/kg (max. 5 mg); 0.25–0.4 mg/kg intranasal (max. 5 mg)

Morphine: 0.1–0.2 mg/kg (max. 15 mg) IM/IV/SC

Pentobarbital 1–2 mg/kg IV (max. 100 mg); 2–4 mg/kg IM (max. 100 mg)

Propofol: 1.5 mg/kg (max. 30 mg), then 0.5 mg/kg (max. 20 mg)

Stridor/Croup

Racemic epi (2.25%) 0.05 mL/kg (max. 0.5 mL) in 3 mL NS via nebulizer q 20 min

Dexamethasone 0.3–0.6 mg/kg (max. 10 mg) IM/IV/PO

Pediatric Cardiac Arrest Algorithm–2015 Update

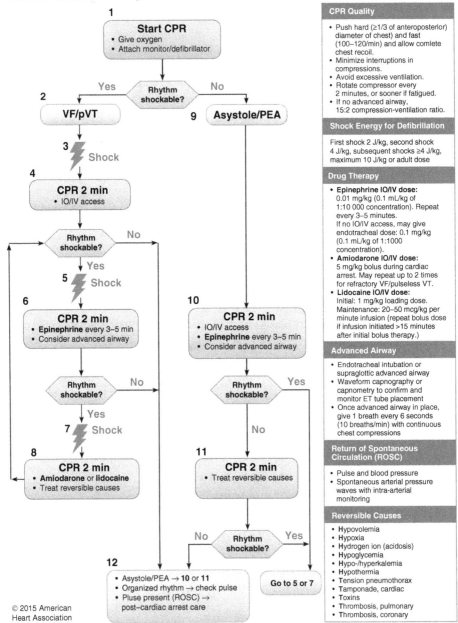

CPR Quality

- Push hard (≥1/3 of anteroposterior) diameter of chest) and fast (100–120/min) and allow comlete chest recoil.
- Minimize interruptions in compressions.
- Avoid excessive ventilation.
- Rotate compressor every 2 minutes, or sooner if fatigued.
- If no advanced airway, 15:2 compression-ventilation ratio.

Shock Energy for Defibrillation

First shock 2 J/kg, second shock 4 J/kg, subsequent shocks ≥4 J/kg, maximum 10 J/kg or adult dose

Drug Therapy

- **Epinephrine IO/IV dose:** 0.01 mg/kg (0.1 mL/kg of 1:10 000 concentration). Repeat every 3–5 minutes. If no IO/IV access, may give endotracheal dose: 0.1 mg/kg (0.1 mL/kg of 1:1000 concentration).
- **Amiodarone IO/IV dose:** 5 mg/kg bolus during cardiac arrest. May repeat up to 2 times for refractory VF/pulseless VT.
- **Lidocaine IO/IV dose:** Initial: 1 mg/kg loading dose. Maintenance: 20–50 mcg/kg per minute infusion (repeat bolus dose if infusion initiated >15 minutes after initial bolus therapy.)

Advanced Airway

- Endotracheal intubation or supraglottic advanced airway
- Waveform capnography or capnometry to confirm and monitor ET tube placement
- Once advanced airway in place, give 1 breath every 6 seconds (10 breaths/min) with continuous chest compressions

Return of Spontaneous Circulation (ROSC)

- Pulse and blood pressure
- Spontaneous arterial pressure waves with intra-arterial monitoring

Reversible Causes

- Hypovolemia
- Hypoxia
- Hydrogen ion (acidosis)
- Hypoglycemia
- Hypo-/hyperkalemia
- Hypothermia
- Tension pneumothorax
- Tamponade, cardiac
- Toxins
- Thrombosis, pulmonary
- Thrombosis, coronary

Score	Glasgow Coma Scale			Modified Glasgow Coma Scale <1 year		
	Eye opening	Verbal	Motor	Eye opening	Verbal	Motor
6	–	–	Obeys	–	–	Normal spontaneous
5	–	Oriented	Localizes	–	Coos/babbles	Withdraws to touch
4	Spontaneous	Confused	Withdraws	Spontaneous	Irritable cries	Withdraws to pain
3	To speech	Inappropriate words	Abnormal flexion	To speech	Cries to pain	Abnormal flexion
2	To pain	Nonspecific sound	Abnormal extension	To pain	Moans to pain	Abnormal extension
1	None	None	None	None	None	None

Newborn resuscitation in the ED

A. Warm, position, clear airway, dry, stimulate, reposition

B. HR <100/min: O_2 by face mask, BVM, or ETT at 40–60/min

C. HR <60/min: Chest compressions at 90/min with 30 breath/min

D. HR <60/min: Epinephrine (1:10,000 = 0.1 mg/mL) IV 0.1 mL/kg; ETT 0.5 mL/kg

Meconium with apnea or HR <100/min or limp or cyanotic: Direct ETT suction

Endotracheal tube size

Uncuffed: (Age +16)/4   Cuffed: (Age +14)/4   Premature: Gestational age (wks)/10

Endotracheal tube depth: 3 × (endotracheal tube size)

Systolic BP

Minimum: 70 + 2 × (age in years)   Maximum: 110 + 2 × (age in years)

Anion gap

= $Na^+ - (Cl^- + HCO_3^-)$; normal = 10–14 mEq/L)

Osmolality

= 2 × (Na^+ + Glucose/18 + BUN/ 2.8); normal = 275–295 mOsm/L

Acid–base

pCO2 ↑ by 10 mmHg → pH ↓ 0.08   HCO3 ↓ by 10 mEq/L → pH ↓ 0.15

Transfusion of pRBC/platelets/fresh frozen plasma/albumin/cryoprecipitate

= 10 mL/kg

Initial ventilator settings

<10 kg: Pressure-limited with IP 20 cm H_2O >10 kg: volume-preset with TV 8–10 mL/kg

Rate: Infant 20–30/min; child 18–24/min; adolescent 14–20/min

PIP =20–30 cm H_2O PEEP = 4–5 cm H_2O Inspiratory time =   I: E = 1:2
0.5–1 second

BiPAP: Initial IPAP = 8–12 cm H_2O EPAP = 4–5 cm H_2O

Chapter

Resuscitation

Waseem Hafeez, Michele Fagan, and Theresa Maldonado

Cardiopulmonary Resuscitation Overview

Cardiopulmonary arrest in infants and children is rarely a sudden event. The usual progression of arrest begins with hypoxia, hypercarbia, and acidosis resulting in respiratory failure, which eventually leads to asystolic cardiac arrest. Etiologies include sudden infant death syndrome (SIDS), respiratory disease, sepsis, major trauma, submersion, poisoning, metabolic/electrolyte imbalance, and congenital anomalies. In contrast, primary cardiac arrest is relatively rare in the pediatric age group and is most frequently caused by congenital heart disease, myocarditis, and chest trauma with myocardial injury. Although asystole and pulseless electrical activity (PEA) are the primary rhythms in pediatric cardiac arrest, patients with sudden cardiac arrest are likely to have ventricular tachycardia (VT) or ventricular fibrillation (VF). *(asystole & PEA), VT & VF*

The outcome of unwitnessed cardiopulmonary arrest in infants and children is poor. Less than 10% of pediatric patients who have out-of-hospital cardiac arrests survive to discharge and most are neurologically impaired. In contrast, about one-third of children with in-hospital cardiac arrest survive to hospital discharge, with a better neurological outcome. *Survival ~ < 10% out, 1/3 in Hospital*

Begin resuscitation with C-A-B: Chest compression, Airway and Breathing, as the key factor in return of spontaneous circulation (ROSC) and survival is the maintenance of adequate coronary artery and cerebral artery perfusion. This is best achieved by starting resuscitation with chest compressions. However, individualize the CPR sequence based upon the location of the arrest and the presumed etiology. *Start c ,Compression,*

CAB - Compression, airway, breathing.

Emergency Department Priorities *Resp Failure & shock*

To optimize outcome, it is essential to recognize early signs and symptoms of impending respiratory failure and circulatory shock prior to the development of full cardiopulmonary arrest. All equipment, supplies, and drugs must be available and organized for easy access. It is imperative that the staff have training in American Heart Association Pediatric Advanced Life Support (PALS), and routinely practice mock pediatric resuscitations. Pediatric Advanced Life Support utilizes a systematic approach to the assessment and treatment of seriously ill or injured pediatric patients.

In order to optimize care in a high-stress situation, use pre-calculated drug sheets or the Broselow tape, a height-based weight system for accurate dosing of resuscitation medication which also offers immediate access to pre-sized emergency equipment. In addition, develop and maintain a comprehensive plan to organize the resuscitation team (Figure 1.1). Assign

$$wgt\ (kg) = (Age\ (yrs) + 4) \times 2$$

$$Kg = (Age + 4) \times 2$$

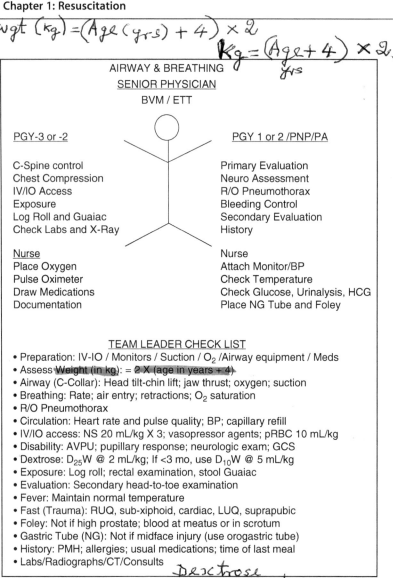

AIRWAY & BREATHING
SENIOR PHYSICIAN
BVM / ETT

PGY-3 or -2

C-Spine control
Chest Compression
IV/IO Access
Exposure
Log Roll and Guaiac
Check Labs and X-Ray

Nurse
Place Oxygen
Pulse Oximeter
Draw Medications
Documentation

PGY 1 or 2 /PNP/PA

Primary Evaluation
Neuro Assessment
R/O Pneumothorax
Bleeding Control
Secondary Evaluation
History

Nurse
Attach Monitor/BP
Check Temperature
Check Glucose, Urinalysis, HCG
Place NG Tube and Foley

TEAM LEADER CHECK LIST
- Preparation: IV-IO / Monitors / Suction / O_2 /Airway equipment / Meds
- Assess Weight (in kg): = 2 X (age in years + 4)
- Airway (C-Collar): Head tilt-chin lift; jaw thrust; oxygen; suction
- Breathing: Rate; air entry; retractions; O_2 saturation
- R/O Pneumothorax
- Circulation: Heart rate and pulse quality; BP; capillary refill
- IV/IO access: NS 20 mL/kg X 3; vasopressor agents; pRBC 10 mL/kg
- Disability: AVPU; pupillary response; neurologic exam; GCS
- Dextrose: $D_{25}W$ @ 2 mL/kg; If <3 mo, use $D_{10}W$ @ 5 mL/kg
- Exposure: Log roll; rectal examination, stool Guaiac
- Evaluation: Secondary head-to-toe examination
- Fever: Maintain normal temperature
- Fast (Trauma): RUQ, sub-xiphoid, cardiac, LUQ, suprapubic
- Foley: Not if high prostate; blood at meatus or in scrotum
- Gastric Tube (NG): Not if midface injury (use orogastric tube)
- History: PMH; allergies; usual medications; time of last meal
- Labs/Radiographs/CT/Consults

Dextrose
D_{25} 2 ml/kg
< 3 mths 5 ml/kg ($D_{10}W$)

Figure 1.1 Resuscitation team roles and preparation

a role to each team member: team leader, airway management, chest compressions, achieving vascular access, obtaining a history, medication administration, recorder, and runner. Identify a team leader early whose sole responsibility is to oversee the resuscitation and coordinate the team dynamics. Ideally, along with the physicians and nurses, a respiratory therapist and pharmacist will assist the team. Prepare the essential equipment needed for resuscitation in advance, using the mnemonic IMSOAPP (Table 1.1).

Rapid Cardiopulmonary Assessment   A A B C

Quickly perform a primary evaluation, which focuses on the Appearance, Airway, Breathing and Circulatory (ABCs) status of the patient. This initial examination provides assessment

Table 1.1 IMSOAPP mnemonic for resuscitation

I	IV fluids/IV catheter/intraosseous needle
M	Monitors: cardiorespiratory; pulse oximeter; blood pressure
S	Suction: tonsil tipped (Yankauer) and flexible catheters
O	100% Oxygen source
A	Airway equipment
	Bag-mask: different size masks
	Oral airway: nasopharyngeal and oral
	Laryngoscope with assorted blades: Miller, Macintosh
	Tracheal tube: cuffed and uncuffed, multiple sizes
	Stylet
P	Pharmacy: medications, either a pre-calculated drug sheet or Broselow tape
P	Personnel: call a code, have resuscitation team available

of the patient's acuity, and prioritizes the urgency and aggressiveness of intervention in response to the degree of physiologic compromise. Following stabilization of the ABCs, the secondary assessment includes a complete head-to-toe examination of the patient, while maintaining normothermia and normoglycemia.

Appearance

Assess the general appearance of the patient. Evaluate the activity level of the child, reaction to painful or unfamiliar stimuli, interaction with the caretaker, consolability, and the strength of cry, relative to the patient's age.

Airway   *Clear, maintainable, Unmaintainable.*

Airway patency is particularly prone to early compromise in pediatric patients, as the airway diameter and length are smaller than in adults. Determine whether the airway is clear (no intervention required), maintainable with noninvasive intervention (positioning, suctioning, oropharyngeal or nasopharyngeal airway placement, bag-mask ventilation) or not maintainable without intubation.

Breathing   *RACE*

Ventilation and oxygenation are reflected in the work of breathing and can be quickly assessed by the mnemonic RACE:

- Rate: age-dependent. Tachypnea is often the first sign of respiratory distress, but it may also be secondary to acidosis.
- Air entry:
  - listen to breath sounds in all areas: anterior and posterior chest, axillae
  - a priority is to rule-out tension pneumothorax: absent breath sounds, tracheal deviation
  - abnormal sounds: rales, rhonchi, wheezing.

5 VS ① RR ② HR ③ BP ④ T ⑤ O_2 sat.

- Color
  - pink, pallid, cyanotic, or mottled
  - pulse oximetry: use the O_2 saturation as the fifth vital sign.

- Effort/mechanics:
  - "Tripod" position, nasal flaring, grunting, stridor, head bobbing;
  - Accessory muscle use: sternocleidomastoid prominence;
  - Retractions: suprasternal, subcostal, intercostal.

The presence of abnormal clinical signs of breathing such as grunting, severe retractions, mottled color, use of accessory muscles, and cyanosis are precursors to impending respiratory failure. Abnormal Breathing - Precursor to Respy failure

Circulation

The circulatory status reflects the effectiveness of cardiac output as well as end-organ perfusion. The rapid assessment includes:

- Cardiovascular function:
  - heart rate: age-dependent
  - central and peripheral pulses: compare the femoral, brachial, and radial pulses
  - blood pressure: age-dependent; use the following guidelines to estimate the lowest acceptable (fifth percentile) systolic BP: SBP 5th perc (70 + (2 × age) yrs)
    - Newborn to 1 month = 60 mm Hg
    - 1 month to 1 year = 70 mm Hg
    - 1–10 years = 70 mm Hg + (2 × age in years)
    - >10 years = 90 mm Hg.

- End-organ perfusion (systemic circulation):
  - skin perfusion: capillary refill (<2 seconds normal), color, extremity temperature (relative to ambient temperature) adult 50 ml/hr.
  - renal perfusion: urinary output = 0.5–1 mL/kg/h (about 30 mL/h for an adolescent)
  - CNS perfusion: mental status, level of consciousness, irritability, consolability, AVPU response:

    A awake
    V responsive to voice
    P responsive to pain
    U unresponsive.

Tachycardia and tachypnea are early signs of cardiorespiratory compromise. Observe for central or peripheral cyanosis and feel the skin temperature and moisture. With the fingers at the level of the heart, apply pressure to the nail bed until it blanches, then release, timing the interval until the fingertip "pinks up." Delayed capillary refill (>2 seconds), and cool, clammy extremities are clinical indicators of poor perfusion. A systolic blood pressure below the fifth percentile (measured with an appropriate-size cuff), loss of central pulses, oliguria, and altered level of consciousness are ominous signs of impending hypotensive/decompensated circulatory shock.

Urine output - 0.5 ml - 1ml / kg / hr
Adolescents - 30ml/hr, Adult - 50ml/hr.

Initial Management

Immediate goals in the emergency department (ED) include supporting ventilation and organ perfusion. After a quick initial assessment, determine if the child is responsive and is breathing with a pulse. If the patient is unresponsive, not breathing or only gasping, without a pulse, immediately start CPR starting with chest compression, open and maintain the airway, support ventilation and perfusion, and identify and treat reversible causes (Table 1.2 and Figure 1.2).   *Start CPR c̄ CHEST Compressions.*

Airway Management

Airway management is always the initial priority. To open the airway, first use simple maneuvers such as repositioning the head, suctioning secretions from the mouth, and placing an oropharyngeal or nasopharyngeal airway.

Head Tilt–Chin Lift

Open the airway using the head tilt–chin lift technique or jaw thrust maneuver. In an unresponsive child, perform the head tilt–chin lift maneuver by placing one hand on the patient's forehead and gently tilting the head back into a neutral position. Curl the fingers of the other hand gently under the jaw near the chin, and lift the mandible upward to open the airway.

Jaw Thrust   *w/o head extension in Trauma patients.*

In a known or suspected trauma victim, use the jaw thrust maneuver without head extension. Protect the cervical spine by providing manual in-line traction. Place one hand on each side of the patient's head to hold it still, since immobilization devices may interfere with maintaining a patent airway. Perform the jaw thrust by keeping the head midline, placing the fingers at the angle of the jaw on both sides, and lifting the mandible upward and forward without extending the neck. If a jaw thrust does not open the airway, protect the C-spine and use a gentle head tilt–chin lift maneuver to open the airway, since maintaining airway patency is critical in providing adequate ventilation.

Suction Catheters   *Size = 2 × ETT size.*

Suction secretions and blood from the nasal passages, oropharynx, and trachea with flexible suction catheters. These must be available in sizes small enough to pass through the smallest endotracheal tube (ETT). A 5 Fr catheter will pass through a 2.5 mm ETT (usually 2 × the ETT size). Large rigid tonsil tip catheters (Yankauer) have rounded tips which are less likely to injure the tonsils and are useful for clearing blood and particulate matter from the mouth and hypopharynx. Limit suctioning to less than ten seconds, while monitoring the pulse oximeter and heart rate, as vigorous suctioning may cause vagal stimulation resulting in bradycardia and hypoxia.   *Limit suctioning to < 10 secs.*

Oropharyngeal Airway   *(unresponsive pt w/o a gag reflex)*

The oropharyngeal airway is an adjunct for ventilating an unresponsive patient with an absent gag reflex. It will keep the base of the tongue away from the posterior pharyngeal wall to maintain airway patency, and it will also serve as a bite block in intubated patients. Do not use in an awake patient as it can precipitate vomiting and laryngospasm.

Corner of mouth – angle of jaw.

Table 1.2 Summary of BLS maneuvers for infants, children, and adolescents

Maneuver	1 month to 1 year	≥1 year to puberty	Adolescent or adult
Scene safety	Make sure environment is safe for rescuer and victim		
Recognition of cardiac arrest	Check for responsive versus unresponsive No breathing or gasping No pulse palpated within 10 seconds Breathing and pulse check performed simultaneously		
Activate	Activate after verifying that victim is unresponsive Unwitnessed arrest: CPR 5 cycles in 2 min then call EMS Witnessed sudden arrest: activate EMS, get AED, start CPR		Activate if victim found unresponsive Activate EMS and get AED, start CPR If asphyxia arrest likely, call after CPR for 5 cycles in 2 min
Emergency Response System If mobile phone – call EMS			
CPR sequence	C – A – B (COMPRESSION – AIRWAY – BREATHING)		
C: CIRCULATION Pulse check in <10 seconds	Brachial or femoral	Femoral or carotid	Carotid
Compression landmark	Just below nipple line One rescuer: 2 fingers Two rescuers: 2-thumb encircling chest	Center of chest, mid-sternum between nipples One hand: heel of one hand only Two hands: heel of one hand with second on top	
Compression depth	At least ⅓ AP diameter About 1½ inches (4 cm)	At least ⅓ AP diameter About 2 inches (5 cm)	At least 2 inches (5 cm) But less than 2.4 inches (6 cm)
Compression rate		100–120/min	
	Push hard and fast; allow complete recoil between compressions		
Compression–ventilation ratio	One rescuer = 30:2 Two rescuers = 15:2		30:2 One or two rescuers
A: AIRWAY		Head tilt–chin lift	
	Suspected trauma: use jaw thrust. If unable, protect C-spine then head tilt–chin lift		

B: BREATHING

Initial	2 effective breaths at 1 second/breath; confirm chest rise		
Rescue breathing without chest compressions		12–20 breaths/min = about 1 breath every 3–5 seconds	10–12 breaths/min = about 1 breath every 5–6 seconds
Rescue breaths with advanced airway	10 breaths/min (1 breath every 6 seconds) with continuous chest compression (100–120/min)		
Foreign body obstruction	Back slaps and chest thrusts		Abdominal thrusts

D: DEFIBRILLATION AED
Witnessed sudden collapse

<1 year of age or weight <10 kg	≥1 to 8 years	≥8 years
Manual defibrillator preferred	Use pediatric dose-attenuator pads	Use adult pads. Do not use child pads.
Give one shock and resume CPR	Give one shock and resume CPR	Witnessed arrest: use AED. Give one shock and resume CPR. Unwitnessed arrest or AED unavailable: start CPR 5 cycles in 2 min shock

Adapted from AHA PALS 2015 Guidelines.

Breathing & Pulse check - simultaneously (10 Secs)
Unwitnessed arrest - CPR 5 cycles in 2 min, Activate EMS, & get AED
Witnessed arrest - Call Ems, get AED & CPR
Rescue Breaths - w/o ett child -10-20, Adolescent 10
c̄ adv airway 10/min, CC 100-120/min.

Defib - ≥8yrs, adult Pads.

App, Airway, Breathing, Circulation

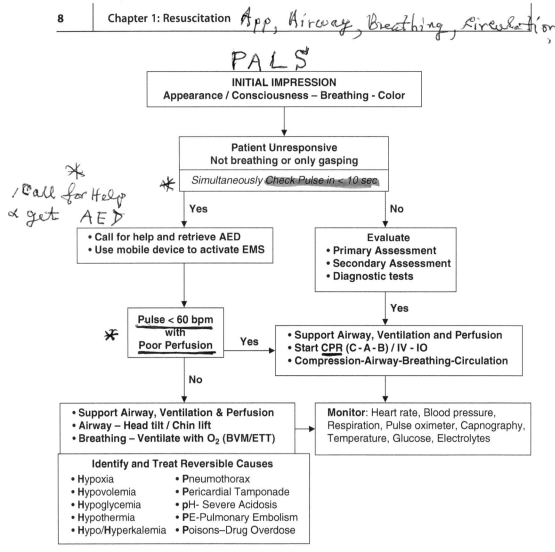

Call for Help & get AED

Figure 1.2 Summary of PALS 2015 Systematic Approach Algorithm. Adapted from AHA PALS 2015 Guidelines

An appropriately sized oral airway extends from the corner of the patient's mouth to the angle of the jaw. Use a tongue depressor to push the tongue down, and insert the oropharyngeal airway with its curvature along the hard palate. In infants and children, avoid inserting an airway that is too large. Do not attempt to insert the airway in an inverted position and then rotate it 180°, as this technique may damage the palate and push the base of the tongue posteriorly, occluding the airway. The proximal part of the oral airway is firm and flat and is designed to be placed between the teeth to prevent biting (the tracheal tube or your finger). Tape the flange to the lips to prevent it from being dislodged.

Nasopharyngeal Airway

Use a nasopharyngeal airway in an obtunded patient with an intact gag reflex to prevent upper airway obstruction secondary to a floppy tongue. Estimate the size by measuring the distance from the tip of the nose to the tragus of the ear; the appropriately sized airway

Tip of Nose to Tragus of ear.

remove only if Visible.

extends from the nostril to the base of the tongue without compressing the epiglottis. Lubricate the device and gently insert it along the floor of the nostril to avoid injuring the nasal mucosa or adenoids. A nasopharyngeal airway is ~~contraindicated~~ in a patient with a ~~suspected basilar skull or nasal bone fracture~~.

Foreign Body Airway Obstruction

If choking or airway obstruction from a foreign body is suspected and the patient is awake and can speak, make no attempts to remove the object. Allow the patient to cough and clear the airway while observing for signs of complete obstruction (i.e., the victim is gagging, struggling to breathe, has high-pitched noise while breathing, is unable to make a sound, or is cyanotic). ~~Remove the foreign body from the mouth only if it is visible.~~ Do not perform blind finger sweeps in any age because the obstructing object may be pushed further into the pharynx and cause complete airway obstruction. If the patient deteriorates, use the following procedures, as summarized in Table 1.2.

Infants <1 Year of Age
(Conscious) *(5 Back Blows, 5 chest Thrusts)*

Lay the infant prone over your thighs, with the head supported in a dependent position. Alternatively, hold the infant over your arm, in the prone position, supporting the head in your hand. Deliver five sharp back slaps, in rapid succession, between the baby's scapulae. Turn the infant over and give five chest thrusts using two fingers on the mid-sternum, as in giving chest compressions. Look into the mouth to see if the foreign body is dislodged. Repeat these maneuvers until the object is expelled or the infant becomes unconscious. ~~Do not perform abdominal thrusts in infants~~ as there is risk of injury to the abdominal organs.

Unconscious Infant
CPR 5 cycle, 30:2 over 2 mtes

First open the mouth wide by grasping the tongue and jaw, and look for the foreign body in the oral cavity. If an object is seen, remove it, but do not perform a blind finger sweep. If there is no improvement, begin cardiopulmonary resuscitation (CPR) ~~providing five cycles (30 compressions and 2 breaths per cycle) over 2 min~~. If breaths cannot be delivered, reposition the head and try again, or proceed with advanced airway maneuvers until respirations have been restored.   *CPR 30:2, 5 cycles, over 2 mtes.*

Children >1 Year of Age to Adolescent

Use the Heimlich abdominal thrust maneuver in this age group. If the patient is awake, stand or kneel behind the child and position the heel of the hand in the midline of the epigastrium with the other hand on top of the first, then give a rapid series of separate and distinct upward thrusts. With each thrust use sufficient force to dislodge the foreign body. For a small child, the heel of one hand is sufficient, as overly vigorous abdominal thrusts may cause damage to internal organs. If the patient loses consciousness, lay the child supine on the floor, reposition the head, and ~~attempt to visualize the object~~. Do not attempt a blind finger sweep. If the object is not visualized, begin CPR, providing five cycles for 2 min.

A foreign body may also be removed under direct visualization with a laryngoscope and Magill forceps. Consult an otolaryngologist to remove more distal tracheal or laryngeal foreign bodies via flexible bronchoscopy.

NC low flow 1-4 L, = FiO₂ 22-60%, Rates >3L poorly Tolerated

Oxygenation, Ventilation, and Intubation

Once the airway has been stabilized and the breathing assessed, the need for oxygenation and ventilation takes priority. Provide supplemental oxygen to all patients with respiratory distress. Reassess breathing effort by physical examination and pulse oximetry. The equipment for airway support is described below.

Nasal Cannula

HFNC Infants 1-8L/mte (FiO₂ Older 50-60L/mte >60%) (NIPPV)

Low — Oxygen can be delivered by a low-flow or high-flow system. The actual oxygen concentration delivered by nasal cannula is unpredictable, so this method is appropriate only for a patient who requires minimal O_2 supplementation. Low-flow oxygen is delivered by nasal cannula at rates of 1–4 L/min and provides O_2 concentrations of 22–60%. However, flow rates >3 L/min are usually poorly tolerated by children, while flow rates >1–2 L/min may inadvertently administer positive pressure to newborns.

High — High-flow nasal cannula (HFNC) delivers an oxygen concentration of >60% at flow rates from 1–8 L/min in infants to 50–60 L/min in children and adults. Titrate the flow for

Cpap? — additional inspiratory and expiratory pressure based on the patient's work of breathing. High-flow nasal cannula uses a special device that warms and humidifies high flows of a combination of room air and oxygen. It can be used as an alternative to standard oxygen therapy or noninvasive positive pressure ventilation in a patient with acute hypoxemic respiratory distress without hypercapnia. Maximum deliverable flow rates vary by device manufacturer.

Simple O_2 Mask

6-10L/mte, FiO₂ 30-60%

This is the most frequently used method for oxygen delivery in spontaneously breathing patients and it is more easily tolerated than nasal cannula. The actual O_2 concentration that the patient receives is dependent on the flow rate and the patient's ventilatory pattern, as room air enters through the ventilation holes on the sides of the mask. Oxygen flow rates of 6–10 L/min will deliver O_2 concentrations of 35-60% and prevent rebreathing of exhaled CO_2.

O_2 Mask With Reservoir

FiO₂ of 65-95%, (10-15L/mte) Possible

A nonrebreather (NRB) mask is another form of high-flow delivery system which consists of a simple mask attached to a reservoir bag that is connected to an oxygen source. The NRB contains one-way valves at the exhalation ports to prevent the entrainment of room air, and a second valve at the reservoir bag to prevent the entry of exhaled gas back into the reservoir bag. The reservoir bag must be larger than the patient's tidal volume (5–7 mL/kg) and remain inflated during inspiration. Oxygen concentrations up to 60% can be achieved in partial rebreathing systems, and >95% is possible if the oxygen flow rate is 10–15 L/min, and a good seal is maintained around the facemask.

Ventilation

For patients with respiratory failure, ventilate with a bag-mask apparatus until all the appropriate equipment and personnel for intubation are assembled. For optimum airway alignment, position the patient so that the auditory meatus is in line with the top of the anterior shoulder. Use the "sniffing" position in an older child by placing a folded towel under the head and elevating it. Due to a relatively larger head in an infant, keep the head

POSITION Ear Canal at level of Anterior shoulder

Infant - Towel under Shoulder, Older - Towel under Head
Large occiput   Sniffing Position.

midline and neck slightly extended with a pad under the shoulder. Flexing or overextending the neck may inadvertently obstruct the airway.

Adequate ventilation results in symmetric movement of the chest wall, with good breath sounds heard on auscultation. If the patient is making any respiratory effort, synchronize the delivered breaths with his or her efforts.

Bag-Mask O_2 10-15 L/min - F_iO_2 60-95%

The most common system used to ventilate an apneic patient consists of a self-inflating bag (Ambu Bag), an O_2 reservoir (corrugated tubing), and mask with a valve. These bags do not need a constant flow of O_2 to refill. Using a reservoir with a supplemental oxygen flow rate of 10–15 L/min delivers 60–95% oxygen to the patient. Ensure that the corrugated tubing is pulled out to its full length to allow for the largest reservoir. If the bag has a pop-off valve set at 35–45 cm H_2O, there must be a way to override it, since ventilatory pressure may be inadequate in patients with increased airway resistance or poor lung compliance.

Adequate ventilation requires an appropriate-size facemask, one that extends from the bridge of the nose to the cleft of the chin. The minimum volume for the bag in newborns, infants, and small children is 450–500 mL; use an adult bag (1000 mL or larger) for adolescents. If the only bags available are larger than the recommended size, ventilate infants and children by using the larger bag with a proper-size face mask and administering only enough volume to cause the chest to rise. Double E-C i 2 people - Better.

Use the E-C clamp technique to achieve proper ventilation with a bag-mask device. Hold the mask snugly to the face with the left thumb and index finger forming a "C." Apply downward pressure over the mask to achieve a good seal, while avoiding pressure to the eyes. Place the remaining three fingers of the left hand, which form an "E," on the mandible to lift the jaw, avoiding compression of the soft tissues of the neck. Using two hands to maintain the mask against the face (double E-C), while having a second provider compress the bag, will provide better ventilation than having a single provider perform bag-valve-mask alone.

Use a rate of 12–20 breaths per minute for an infant or child (Figure 1.2) (approximately one breath every 3–5 seconds). Squeeze the bag gently and deliver the breath over one second. Observe the chest rise, listen for breath sounds, and monitor the O_2 saturation. Bagging too rapidly or using excessive pressure causes inflation of the stomach and barotrauma to the airways. If ventilation is difficult or breath sounds are unequal, reposition the head, suction the airway, switch to two-person bag-mask ventilation, and consider foreign body aspiration or pneumothorax. An oral or nasopharyngeal airway may help to maintain a patent airway during bag-mask resuscitation, and if the patient is ventilated for more than a few minutes, place a nasogastric tube to decompress air from the stomach to minimize the risk of aspiration from vomiting.

Ventilation for > few mins in sert a NGT.

Intubation Difficult Ventilation - think FB or pneumothx,

Tracheal intubation is the best way to manage the airway during cardiopulmonary resuscitation. The indications for tracheal intubation include:

- apnea
- respiratory failure despite effective initial intervention
- lack of airway protective reflexes (gag, cough)
- complete airway obstruction unrelieved by foreign body airway obstruction maneuvers
- CNS disorder (increased intracranial pressure, inadequate control of ventilation)

Table 1.3 Laryngoscope blade size

Age	Blade sizes
Premature to newborn	Miller 00–0
One month to toddler	Miller 1
18 months to 8 years	Miller 2, Macintosh 2
≥8 years	Macintosh 3

Table 1.4 Tracheal tube size and depth

Age	Uncuffed ETT	Cuffed ETT	Depth
Premature	2.5 mm	–	6–7 mm
Newborn	3.0–3.5	–	8–10 mm
1 month to 1 year	3.5–4.0 mm	3.0 mm	10–11 mm
Older	4 + (age in years/4)	3 + (age in years/4)	3 × ETT size

Before attempting intubation, ensure that all necessary supplies, medications, and personnel are available. All equipment must be available in various sizes along with spare laryngoscope handles, bulbs, and batteries. A Broselow tape, which accurately correlates weight with length (for patients <35 kg), gives precise sizes of airway equipment, as well as appropriate drug doses. "Straight blades" (Miller) are often easier to use than "curved blades" (Macintosh) in infants and young children. Estimate laryngoscope blade size by measuring the distance from the incisors to the angle of the mandible. If the patient is between sizes, use a blade that is larger and then pull back to visualize the cords. See Table 1.3 for the most popular age-appropriate blade sizes.

ETT Tubes

Estimate the tracheal tube size by matching the diameter of the endotracheal tube (ETT) to the width of the nail of the patient's fifth finger or the diameter of the nares. Tracheal tube size for different age groups is listed in Table 1.4. Alternatively, use the following formulas, but always have available tracheal tubes 0.5 mm larger and smaller than the calculated size:

$$\text{Uncuffed ETT size} = 4 + (\text{age in years}/4)$$

$$\text{Cuffed ETT size} = 3.5 + (\text{age in years}/4)$$

Previously, cuffed tracheal tubes were indicated only in children >8 years of age. Now, low-pressure cuffed tracheal tubes may be used in all ages (except newborns), provided the cuff inflation pressure is kept <20 cm H_2O.

Prepare the tracheal tube with a stylet tip placed 1 cm from the distal end of the tube and bent in a gradual anterior curve at the distal third. The tip and cuff of the tube may be lubricated with viscous lidocaine or a water-soluble gel for easy passage.

Intubation Procedure

In an emergency situation, perform oral intubation, which is easier than nasal intubation. In general, use a straight Miller laryngoscope blade for pediatric intubations. Have a tonsil tipped suction (Yankauer) and an appropriately sized flexible suction catheter readily available. To intubate the patient, keep the head midline in the "sniffing" position. If cervical spine trauma is a concern, have an assistant maintain manual in-line stabilization during the intubation, avoiding traction or movement of the neck. Continuously monitor the heart rate and pulse oximeter throughout the procedure.

Place the thumb and index finger of the (gloved) right hand into the right side of the patient's mouth. Place the index finger on the patient's upper teeth and the thumb on the lower teeth, using the scissor technique to open the mouth as wide as possible. Hold the laryngoscope in the left hand and introduce the blade into the right edge of the mouth, sweeping the tongue toward the left and out of the line of vision. Position a straight blade under the epiglottis and place a curved blade into the vallecula. Lift by pulling the handle of the laryngoscope up and away at a 45° angle to the floor, in the direction of the long axis of the handle. If the blade is in too deep, slowly withdraw it until the glottis pops into view. Be careful not to tilt the handle or blade, which may risk breaking or damaging the teeth.

The routine use of cricoid pressure (Sellick maneuver) during tracheal intubation in cardiac arrest is not recommended, as it may not prevent aspiration, while potentially interfering with the delivery of positive pressure breaths.

Once the vocal cords are exposed, introduce the ETT from the right side of the mouth (not down the barrel of the blade). Advance the ETT until the cuff just passes beyond the vocal cords. Uncuffed tubes often have a mark at the distal end of the tube, which when placed at the level of the cords will position the distal tip in the mid-trachea. As an alternative, estimate the tube depth to be equal to 3 × ETT size. A proper-size ETT easily passes through the cords. If it meets resistance in the subglottic area, do not try to force it through. Rather, replace it with a smaller tube. Hold the tube securely against the upper teeth or gums and carefully withdraw the laryngoscope first, and then remove the stylet from the ETT. If the patient was intubated with a cuffed tube, inflate the cuff to a pressure of <20 cm H_2O.

Confirming Position *Sym - /chest rise, Equal BS, CO_2, O_2.*

Verify proper tube placement by listening for equal breath sounds and observing symmetrical rise of the chest. Confirm the presence of exhaled CO_2 from the tracheal tube with either a colorimetric CO_2 detector or capnography, and use a pulse oximeter to monitor oxygen saturation. Colorimetric devices are inaccurate if the patient does not have a perfusing rhythm (even with appropriate chest compressions) or the patient weighs <2 kg. Use continuous quantitative waveform capnography (PetCO$_2$) to confirm correct placement of the ETT and to monitor intubated patients throughout the periarrest period. If breath sounds are louder over the stomach than the chest, or if it is unclear that the tube is in the trachea, remove the tracheal tube and ventilate by bag-mask. An audible air leak is expected with an uncuffed tube, but if there is a large air leak or none at all, the tube size may be inadequate; replace with an appropriately sized ETT. Secure the ETT to the patient's face with tape or use a tracheal tube holder. Obtain a chest radiograph to confirm that the tip of the tube is opposite T2 (one fingerbreadth above the carina). Be aware that neck extension or head movement brings the tube higher, while neck flexion pushes the ETT deeper.

Complications

If the patient deteriorates after endotracheal intubation, use the mnemonic DOPE to reassess: Displacement of the tube into the esophagus or down the right mainstem bronchus; Obstruction of the tube with blood, secretions or kinking; Pneumothorax with decreased breath sounds and chest expansion on the affected side and deviation of trachea to the opposite side; or Equipment malfunction. If the patient is on a ventilator, disconnect and either attempt to ventilate with a bag or replace the ETT.

Rapid-Sequence Intubation

The goals of rapid-sequence intubation (RSI) are to create ideal intubating conditions by attenuating airway reflexes while minimizing elevations of intracranial pressure and maintaining adequate blood pressure. Rapid-sequence intubation is indicated for patients who require emergent tracheal intubation but are at high risk for pulmonary aspiration of gastric contents. Medications to facilitate intubation are rarely needed for patients who are moribund or in cardiac arrest, or for newborns within a few hours of delivery.

Anticipate the possibility of an unsuccessful intubation and prepare for alternate airway techniques before initiating sedation. Also, expect a difficult intubation and request help for patients with significant facial trauma, restricted neck extension, or if the tip of the uvula is not visible when the mouth is opened. Do not use sedation or muscle relaxation if there is any concern that bag-mask ventilation will be inadequate.

> ✴ NEVER sedate or paralyze a patient whom you may not be able to ventilate!

Procedure

Rapid-sequence intubation involves the use of premedications to minimize adverse events; sedative/hypnotic agents with rapid onset and short duration of activity; and neuromuscular blocking agents, with the goal of gaining immediate control of the airway, all performed in rapid sequence. Calculate and prepare all of the medications before beginning RSI.

Pre-Oxygenation

While preparing for RSI, have the patient breathe 100% oxygen via a nonrebreather face mask for at least 3 min. If the patient is apneic or has inadequate respiratory effort, deliver 4–5 breaths by bag-mask in 30 seconds, which establishes an oxygen reserve that will last up to 4 min in an infant and longer in older children and adolescents. Providing continuous oxygen via nasal cannula during intubation (apneic oxygenation) may allow for a longer interval for attempting intubation before the patient experiences oxygen desaturation. During the period of pre-oxygenation, determine the likelihood of a difficult intubation, establish intravenous access, place the patient on cardiac and pulse oximeter monitors, and assemble all necessary equipment and personnel for tracheal intubation.

History and Physical Examination

No single feature on physical examination accurately predicts a difficult intubation. Therefore, perform a detailed pre-sedation assessment, including the SAMPLE history and a focused physical examination. A SAMPLE history is:

Signs and symptoms

Allergy: allergy to drugs, latex, foods

Medications: current prescription and nonprescription drugs

Past medical history: significant past medical and surgical history including asthma or bronchospasm, neuromuscular disease, previous difficult intubation(s), micrognathia, poor neck mobility

Last meal time: last oral intake and type of food

Event: recent events or history of present illness.

Upper Airway Examination

Ask a cooperative patient to open the mouth as wide as possible, with the tongue fully protruded. The Mallampati airway class I and II (visible faucial pillars and uvula) indicates relatively easier airway management (Figure 1.3). Use the "3–3–2 rule," which is a predictor of difficult intubation in adults. The patient should be able to place three fingers between the open incisors, three fingers from the mental tubercle of the mandible to the thyroid (two fingers in children, one finger in infants), and two fingers from the laryngeal prominence to the floor of the mouth.

If the patient cannot cooperate, gently open the mouth (if possible) and use a direct laryngoscope blade in the manner of a conventional tongue blade to assess the size of the tongue compared with that of the oropharynx. If this assessment reveals a large tongue to oropharynx ratio or it cannot be done, assume that direct laryngoscopy will be difficult.

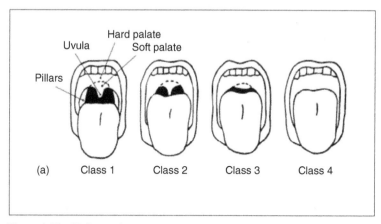

Figure 1. The Mallampati score:
 Class 1. Complete visualization of the soft palate
 Class 2. Complete visualization of the uvula
 Class 3. Visualization of only the base of the uvula
 Class 4. Soft palate is not visible at all

Figure 1.3 Mallampati classification.
From: Mallampati SR, et al: A clinical sign to predict difficult tracheal intubation: a prospective study. *Can Anaesth Soc J* 1985; 32:429.

Table 1.5 Sedative agents for rapid-sequence intubation

Clinical status	Agents
Normotensive	Etomidate 0.3 mg/kg
	or Midazolam 0.3 mg/kg
	or Propofol 1.5–3 mg/kg
Mild hypotension/no head injury	Etomidate 0.3 mg/kg
	or Ketamine 1–2 mg/kg
	or Fentanyl 1–4 mcg/kg
Severe hypotension/no head injury	None
	or Etomidate 0.2–0.3 mg/kg
	or Fentanyl 1–2 mcg/kg
Head injury/no hypotension	Etomidate 0.3 mg/kg
Head injury with mild hypotension	Etomidate 0.3 mg/kg
	or Midazolam 0.1–0.2 mg/kg
Status asthmaticus	Ketamine 1–2 mg/kg
Status epilepticus	Midazolam 0.1–0.3 mg/kg

Premedications, Sedative/Hypnotics and Paralytics (Table 1.5)

The choice of premedication drugs for RSI will depend on the clinical situation as well as individual experience of the provider with these agents. The patient may be given a premedication agent (e.g., atropine or lidocaine), then a short-acting sedative/analgesic (e.g., etomidate, thiopental, midazolam, ketamine, fentanyl, or propofol) followed immediately by a short-acting muscle relaxant (e.g., succinylcholine or rocuronium).

Premedication

Atropine (0.02 mg/kg; No Minimum Dose When Used as a Premedication for Emergency Intubation). Atropine as a premedication to prevent bradycardia is not routinely indicated. However, it may be useful in specific emergency intubations: when drugs (e.g., succinylcholine or fentanyl) which cause bradycardia are used; when the patient is already bradycardic at the time of intubation; or when there is a need to dry excessive secretions, permitting easier airway visualization during intubation.

Lidocaine (1–1.5 mg/kg). Lidocaine will attenuate the hypertension, tachycardia, and gagging response which occur during manipulation of the airway during laryngoscopy, when given 1–3 min prior. It may be useful for patients with head injuries and suspected raised intracranial pressure.

Analgesia-Sedation

Etomidate (0.3 mg/kg). Etomidate is a short-acting anesthetic that decreases intracranial pressure but has minimal hemodynamic effects. It is the drug of choice for RSI in most clinical situations. Do not use etomidate if there is evidence of septic shock, since even a single dose can cause adrenal suppression, which is associated with a higher mortality rate in children. Since etomidate has no analgesic properties, small doses of fentanyl (1–2 mcg/kg) may also be needed.

Midazolam (0.1–0.3 mg/kg). This rapid-acting benzodiazepine produces potent amnesia and sedation. At RSI doses, which are higher than that used in procedural sedation, side effects include respiratory and myocardial depression.

Ketamine (1–2 mg/kg). Ketamine is a short-acting dissociative anesthetic agent that causes rapid sedation, amnesia, and analgesia. Ketamine maintains blood pressure and increases intracranial blood flow, which makes it useful for hypovolemic patients. It is also beneficial in patients with status asthmaticus, in whom it has been shown to decrease bronchospasm. Side effects include ICP elevation, emergence phenomenon, laryngospasm, and excessive airway secretions. Its use is relatively contraindicated in patients with hypertension, head injury, and psychiatric disorders. Excessive airway secretions may be controlled by pretreatment with atropine, and emergence reaction may be attenuated with midazolam.

Fentanyl (1–4 mcg/kg). Fentanyl is a rapid-acting narcotic analgesic with minimal cardiovascular effects, but it may cause respiratory depression. A significant side effect is chest wall rigidity, which usually occurs with rapid injection or using higher doses (10 mcg/kg). The combined use of opioid medications with benzodiazepines or other drugs that depress the CNS increase the risk of serious adverse reactions, including respiratory failure.

Propofol (1.5–3 mg/kg). Propofol is an extremely rapid-acting non-barbiturate sedative-hypnotic agent with no analgesic properties that produces general anesthesia. The onset of effect is extremely rapid, with short duration of action, and is an excellent induction agent in hemodynamically stable patients. It decreases ICP and cerebral metabolism, but also causes bradycardia and significant decrease in mean arterial blood pressure. This hypotensive effect limits its use in trauma patients. A pre-induction fluid bolus with normal saline may minimize its hypotensive effect. It is contraindicated in patients with egg or soy allergies.

Muscle Relaxants

Neuromuscular blocking agents (NMBs) rapidly cause paralysis and relaxation of the airway muscles by blocking the neuromuscular junction. Their use has been shown to significantly improve success of tracheal intubation and reduce complications. Use an NMB agent for all intubations unless there are contraindications, or if a difficult airway is anticipated. In such cases, use light sedation only.

Succinylcholine (infants: 1–2 mg/kg; children and adolescents 1–1.5 mg/kg). This is the most rapid-onset and shortest-acting muscle relaxant available. It is widely used because of its fast onset of action (<1 minute) and recovery (within 5–10 minute). Pretreatment with atropine may prevent potential serious bradyarrhythmias and excessive bronchial secretions (especially in children). Succinylcholine may cause an acute rise in intracranial pressure. Contraindications to using succinylcholine include: patients with chronic myopathy; increased intracranial and intraocular pressure; rhabdomyolysis (burn and crush injuries); preexisting hyperkalemia; and history of malignant hyperthermia.

[handwritten top margin: Presure *, PIP 20-25 cm H₂O, Both, <10kg <1yr, PIP NB 15-25, infants 20-25 cm H₂O start 100% O₂, Peep 3-5 cm, RR 20-40, IT 0.8-1 sec, I/E 1:2]*

Rocuronium (0.9–1.2 mg/kg). Rocuronium is a nondepolarizing muscle relaxant with a rapid onset of action (30–60 seconds) and minimal hemodynamic side effects. Myasthenia gravis is the only specific contraindication for this class of NMB agents. Rocuronium produces intubating conditions similar to succinylcholine, but with a longer duration of action (45 minutes versus 5–10 minutes).

Post-Intubation Monitoring *[handwritten: Insert NGT]*

Once the ETT is secured and the position is radiographically confirmed, provide adequate sedation and analgesia, and continue muscle paralysis with a long-acting agent (vecuronium or rocuronium) if indicated. To reduce the risk of aspiration, insert a nasogastric tube as soon as possible to decompress the stomach, especially in infants and children. However, use an orogastric tube if a basilar skull fracture or nasal fracture is suspected.

Initial Mechanical Ventilator Settings

The two modes of mechanical ventilation for emergency ventilation in children are pressure-limited and volume-limited support. For newborns and infants <10 kg, pressure-limited ventilators are most often used, while volume-limited ventilators are indicated for older children. When using pressure-limited ventilators, start with peak inspiratory pressures (PIP) of 15–25 cm H_2O for newborns and 20–25 cm H_2O for infants <1year of age, with a positive end-expiratory pressure (PEEP) of 3–5 cm H_2O. Set the respiratory rate appropriate for age (20–40/min). For volume control ventilation, begin with tidal volumes of 6–8 mL/kg. Set an initial PEEP of 5 cm H_2O, unless contraindicated, with respiratory rates of 20–30/min in children, and 12–20/min in adolescents. For both types of ventilators, initially use 100% O_2, an inspiratory time of 0.8–1 second, and the inhale/exhale (I/E) ratio set at 1:2. Once the initial settings have been established, monitor continuously, making appropriate adjustments as dictated by the patient's clinical condition.

Alternate/Adjunctive Airway Techniques *[handwritten: HFNC, NIPPV, LMA]*

Alternate advanced airway techniques are useful for securing a difficult airway when intubation is not feasible or unsuccessful. The presence of certain congenital anomalies (Pierre Robin, Beckwith–Wiedemann, Down syndrome), anatomical defects (neck mass, laryngeal hemangioma, subglottic stenosis), or disease states (epiglottitis, angioedema, facial/neck trauma) may necessitate the use of advanced airway techniques. These include HFNC, noninvasive positive pressure ventilation (NIPPV), Heliox, and laryngeal mask airways (LMA). Other advanced airway techniques, such as fiberoptic laryngoscopy, lighted stylet, needle cricothyrotomy, or surgical cricothyrotomy, require training and experience to perform successfully.

Noninvasive Ventilation

Noninvasive ventilation (NIV) provides short-term mechanical ventilation without placement of a tracheal tube in stable, spontaneously breathing, alert, and cooperative patients. Although tracheal intubation is often a life-saving procedure, NIV functions to bridge the gap between maximal medical management and intubation. Benefits include decreasing the work of breathing, improving oxygenation, and avoiding common complications of intubation. It is important to note that NIV is not a replacement for tracheal intubation in patients

Volume >10 kg >1 yr.

TV 6-8 ml/kg, Initial peep ~5 cm H₂0   RR - 20-30 - y
12 - 20 - Adolesc

who have life-threatening respiratory failure or require airway protection. It is contra-indicated in patients who are hemodynamically unstable, lethargic, vomiting, or have cardiac dysrhythmias. The decision to use NIV is dependent on the patient (conscious and cooperative), specific disease (status asthmaticus, bronchiolitis, acute pulmonary edema, and neuromuscular disease), and whether airway protection is required. *HFNC - 2L/mt*

The common NIPPV methods include HFNC, continuous positive airway pressure *× ↑* (CPAP), and bilevel positive airway pressure (BiPAP). CPAP and BiPAP are delivered via a nasal or full-face mask in children and by nasal prongs in infants. Straps hold the BiPAP face mask firmly to the patient's face to create a tight seal. Neonates, who are obligate nose breathers, generally do not tolerate BiPAP, but may benefit from nasal prong CPAP or HFNC. Typical initial settings for CPAP include an inspiratory positive airway pressure (IPAP) of 5 cm H_2O, and for BiPAP 8–10 cm H_2O, with an expiratory positive airway pressure (EPAP) of 5 cm H_2O. Titrate these settings upwards in 2 cm H_2O increments until the desired effects are achieved. Adjust the FiO_2 to maintain a target oxygen saturation of > 92–95%. Start HFNC at 1–2 L/kg/min, and titrate up based on patient response.

Monitor the patient closely for worsening respiratory failure with serial lung exams, vital signs and oxygen saturation measurements. If the patient's respiratory status worsens or does not improve, discontinue NIPPV and perform tracheal intubation. *(Titrate 2 cm increments)*

Infants, .   older - CPAP - 5 cm H₂O

Heliox   *Nasal prongs. masks. Bipap - 8 - 10 cm H₂0 Iy, Exp 5 cm*

Helium is a biologically inert gas that decreases turbulent gas flow when mixed with oxygen. Heliox improves delivery of oxygen and aerosolized medications to constricted peripheral airways, thus reducing the work of breathing. It has been used in conditions that are *CPAP 5* refractory to medical measures, such as status asthmaticus, moderate to severe bronchiolitis, and severe croup. Heliox is delivered in mixtures of 80% helium and 20% oxygen (80/20 *Bipap* Heliox) or 70% helium and 30% oxygen (70/30 Heliox). The low FiO_2 in the gas mixture is *10/5* an important limitation of Heliox use, so that it may not be adequate to use for patients with hypoxemia. Administer to spontaneously breathing patients by using a facemask and reservoir bag. Improvement of oxygenation and reduction of respiratory distress generally occurs within several minutes of Heliox initiation. If there is no improvement, or worsening of the patient's clinical status, change to an alternate method of ventilation. *Heliox 80/20 or 70/30.*

Laryngeal Mask Airway   *risk - aspiration,*

The laryngeal mask airway (LMA) is a supraglottic airway that is indicated for patients who require an airway but cannot be tracheally intubated or adequately ventilated with a bag-mask. It can be used in patients with decreased airway reflexes (i.e., obtunded or comatose). The LMA consists of a tube attached to a mask, rimmed with a soft, inflatable cuff. When properly placed, the LMA sits in the hypopharynx around the glottic opening and directs air into the trachea. Unlike a tracheal tube, it will not fully prevent aspiration of gastric contents into the trachea. *opening - faces the Tongue.*

Select the appropriate-size LMA (Table 1.6) and check for possible air leaks by inflating the cuff. Hold the LMA like a pen, with the index finger of the dominant hand placed at the junction of the tube and proximal aspect of the mask. Lubricate the posterior surface of the deflated mask, and orient it so that the opening is directed toward the tongue. With one smooth motion, insert the mask firmly along the hard palate and advance until resistance is *✶* encountered. With the tip of the mask placed in the hypopharynx, inflate the cuff. Auscultate the lungs to confirm correct placement. If endotracheal intubation is

Lubricate the posterior surface.
Insertion - opening should face the Tongue.

You may intubate through the LMA.

Table 1.6 Laryngeal mask airway sizes (LMA North America, Inc.)

Mask size	Patient size	Maximum cuff volume
1	Neonates/infants up to 5 kg	Up to 4 mL
1½	Infants 5–10 kg	Up to 7 mL
2	Infants/children 10–20 kg	Up to 10 mL
2½	Children 20–30 kg	Up to 14 mL
3	Children 30–50 kg	Up to 20 mL
4	Adults 50–70 kg	Up to 30 mL
5	Adults 70–100 kg	Up to 40 mL
6	Adults >100 kg	Up to 50 mL

subsequently necessary, insert the ETT blindly through the properly placed LMA as it will be directed into the trachea.

There are newer LMAs available for specific situations. One version (Proseal LMA) has a parallel drainage tube attached to the airway tube to allow passage of a nasogastric tube, potentially decreasing the risk of aspiration. Other variations include the intubating LMA (Fastrach LMA), which is designed to facilitate blind tracheal intubation while allowing for continuous positive pressure ventilation, and the LMA CTrach, which has a built-in fiberoptic video screen for ease of intubation.

Circulation

Chest Compressions

After beginning chest compression and stabilization of ventilation, the next priority is establishing cardiovascular perfusion. However, in a real-life scenario, the code team, with assigned roles (Figure 1.1), will be performing all tasks simultaneously. Begin chest compressions in patients with cardiac arrest or in an unresponsive child with gasping respirations and a heart rate <60 bpm, associated with signs of poor perfusion (altered mental status, delayed capillary refill, thready or absent pulses, cool extremities, hypotension). To be effective, deliver chest compressions on a firm surface. Components of high-quality CPR include the following:

- "Push fast." Perform chest compressions at a rate of 100–120 compressions per minute. For the lone rescuer, use a compression–ventilation ratio of 30:2 for all ages. After giving 30 compressions, provide 2 breaths then immediately resume compressions, providing 5 cycles in about 2 minutes. For two-rescuer infant and child CPR, one provider performs 15 chest compressions while the second rescuer opens the airway with a head tilt–chin lift maneuver and delivers two breaths. A compression–ventilation ratio of 15:2 provides more ventilations per minute, which is appropriate for most hypoxic, hypercarbic pediatric arrests.
- "Push hard." For an infant, depress the chest at least one-third the anterior–posterior (AP) diameter of the chest, or approximately 1.5 inches (4 cm). For children and adolescents, depress the chest 2 inches (5 cm). Adequate compressions usually generate

Single – 30:2 – all cases & ages.
Two – 15:2 – one compresses, other ventilates.
5 cycles in 2 mts – then rotate.

HR 100-120/mte, Pulse check < 10 secs.

C:V w/o airway, Coordinate; i airway - asynchronous

a pulse. Coordinate compressions with ventilations to avoid simultaneous delivery and minimize interruptions in chest compressions. However, once the airway is secured by tracheal intubation, compressions and ventilation may be asynchronous and still be effective.

- Compression landmarks. In infants, the lone rescuer should compress the sternum with two fingers placed just below the intermammary line. Push straight down, making sure to make the compressions smooth, not jerky. Avoid compression over the xiphoid or ribs, which may damage internal organs. When CPR is provided by two rescuers, the two-thumb encircling hands technique is recommended. Place both the thumbs together over the lower third of the sternum and encircle the infant's chest with both hands. Forcefully compress the sternum with the thumbs, being careful to not compress the lateral walls of the chest with the hands. In children, compress the lower half of the sternum with the heel of one or two hands. For adolescents, compress the lower half of the sternum with the heel of two hands. The long axis of both heels should be placed parallel with the long axis of the sternum; straighten the arms, lock the elbows, and position the shoulders over the arms so that the body weight is added to the force of the compressions.

- Allow complete chest recoil. After each compression, allow the chest wall to recoil completely, which permits the heart to refill with blood and improves the blood flow to the body during CPR. Do not lean on the chest. *Pulse check < 10 secs.*

- Minimize interruptions of chest compressions. Limit pulse check to under ten seconds. When chest compressions are interrupted, coronary perfusion pressure rapidly declines, which may require several chest compressions to restore adequate coronary pressure once compressions are resumed. *Rotate roles every 2 mtes.*

- Rotate the compressor role approximately every two minutes, as rescuer fatigue is common and can lead to inadequate compression rate and depth, with deterioration in CPR quality. To prevent compressor fatigue, rescuers should switch compressor and ventilation roles approximately every five cycles (about two minutes). To minimize interruptions in chest compressions, the switch should be anticipated by the providers and accomplished as quickly as possible, ideally in under five seconds.

The level of end-tidal carbon dioxide tension ($PetCO_2$) correlates with coronary and cerebral perfusion pressures and is predictive of the outcomes of cardiopulmonary resuscitation. The use of $PetCO_2$ measurement may help guide therapy especially for monitoring cardiac output and the effectiveness of chest compressions during CPR or shock.

Vascular Access

Spend no more than 1–2 minutes attempting peripheral vascular access in cardiac arrest or other emergent situations. Intraosseous access (IO) may be easily established and more rapidly achieved than IV access. In any patient requiring resuscitation, make sure to have two functioning lines. *2 lines.*

Intraosseous Approach   *all ages.*

The IO approach allows for rapid vascular access for patients of all ages. Any drug or fluid normally given through the IV route, including blood products, can be given via the IO needle, although high flow rates are not possible without using an infusion pump. The IO needle is an emergency access device only. Replace it with another secure intravascular catheter or central line as soon as possible to prevent complications, such as infection, or compartment syndrome from fluid extravasation.

Intraosseous Technique

The primary site for IO insertion is the proximal tibia. Other acceptable sites are the distal tibia, proximal humerus, and anterior superior iliac spine. Position the leg in external rotation, locate the tibial tuberosity, and palpate approximately two fingerbreadths (one fingerbreadth in infants) distally on the medial flat portion of the tibia. Prepare the puncture site with a topical antiseptic (e.g., povidone-iodine). In a conscious patient, anesthetize the puncture site with 1–2 mL of 1% lidocaine. Contraindications to IO needle placement include a fracture or overlying skin infection at the site.

Intraosseous Needle

The Jamshidi IO needle is available in 18 G for infants and 15 G for all others, while the Cook IO needle is available in 16 G and 18 G sizes. Select the appropriate site and direct the IO needle perpendicular to the bone. Puncture the skin first, so that the needle is touching the bone. For manual IO insertion, use steady pressure with a screwing motion until a sudden loss of resistance is felt, indicating that the needle has entered the marrow cavity. If placed correctly, the needle will stand freely and upright without support. Remove the stylet and aspirate with a syringe. Inability to aspirate blood does not indicate improper placement, while infusion of fluid easily without extravasation or resistance confirms proper placement. After proper placement is determined, tape the needle in place to prevent accidental dislodgement. If fluid does extravasate (the calf expands or feels cold), remove the needle and make an attempt on the other side. Do not attempt more than once in the same bone.

Automated IO Infusion (IO Gun)

There are various automated IO infusion devices on the market that are designed for use in children and adolescents. If your ED stocks one of these automated devices, become familiar with it and follow the specific product directions.

Fluid Resuscitation

Critically ill
Shock or Arrest } *Use a Syringe .*
infuse rapidly in mls,

Shock and circulatory collapse may be the primary cause of cardiopulmonary arrest, and restoration of the circulating blood volume by fluid therapy is a mainstay of shock resuscitation. Once vascular access (peripheral IV, IO, central line) is established, give an initial fluid bolus of 20 mL/kg of an isotonic crystalloid solution. In patients who are critically ill or in cardiopulmonary arrest, use a syringe to infuse the fluid rapidly over a few minutes. If cardiogenic shock is suspected, give smaller fluid boluses of 5–10 mL/kg over 10–20 minutes and reassess after each bolus. For hypovolemic trauma victims, consider giving 10 mL/kg of O-negative packed red blood cells, if readily available.

Rapid infusion of dextrose-containing solutions results in an osmotic diuresis and is contraindicated in the initial phase of fluid resuscitation. Fluid resuscitation is particularly challenging in patients with cardiac disease, diabetic ketoacidosis (DKA), calcium channel or beta-blocker ingestion, or head injury, as restoring and maintaining adequate tissue perfusion must be balanced with the risk of worsening cardiac output or cerebral edema.

Base the decision to give additional IV fluids on frequent reassessments of perfusion: mental status, quality of pulses, blood pressure, heart rate, capillary refill, and urine output. In severe shock, give additional isotonic crystalloid solution boluses of 20 mL/kg, up to a total of 60 mL/kg, until the vital signs and perfusion are restored, while monitoring for signs of fluid overload. If further fluid is required, add pressors (see below) to increase myocardial contractility and maintain adequate vascular tone. If the patient is in septic shock, there may be significant capillary leakage. Large fluid volumes >60 mL/kg or 5% albumin given in 10 mL/kg doses may be required.

cold shock - Epi

Vasoactive Infusions   *warm shock - Norepi.*

Vasoactive agents (Figure 1.4) are the drugs of choice for improving myocardial contractility and cardiac output in patients with shock who have received adequate fluid administration. Because of their short half-life and potency, they are given as an infusion. The choice of agent is determined by the etiology contributing to shock; they include epinephrine, norepinephrine, dopamine, dobutamine, milrinone, or inamrinone. In patients who remain hypotensive despite adequate fluid resuscitation, epinephrine infusion is preferable for children with hypodynamic cold shock (low cardiac output states). Norepinephrine is the agent of choice for fluid-refractory warm septic shock (hyperdynamic cardiac output, bounding pulses, vasodilation, and wide pulse pressure). Dobutamine improves systolic function and decreases systemic vascular resistance without significantly increasing heart rate, and is effective for patients with cardiomyopathy and congestive heart failure. For patients with adequate blood pressure but with persistent signs of shock, use milrinone or inamrinone to improve cardiac output by reducing afterload due to its vasodilator effects. If the desired effect is not achieved with one agent, combinations of several agents may be necessary.

Epinephrine (0.1–1 mcg/kg/min)

Epinephrine is a potent inotropic agent that effectively increases myocardial perfusion pressure. Low-dose epinephrine (<0.2 mcg/kg/min) stimulates both beta-1 cardiac and beta-2 peripheral vascular receptors, which results in increased heart rate and contractility, decreased systemic vascular resistance (SVR), and decreased diastolic blood pressure. At doses >0.3 mcg/kg/min, alpha-adrenergic vasoconstriction leads to an increase in blood pressure. Epinephrine causes increased myocardial oxygen demand and may lead to myocardial ischemia; however, this is rare in children. An epinephrine infusion is useful for persistent hypotension after cardiopulmonary resuscitation and in low-output septic shock, and its bronchodilator effects are also useful in anaphylactic shock. Since infants are less responsive to dopamine and dobutamine, epinephrine may be superior at maintaining blood pressure and cardiac output. Infuse at an initial rate of 0.1 mcg/kg/min, and titrate to the desired effect.

Norepinephrine (0.1–2 mcg/kg/min)

Norepinephrine acts on both alpha- and beta-adrenergic receptors, producing potent inotropic effects and peripheral vasoconstriction, significantly increasing mean arterial pressure and cardiac contractility, without causing tachycardia. The increased blood pressure also improves renal perfusion in patients with septic shock. Norepinephrine is effective in persistent hypotension after cardiopulmonary resuscitation in patients with low SVR, as

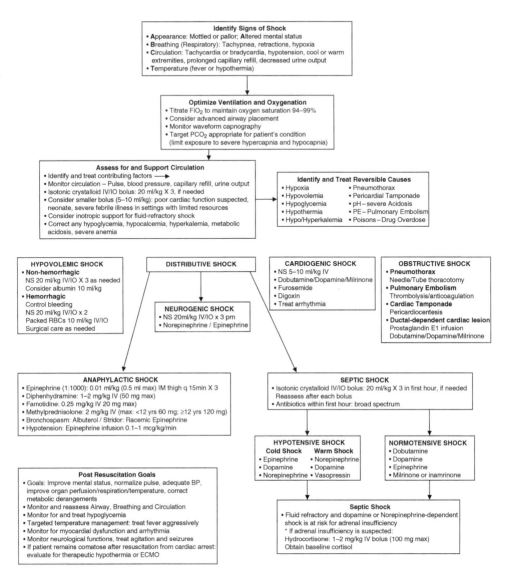

Identify Signs of Shock
- Appearance: Mottled or pallor; Altered mental status
- Breathing (Respiratory): Tachypnea, retractions, hypoxia
- Circulation: Tachycardia or bradycardia, hypotension, cool or warm extremities, prolonged capillary refill, decreased urine output
- Temperature (fever or hypothermia)

Optimize Ventilation and Oxygenation
- Titrate FiO_2 to maintain oxygen saturation 94–99%
- Consider advanced airway placement
- Monitor waveform capnography
- Target PCO_2 appropriate for patient's condition (limit exposure to severe hypercapnia and hypocapnia)

Assess for and Support Circulation
- Identify and treat contributing factors →
- Monitor circulation – Pulse, blood pressure, capillary refill, urine output
- Isotonic crystalloid IV/IO bolus: 20 ml/kg X 3, if needed
- Consider smaller bolus (5–10 ml/kg): poor cardiac function suspected, neonate, severe febrile illness in settings with limited resources
- Consider inotropic support for fluid-refractory shock
- Correct any hypoglycemia, hypocalcemia, hyperkalemia, metabolic acidosis, severe anemia

Identify and Treat Reversible Causes
- Hypoxia
- Hypovolemia
- Hypoglycemia
- Hypothermia
- Hypo/Hyperkalemia
- Pneumothorax
- Pericardial Tamponade
- pH – severe Acidosis
- PE – Pulmonary Embolism
- Poisons – Drug Overdose

HYPOVOLEMIC SHOCK
- **Non-hemorrhagic**
  NS 20 ml/kg IV/IO X 3 as needed
  Consider albumin 10 ml/kg
- **Hemorrhagic**
  Control bleeding
  NS 20 ml/kg IV/IO x 2
  Packed RBCs 10 ml/kg IV/IO
  Surgical care as needed

DISTRIBUTIVE SHOCK

NEUROGENIC SHOCK
- NS 20ml/kg IV/IO x 3 prn
- Norepinephrine / Epinephrine

CARDIOGENIC SHOCK
- NS 5–10 ml/kg IV
- Dobutamine/Dopamine/Milrinone
- Furosemide
- Digoxin
- Treat arrhythmia

OBSTRUCTIVE SHOCK
- **Pneumothorax**
  Needle/Tube thoracotomy
- **Pulmonary Embolism**
  Thrombolysis/anticoagulation
- **Cardiac Tamponade**
  Pericardiocentesis
- **Ductal-dependent cardiac lesion**
  Prostaglandin E1 infusion
  Dobutamine/Dopamine/Milrinone

ANAPHYLACTIC SHOCK
- Epinephrine (1:1000): 0.01 ml/kg (0.5 ml max) IM thigh q 15min X 3
- Diphenhydramine: 1–2 mg/kg IV (50 mg max)
- Famotidine: 0.25 mg/kg IV 20 mg max)
- Methylprednisolone: 2 mg/kg IV (max: <12 yrs 60 mg; ≥12 yrs 120 mg)
- Bronchospasm: Albuterol / Stridor: Racemic Epinephrine
- Hypotension: Epinephrine infusion 0.1–1 mcg/kg/min

SEPTIC SHOCK
- Isotonic crystalloid IV/IO bolus: 20 ml/kg X 3 in first hour, if needed
  Reassess after each bolus
- Antibiotics within first hour: broad spectrum

HYPOTENSIVE SHOCK
Cold Shock	Warm Shock
• Epinephrine	• Norepinephrine
• Dopamine	• Dopamine
• Norepinephrine	• Vasopressin

NORMOTENSIVE SHOCK
- Dobutamine
- Dopamine
- Epinephrine
- Milrinone or inamrinone

Post Resuscitation Goals
- Goals: Improve mental status, normalize pulse, adequate BP, improve organ perfusion/respiration/temperature, correct metabolic derangements
- Monitor and reassess Airway, Breathing and Circulation
- Monitor for and treat hypoglycemia
- Targeted temperature management: treat fever aggressively
- Monitor for myocardial dysfunction and arrhythmia
- Monitor neurological functions, treat agitation and seizures
- If patient remains comatose after resuscitation from cardiac arrest: evaluate for therapeutic hypothermia or ECMO

Septic Shock
- Fluid refractory and dopamine or Norepinephrine-dependent shock is at risk for adrenal insufficiency
- * If adrenal insufficiency is suspected:
  Hydrocortisone: 1–2 mg/kg IV bolus (100 mg max)
  Obtain baseline cortisol

Figure 1.4 Management of shock.
Adapted from AHA PALS 2015 Guidelines.

in high-output warm shock, anaphylactic shock, and spinal shock. Infuse at an initial rate of 0.1 mcg/kg/min, and titrate to the desired effect.

Dopamine (2 – 20 mcg/kg/min)

Dopamine is an endogenous catecholamine with complex effects on the heart and circulation. At low doses (2 mcg/kg/min) dopamine has relatively little chronotropic effects; the primary result is an increase in renal and splanchnic perfusion. At higher infusion rates, it has positive inotropic and chronotropic effects and tends to increase cardiac output and systemic vascular resistance. Infuse at an initial rate of 5–10 mcg/kg/min and titrate to the desired effect.

Dobutamine (2–20 mcg/kg/min)

Dobutamine has selective action on beta-1 and -2 adrenergic receptors with chronotropic and inotropic actions, along with alpha-adrenergic blocking activity. It is an effective inotrope for the normotensive post-arrest patient with poor perfusion. Dobutamine is particularly useful for patients with congestive heart failure or cardiogenic shock, since it increases cardiac output without significantly increasing heart rate. At a dose >10 mcg/kg/min, dobutamine tends to produce hypotension due to afterload reduction and decreased SVR. The hypotension may then require dopamine or epinephrine to increase the SVR. An alternate approach is to start the patient on norepinephrine or dopamine to stabilize the blood pressure and then switch to dobutamine. Infuse dobutamine at an initial rate of 2–10 mcg/kg/min, and titrate to the desired effect.

[handwritten: Milrinone ↑ Contractility / afterload reduction (myocardium) (DILATION)]

Phosphodiesterase Inhibitors

[handwritten: Inaminone]

Phosphodiesterase inhibitors combine inotropic effects on the myocardium (improved cardiac contractility) with systemic arterial and venous dilation (afterload reduction). They increase cardiac output without causing tachycardia or increasing myocardial oxygen demand. They are beneficial in normotensive fluid-resistant shock in patients with myocardial dysfunction associated with increased systemic and pulmonary vascular resistance. Use either: milrinone 50 mcg/kg loading dose over 10–60 minutes, then infuse at 0.25–0.75 mcg/kg/min; or inamrinone 0.75–1 mg/kg loading dose over 5 minutes, may repeat twice; 3 mg/kg total maximum, then infuse at 5–10 mcg/kg/min.

[handwritten: ETT - Flush 5 ml Saline, all drugs (except Epi) 2-3 × dose]

Medications and Electrical Therapy in Resuscitation

The preferred routes of drug administration are IV or IO. However, if an ETT is placed prior to IV or IO insertion, the following medications can be administered via the ETT: lidocaine, epinephrine, atropine, naloxone (LEAN). Instill the drug directly into the ETT or through a 5 Fr feeding tube that extends beyond the tip of the ETT and follow with a 5 mL normal saline flush.

Provide five manual positive pressure ventilations after drug administration to facilitate drug delivery. Drug absorption via the ETT route is unpredictable, so higher doses are required to achieve appropriate therapeutic levels. For epinephrine, use 0.1 mg/kg (0.1 mL/kg) of the 1:1000 concentration; for other drugs, administer 2–3 times the usual IV dose.

[handwritten: ET drugs - 5 Fr feeding tube, 5 ml saline, 5 puffs]

Epinephrine

[handwritten: Epi 0.1 ml = 0.1mg/kg of 1:1000. other drugs 3 times the IV dose.]

Epinephrine is indicated in cardiac arrest (asystole and pulseless electric activity), and in patients with symptomatic bradycardia who are still hypotensive after volume resuscitation. It increases heart rate, myocardial contractility, systemic vascular resistance, and cardiac automaticity, although it also increases myocardial oxygen demand. The increase in coronary perfusion pressure correlates directly with myocardial blood flow, which is a good predictor of return of spontaneous circulation. With ventricular arrhythmias, epinephrine makes the myocardium more susceptible to successful defibrillation.

[handwritten: Helps-defibrillation]

[handwritten: Asystole, PEA   Epinephrine
Symptomatic Bradycardia   ↑HR, Contractility, SVR
Ventricular arrythmia   , Cardiac automacity
*   Coronary perfusion pressure*
*   also ↑ Myocardial O₂ demand]*

Atropine indications

① Sympt. Bradycardia, ② A-V Block ③ Cholinergic toxicity.

The IV/IO dose is 0.01 mg/kg (0.1 mL/kg) of the 1:10,000 concentration every 3–5 minutes as needed (1 mg = 10 mL maximum). The ETT dose is 0.1 mg/kg (0.1 mL/kg) of the 1:1000 concentration every 3–5 minutes. For specific toxins or drug overdoses such as beta-blocker (pp. 462–463) or calcium channel blocker (pp. 464–465), high-dose epinephrine may be used if there is no response after the usual IV/IO dose.

Atropine *Parasympatholytic* *Accelerates* *enhances*
Inhibits Vagal activity, pace maker, A-V Conduction.

Atropine is a parasympatholytic drug that inhibits vagal activity, accelerates sinoatrial pacemaker, and enhances atrioventricular conduction. Atropine is indicated for symptomatic bradycardia with evidence of poor perfusion or hypotension, secondary to increased vagal tone, cholinergic drug toxicity, or AV heart block. However, since hypoxia is commonly the underlying cause for bradycardia, particularly in infants, efforts to improve oxygenation and perfusion must precede the administration of atropine. If the patient does not respond to atropine despite adequate oxygenation and ventilation, use epinephrine. Give 0.02 mg/kg IV/IO (maximum single dose: 0.5 mg in children, 1 mg in adolescents). Atropine may be repeated once in five minutes. For ETT, use 2–3 times the IV dose.

Minimum dose 0.1mg to avoid Paradoxical reaction.

Glucose *DOSE: 0.5 - 1 G/kg.*

Check the blood glucose concentration at the bedside with a glucometer, during and after an arrest. Promptly give dextrose if the glucose level is <45 mg/dL in a neonate or <60 mg/dL in an infant or child. Recheck the blood glucose concentration after each administration, and try to avoid excessive hyperglycemia, which is related to increased mortality in critically ill children.

The dose is 0.5–1 g/kg. In neonates, infants, and children under five years of age, use 5 mL/kg of a 10% dextrose solution prepared by diluting D_{50} W 1:4 with sterile water. For older children, use 2 mL/kg of a 25% dextrose solution or 5 mL/kg of a 10% dextrose solution.

Calcium Chloride 10%, Calcium Gluconate 10%

Routine administration of calcium does not improve outcomes of cardiac arrest, and can antagonize the action of epinephrine and other adrenergic agents. However, calcium is indicated for documented hypocalcemia, hyperkalemia, hypermagnesemia, and calcium channel blocker overdose. Use the measured ionized calcium concentration to determine the need for subsequent doses. Avoid rapid calcium administration, which can cause bradycardia or sinus arrest. In the setting of imminent or ongoing cardiac arrest, calcium chloride is preferred over calcium gluconate because it provides greater bioavailability of calcium. Due to the risk of skin sclerosis, if there is extravasation through a peripheral venous line, administer calcium chloride via a central venous catheter, if possible. Calcium gluconate is otherwise preferred for all non-arrest situations, and it can be administered by peripheral or central venous access.

The dose for calcium chloride is 20 mg/kg (0.2 mL/kg) IV slow; this dose may be repeated once in ten minutes. The dose for calcium gluconate is 60 mg/kg (0.6 mL/kg) IV slow. Flush the line with normal saline before and after calcium administration.

Sodium Bicarbonate

Do not use sodium bicarbonate routinely during cardiopulmonary resuscitation, as it may further depress cardiac contractility and inactivate simultaneously administered catecholamines. Sodium bicarbonate is recommended for symptomatic hyperkalemia, tricyclic antidepressant or sodium channel blocker overdose, or for severe metabolic acidosis or prolonged cardiopulmonary arrest after appropriate ventilation and volume restoration is provided. The dose is 1 mEq/kg (1 mL/kg) slow IV or IO; it cannot be given through ETT. Use a 4.2% solution in infants under six months of age. Sodium bicarbonate causes hypernatremia and hyperosmolarity and, if it extravasates, may cause skin necrosis. IV/IO tubing must be flushed with normal saline before and after giving sodium bicarbonate to prevent precipitation with administered calcium chloride or inactivation of administered epinephrine.

Adenosine   *IV Close to Heart, Flush: 5-10 ml saline, use 3-way*

Adenosine is the drug of choice for the treatment of stable supraventricular tachycardia (SVT) (pp. 52–53) if vagal maneuvers are unsuccessful or in unstable SVT while preparations are being made for cardioversion. Administer adenosine rapidly and follow with a rapid push of normal saline using a three-way stopcock through an IV placed as close to the heart as accessible. After a brief period (15–30 seconds) of asystole or heart block, the rhythm either converts to sinus or reverts to SVT. The first dose is 0.1 mg/kg IV/IO (rapid) to a maximum of 6 mg, followed by a 5–10 mL normal saline flush. If needed, the second dose is 0.2 mg/kg IV/IO (12 mg maximum). This dose may be repeated once (total of three doses). If the patient has unstable SVT or deteriorates, immediately attempt synchronized cardioversion. Adenosine is contraindicated in patients with Wolff–Parkinson–White (WPW) syndrome and preexisting second- or third-degree heart block.

2nd dose may be repeated once (total 3 doses)

Amiodarone   *V-TACHYCARDIA a SVT.*

Amiodarone (pp. 57–58) is indicated for shock-refractory ventricular tachycardia (VT) or pulseless VT, hemodynamically unstable VT, and stable SVT refractory to adenosine. Avoid administering amiodarone with any other drug that causes QT prolongation (procainamide) or in patients with prolonged QT syndrome, as it may precipitate polymorphic VT.

The loading dose for SVT, VT (with and without pulses), and ventricular fibrillation is 5 mg/kg IV (300 mg maximum) over 20–60 minutes. Repeat this dose every 10 minutes to a maximum total dose of 15 mg/kg/day (2.2 g/day).   *30-60 mts IV,*

Dose - 5 mg/kg IV max 300mg over 30-60 mts IV, repeat q 10 mtes, Max Total 15 mg/kg/day.

Lidocaine

Lidocaine (pp. 58–59) is an alternative to amiodarone for VT with pulses and pulseless shock-resistant VF or VT. The initial IV/IO dose is 1 mg/kg (ETT 2–3 mg/kg). This dose may be repeated in 10–15 minutes. If maintenance infusion is required, infuse at 20–50 mcg/kg/min. Lidocaine is contraindicated in WPW syndrome and may cause seizures, myocardial depression, and circulatory shock.

Procainamide

Procainamide (p. 58) is effective in the treatment of atrial fibrillation, atrial flutter, and adenosine-refractory stable SVT (including WPW syndrome) and can be used as an alternative therapy for refractory or recurrent stable VT with pulse. Infuse medication slowly to avoid heart block, myocardial depression, hypotension, or prolongation of the QT interval. Monitor blood pressure and the ECG continuously. If the QRS widens by more than 50% or hypotension develops, stop the infusion. Do not administer concurrently with other

Cardio Version

unstable AF, AFL, VT c̄ Pulse   1st dose 0.5-1 J/kg, Max 50-100 J
SVT)   in shock. Subsequent - 2 J/kg

medications that prolong the QT interval (amiodarone). The dose is 15 mg/kg IV/IO (1000 mg maximum) over 30–60 minutes followed by a continuous IV infusion at 40–50 mcg/kg/min.

Cardioversion and Defibrillation

Cardioversion is the synchronized electrical conversion of a rhythm disturbance. Synchronized cardioversion is timed with the QRS complex to avoid delivery during the relative refractory period of the cardiac cycle, during which a shock could induce potentially lethal VF. It is indicated for unstable SVT, atrial fibrillation, atrial flutter, monomorphic VT with a pulse, and clinical signs of shock. The first dose is 0.5–1 J/kg (50–100 J maximum). If the initial dose is ineffective, increase subsequent doses to 2 J/kg.

Defibrillation is the delivery of electricity asynchronous to the cardiac cycle, indicated for VF or pulseless VT. Defibrillators are either manual or automated (AED), and deliver monophasic or biphasic waveforms. Place the paddles or self-adhering electrodes on the chest wall, leaving about two fingerbreadths between the paddles. Use infant paddles for children <1 year of age or those weighing <10 kg. Place one paddle over the right side of the upper chest and the other to the left of the nipple on the left lower ribs. Alternatively, apply one electrode on the front of the chest just to the left of the sternum and the other over the upper back below the scapula. Immediately after the shock, resume high-quality CPR for two minutes or five cycles, beginning with chest compressions. Try to limit interruption of CPR for rhythm checks to <10 seconds. If one shock does not convert the rhythm to normal, repeat the process. If VF or VT persists despite delivery of one shock followed by two minutes of CPR, give epinephrine as soon as IV or IO access is available. The first dose for defibrillation is 2 J/kg, then deliver subsequent doses at 4 J/kg. *Defibrillation - VF, Pulseless VT*

Dose - 1st 2J/kg, then 4J/kg. (Also Epi)

Shock

Shock is defined as a physiologic state characterized by inadequate tissue perfusion to meet metabolic demands and tissue oxygenation. Shock is categorized as hypovolemic, distributive, cardiogenic, and obstructive (Table 1.7). It can be further classified by severity, as compensated or decompensated (hypotensive) shock. In the early phases of shock, multiple compensatory physiologic mechanisms act to maintain blood pressure and perfusion of vital organs (brain, heart, kidneys). If compensatory mechanisms fail and are unable to maintain a systolic blood pressure within a normal range (greater than fifth percentile systolic blood pressure for age), shock is classified as hypotensive. The earlier shock is recognized and treated, the better the patient's prognosis.

Clinical Presentation

The clinical presentation of patients in compensated shock depends on the cardiac output relative to end-organ demand. In infants and children, cardiac output is initially maintained by changes in heart rate, so that the blood pressure may be normal, although there may be tachycardia and irritability. Poor tissue perfusion leads to metabolic acidosis, so that the respiratory rate is increased to promote the excretion of CO_2. Therefore, unexplained tachycardia and tachypnea, with a normal blood pressure, and without other signs of

Table 1.7 Classification and etiologies of shock

Type of shock	Etiology
Hypovolemic: pump is empty	
	Dehydration (vomiting, diarrhea, poor intake, heat stroke)
	Hemorrhage (trauma, GI bleed)
	Metabolic disease (diabetes, adrenal insufficiency)
	Plasma losses (burns, peritonitis, hypoproteinemia)
Cardiogenic: weak/sick pump	
	Rhythm disturbances
	Congestive heart failure
	Cardiomyopathy
	Post-resuscitation
Distributive: fluid distribution problem	
	Sepsis
	Anaphylaxis
	Neurogenic shock (head trauma, spinal cord injury)
Obstructive: obstruction of outflow	
	Tension pneumothorax
	Cardiac tamponade
	Pulmonary embolism
	Ductal-dependent cardiac disease

Table 1.8 Signs of shock

Early	Late
Tachycardia	Hypotension
Orthostatic changes	Altered mental status
Delayed capillary filling >2 seconds	Markedly delayed capillary filling >4 seconds
Adequate central pulse	Weak or absent peripheral pulse
Tachypnea	Cold, pale mottled skin
Normal blood pressure	Oliguria

shock, may be the earliest signs of cardiorespiratory compromise. Bradycardia and hypotension are ominous, and occur in advanced stages of shock, which can rapidly progress to irreversible multiple organ damage and cardiorespiratory arrest. The signs of shock are summarized in Table 1.8.

Hypovolemic Shock (M C)

Hypovolemic shock is the most common etiology of shock and refers to a clinical state of reduced intravascular volume. It can be caused by extravascular fluid loss (e.g., diarrhea, dehydration) or intravascular volume loss (e.g., hemorrhage) and results in decreased preload leading to reduced stroke volume and low cardiac output. Tachycardia, increased SVR, and increased cardiac contractility are the primary compensatory mechanisms, resulting in redistribution of intravascular perfusion to the heart, brain, and kidneys. The shunting of blood flow away from the skin causes the changes in skin color, temperature, and moisture seen in compensated shock. Tachypnea is an early finding, as a partial compensation for the metabolic acidosis that accompanies shock. Compensatory mechanisms cannot be maintained indefinitely and bradycardia, myocardial ischemia, hypoxia, and subsequent cardiopulmonary arrest will occur without timely intervention.

Distributive Shock

Distributive shock refers to a clinical state characterized by reduced SVR leading to maldistribution of blood flow and tissue hypoperfusion. Causes include: septic shock, anaphylactic shock, and neurogenic/spinal shock.

Septic Shock   *M C distributive shock.*

Septic shock is the most common cause of distributive shock. It may evolve over a few hours (particularly in young infants) or days. There is wide variability in clinical presentation and progression, as the cardiac output may be high, normal, or low. Early phases of "warm" septic shock may not be clinically apparent since the skin may be warm and dry without an increase in capillary refill time. This is due to low SVR and cutaneous vasodilation, which result in hyperdynamic cardiac output. Pulses will be rapid, full, and bounding, and the pulse pressure is wide. Normal- or low-output "cold" septic shock is characterized by high SVR and peripheral vasoconstriction, resulting in cold extremities, with weak pulses and delayed capillary refill time.

Anaphylaxis   *Mostly Vasodilation c̄ Pulmonary Vaso Constriction*

Anaphylactic shock (pp. 37–41) is an acute multisystem potentially life-threatening response to an allergen involving two or more body systems (cutaneous, respiratory, gastrointestinal, cardiovascular, or neurologic). The reaction is characterized by venodilation, arterial vasodilation, increased capillary permeability, and pulmonary vasoconstriction. The patient presents with some combination of anxiety or agitation, urticaria, nausea and vomiting, wheezing and respiratory distress, angioedema resulting in stridor, and hypotension. Anaphylaxis can progress rapidly (seconds to minutes) to cardiovascular collapse and death.

Neurogenic Shock   *Loss of Sympathetic tone.*

Neurogenic shock is caused by an acute high spinal cord injury with sudden loss of sympathetic vascular tone, resulting in peripheral vasodilation. Signs of neurogenic shock include: hypotension with a wide pulse pressure, paradoxical bradycardia (absence of compensatory tachycardia), and respiratory distress if the diaphragm is involved. Neurogenic shock may present with flaccid paralysis and loss of bladder and rectal tone.

A careful assessment is necessary to differentiate neurogenic shock from other causes of shock. Although patients in neurogenic shock may be warm and well-perfused, they may not respond to either fluid boluses or pressor support. *may not respond to Fluids or Vasopressors.*

Cardiogenic Shock

Cardiogenic shock occurs when cardiac output is compromised secondary to myocardial dysfunction. Common causes include congenital heart disease, arrhythmias, myocarditis, cardiomyopathy, sepsis, toxins, and myocardial injury. Cardiogenic shock is also a terminal complication of virtually all types of shock as a result of high myocardial oxygen requirement and decreased cardiac contractility. Findings consistent with cardiogenic shock are marked tachycardia, normal or low blood pressure with narrow pulse pressure, weak central and peripheral pulses, signs of congestive heart failure (pulmonary edema, hepatomegaly, jugular venous distention), cyanosis, cold, mottled skin, change in level of consciousness, and oliguria. A 12-lead ECG may show low-voltage tachycardia or ST changes, and a chest radiograph reveals cardiomegaly and pulmonary edema. An urgent echocardiogram will determine cardiac function as well as any underlying anatomic defects that may be contributing to the condition.

Obstructive Shock

Obstructive shock refers to conditions that physically impair cardiac output as a result of reduced venous return or limited cardiac contractility. Causes include pericardial tamponade, tension pneumothorax, massive pulmonary embolism, and ductal-dependent congenital heart defects (e.g., coarctation of the aorta, hypoplastic left ventricle). In pericardial tamponade (pp. 758–759), fluid accumulates within the pericardial sac, resulting in increased pericardial pressure and decreased cardiac compliance and cardiac output. Classic signs of cardiac tamponade are tachycardia, poor peripheral perfusion, cool extremities, muffled or diminished heart sounds, narrowed pulse pressure with pulsus paradoxus (decrease in systolic blood pressure by >10 mm Hg during inspiration), and changes in level of consciousness. *Pulsus Paradoxus - ↓ SBP, >10 mm Hg i inspiration*

In tension pneumothorax (pp. 760–761) free air accumulates within the pleural cavity, causing a mediastinal shift toward the opposite side, collapsing the lung and compromising cardiac output. Patients present with severe respiratory distress, decreased breath sounds on the affected side, tracheal deviation to the contralateral side, shift in the apical cardiac impulse, tachycardia, distended neck veins, pulsus paradoxus, and rapid deterioration in perfusion with cool extremities.

Findings consistent with massive pulmonary embolism are respiratory distress with hypoxia (as a result of ventilation–perfusion mismatch), chest pain, cough with hemoptysis, tachypnea, tachycardia, and hypotension.

Ductal-dependent congenital cardiac anomalies usually present in the first days to weeks of life when the ductus arteriosus closes. Common lesions include coarctation of the aorta, interrupted aortic arch, coarctation, and hypoplastic left heart syndrome. Restoring patency of the ductus arteriosus is critical for survival until surgical intervention is achieved. Neonates present with cyanosis, tachypnea, congestive heart failure, higher preductal versus postductal blood pressure and O_2 saturation, absence of femoral pulses (coarctation and interrupted aortic arch), metabolic acidosis, and shock.

(1) AABC, (2) RACE (3) VS (4) SAMPLE

Diagnosis   Signs of early shock, can be subtle. High index of suspicion. maintain

Perform an initial assessment of the patient, including the general appearance, mental status and ABCs (see pp. 2–4, Rapid Cardiopulmonary Assessment), a SAMPLE history, and a complete set of vital signs. During the initial assessment, do not delay providing critical interventions, properly position the head, provide supplemental oxygen, and establish IV or IO access.

   Since the signs of early shock are subtle, maintain a high index of suspicion. Be alert to tachycardia, tachypnea, delayed capillary refill (>2 seconds), orthostatic changes in blood pressure or pulse, and irritability. Patients with septic shock may have hypothermia or hyperthermia, altered mental status, irritability or lethargy, and peripheral vasodilation with bounding pulses (warm shock) or mottled cool extremities with thready pulses (cold shock).

If cardiogenic shock is suspected, obtain a 12-lead ECG, which may show low-voltage tachycardia or ST changes; a chest radiograph reveals cardiomegaly and pulmonary edema. An urgent echocardiogram will determine cardiac function as well as any underlying anatomic defects that may be contributing to the condition.

Warning signs that indicate progression from compensated to decompensated (hypotensive) shock include increasing tachycardia, diminishing or absent peripheral pulses, weakening central pulses, narrowing pulse pressure, cold distal extremities with prolonged capillary refill, and decreasing level of consciousness.

ED Management (Figure 1.4)

The most common error in treating shock is underestimating the severity of the condition. Tachycardia that is unexplained by pain or fever is always concerning. If compensated shock is suspected, treat promptly and aggressively to prevent progression to hypovolemic shock. All patients require secure vascular access, oxygen therapy, and cardiopulmonary monitoring. The goals of initial management are to restore normal mental status, heart rate and blood pressure, good peripheral perfusion, and adequate urine output. Early identification of the etiology will help to treat reversible causes.

Position. Allow a conscious patient to assume a position of comfort. If hypotensive, place the child in the Trendelenburg position, unless breathing is compromised.

Oxygenation and Ventilation. For spontaneously breathing patients, administer high-concentration oxygen via nonrebreather mask. Other interventions may include non-invasive positive airway pressure (BiPAP, CPAP) in awake and cooperative patients, or assisted ventilation with a bag-mask device or mechanical ventilation with PEEP if there is evidence of airway compromise. If no IV in 2 mins start IO

Establish Vascular Access. Establish two large-bore peripheral IV lines or place a central catheter. If venous access is not possible or delayed, use an IO needle. In critically ill or injured patients, do not spend more than 1–2 minutes attempting to establish peripheral vascular access. The effort may be resumed after the IO line is secured.

Fluid Resuscitation. Give isotonic crystalloid (NS or LR) 20 mL/kg IV bolus over 5–20 minutes, and repeat as needed to restore blood pressure and tissue perfusion. If there is a concern for cardiogenic shock, use smaller fluid boluses of 5–10 mL/kg given over 10–20

Check glucose 45/60 in all ill children .. Neonate <45mg, others <60mg%

minutes. Carefully monitor for signs of pulmonary edema or worsening tissue perfusion, and stop the infusion if any of these occur. *Keep glucose <150mg%*

Consider blood transfusion in cases of blood loss or other causes of severe anemia. Trauma victims may require blood transfusion of packed RBCs (10 mL/kg) to replace ongoing losses; use cross-matched, type-specific or O-negative blood. Trauma patients who remain hypotensive despite fluid resuscitation require immediate operative intervention. *>60ml/kg Total, Consider Vasopressors.*

Medication and Pressor Infusion. The patient might need pharmacologic support to improve cardiac output, correct metabolic derangements, and/or manage pain and anxiety. If the patient remains hypotensive after initial fluid resuscitation of 40–60 mL/kg, an inotropic agent or a combination of several agents may be necessary to stabilize blood pressure (pp. 23–25). Titrate the dose to the desired effect. Monitor the patient carefully and wean off pressors once blood pressure has improved.

Laboratory Studies. Laboratory studies (i.e., CBC, glucose, potassium, calcium, lactate, blood gas analysis) provide important information to help identify the etiology and severity of shock, evaluate organ dysfunction and metabolic derangements, and assess the response to therapy. Check bedside glucose and treat hypoglycemia (neonate <45 mg/dL; infant, child, and adolescent <60 mg/dL) with an IV glucose bolus.

Monitoring and Reassessment. Assess and continuously reassess the effectiveness of fluid resuscitation and medication therapy. Initiate noninvasive monitoring, including the level of consciousness, heart rate, blood pressure, SpO$_2$, and temperature. Insert a Foley catheter and monitor urine output; the goal is 0.5–1 mL/kg/h, or about 30 mL/h in adolescents. Recognize any limitations in the care and call for help when needed. Early subspecialty consultation (e.g., pediatric critical care, pediatric cardiology, pediatric surgery) is an essential component of shock management and may influence outcome.

Management of Shock According to Cause (Figure 1.5)

Hypovolemia Shock

Non-hemorrhagic. Give an isotonic crystalloid 20 mL/kg bolus, and repeat as needed. Colloid may be necessary

Hemorrhagic. Control the external bleeding and initially give 3 mL of isotonic crystalloid for every 1 mL of estimated blood lost. Once blood is available, transfuse packed RBCs (10 mL/kg) to replace ongoing losses; use cross-matched, type-specific, or O-negative blood.

Distributive Shock *Septic > Fluids upto 60ml/kg. ATB <1hr even w/o C&S*

Septic Shock. Administer isotonic crystalloid, 20 mL/kg bolus rapidly, up to 60mL/kg in the first hour. Administer antibiotic therapy as soon as possible, preferably within the first 60 minutes. Send the appropriate cultures, but do not delay antibiotic therapy if cultures are not readily obtained. See pp. 391–393 for empiric antibiotic choices and doses.

Anaphylactic Shock. The management is summarized on pp. 38–40. Effective treatment involves early recognition of symptoms of anaphylaxis and anticipating the need for advanced airway techniques. *Anticipate need for airway management.*

1. Assess patient and check pulse
2. Analyze rate
3. Rhythm: P-wave and QRS
4. Treat patient

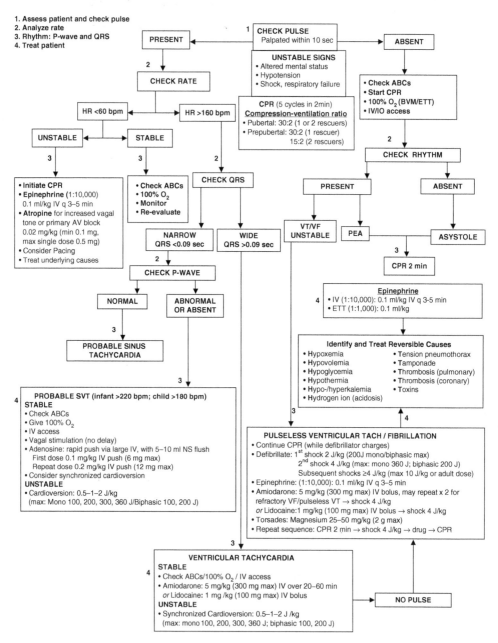

Figure 1.5 Pediatric cardiac arrest and dysrhythmia algorithm
Adapted from AHA PALS 2015 Guidelines.

Neurogenic Shock. Position the patient child flat or head-down. Administer a trial of bolus of isotonic crystalloid (20 mL/kg) and repeat as necessary. For fluid-refractory hypotension, use vasopressors. Provide supplementary warming or cooling as needed.

Cardiogenic Shock

Rapid volume resuscitation of cardiogenic shock in the setting of poor myocardial function can aggravate pulmonary edema and further impair myocardial function, compromising oxygenation, ventilation, and cardiac output. Administer gradual volume resuscitation with 5–10 mL/kg boluses of isotonic crystalloid delivered over a longer period of time. Carefully monitor hemodynamic parameters during fluid infusion, and repeat the infusion as needed to maintain tissue perfusion. Children with cardiogenic shock often require vasopressor medications to increase and redistribute cardiac output, improve myocardial function, and reduce SVR. The treatment of congestive heart failure (pp. 68–69) and dysrhythmias (pp. 47–62) is detailed elsewhere.

Obstructive Shock

The treatment of pericardial tamponade (pp. 758–759), tension pneumothorax (pp. 760–761), ductal-dependent cardiac defects (p. 802), and pulmonary embolism (p. 377) are detailed elsewhere.

Post-Resuscitation Care

The goals of post-resuscitation care (Figure 1.4) are to preserve brain function, avoid secondary organ injury, and to diagnose and treat the cause of illness. Ultimate outcome after resuscitation is often determined by the subsequent care the child receives. The first phase in post-resuscitative management is to continue to provide advanced life support for immediate life-threatening conditions and focus on the ABCs. The second phase provides broader multiorgan supportive care. When the patient is stable, transfer to a pediatric center if locally there is inadequate pediatric emergency and critical care expertise.

Providing Adequate Oxygenation and Ventilation. Titrate the inspired oxygen to maintain an O_2 saturation ≥94–99%) and maintain acceptable $PaCO_2$ levels (<45 mm Hg). For an intubated patient, verify tube position, obtain ABGs, and adjust ventilatory settings as necessary. Use the DOPE mnemonic (Displaced, Obstructed, Pneumothorax, Equipment failure) to assess clinical deterioration in an intubated patient. $O_2 > 94$, $CO_2 < 45$.

Supporting Tissue Perfusion and Cardiovascular Function. Post-resuscitation patients are often poorly perfused as a result of ongoing fluid loss, decreased cardiac function, and alterations in SVR. Give parental fluids and vasoactive agents to maintain the systolic blood pressure above the fifth percentile for age. Monitor mental status, skin perfusion, pulse quality, and blood pressure. Place a urinary catheter to monitor urine output (>0.5–1 mL/kg/h in infants and children; >30 mL/h in adolescents).

Maintaining Adequate Glucose Concentration. Check glucose early and treat as needed. Avoid hyperglycemia and use a target glucose level of <150 mg/dL.

Correcting Acid–Base and Electrolyte Imbalances. Patients usually have metabolic acidosis, which responds to adequate fluid therapy. The routine use of sodium bicarbonate is not indicated.

Temperature Regulation. Maintain a normal temperature and avoid hyperthermia by treating fever (>38 °C). Provide warming devices for hypothermic infants. For a comatose patient resuscitated from an out-of-hospital cardiac arrest, maintain either five days of normothermia

(36–37.5 °C) or two days of initial continuous hypothermia (32–34 °C) followed by three days of normothermia. For a patient who remains comatose after in-hospital cardiac arrest, there is insufficient data to recommend hypothermia over normothermia.

Ensure Adequate Analgesia and Sedation (pp. 715–722). Control pain and discomfort with analgesics (fentanyl or morphine) and sedatives (lorazepam or midazolam).

Family Presence During Resuscitation

Presence of family members during in-hospital resuscitation appears to be beneficial and helps in their own adjustment and grieving process, and does not negatively impact staff performance. Healthcare providers should offer the opportunity to be present, whenever possible. However, gently ask family members to leave if they become disruptive to the resuscitation team. Have a member of the resuscitation team stay with the family to inform them of the progress of resuscitation efforts, offer an explanation of events, answer questions, and offer comfort.

Termination of Resuscitation

There are no reliable predictors of when to stop resuscitative efforts after in-hospital pediatric cardiac arrest. In the past, children who underwent prolonged resuscitation without return of spontaneous circulation after two doses of epinephrine were considered unlikely to survive, although neurologically intact survival has been documented. Offer prolonged resuscitative efforts for patients with recurring or refractory VF/VT, drug toxicity, or a primary hypothermic insult. Witnessed collapse, bystander CPR, and a short interval from collapse to arrival of EMS improve the chance of survival. Some predictors of poor outcome in infants and children with out-of-hospital cardiac arrest are: age <1 year, longer duration of cardiac arrest, and presentation with a nonshockable rhythm.

When resuscitation efforts are terminated, arrange for the team leader to meet with family members in order to comfort and apprise them of the resuscitation efforts. Soon afterwards, have the senior members organize a debriefing of the resuscitation team in order to acknowledge the contributions of the team and review the resuscitation efforts.

Bibliography

Bhanji F, Topjian AA, Nadkarni VM, et al. American Heart Association's Get With the Guidelines: Survival Rates Following Pediatric In-Hospital Cardiac Arrests During Nights and Weekends. *JAMA Pediatr.* 2017;**171**(1):39–45.

de Caen AR, Berg MD, Chameides L, et al. Part 12: Pediatric Advanced Life Support: 2015 American Heart Association Guidelines Update for Cardiopulmonary Resuscitation and Emergency Cardiovascular Care. *Circulation.* 2015;**132**(18 Suppl. 2):S526–S542

Hafeez W, Ronca L, Maldonado T. Pediatric Advanced Life Support Update for the Emergency Physician: Review of 2010 Guideline Changes. *CPEM.* 2011;**12**(4): 255–265.

Samson RA, Schexnayder SM, Hazinski MF, eds. *Pediatric Advanced Life Support (PALS) Provider Manual: 2015 American Heart Association Guidelines for CPR and ECC* American Heart Association, 2016.

Tay ET, Hafeez W: Intraosseous Access. *E-Medicine Journal*, April 4, 2007, updated 2009, 2011, 2013, 2014; www.emedicine.com/proc/topic80431.htm (accessed May 24, 2017).

Chapter 2

Allergic Emergencies

Stephanie Jennings

Anaphylaxis

Anaphylaxis is a potentially life-threatening multisystem allergic reaction that can be triggered by a variety of agents (Table 2.1). The mechanism may be either IgE-mediated (anaphylactic reaction) or non-IgE-mediated (anaphylactoid reaction). Each process, however, leads to the release of immune mediators from mast cells and basophils, so the clinical presentation and treatment is similar and the term "anaphylaxis" is often applied to both.

Clinical Presentation

Anaphylaxis can present with a variety of signs and symptoms (Table 2.2). It involves at least two organ systems, most commonly cutaneous, respiratory, gastrointestinal, and/or

Table 2.1 Agents that can trigger anaphylaxis

Anaphylactic (IgE dependent)

Animal dander

Antibiotics: beta-lactams, sulfonamides

Colorants (carmine dye)

Foods: shellfish (crustaceans, mollusks), peanuts, tree nuts (pecans, pistachios, walnuts), egg whites, fish, wheat, milk, soy, sesame

Hormones (estrogen, progesterone)

Hymenoptera sting (yellow jacket, hornet, wasp, honeybee, fire ant)

Latex

Anaphylactoid (IgE-independent)

Immune aggregates

IV Immunoglobulin

Medications: opioids, muscle relaxants, nonsteroidal anti-inflammatories, aspirin

Physiologic factors: exercise, cold temperature, heat, pressure, sunlight

Radiocontrast material (any)

Transfusion reaction

Idiopathic

Table 2.2 Clinical manifestations of anaphylaxis

Organ system	Signs and symptoms	Frequency (%)
Cutaneous	Urticaria, angioedema	88
Cutaneous	Flushing	46
Cutaneous	Pruritus (no rash)	5
Respiratory	Wheezing, dyspnea, stridor	50
Gastrointestinal	Nausea, vomiting, diarrhea, abdominal pain	30
Cardiovascular	Syncope, hypotension, arrhythmias	30
Miscellaneous	Sense of impending doom, seizure, diaphoresis, rhinitis, headache, metallic taste	1–20

cardiovascular. A reaction can occur as rapidly as seconds after exposure or it may be delayed for hours. Up to 20% of patients with a severe allergic reaction will have a biphasic response, with symptoms recurring 1–72 hours (average eight hours) after the initial reaction has remitted. In protracted anaphylaxis, symptoms may persist for up to 32 hours.

Diagnosis

The diagnosis of anaphylaxis is based on clinical manifestations fulfilling one of the following three criteria:

1. Acute onset with involvement of skin and/or mucosal tissues *and* at least one of the following:
   a. respiratory compromise
   b. hypotension
   c. evidence of end-organ dysfunction.

2. Rapid onset of involvement in two or more organ systems after exposure to a known allergen.
3. Hypotension after exposure to a known allergen.

The differential diagnosis of anaphylaxis is summarized in Table 2.3.

ED Management

Anaphylaxis is a *medical emergency* requiring *immediate attention*. Institute the ABCs of emergency care. Limit any continued exposure and discontinue any intravenous agents immediately. Avoid using latex products when caring for a latex-allergic patient. If the affected patient is taking beta-blocking medication, be prepared for a difficult recovery; sometimes extraordinary efforts are required to overcome beta-blockade associated with anaphylaxis.

The first priority is to maintain airway patency. If adequate ventilation and oxygenation are documented by pulse oximetry, do not change the patient's position, but administer 100% oxygen as tolerated. Place a hypotensive patient in the recumbent position and elevate

Table 2.3 Differential diagnosis of anaphylaxis

Diagnosis	Differentiating features
Airway foreign body	Aspiration history
	Auscultatory findings may be localized
Angioedema	No respiratory symptoms
Asthma	Involves only the respiratory system
Cardiac tamponade	Muffled heart sounds, pericardial rub, pulsus paradoxus
Croup	Barking cough
Food poisoning	Scombroid
Flushing syndromes	Catecholamine excreting tumors; carcinoid
Globus hystericus	Sensation of a lump in the throat
Hereditary angioedema	May have a history of previous similar episodes
Panic attack	Precipitating event
	No cutaneous findings
Pulmonary embolism	Pleuritic pain, fourth heart sound
	Jugular venous distension
Red man syndrome	History of vancomycin exposure
Serum sickness	Fever, lymphadenopathy, arthralgias/arthritis
Urticaria	Skin is sole organ system involved
Vasovagal episode	Gradual onset after precipitating event
Vocal cord dysfunction	Onset is not acute

the lower extremities. If stridor is present, prepare to intubate the patient if initial therapy with epinephrine (see below) is not effective. Monitor the ECG and oxygen saturation continuously, and if the patient is tachycardic or hypotensive, establish IV access and give a 20 mL/kg normal saline bolus. Make a rapid assessment of the rate of progression and the extent of the reaction.

Epinephrine

Epinephrine is the mainstay of treatment of anaphylaxis. The alpha-adrenergic effects reverse peripheral vasodilation, decreasing hypotension and reducing angioedema and urticaria; the beta-adrenergic effects cause bronchodilation, increase myocardial contractility, and suppress further release of mast cells and basophils.

For a normotensive patient, give 0.01 mL/kg (0.5 mL maximum) of *1:1000* epinephrine *intramuscularly*. Repeat the dose every 5–15 minutes, as needed.

Give a hypotensive patient 0.01 mg/kg (0.1 mL/kg, 10 mL maximum) of *1:10,000* epinephrine *intravenously*. Repeat every 3–5 minutes. If venous access is not available, administer epinephrine (0.1 mL/kg of 1:1000) via the endotracheal tube. If the initial response to epinephrine is inadequate, use an intravenous drip, starting with 0.1 mcg/kg/min (1.5 mcg/kg/min maximum).

Vasopressor Infusion

A vasopressor infusion is indicated for hypotension refractory to epinephrine and volume repletion. Give dopamine at 2–20 mcg/kg/min.

Antihistamines

H_1 and H_2 antihistamines block the effect of circulating histamines but do not decrease mediator release. H_2 blockers may also inhibit the histamine effects on peripheral vasculature and myocardial tissues. The onset of action of antihistamines is delayed, so epinephrine is still necessary. Give diphenhydramine (H_1), 1–2 mg/kg IV or PO q 6h (50 mg/dose maximum, 200 mg/day maximum) *and* ranitidine (H_2), 2 mg/kg q 6–8h IV or PO (50 mg/dose maximum).

Albuterol

Treat bronchospasm resistant to epinephrine with nebulized albuterol 0.15 mg/kg/dose, either hourly or continuously (2.5 mg minimum, 10 mg maximum). See Asthma (p. 625) for the treatment of bronchospasm not responsive to albuterol.

Corticosteroids

Give systemic corticosteroids to a patient with a history of asthma, idiopathic anaphylaxis, or severe or prolonged symptoms. Steroids may also reduce the risk of recurrent or protracted anaphylaxis. Use methylprednisolone 1–2 mg/kg/day divided q 6h IV (60 mg/day maximum) or prednisone 1–2 mg/kg/day PO (60 mg/day maximum), for three days.

Glucagon

Anaphylaxis may be very difficult to treat in a patient taking beta-adrenergic blockers, which blunt the response to epinephrine. The patient is at increased risk for bronchospasm, hypotension, and paradoxical bradycardia. Glucagon has both inotropic and chronotropic effects that are mediated independently of alpha- and beta-receptors and therefore can reverse refractory hypotension and bradycardia. Give a loading dose of 20–30 mcg/kg IV (1 mg maximum) over five minutes, followed by a continuous infusion of 5–15 mcg/min, titrating the dose to the desired blood pressure. Glucagon may cause emesis; therefore, protect the airway if the patient is drowsy or obtunded.

Discharge Considerations

1. Observe for 6–8 hours. Most late-phase reactions occur within this time period.
2. Give prednisone 1–2 mg/kg/day (60 mg/day maximum) for three days.
3. Give diphenhydramine (5 mg/kg/day div q 6h, 50 mg/dose maximum) for 2–3 days to treat urticaria.
4. Give an H_2 antihistamine, ranitidine (2 mg/kg q 6–8h, 50 mg/dose maximum) for 2–3 days.
5. Prescribe injectable epinephrine (EpiPen Jr. <30 kg, EpiPen >30 kg) and instruct the parent and/or child when and how to administer it in the anterolateral aspect of the thigh, through the clothing, while avoiding placing the thumb over the tip.
6. Educate the family regarding avoidance of the trigger(s).
7. Inform the family about MedicAlert bracelets (1-888-633-4298 or www.medicalert.org).
8. Refer all patients with an episode of anaphylaxis to an allergist.

Indications for Admission

- Severe anaphylaxis
- Hypotension
- Persistent bronchospasm or hypoxia
- Patient resides some distance from medical facilities

Follow-up

- Primary care 2–3 days
- Allergist 2–3 weeks

Bibliography

Alqurashi W, Stiell I, Chan K, et al. Epidemiology and clinical predictors of biphasic reactions in children. *Ann Allergy Asthma Immunol.* 2015;**115**(3):217–223.

Brown SG, Stone SF, Fatovich DM, et al. Anaphylaxis: clinical patterns, mediator release, and severity. *J Allergy Clin Immunol.* 2013;**132**(5):1141–1149.

Lieberman P, Nicklas RA, Randolph C, et al. Anaphylaxis: a practice parameter update 2015. *Ann Allergy Asthma Immunol.* 2015;**115**(5):341–384.

Simons FE, Ardusso LR, Bilò MB, et al.2012 update: World Allergy Organization Guidelines for the assessment and management of anaphylaxis. *Curr Opin Allergy Clin Immunol.* 2012;**12**(4):389–399.

Angioedema

Angioedema is swelling of the deeper layers of skin and/or submucosal tissue. It often occurs simultaneously with urticaria.

Clinical Presentation

The face, neck, and extremities are most commonly affected, although angioedema may occur anywhere on the body. The swelling is most evident where the skin is loose, such as the scrotum, lips, and eyelids. There is usually accompanying erythema, warmth, and a sensation of pressure or pain, but pruritus is rare. Angioedema may also present as unexplained abdominal pain secondary to the swelling of any portion of the gastrointestinal tract.

The etiologies of angioedema are the same as for urticaria (p. 44). In addition, hereditary angioedema (HAE) is an autosomal dominant condition that affects the gene for the plasma protein C_1 inhibitor, leading to uncontrolled generation of bradykinin. The patient will have recurrent episodes of angioedema, usually beginning in childhood and worsening during puberty. Attacks of HAE are often sporadic, although about one-third are triggered by injury or trauma. Most episodes are of 1–2 days' duration and are preceded by a prodrome of numbness, tingling, and pressure. The edema of HAE most commonly involves the hands and feet, although other sites can be affected as well. In addition, life-threatening swelling of the airway can occur.

Diagnosis

Angioedema is most often confused with edema, although angioedema is non-pitting and is not limited to dependent areas. It may also be difficult to distinguish angioedema

Table 2.4 Differential diagnosis of angioedema

Diagnosis	Differentiating features
Anaphylaxis	Other organ systems involved (respiratory, gastrointestinal, etc.)
Cellulitis	Usually localized, on exposed areas of skin
	May have fever and/or chills
Edema	Occurs in dependent areas, may be pitting
Erysipelas	Raised above the level of the skin
	Sharply demarcated borders
Lymphedema	Usually involves one extremity including digits
Vasculitis	Fever, weight loss
	Paresthesias, joint/muscle pain

from anaphylaxis, especially since angioedema can be the primary manifestation of anaphylaxis. Anaphylaxis, however, involves at least two organ systems, while angioedema is solely an edema of the deeper tissues. Angioedema can present as abdominal pain from swelling in the GI tract as well, but again this can be differentiated from anaphylaxis by the absence of other system involvement. The differential diagnosis is summarized in Table 2.4.

Once it is clear that the patient has angioedema, and not anaphylaxis, obtain a complete history, seeking a possible offending agent, as well as a family history of similar episodes. Obtain blood for a CBC with differential, ESR, total serum IgE, and C_1-inhibitor level (low in 85% of cases). A more extensive evaluation is indicated for severe or recurrent cases of angioedema, although this can be deferred to a primary care setting.

ED Management

The priority is to ensure an adequate airway, as laryngeal edema can be rapidly progressive (see Anaphylaxis, pp. 37–41, for the treatment of airway edema). If the patient is known to have hereditary angioedema, give C_1-inhibitor concentrate as soon as possible for significant edematous attacks (i.e., laryngeal edema, extensive facial edema, and severe abdominal attacks). Use 10–20 units/kg (500 units maximum <50 kg; 1000 units maximum 50–100 kg) and repeat if needed in one hour.

The best treatment is prevention and education of the family and patient. Remove the offending agent, if identified. Advise the patient to avoid dry skin or harsh soaps/creams, as well as aspirin and oral contraceptives, which can precipitate an attack.

If the etiology is unknown, prescribe an H_1 antihistamine such as diphenhydramine (5 mg/kg/day div q 6h, 50 mg/dose maximum) or hydroxyzine (2 mg/kg/day div q 8h, 100 mg/day maximum). Reserve corticosteroids for severe cases (prednisone or prednisolone, 2 mg/kg/day, 60 mg/day maximum, for five days).

Follow-up

- Primary care follow-up in 1–2 weeks
- Dermatology or allergy follow-up in 2–4 weeks

Bibliography

Cicardi M, Aberer W, Banerji A, et al. Classification, diagnosis, and approach to treatment for angioedema: consensus report from the Hereditary Angioedema International Working Group. *Allergy*. 2014;**69**(5):602–616.

Cicardi M, Craig TJ, Martinez-Saguer I, Hébert J, Longhurst HJ. Review of recent guidelines and consensus statements on hereditary angioedema therapy with focus on self-administration. *Int Arch Allergy Immunol*. 2013;**161**(Suppl. 1):3–9.

Hsu D, Shaker M. An update on hereditary angioedema. *Curr Opin Pediatr*. 2012;**24**(5):638–646.

MacGinnitie AJ. Pediatric hereditary angioedema. *Pediatr Allergy Immunol*. 2014;**25**(5):420–427.

Urticaria

Urticaria, or hives, is a common cutaneous reaction caused by release of chemical mediators, especially histamine, from mast cells or basophils. Urticaria may occur at any age and up to 25% of the population will have at least one episode in their lifetime.

Acute urticaria lasts less than 6–8 weeks in duration, while chronic urticaria is defined as hives persisting beyond this time frame. In 80% of cases the etiology is unknown, although chronic urticaria can be associated with systemic illnesses such as juvenile idiopathic arthritis (JIA), systemic lupus erythematosus (SLE), viral hepatitis, lymphomas, and thyroid disease. The most common causes are listed in Table 2.5.

Clinical Presentation

Hives are pruritic, well-circumscribed, raised, evanescent areas of skin edema on an erythematous base. They are usually circular or annular in shape, found most commonly on the trunk and extremities, and vary in size from a few millimeters to centimeters (giant urticaria). Acute urticaria usually develops within minutes of exposure to the causative agent and is virtually always pruritic. Simple hives tend to come and go in crops, with individual lesions usually lasting for less than one day, although new lesions tend to evolve as older ones resolve. On rare occasions a hive will persist for up to 48 hours.

Diagnosis

The key feature in making the diagnosis of urticaria is the duration of the lesions. Hives that remain fixed in place for longer than 24–48 hours are not typical. A violet hue within the lesions, or the absence of pruritus, also suggests alternative etiologies. Obtain a history looking for a possible offending agent. Determine the time of onset, site, duration, and frequency of the lesions. Inquire about recent medication use, injections, insect bites, illness, and other triggers or provoking factors. Examine the distribution of lesions to check for temperature-exposed regions or contact etiologies. Stroke the skin to assess for dermatographism, which is caused by histamine release from mast cells. The differential diagnosis of urticaria is summarized in Table 2.6.

For patients with chronic urticaria, ascertain if there are any related symptoms, such as fever, joint pain, abdominal pain, weight loss, or poor circulation in the hands or feet.

A priority is to assess for signs of associated respiratory, cardiovascular, or gastrointestinal involvement, which would imply that the urticaria is a manifestation of an anaphylactic episode. Similarly, look for the presence of associated angioedema on physical examination.

Table 2.5 Causes of urticaria

Acute urticaria

Contact urticaria: latex, animal saliva

Hypersensitivity

   Foods: eggs, milk, wheat, soy, peanuts

   Antibiotics: beta-lactam, sulfa

   Stings and bites: bees, wasps, scorpions, spiders, jellyfish

Idiopathic

Immune complex mediated: serum sickness, post-transfusion, post-viral

Infectious: viral, bacterial (strep), parasitic, fungal

Pseudoallergic reactions: medications, radiocontrast, foods

Toxin mediated

Chronic urticaria

Adrenergic

Autoimmune

Cholinergic

Cold/solar (sun exposure)

Dermographism

Exercise-induced

Hypersensitivity reactions

Idiopathic

Presumed immune complex mediated

   Thyroid disease

   Urticarial vasculitis

   Malignancy

   Collagen vascular disease: acute rheumatic fever, dermatomyositis, juvenile idiopathic arthritis, systemic lupus erythematosus

   Inflammatory bowel disease

   Behçet's disease

In general, for acute urticaria, no laboratory testing is required and it is not necessary to identify the trigger for a patient who is otherwise well, and in whom the history and physical examination do not suggest a cause. When a patient presents with chronic urticaria, and the history and physical examination do not suggest an etiology, obtain a CBC with differential, ESR and/or CRP, liver function tests, urinalysis, antinuclear antibody, thyroid function, antithyroid antibodies, and a chest x-ray.

Table 2.6 Differential diagnosis of urticaria

Diagnosis	Differentiating features
Anaphylaxis	Involves more than one organ system
Erythema multiforme	Symmetrical target lesions
	Mucosal involvement with erythema multiforme major
Guttate psoriasis	Small salmon-pink drop-like papules
Henoch–Schönlein purpura	Abdominal pain, hematochezia, joint pain, purpura
Mastocytosis	Widespread symmetric lesion
	Macules, papules, nodules, plaques, bullae, and vesicles
	Darrier sign (wheal develops after rubbing)
	Hepatosplenomegaly
Pityriasis rosea	Herald patch precedes general eruption
	Christmas tree pattern of pruritic lesions on the back

ED Management

The priority for all patients with urticaria is to rule-out anaphylaxis.

Acute Urticaria

Remove or avoid the offending agent, if it can be identified. If there is airway involvement, give epinephrine as for anaphylaxis (p. 39). Treat severe pruritus with 1:1000 epinephrine subcutaneously (0.01 mL/kg, 0.5 mL maximum). Otherwise, prescribe a non-sedating oral H_1-antihistamine for 3–4 days. Choices include loratadine, cetirizine, or fexofenadine. Also prescribe an H_2 antihistamine, such as ranitidine, cimetidine, or famotidine (see Table 2.7). For breakthrough itching, prescribe either diphenhydramine or hydroxyzine.

Chronic Urticaria

In addition to the treatment listed for acute urticaria, in severe cases add an antileukotriene, montelukast (6 months to 6 years old: 4 mg/day; 6–14 years old: 5 mg/day; ≥15 years old: 10 mg/day) in combination with the antihistamines. Refer patients with chronic urticaria to either an allergist or primary care provider for further evaluation.

Follow-up

- Acute urticaria: if no improvement; primary care in 3–5 days
- Allergy referral in 1–2 weeks: peanut- or latex-induced urticaria, urticarial vasculitis, urticaria with systemic manifestations, urticaria with angioedema, urticaria that responds poorly to therapy, or if the results of the ED evaluation do not suggest an etiology for chronic urticaria

Table 2.7 Antihistamines for urticaria

Drug	Dose
Traditional H$_1$ antihistamines	
Diphenhydramine	5 mg/day div q 6h, 50 mg/dose maximum
Hydroxyzine	2 mg/kg/day div q 8h, 100 mg/day maximum
Non-sedating H$_1$ antihistamines	
Loratadine	2–12 years old: 5 mg/day >12 years old: 10 mg/day
Cetirizine	6 months to 1 year old: 2.5 mg/day ≥1–5 years old: 2.5 mg/day (may increase to 5 mg/day if needed) ≥6 years old: 5–10 mg/day
Fexofenadine	6 months to 2 years old: 15 mg/dose bid ≥2–11 years old: 30 mg bid ≥12 years old: extended-release 180 mg daily
H$_2$ antihistamines	
Ranitidine	2 mg/kg/day div q 12h, 300 mg/day maximum
Cimetidine	20–40 mg/kg/day div q 6h, 800 mg/day maximum
Famotidine	0.5–1 mg/kg q 12h, 40 mg/day maximum

Bibliography

Confino-Cohen R, Chodick G, Shalev V, et al. Chronic urticaria and autoimmunity: associations found in a large population study. *J Allergy Clin Immunol.* 2012;**129**(5):1307–1313.

Mathur AN, Mathes EF. Urticaria mimickers in children. *Dermatol Ther.* 2013;**26**(6):467–475.

Tsakok T, Du Toit G, Flohr C. Pediatric urticaria. *Immunol Allergy Clin North Am.* 2014;**34**(1):117–139.

Zuberbier T. A summary of the new international EAACI/GA(2)LEN/EDF/WAO guidelines in Urticaria. *World Allergy Organ J.* 2012;**5**(Suppl. 1):S1–S5.

Cardiac Emergencies

Irfan Warsy and Michael H. Gewitz

Arrhythmias

Pediatric arrhythmias are increasing in prevalence secondary to improved patient survival following cardiac surgery, more extensive use of ECG monitoring, and the epidemic of childhood obesity. Proper management includes accurate electrocardiographic diagnosis, careful clinical evaluation, and initiation of appropriate therapy. With all rhythm disturbances, the approach to the patient begins with a 12-lead ECG, but if there is hemodynamic instability, a single-lead ECG will suffice.

Cardiac arrhythmias requiring emergency therapy can be classified simply into tachyarrhythmias and bradyarrhythmias. The tachyarrhythmias can be further divided into narrow and wide QRS complex groups. Narrow complex rhythms can be subdivided into the various forms of supraventricular tachycardia (SVT), including non-preexcited atrial fibrillation, atrial flutter, ectopic atrial tachycardia, junctional ectopic tachycardia, and microreentrant and macroreentrant SVT. However, the most common cause is sinus tachycardia.

Atrial Fibrillation

Atrial fibrillation is rare in children. It most commonly occurs in patients with congenital heart disease, chronic atrioventricular (AV) valve insufficiency, cardiomyopathy, and Wolff–Parkinson–White (WPW) syndrome, or following the Fontan procedure in patients with only one functional ventricle. Other associations include hyperthyroidism, hypertension, Ebstein's anomaly, atrial septal defect, and atrial tumor. Atrial fibrillation suggests significant atrial conduction system disease and is usually a chronic problem. "Lone" atrial fibrillation, in the absence of other cardiac abnormalities, is rare in children.

Clinical Presentation and Diagnosis

Suspect atrial fibrillation when the pulse is "irregularly irregular." Heart sounds may vary in intensity, a pulse deficit may be present, and the cardiac impulse is markedly variable. The ECG shows chaotic fibrillatory waves of varying amplitude, morphology, and duration, causing variation of the baseline. The RR interval is irregularly irregular. The atrial rate is generally >350 bpm, while the ventricular rate varies between 100 and 200 bpm (Figure 3.1). Sporadic aberrant ventricular conduction can result in random wide QRS complexes.

rate - Atrial > 350 , Ventricls 150 - 200 r

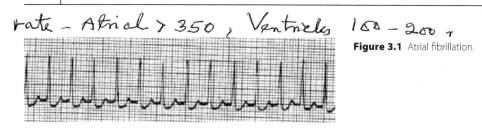

Figure 3.1 Atrial fibrillation.

ED Management

Treatment can usually be delayed until the patient is admitted to an intensive care setting, where therapy is aimed at control of ventricular rate, conversion to sinus rhythm, and prevention of stroke. However, in the ED, treat acute atrial fibrillation associated with a rapid ventricular rate and signs of hemodynamic compromise with synchronized cardioversion (0.5–2 J/kg).

If the patient is hemodynamically stable, consult a pediatric cardiologist before initiating pharmacologic cardioversion, which can most frequently be accomplished with amiodarone, sotalol, or procainamide. Rate control is best accomplished with diltiazem, digitalis, or esmolol. However, digitalis and verapamil are contraindicated if the patient is known to have WPW syndrome, since they may facilitate conduction through an accessory AV connection, leading to ventricular fibrillation.

Although atrial thrombus is uncommon in children with atrial fibrillation, give anticoagulation prior to cardioversion if the fibrillation has lasted for >48 hours. To document the presence of a thrombus, obtain a standard transthoracic echocardiogram, and if no thrombus is detected, a transesophageal study.

Indications for Admission

- Acute onset of atrial fibrillation
- Chronic atrial fibrillation with an increase in ventricular rate requiring treatment with a new anti-arrhythmic medication
- Intracardiac thrombus documented on echocardiogram

Bibliography

Agrawal H, Shakya N, Naheed Z. Atrial fibrillation in two adolescents. *Pediatr Cardiol.* 2012;**33** (5):850–853.

Cannon, BC, Snyder, CS. Disorders of cardiac rhythm and conduction. In Allen HD, Shaddy RE, Penny DJ, Feltes TF, Cetta F (eds.) *Moss and Adams' Heart Disease in Infants, Children, and Adolescents, Including the Fetus and Young Adult* (9th edn.). Philadelphia, PA: Lippincott Williams & Wilkins, 2016; 623–654.

Ceresnak SR, Liberman L, Silver ES, et al. Lone atrial fibrillation in the young: perhaps not so "lone"? *J Pediatr.* 2013;**162**:827–831

Fazio G, Visconti C, D'Angelo L, et al. Pharmacological therapy in children with atrial fibrillation and atrial flutter. *Curr Pharm Des.* 2008;**14**:770–775.

January CT, Wann LS, Alpert JS, et al. 2014 AHA/ACC/HRS guideline for the management of patients with atrial fibrillation: a report of the American College of Cardiology/American Heart Association Task Force on Practice Guidelines and the Heart Rhythm Society. *J Am Coll Cardiol*. 2014;**64**(21): e1–76.

[handwritten: (10) Anxiety, Fear, Pain, Fever, Exercise, Anemia, Hypovolemia, Hyperthyroidism, Congestive Ht failure, Medications]

Sinus Tachycardia

Sinus tachycardia (ST) is a physiologically increased heart rate for age that originates from the sinus node. The most common causes of ST are anxiety, fever, pain, hypovolemia, anemia, congestive heart failure, exercise, hyperthyroidism, and medications (stimulants, bronchodilators, decongestants). *[handwritten: DD - SVT (myocarditis)]*

Clinical Presentation and Diagnosis *[handwritten: rate 100–180, Infants upto 240]*

Since normal hemodynamics are generally maintained, ST is usually an incidental finding in a patient with a noncardiac disease process. The rate is generally between 100 and 180 bpm, although in infants the rate may reach 240 bpm.

Sinus tachycardia must be differentiated from supraventricular tachycardia, in which the rates are generally faster with little to no variability and the QRS complexes may not be preceded by recognizable P-waves of sinus origin. In some cases of SVT, the QRS complexes may follow abnormally directed P-waves. Increasing the ECG paper speed to 50 mm/second may help to identify normal P-waves.

ED Management

Most often, ST is encountered in the settings mentioned above, so therapy is directed toward identifying and treating these conditions.

Bibliography

Sedaghat-Yazdi F, Koenig PR. The teenager with palpitations. *Pediatr Clin North Am*. 2014;**61**(1):63–79.

Sowinski H, Karpawich PP. Management of a hyperactive teen and cardiac safety. *Pediatr Clin North Am*. 2014;**61**(1):81–90.

Vignati G, Annoni G. Characterization of supraventricular tachycardia in infants: clinical and instrumental diagnosis. *Curr Pharm Des*. 2008;**14**:729–735.

Supraventricular Tachycardia *[handwritten: HR 150 - 300.]*

Supraventricular tachycardia is the most common significant pediatric cardiac arrhythmia. The mechanism of SVT is usually reentry, secondary to microreentrant or macroreentrant circuits. In 20% of patients there is a trigger, such as infection or the use of cold remedies containing sympathomimetics (Table 3.1).

[handwritten: Trigger - Infection, Sympathomimetics.]

Clinical Presentation

The presentation depends on the age of the patient, the rate and duration of the tachycardia, and whether there is associated heart disease. Common clinical findings include palpitations, shortness of breath, chest pain, respiratory distress, dizziness, syncope, irritability, pallor, and poor feeding in infants. The heart rate is usually between 150 and 300 bpm.

Table 3.1 Factors predisposing to supraventricular tachycardia

Cardiomyopathy

Drugs

    Decongestants

    Ephedrine

    Epinephrine

    Methylphenidate

Ebstein's anomaly

Fever

Hyperthyroidism

Mitral valve prolapse

Myocarditis

Previous cardiac surgery

    Mustard or Senning procedure for transposition

    Fontan

Primary electrical disease

Atrioventricular bypass tract (WPW)

Dual AV nodal pathways

Sepsis

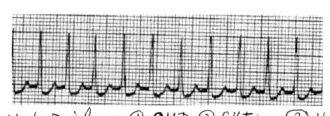

Figure 3.2 Supraventricular tachycardia.

Heart Failure ① CHD ② SVT ③ HR >200,
>24hrs

Heart failure is uncommon in patients >1 year of age and is usually associated with congenital heart disease, SVT for >24 hours, and heart rates >200 bpm.

Diagnosis

The electrocardiogram in SVT typically reveals a narrow complex tachycardia at a rate of 150–300 bpm. The P-wave may not be seen; it may be inverted just after the QRS complex; or it may precede the QRS, but have an abnormal axis (negative in leads I or AVF). The ventricular complexes are usually normal in contour, although aberrant rate-dependent conduction can cause slight widening. In SVT the atrial rate is 180–240 bpm, with 1:1 AV conduction and a fixed RR interval (Figure 3.2).

EKG HR 150-300, absent P waves, Narrow Complexes
RR interval is fixed.
No beat to beat Variation.

assume VT unless Dx SVT is absolutely certain,

Supraventricular tachycardia must be differentiated from ST. In the latter, the rate is usually <180 bpm (240 bpm in infants), a P-wave with normal axis precedes the QRS complex, and some variation in the RR interval may be present.

Supraventricular tachycardia with wide QRS complexes due to aberrant conduction may be difficult to differentiate from ventricular tachycardia. Ventricular tachycardia is suggested by the presence of atrioventricular dissociation, "fusion beats" (when the sinus and ventricular beats coincide to produce a hybrid beat), "capture beats" (when a conducted sinus beat transiently captures the ventricles to produce a narrow QRS complex beat), and very broad QRS complexes (>160 ms). In addition the patient will appear sicker, and possibly the tachycardia will be slower. *Assume that all wide complex tachycardias in children are ventricular tachycardia unless the diagnosis of SVT is absolutely* ✳ *certain.*

ED Management CHF Hemodynamic → Cardio Version•
compromise

Perform a history and physical examination, carefully evaluate the patient's hemodynamic status, and continuously monitor the ECG and blood pressure. Congestive heart failure or hemodynamic compromise are indications for rapid termination of the arrhythmia with DC cardioversion. After successful conversion to a sinus rhythm, obtain a complete ECG looking for WPW and refer the patient to a pediatric cardiologist.

Vagal Maneuvers

Vagal nerve stimulation increases the effective refractory period of the AV node, thus interrupting the reentrant circuit. Continuously monitor the ECG when vagal maneuvers are attempted. If successful, the tachycardia breaks abruptly and is replaced by a normal sinus rhythm (Figure 3.3). Transient slowing of the ventricular rate suggests that either sinus tachycardia or atrial flutter (Figure 3.4) was misdiagnosed as SVT. Do not use eyeball pressure, which can cause retinal detachment. Gagging and inducing vomiting can be effective, but may lead to aspiration in infants or agitated patients. Commonly employed vagal techniques include the following.

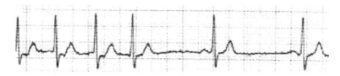

Figure 3.3 SVT response to treatment.

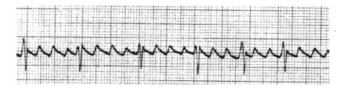

Figure 3.4 Atrial flutter.

Eliciting the Diving Reflex. Submerge the face of an older child in ice-cold water or place an ice bag with equal volumes of ice and water over the entire face for 10–20 seconds.

Unilateral Carotid Massage. Perform the massage at the junction of the carotid artery and the mandible. This is much more likely to be successful in the older child or adolescent.

Valsalva Maneuver. Ask the patient to "bear down," or "strain," as if attempting to move his or her bowels. If this is unsuccessful, have the patient stand on his or her head for 15–30 seconds.

Pharmacotherapy

Adenosine

Adenosine is the drug of choice for the treatment of SVT. It terminates SVT by slowing or blocking conduction in the AV node, thus breaking the reentry circuit. Give an initial dose of 0.1 mg/kg (6 mg maximum) as a rapid IV bolus, followed by a rapid saline bolus, preferably at a proximal IV site. The use of a three-way stopcock facilitates effective delivery. If ineffective in 2–3 minutes, double the dose (12 mg maximum). The onset of action is within 10–15 seconds and the half-life is about 15 seconds. Bradycardia, transient asystole, or atrial fibrillation may occur after termination of the arrhythmia. Flushing, wheezing, cough, and chest tightness are transient side effects.

Verapamil

Verapamil is a calcium slow channel blocker which is extremely effective in treating SVT. The dose is 0.075–0.15 mg/kg, slowly IV. This can be repeated twice at 15-minute intervals. Verapamil is contraindicated in patients <1 year of age because of possible cardiovascular collapse. Other contraindications include WPW (shortens the refractory period of a bypass tract), congestive heart failure, and beta-blocker (propranolol) use. Side effects may include bradycardia and hypotension; treat with atropine (0.01–0.04 mg/kg), isoproterenol (0.1 mcg/kg/min infusion), and calcium chloride (5–7 mg/kg of elemental calcium = 0.2–0.25 mL/kg of calcium chloride).

Digoxin   *for chronic therapy.*

Digoxin has a delayed onset of action (6–24 hours), so it is useful for the chronic therapy of SVT. The IV total digitalizing dose (TDD) is 30 mcg/kg. Give one-half of the TDD initially, then one-quarter of the TDD at 6–8-hour intervals. Digoxin is contraindicated in patients with WPW as it can shorten the refractory period of a bypass tract.

Cardioversion   *Synchronised, 0.5 – 1 J/kg, double upto 2J/kg*

Synchronous cardioversion is indicated when there is hemodynamic compromise (heart failure, shock, acidosis) or, rarely, if other treatment modalities have failed. The dose is 0.5–1 J/kg, which can be repeated, doubling the dose to a maximum of 2 J/kg. Sedate older patients with midazolam (0.1 mg/kg IV) prior to cardioversion. To prevent ventricular dysrhythmias, give lidocaine (1 mg/kg IV) to digitalized patients prior to attempting cardioversion. Prior to cardioversion, *be certain of synchronized mode setting*, to avoid precipitating a potentially lethal ventricular arrhythmia.

   Conversion to sinus rhythm using vagal maneuvers, adenosine, verapamil, and/or cardioversion is within the realm of the ED physician. If the SVT is refractory, consult

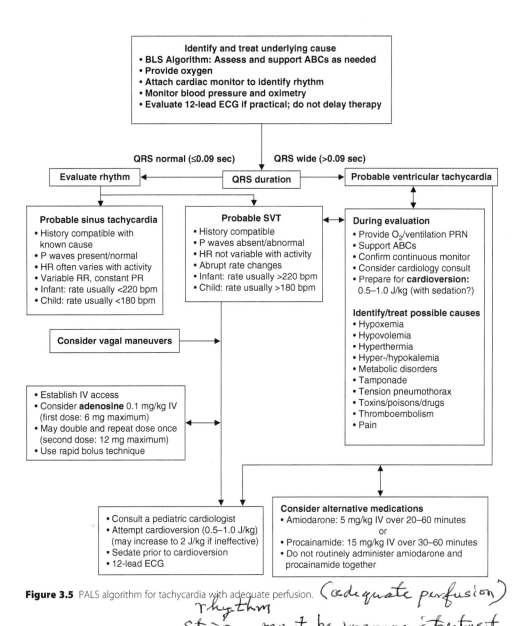

Figure 3.5 PALS algorithm for tachycardia with adequate perfusion. *(adequate perfusion)*
rhythm
strip — must be running ē treatment.

with a pediatric cardiologist who will determine the choice of second-line medications. Also consult after conversion is accomplished, to arrange appropriate evaluation and follow-up. It is imperative that a rhythm strip be running at the time of either adenosine infusion or cardioversion to document termination of the SVT, as this will aid in the categorization of the SVT subtype and is crucial in the prompt detection of degeneration of the rhythm. The Pediatric Advanced Life Support algorithms for tachycardia with adequate and poor perfusion are summarized in Figures 3.5 and 3.6.

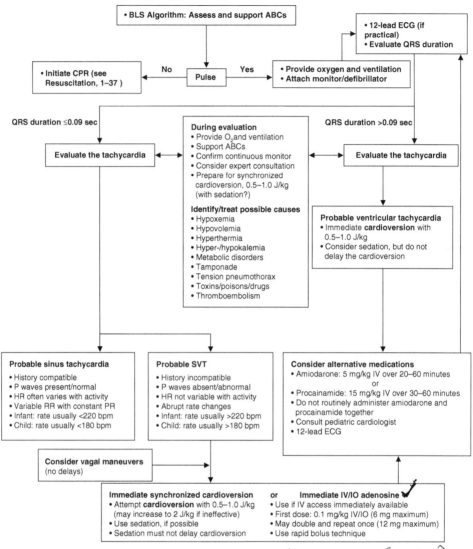

Figure 3.6 PALS algorithm for tachycardia with poor perfusion. (poor perfusion)

Follow-up

- SVT without hemodynamic compromise, terminated in ED: consult a pediatric cardiologist to determine appropriate follow-up

Indications for Admission

- SVT causing hemodynamic compromise
- Initiation of a medication with proarrhythmia potential (flecainide, sotalol, amiodarone)

Emergent - SCV (Collapse c Pulse) Defibrillation (Collapse w/o Pulse)

Rx

V. Tach Meds - Adenosine, Amiodarone or Procainamide.

Bibliography

Campbell M, Buitrago SR. BET 2: ice water immersion, other vagal manoeuvres or adenosine for SVT in children. *Emerg Med J.* 2017;**34**(1):58–60.

Cannon, BC, Snyder, CS. Disorders of cardiac rhythm and conduction. In Allen HD, Shaddy RE, Penny DJ, Feltes TF, Cetta F (eds.) *Moss and Adams' Heart Disease in Infants, Children, and Adolescents, Including the Fetus and Young Adult* (9th edn.). Philadelphia, PA: Lippincott Williams & Wilkins, 2016; 623–654.

Díaz-Parra S, Sánchez-Yañez P, Zabala-Argüelles I, et al. Use of adenosine in the treatment of supraventricular tachycardia in a pediatric emergency department. *Pediatr Emerg Care.* 2014;**30**(6):388–393.

Hanash CR, Crosson JE. Emergency diagnosis and management of pediatric arrhythmias. *J Emerg Trauma Shock.* 2010;3(3):251–260

Sedaghat-Yazdi F, Koenig PR. The teenager with palpitations. *Pediatr Clin North Am.* 2014;**61**(1):63–79.

Ventricular Premature Contractions

Ventricular premature contractions (VPCs) most commonly occur due to primary electrical disease in asymptomatic adolescents without structural heart disease. Other etiologies include ingestions (tobacco, sympathomimetic agents, tricyclic antidepressants, digoxin, caffeine), electrolyte imbalances (hypokalemia, hypocalcemia), anesthesia, and underlying heart disease (mitral valve prolapse, myocarditis, cardiomyopathy, coronary artery malformation, status-post ventricular surgery).

Clinical Presentation

Most cases are discovered during the routine examination of an asymptomatic patient, when an irregular heart beat is noted. However, some patients complain of chest discomfort, palpitations, chest pain, or syncope.

Diagnosis

Ventricular premature contractions are characterized by bizarre, widened QRS complexes which are not preceded by a P-wave (Figure 3.7). They may occur in a fixed ratio with normal beats (bigeminy 1:1; trigeminy 2:1) (Figure 3.8). They can be uniform (identical electrocardiographic appearance with consistent interval from the preceding QRS) or multiform (dissimilar ECG appearances with varying coupling intervals with the preceding

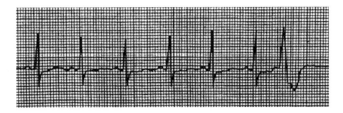

Figure 3.7 Ventricular premature contraction.

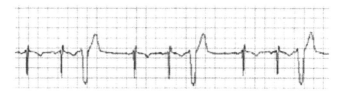

Figure 3.8 VPC in trigeminal pattern.

QRS). It is possible for a VPC with a short coupling interval to fall on the T-wave of the preceding normal complex (R-on-T phenomenon) and initiate ventricular tachycardia.

Ventricular premature contractions can also be divided into benign and ominous categories. *Benign VPCs* are uniform in morphology, with an otherwise normal resting ECG, including the QTc interval, and are not associated with an R-on-T phenomenon or structural heart disease. Benign VPCs can normally be suppressed by exercise, such as 20 seconds of jumping jacks.

Ominous VPCs may be multiform or short-coupled, and may be associated with a prolonged QTc interval, an R-on-T phenomenon, or structural heart disease. Exercise either has no effect or increases the VPC frequency and the number of VPCs can worsen during the recovery phase of activity. Ominous VPCs indicate an increased risk of ventricular tachycardia (three or more consecutive VPCs).

ED Management

Benign VPCs
No treatment is necessary. However, for reassurance, elective referral to a pediatric cardiologist may be indicated.

Ominous VPCs
Consult with a pediatric cardiologist, who may recommend admission and/or treatment.

Follow-up
- Benign VPCs: primary care follow-up in 1–2 weeks

Indications for Admission
- Ominous VPCs

Bibliography

Cannon, BC, Snyder, CS. Disorders of cardiac rhythm and conduction. In Allen HD, Shaddy RE, Penny DJ, Feltes TF, Cetta F (eds.) *Moss and Adams' Heart Disease in Infants, Children, and Adolescents, Including the Fetus and Young Adult* (9th edn.). Philadelphia, PA: Lippincott Williams & Wilkins, 2016; 623–654.

Crosson JE, Callans DJ, Bradley DJ, et al. PACES/HRS expert consensus statement on the evaluation and management of ventricular arrhythmias in the child with a structurally normal heart. *Heart Rhythm.* 2014;**11**(9):e55–78.

Spector ZZ, Seslar SP. Premature ventricular contraction-induced cardiomyopathy in children. *Cardiol Young*. 2016;**26**(4):711–717.

Tanel RE. ECGs in the ED. *Pediatr Emerg Care*. 2015;**31**(7):542–543.

Ventricular Tachycardia   *Can degenerate to V. fib.*

Wide complex tachycardias are uncommon in children, but they are potentially more dangerous than narrow complex tachycardias. Wide complex tachycardias may be ventricular or supraventricular (with aberrancy secondary to a bundle branch block or WPW syndrome) in origin. However, in the ED, *assume that a wide complex tachycardia is ventricular tachycardia* and treat accordingly. Erroneously treating ventricular tachycardia as SVT can be devastating. Also, ventricular tachycardia can degenerate into ventricular fibrillation, either as a terminal event or in the setting of a prolonged QT interval.

It is important to remember that the upper limit of normal QRS duration varies with age. For example, a tachycardia with a QRS duration of 0.10 seconds is wide complex in a newborn, but narrow complex in a ten-year-old.

Ventricular tachycardia (VT) is defined as a series of three or more consecutive ectopic beats originating from the ventricles. Etiologies include a heterogeneous group of disorders, including primary electrical disease (long QTc syndrome), hypoxemia, electrolyte imbalance (hyperkalemia), and ingestions (tricyclics, digoxin). More than 50% of children with VT have evidence for organic heart disease such as cardiomyopathy (including arrhythmogenic right ventricular dysplasia) and myocarditis.

Clinical Presentation

The symptomatology depends on the rate and duration of the tachycardia and the presence or absence of underlying structural heart disease. Occasional patients are asymptomatic, although chest pain, syncope, and palpitations are common, and lethargy, disorientation, hypotension, and sudden death with hemodynamic collapse can occur.

Diagnosis

Ventricular tachycardia is a wide QRS complex tachycardia. The rate of VT (Figure 3.9) is 120–200 bpm, which is slower than SVT with aberrant conduction. Ventricular tachycardia is suggested by AV dissociation, or QRS morphology that resembles a single VPC present during sinus rhythm elsewhere on the ECG.

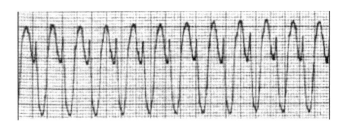

Figure 3.9 Ventricular tachycardia.

ED Management

Regardless of the patient's status, consult a pediatric cardiologist.

Hemodynamically Stable

Treat stable monomorphic VT and polymorphic VT in a patient with a normal baseline QTc interval with intravenous amiodarone (5 mg/kg over 20–60 min) or intravenous procainamide (15 mg/kg over 30–60 min). Consult a pediatric cardiologist for further management in an intensive care setting. In patients with digitalis toxicity, use antidigitalis antibody. For polymorphic VT in a patient with QTc prolongation on baseline EKG, give magnesium sulfate (10–25 mg/kg infusion over 30–60 min).

Hemodynamically Compromised With Palpable Pulses

The treatment of choice is synchronized cardioversion at an initial dose of 0.5 J/kg; double the dose and repeat if not successful. If the rhythm does not convert, give an IV lidocaine bolus (1 mg/kg), followed by a third attempt at cardioversion. Ventricular pacing by a cardiologist may be required. The treatment is summarized in Figure 1.5.

Hemodynamically Compromised Without Pulses

Defibrillate with 2 J/kg; double to 4 J/kg for a maximum of three consecutive defibrillations or until conversion to sinus rhythm. The treatment is summarized in Figure 3.6.

Indications for Admission

- Newly diagnosed or difficult to control VT
- Presumed or documented VT with long QT syndrome

Bibliography

Cannon, BC, Snyder CS. Disorders of cardiac rhythm and conduction. In Allen HD, Shaddy RE, Penny DJ Feltes TF, Cetta F (eds.) *Moss and Adams' Heart Disease in Infants, Children, and Adolescents, Including the Fetus and Young Adult* (9th edn.). Philadelphia, PA: Lippincott Williams & Wilkins, 2016; 623–654.

Denjoy I, Lupoglazoff JM, Crosson JE, et al. PACES/HRS expert consensus statement on the evaluation and management of ventricular arrhythmias in the child with a structurally normal heart. *Heart Rhythm*. 2014;**11**(9):e55–78

Priori SG, Blomström-Lundqvist C, Mazzanti A, et al. 2015 ESC guidelines for the management of patients with ventricular arrhythmias and the prevention of sudden cardiac death: The Task Force for the Management of Patients with Ventricular Arrhythmias and the Prevention of Sudden Cardiac Death of the European Society of Cardiology (ESC). Endorsed by: Association for European Paediatric and Congenital Cardiology (AEPC). *Eur Heart J*. 2015;**36**(41):2793–2867.

Swayampakula AK, Fong J, Kulkarni A. Arrhythmogenic causes of syncope. *Pediatr Emerg Care*. 2014;**30**(12):894–895.

Ventricular Fibrillation

Ventricular tachycardia can degenerate into ventricular fibrillation, either as a terminal event or when there is a prolonged QT interval or R-on-T phenomenon.

℞ Defibrillation 2J/kg, 4J/kg consecutive × 3 times,
then IV - alternate Lidocaine & Epinephrine -
& Cont defibrillation.

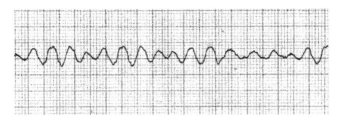

Figure 3.10 Ventricular fibrillation.

Clinical Presentation

Patients with ventricular fibrillation are generally unresponsive and pulseless.

Diagnosis

In ventricular fibrillation (Figure 3.10) there is a wavy, sinusoidal line, without any true QRS complexes.

ED Management

If the VT degenerates into ventricular fibrillation, immediately defibrillate using 2 J/kg. If unsuccessful, double to 4 J/kg for three consecutive defibrillations. If unsuccessful, also give IV lidocaine (1 mg/kg) alternating with epinephrine (0.1 mL/kg of 1:10,000 IV or 0.1 mL/kg of 1:1000 ET). If fibrillation recurs, start a lidocaine continuous infusion (20–50 mcg/kg/min).

Indications for Admission

- Any patient who survives after treatment for ventricular fibrillation

Bibliography

Cannon BC, Snyder CS. Disorders of cardiac rhythm and conduction. In Allen HD, Shaddy RE, Penny DJ, Feltes TF, Cetta F (eds.) *Moss and Adams' Heart Disease in Infants, Children, and Adolescents, Including the Fetus and Young Adult* (9th edn.). Philadelphia, PA: Lippincott Williams & Wilkins, 2016; 623–654.

de Caen AR, Berg MD, Chameides L, et al. Part 12: Pediatric Advanced Life Support: 2015 American Heart Association Guidelines Update for Cardiopulmonary Resuscitation and Emergency Cardiovascular Care. *Circulation.* 2015;**132**(18 Suppl. 2):S526–S542.

Lichtenfeld J, Deal BJ, Crawford S. Sudden cardiac arrest following ventricular fibrillation attributed to anabolic steroid use in an adolescent. *Cardiol Young.* 2016;**26**(5):996–998.

Shah AJ, Hocini M, Denis A, et al. Polymorphic ventricular tachycardia ventricular fibrillation and sudden cardiac death in the normal heart. *Card Electrophysiol Clin.* 2016;**8**(3):581–591.

Heart Block (Atrioventricular Block)

Heart block is secondary to delayed atrioventricular (AV) conduction. It can be primary, as in patients with congenital complete heart block, or secondary, as with myocarditis or Lyme disease.

Clinical Presentation and Diagnosis

First-Degree AV Block

First-degree block is defined as prolongation of the PR interval (Figure 3.11). Patients are asymptomatic. It may be seen with increased vagal tone, digoxin administration, myocarditis, acute rheumatic fever, or diphtheria, or it may be a primary electrical phenomenon. The location of the delay is supranodal (above the level of the AV node), and thus does not represent malignant AV conduction system disease.

Second-Degree AV Block *Mobitz II can progress to 3° A-V Block.*

Second-degree block may be secondary to acute or chronic heart disease, or it may occasionally occur in otherwise normal children. With *Mobitz type I* (Wenckebach) there is progressive lengthening of the PR interval until the impulse is not conducted and a ventricular beat is dropped (Figure 3.12). Mobitz type I is thought to occur at the AV node and it can present in otherwise normal patients, usually during periods of hypervagotonia. In *Mobitz type II*, ventricular beats are dropped without prior prolongation of the PR interval (Figure 3.13). The site of block is in the more distal AV conduction system. Therefore, with type II there is a greater chance of progression to complete (third-degree) heart block, while type I is more likely to be benign.

Third-Degree AV Block *A-V dissociation, Atrial rate > Vent. rate*

Third-degree AV block represents complete failure of conduction of the atrial impulses to the ventricles. There is AV dissociation; the atria and ventricles beat completely independently (Figure 3.14) and the atrial rate is faster than the ventricular rate. Generally, the lower the location of the pacemaker within the ventricular conduction system, the slower the rate

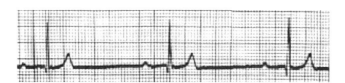

Figure 3.11 First-degree heart block.

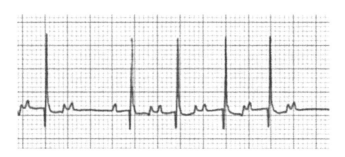

Figure 3.12 Mobitz I second-degree heart block.

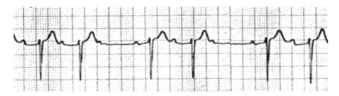

Figure 3.13 Mobitz II Second-degree heart block.

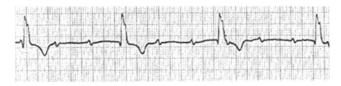

Figure 3.14 Third-degree heart block.

and the wider the QRS complexes. The etiology may be congenital (isolated or associated with congenital heart disease) or acquired (postoperative, acute rheumatic fever, Lyme disease, streptococcal infection, digoxin toxicity, or hyper- and hypocalcemia).

Many patients with congenital third-degree heart block are asymptomatic. However, a patient may exhibit decreased exercise tolerance, congestive heart failure, dizziness, or syncope. Acquired complete heart block is usually symptomatic, with syncope, congestive heart failure, shock, or sudden death. These are more likely in a patient with an awake pulse <50 bpm, a wide complex escape rhythm, and structural heart disease.

ED Management

First-Degree AV Block

No treatment is required other than determining the etiology of the disturbance. If no pathologic mechanism is identified, the patient may be discharged.

Second-Degree AV Block *Type I – no Rx, Type II – admit, pacemaker.*

No intervention is needed for type I block. For type II, attempt to determine the etiology, admit the patient, and consult a pediatric cardiologist to evaluate for possible pacemaker implantation.

Third-Degree AV Block *will need pacing*

Congenital complete heart block usually requires pacemaker insertion eventually. Infants with congestive heart failure, hydrops, ventricular rates <55 bpm, wide complex escape rhythms, pauses >3 seconds, or premature ventricular contractions require pacing. Older children or adolescents with heart rates <50 bpm, prolonged pauses >3 seconds, sinus tachycardia (short P–P-wave intervals), congenital complete AV block and dizziness, syncope, exercise intolerance, or VPCs also require pacing.

Patients with acquired third-degree block require temporary or permanent pacing. The ventricular rate may occasionally be increased by beta-adrenergic agents (isoproterenol) or vagolytics (atropine) in patients with reversible AV block (Lyme disease or ingestion) or while awaiting permanent pacemaker placement. Consult a pediatric cardiologist prior to instituting pharmacotherapy.

Follow-up
- Cardiology follow-up of newly diagnosed first- or Mobitz type I second-degree AV block within one week

Indications for Admission
- First degree: marked PR interval prolongation (>400 ms)
- Second degree: newly diagnosed, postoperative, or symptomatic
- Third degree: newly diagnosed, congestive failure, or syncope

Bibliography
Cannon BC, Snyder CS. Disorders of cardiac rhythm and conduction. In Allen HD, Shaddy RE, Penny DJ, Feltes TF, Cetta F. (eds.) *Moss and Adams' Heart Disease in Infants, Children, and Adolescents, Including the Fetus and Young Adult* (9th edn.). Philadelphia, PA: Lippincott Williams & Wilkins, 2016; 623–654.

Pacemaker and Defibrillator Assessment
An increasing number of children have permanent pacemakers or implanted defibrillators. These patients may have congenital complete heart block, cardiac channelopathy, or congenital or acquired cardiomyopathy, or may have had cardiac surgery.

Clinical Presentation and Diagnosis
Patients may present with palpitations, dizziness, syncope, or collapse, and may report the sensation of receiving a therapeutic shock. Obtain an ECG or place the patient on a monitor to determine the cardiac rhythm, but interrogation of the implanted device using a manufacturer-specific interrogation/programming device is also necessary for the accurate diagnosis of device function.

ED Management

Pacemaker
Assess the ECG for pacemaker activity, rhythm and rate (Figure 3.15). If heart rate is inadequate for cardiac output, emergency external pacing may be necessary. Contact a pediatric cardiologist or the local manufacturer's representative for interrogation of pacemaker parameters. Some pacemaker issues can be solved with reprogramming, while others will require change of lead and/or device.

Defibrillator
If the patient is stable, consult a pediatric cardiologist to assess the urgency of interrogation of the device and advisability of adjustments in medical therapy.

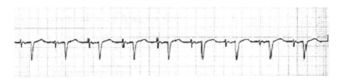

Figure 3.15 Pacemaker spikes.

Follow-up

- As per the pediatric cardiologist, based upon the nature of the device problem and whether it can be solved by reprogramming

Indications for Admission

- Significant problem with pacemaker, defibrillator, or lead that cannot be solved with reprogramming
- Ongoing symptoms that indicate either continuous or intermittent hemodynamic instability or the potential for life-threatening dysrhythmia

Bibliography

Bordachar P, Marquié C, Pospiech T, et al. Subcutaneous implantable cardioverter defibrillators in children, young adults and patients with congenital heart disease. *Int J Cardiol.* 2016;**203**:251–258.

Chiu-Man C. How pacemakers work and simple programming: a primer for the non-electrophysiologist. *Cardiol Young.* 2017;**27**(S1):S115–S120.

Janoušek J, Kubuš P. What's new in cardiac pacing in children? *Curr Opin Cardiol.* 2014;**29**(1):76–82.

Chest Pain

Chest pain is a common complaint in late childhood and adolescence. While it is often a manifestation of underlying cardiac disease in the adult population, it is relatively infrequently associated with cardiac disease in younger patients. In children, chest pain is commonly associated with asthma and musculoskeletal conditions. Nonetheless, it is important to rule-out a cardiac etiology.

Clinical Presentation and Diagnosis

Note the characteristics of the pain, including the subjective quality (e.g., sharp, dull, aching), the position in which it is greatest, radiation, duration, and alleviating or exacerbating factors. Cardiac pain is typically associated with exercise and improves with rest. Associated symptoms may be especially useful in determining the etiology of the pain. Also ask about a family history of sudden death (particularly during exercise), cardiomyopathy, or "heart attacks" at early ages.

Noncardiac Etiologies

Musculoskeletal Problems

Musculoskeletal problems are common causes of chest pain in the pediatric population. Tietze's syndrome (costochondritis) is characterized by anterior chest pain and tenderness to palpation over the sternocostal or costochondral junctions. Reproduction of the patient's pain on palpation is the most helpful sign. Intercostal muscle cramping (precordial catch syndrome) in the left substernal area may mimic this condition.

Psychogenic Causes

Although psychogenic causes are the second most frequent, always consider them to be diagnoses of exclusion. Adolescents with hyperventilation or anxiety can present with chest pain. The history may reveal repeated episodes of hysterical behavior, recent personal or family stresses, or a relative with heart disease. Typical complaints include shortness of breath, palpitations, or tingling of the extremities. The pain often mimics one or more organic conditions, but usually it suggests several conditions in the differential diagnosis.

Pulmonary Chest Pain

Chest pain can be pleuritic in nature, exacerbated by deep inspiration, swallowing, and coughing. It is caused by inflammation or irritation of the pleura, and is seen most commonly in pneumonia, pleurodynia (Coxsackievirus), or pneumothorax. Pulmonary embolism or infarction can present similarly. Bronchospasm may be the most common pulmonary cause of chest pain. A careful history of associated symptoms (fever, cough, preceding upper respiratory infection), oral contraceptive use, and underlying chronic disease (sickle cell anemia, cystic fibrosis, asthma, systemic lupus erythematosus) is useful for differentiating among these etiologies.

Gastroesophageal Disease

Gastrointestinal reflux (GERD), esophagitis, gastritis, and gastrointestinal spasm can all cause precordial pain. While upper esophageal pain is usually well localized, mid- and lower esophageal pain may be noted from the epigastrium to the suprasternal notch and radiate to the back or arms. The heart and esophagus have similar segmental innervation, so the substernal "burning" pain of GERD may mimic angina pectoris, which is distinctly uncommon in the pediatric age group. The discomfort may be associated with eating (postprandially or in the early morning before breakfast), accentuated in the recumbent position and with straining, and relieved with antacids or cold milk.

Cardiac Etiologies

Pericarditis

Pericarditis can present with pleuritic-type chest pain that is relieved by sitting up. Patients are often unable to assume the supine position, and the pain is frequently referred to the neck, shoulders, and abdomen. On physical examination a pericardial friction rub may be noted in the midprecordial area with the patient supine or in the left lateral decubitus position. The ECG typically shows ST segment elevation, and a chest x-ray may reveal cardiomegaly if there is a moderately large pericardial effusion. An echocardiogram is diagnostic in excluding a significant pericardial effusion, but may not be definitive if there is pericarditis without effusion.

Arrhythmias

Inadequate coronary blood flow secondary to an arrhythmia can cause chest pain (see Arrhythmias, pp. 47–62).

Aortic Dissection

Although aortic dissection is extremely rare in childhood, consider it in patients with connective tissue disorders (Marfan syndrome, Ehlers–Danlos syndrome). The severe pain is typically sudden in onset and "tearing" in quality. Radiation is from the anterior chest to the neck and back.

Coronary Artery Disease

Coronary artery disease (myocardial ischemia, angina pectoris, myocardial infarction) is extremely rare in the pediatric population. Arteritis and cocaine use may present with the pain of myocardial ischemia or infarction. Severe persistent irritability has been noted in infants with aberrant origin of the left coronary artery from the pulmonary artery; only very rarely do older children present with recurrent episodes of chest pain after exercise. Patients with a history of Kawasaki disease, who can be at risk for coronary artery thrombosis and aneurysm, may present with pallor, diaphoresis, or irritability, in addition to precordial discomfort. Coronary artery spasm leading to myocardial ischemia can also be seen, most commonly in teenagers, particularly with a history of cocaine use.

ED Management

Most cases of chest pain are either musculoskeletal, gastroesophageal, pulmonary, or psychogenic in origin. Therefore, a careful history, palpation of the chest wall, and pulmonary and cardiac auscultation usually suffice to determine the etiology and initiate appropriate therapy. Ask an adolescent about the possibility of recent cocaine use. Treat costochondritis with ibuprofen 10 mg/kg q 6h.

If a cardiac etiology is suspected (irregular pulse, auscultation of an organic murmur, a systolic click, or a friction rub), obtain an ECG and check for ST- or T-wave abnormalities, chamber enlargement or hypertrophy, conduction, abnormality, or arrhythmia. Many patients with noncardiac chest pain are concerned about the possibility of heart disease and are reassured by a normal ECG.

Further evaluation is dictated by the history and physical findings. A chest x-ray is indicated for patients with pleuritic chest pain, dyspnea, tachycardia, or cyanosis. Obtain a CBC, ESR, CRP, and ECG if acute pericarditis or myocarditis is suspected, and serial troponins if myocardial infarction is a possibility. An echocardiogram, while usually not required for assessment of chest pain in children, can be helpful if these specific conditions are being considered. If an intermittent arrhythmia is suspected, refer the patient to a cardiologist for a non-emergent evaluation.

Follow-up

- Stable patient with noncardiac chest pain: primary care follow-up in 1–2 weeks

Indications for Admission

- Suspected coronary artery disease, pleural effusion, myocarditis, pericarditis, or aortic dissection
- Severe chest pain of unknown etiology

Bibliography

Blake JM. A teen with chest pain. *Pediatr Clin North Am*. 2014;**61**(1):17–28.

Collins SA, Griksaitis MJ, Legg JP. 15-minute consultation: a structured approach to the assessment of chest pain in a child. *Arch Dis Child Educ Pract Ed*. 2014;**99**(4):122–126.

Friedman KG, Alexander ME. Chest pain and syncope in children: a practical approach to the diagnosis of cardiac disease. *J Pediatr*. 2013;**163**(3):896–901.e1–3.

Yeh TK, Yeh J. Chest pain in pediatrics. *Pediatr Ann*. 2015;**44**(12):e274–278.

Congestive Heart Failure

By definition, congestive heart failure (CHF) occurs when the heart cannot maintain adequate tissue perfusion to meet the body's basal metabolic requirements, which in children includes growth.

Four principal factors determine cardiac function: preload (ventricular end diastolic volume), contractility (force of ventricular contraction), afterload (force opposing ventricular ejection or intramyocardial tension during ejection), and heart rate. The first three factors are responsible for generating the stroke volume of the heart (i.e., the volume of blood pumped from the left ventricle with each heart beat). Changes in heart rate or stroke volume directly affect cardiac output, which, in turn, is a major determinant of blood pressure.

In general, physiologic problems include excessive pressure loads (increased afterload), excessive volume loads (increased preload), inotropic depression from impaired muscle, and rhythm disturbances. Either congenital structural heart defects and/or acquired diseases affecting the strength of the heart muscle can lead to CHF (Table 3.2).

Table 3.2 Etiologies of congestive heart failure

Acquired heart diseases

Cardiomyopathy

Endocarditis

Inflammatory conditions

  Kawasaki disease

  Myocarditis

  Rheumatic fever

Rhythm disorders

Congenital heart disease

Rhythm disorders

  Structural problems

  Coarctation of the aorta

  Critical aortic stenosis

  Large shunt lesions

  Left ventricular outflow obstruction

  Severe valvular regurgitation

Table 3.2 (cont.)

Postoperative cardiac problems

AV valve regurgitation

Ischemic cardiomyopathy

Extracardiac diseases

Lipid disorders (severe)

Metabolic-endocrine diseases

   Electrolyte disorders

   Hypocalcemia

   Hypoglycemia

   Hypothyroidism and thyroid storm

Sepsis

Toxins

Anti-arrhythmics

Cancer chemotherapy (adriamycin)

Cardiac depressants

   Phenytoin

   Lidocaine

Cocaine

Digoxin

Primary cardiac medicines

Clinical Presentation

The clinical manifestations of CHF reflect physiologic adjustments to reduced cardiac function. These include mechanical (hypertrophy and dilatation), biochemical (cardiac cellular energetic changes), neurohumoral (adrenergic nervous system), hematologic (oxygen transport effects), and pulmonary (tachypnea) responses.

On examination, the patient is usually tachycardic and tachypneic. Pulmonary congestion causes rales, rhonchi, and wheezing, which may be confused with primary pulmonary disease. In infants, rales may be absent despite considerable tachypnea and intercostal/subcostal retractions, while in older children dyspnea on exertion or orthopnea may be present. A chronic cough may also be associated with pulmonary congestion.

On cardiac auscultation, there may be a third heart sound (S_3), the ventricular gallop, which is a sign of poor ventricular compliance and increased resistance to filling. A fourth heart sound (S_4), the atrial gallop, can also be heard, particularly in older children, although sometimes both of these can be present with otherwise normal cardiac findings. Not infrequently, a holosystolic, blowing murmur associated with mitral regurgitation can be heard, associated with left ventricular dilatation.

There may also be central and peripheral edema, although this is unusual in infants. Liver enlargement, jugular venous distension, and other signs of tissue fluid accumulation may be seen. The extremities may be pale and cool secondary to compensatory vasoconstriction. Pulsus alternans (beat-to-beat variability in pulse strength) is a palpable sign of poor myocardial strength. With chronic CHF, growth failure, especially in young infants, reflects increased caloric expenditure as well as undernutrition associated with feeding difficulties. Congestive heart failure can also be associated with tachypnea and diaphoresis, particularly during feeding in the infant.

Cardiac enlargement results from ventricular dilatation and is usually readily apparent, along with pulmonary congestion, on the chest x-ray. Often, cardiomegaly can also be detected by palpation of a laterally displaced cardiac impulse. Cardiac hypertrophy is usually easily noted on an ECG (left or combined ventricular hypertrophy).

Diagnosis

Obtain a thorough history, as the presence of preexisting cardiac disease or of conditions related to myocardial dysfunction can be important indicators of the possibility of CHF. Ask about a history of thalassemia or other chronic anemia; systemic infections such as HIV; systemic illnesses such as collagen vascular disease or metabolic diseases; or other acquired diseases such as rheumatic fever or Kawasaki disease. Ask about recent history of upper respiratory tract illness, as respiratory viruses are often the most frequent causes of myocarditis in children.

Often, an older child with overt CHF presents with a combination of wheezing, respiratory distress, bibasilar rales, and hepatomegaly. In general, however, wheezing is most often secondary to asthma. There may be a history of asthma and allergies, or a family history of allergies, or the patient may have eczema. Bronchiolitis also causes similar findings during seasonal epidemics. The patient may have fever, rhonchi, and rales in addition to wheezing.

Other causes of tachypnea, respiratory distress, and cough are pneumonia (fever, localized fine end-inspiratory rales, no hepatomegaly), croup (fever, inspiratory stridor), and foreign body aspiration (sudden onset of inspiratory stridor). Most etiologies of hepatomegaly (pp. 272–273) are not associated with tachypnea or respiratory distress. When the diagnosis is in doubt, obtain a chest x-ray to look for cardiomegaly and pulmonary vascular congestion.

ED Management

Although the etiology dictates the specific therapy, begin with general treatment. Give supplemental humidified oxygen and elevate the head and shoulders. Start an IV and obtain blood for an ABG, electrolytes, and a CBC. Obtain an ECG early in the course, as therapy for an underlying arrhythmia may be necessary. Inquire about the chronic use of cardiac medications. Consult with a cardiologist to help confirm the diagnosis and develop a specific treatment strategy.

Give IV diuretics (furosemide 1–2 mg/kg), unless pericardial tamponade (pp. 758–759) is suspected. Give morphine sulfate (0.05–0.1 mg/kg subcutaneously) if there is pulmonary edema and consequent air hunger and restlessness. A slow transfusion of packed RBCs (10 mL/kg) is indicated for severe anemia (hematocrit <28%). Give sodium bicarbonate (1–2 mEq/kg) only for severe acidosis (pH <7.2); the airway must be secure since respiratory decompensation may elevate the pCO_2 and cerebral edema can develop.

Table 3.3 Treatment of congestive heart failure

Preload reduction (diuretics)	
Furosemide	1 mg/kg PO or IV, up to qid
Hydrochlorothiazide	2 mg/kg PO, up to bid
Metalozone	0.2 mg/kg PO, up to bid
Afterload reduction	
Captopril	0.1–0.5 mg/kg PO q 8h
Enalapril	0.1 mg/kg PO q day or bid (0.5 mg/kg/day maximum)
Milrinone	0.5–1 mcg/kg/min IV
Nitroprusside	0.5–10 mcg/kg/min IV
Inotropic agents	
Digoxin (IV doses are 75% of PO)	
Premature babies	5 mcg/kg/day div bid
0–10 years	10 mcg/kg/day PO div bid
>10 years	5 mcg/kg/day PO per day
Dobutamine	5–25 mcg/kg/min IV
Dopamine	5–25 mcg/kg/min IV

Occasionally, respiratory support including intubation and mechanical ventilation may be required; inotropic support is then usually needed also. In the acute setting, dobutamine or dopamine (start with 3–5 mcg/kg/min) is preferred. Digoxin may also be given, but its onset of action is longer and specific control over dosage is less precise. In severe cases, addition of afterload reducing agents (milrinone or enalapril) may be required, once indwelling pressure monitoring has been secured and a cardiologist is present (Table 3.3).

Two-dimensional echocardiography may help identify the cause of the CHF and document the magnitude of the decrease in ventricular function (ejection fraction), as well as the extent of cardiac chamber enlargement and valvar regurgitation. Long-term management usually includes an ACE inhibitor or beta-blocker.

Follow-up
- CHF successfully treated in the ED: 1–2 days

Indications for Admission
- Newly diagnosed or worsening CHF
- New arrhythmia or a newly acquired complication, such as endocarditis, which requires urgent attention

Bibliography

Atallah J, Buchholz H, Chant-Gambacort C, et al. Presentation, diagnosis, and medical management of heart failure in children: Canadian Cardiovascular Society guidelines. *Can J Cardiol.* 2013;**29** (12):1535–1552.

O'Connor, MJ, Shaddy, RE. Chronic heart failure in children. In Allen HD, Shaddy RE, Penny DJ, Feltes TF, Cetta F. (eds.) *Moss and Adams' Heart Disease in Infants, Children, and Adolescents, Including the Fetus and Young Adult* (9th edn.). Philadelphia, PA: Lippincott Williams & Wilkins, 2016; 1687–1706.

Park MK. Congestive heart failure. In *Park's Pediatric Cardiology for Practitioners* (6th edn.). Philadelphia, PA: Elsevier Saunders, 2014; 451–464.

Rossano JW, Cabrera AG, Jefferies JL, Naim MP, Humlicek T. Pediatric Cardiac Intensive Care Society 2014 consensus statement: pharmacotherapies in cardiac critical care chronic heart failure. *Pediatr Crit Care Med.* 2016;**17**(3 Suppl. 1):S20–S34.

Cyanosis

Cyanosis specifically refers to a bluish tone visible in the mucous membranes and skin when desaturated or abnormal hemoglobin is present in the peripheral circulation. At least 5 g/dL of reduced hemoglobin is required for cyanosis to be visible. Thus, systemic desaturation may be substantial but not apparent to the eye if there is an associated anemia. Conversely, abnormal hemoglobins may be fully saturated with oxygen, yet unable to release it to the tissues, so cyanosis will also be visible. Methemoglobinemia is the classic example of this situation.

Central cyanosis occurs when poorly oxygenated blood enters the systemic circulation. This usually occurs through a cardiac defect allowing systemic venous blood to bypass the pulmonary capillary bed. This is termed a "right-to-left" shunt and may occur within the heart or in the pulmonary circulation itself. When there is primary parenchymal lung disease or neurologic disease causing alveolar hypoventilation an "intrapulmonary" right-to-left shunt can occur.

Typical cyanotic lesions are the "five Ts" of congenital heart disease (*t*etralogy of Fallot, *t*ransposition of the great vessels, *t*otal anomalous pulmonary venous return, *t*ricuspid atresia, and *t*runcus arteriosus), but others may also be present. Pulmonary diseases causing cyanosis can occur anywhere along the airway, from upper airway obstructive problems (croup, epiglottitis) to lower airway diseases (asthma, cystic fibrosis, pneumonia with lobar consolidation).

Peripheral cyanosis, on the other hand, usually does not reflect reduced systemic arterial oxygenation but is typically found in otherwise healthy patients who are exposed to cold or who have a vasoconstrictor response to fever. This will be visible in the nail beds, but absent from the perioral mucous membranes or conjunctivae. Peripheral cyanosis can also occur as a result of circulatory insufficiency or chronic neuromuscular disease with changes in peripheral vasomotor tone.

Clinical Presentation and Diagnosis

Observation for the presence of cyanosis requires proper ambient conditions. Neon lighting, for example, may cause a false bluish tint, while cyanosis may be difficult to discern in a dark-skinned patient unless there is a strong light source.

Respiratory findings are of vital importance and may help to differentiate among the possible causes of cyanosis. Tachypnea may be present with most pulmonary diseases or with cardiac conditions associated with excess pulmonary blood flow. Shallow respirations, not necessarily associated with an increase in rate, may indicate a neurologic problem. Hyperpnea, or deep breathing with only a mild increase in rate, is more characteristic of a primary cardiac disorder where alveolar ventilation is maximized but pulmonary blood flow is reduced. Hyperpnea can also reflect metabolic acidosis or elevated intracranial pressure.

Differentiating cardiac from pulmonary etiologies is critical. In many, though not all, cases of cardiac disease the breath sounds will be normal and the pattern of chest excursions symmetric, while wheezes, rhonchi, and chest wall abnormalities usually accompany a pulmonary process. In either case there is reduced oxygen saturation, but the patient with cyanotic cardiac disease has little response to increased ambient oxygen, whereas with pulmonary disease the saturation increase may be dramatic (hyperoxia test). An ABG may also be useful, since an elevated pCO_2 indicating impaired ventilatory status is usually not seen with cyanotic congenital heart disease unless there is associated pulmonary congestion. The chest x-ray may reveal cardiomegaly, an abnormal pulmonary circulatory pattern, or overt pulmonary parenchymal abnormalities such as atelectasis or pneumothorax.

The absence of a heart murmur does not rule-out cyanotic cardiac disease, as in most conditions with right-to-left shunting there is no murmur. Also, in some conditions, such as tetralogy of Fallot, the murmur may lessen as the cyanosis becomes more intense secondary to decreased pulmonary blood flow.

ED Management

See *Cyanotic (Tet) Spells* (pp. 72–73) for the treatment of an acute hypoxemic attack ("spell"). For chronic cyanotic congenital heart conditions, supportive treatment is all that can be done until a surgical or catheter-directed intervention can be accomplished. Give supplemental oxygen, even though dramatic changes in saturation will not occur with oxygen alone. Secure IV access and give fluid to maintain an adequate circulating volume. Treat systemic acidosis once adequate ventilation is assured. Most of all, immediately consult with a cardiologist to arrange for more definitive treatment and to prevent unnecessary interventions.

Indications for Admission

• Central cyanosis

Bibliography

Hiremath G, Kamat D. Diagnostic considerations in infants and children with cyanosis. *Pediatr Ann.* 2015;**44**(2):76–80.

Judge P, Meckler MG. Congenital heart disease in pediatric patients: recognizing the undiagnosed and managing complications in the emergency department. *Pediatr Emerg Med Pract.* 2016;**13**(5):1–28.

Strobel AM, Lu le N. The critically ill infant with congenital heart disease. *Emerg Med Clin North Am.* 2015;**33**(3):501–518.

Cyanotic (Tet) Spells

Acute hypoxemic attacks represent a true emergency and initial treatment is crucial to long-term outcome. Usually, the underlying diagnosis is tetralogy of Fallot, or a variant, and hence the pseudonym for these attacks is *Tet spells*.

In a Tet spell, an acute increase in obstruction to pulmonary blood flow has occurred, either at the level of the right ventricular outflow tract within the heart or at the level of the pulmonary circulation, with a consequent increase in right-to-left shunting through an intracardiac septal defect. Alternatively, if systemic perfusion is reduced, as with hypovolemia or the development of a tachyarrhythmia, right-to-left shunting will also increase and a cyanotic spell will develop.

Clinical Presentation and Diagnosis

Spells are particularly common in the early morning, shortly after the patient awakens, when there is a rapid shift in circulatory dynamics from the recumbent sleeping state. Prolonged agitation and crying are also cited as precipitants, but it is sometimes unclear whether the developing hypoxemia itself has caused the agitated state, which is then first noticed by the parent. Also, noxious stimuli, such as phlebotomy or a bee sting, or any circumstance that leads to enhanced catecholamine output can precipitate a spell in a susceptible child.

When caring for an acutely hypoxemic infant or child, inquire about a history of congenital heart disease, which raises the possibility that a spell has occurred. Rapid diagnosis of the presence of any form of tetralogy of Fallot is a priority. Obtain a chest x-ray, which may reveal poor pulmonary blood flow and the typical "coeur en sabot" (boot-shaped heart), while the pulmonary parenchyma will be normal. Obtain an ECG to document right ventricular hypertrophy and a rightward axis and to rule-out an underlying tachyarrhythmia. In such cases, the absence of a heart murmur is a worrisome indicator that pulmonary blood flow is severely compromised.

ED Management

Management is directed at manipulating the relative resistances of the systemic and pulmonary vascular beds, as well as maintenance of appropriate circulating volume and heart rate. Flex the child's knees to the chest to help raise systemic tone. Some older patients will instinctively squat to achieve the same result. Give 100% oxygen, which also increases systemic resistance and may help enhance oxygen delivery. Treat any underlying arrhythmia and correct hypovolemia.

If oxygen and position changes do not break the spell, establish IV access and give morphine sulfate (0.1 mg/kg IV or subcutaneously). Although the precise mechanism of action is unclear, morphine may cause pulmonary vasodilation and also provide a beneficial sedative effect, with consequent reduction of catecholamine secretion.

If the patient fails to demonstrate improved oxygen saturation promptly or is obtunded, give an IV fluid bolus of 20 mL/kg normal saline and obtain an ABG. Treat metabolic acidosis with sodium bicarbonate, 1–2 mEq/kg by *slow IV, only if ventilation is adequate* (low or normal pCO_2). If cyanosis persists, give phenylephrine (10 mcg/kg by slow IV push) to pharmacologically increase the systemic vascular resistance. Intubation and mechanical ventilation may also be necessary in severe, protracted spells.

Follow-up

- Tet spell not requiring admission: 24–48 hours

Indication for Admission

- Any hypoxemic attack requiring medical attention (not responding to simple position maneuvers)

Bibliography

Hiremath G, Kamat D. Diagnostic considerations in infants and children with cyanosis. *Pediatr Ann.* 2015;**44**(2):76–80.

Judge P, Meckler MG. Congenital heart disease in pediatric patients: recognizing the undiagnosed and managing complications in the emergency department. *Pediatr Emerg Med Pract.* 2016;**13**(5):1–28.

Strobel AM, Lu le N. The critically ill infant with congenital heart disease. *Emerg Med Clin North Am.* 2015;**33**(3):501–518.

Heart Murmurs

Although congenital heart disease is present in only about 0.8% of the general population, the prevalence of heart murmurs in children approaches 50–60% or more. Most murmurs, therefore, are "innocent" or "functional," and not pathologic.

Clinical Presentation and Diagnosis

Innocent (Functional) Murmur

Most innocent murmurs are midsystolic, short in duration (end well before the second heart sound), and mid-frequency or "vibratory" in quality. The intensity is below grade VI and changes with position or Valsalva maneuver. They may be heard at the apex or the base and are not associated with other findings suggestive of cardiovascular disease (wide, fixed, or paradoxical splitting of S_2; ejection click). Innocent murmurs may be increased in intensity with conditions associated with increased stroke volume, such as fever, anemia and hyperthyroidism. Types of innocent murmurs include the following.

Still's Murmur

Still's murmur occurs in over 50% of children 4–10 years of age. It is vibratory, musical, or twanging, heard best in the midprecordium between the lower left sternal border and the apex; it is generally grade II–III/VI in intensity. There is a normal S_2, no ejection click, and no thrill.

Pulmonic Ejection Murmur

A pulmonic ejection murmur is noted most often in older children and young adolescents. It is early to midsystolic, diamond-shaped, grade I–III/VI in intensity, and vibratory in quality. It is best detected in the second left intercostal space. There is a normal S_2, and no thrill, click, or diastolic murmur.

Venous Hum

A venous hum can be appreciated in over 60% of children 3–6 years of age. It is heard best in the infraclavicular area, especially on the right. It is continuous in timing with diastolic accentuation, vibratory and generally grade I–II/VI in intensity. The loudness changes with rotation of the head and generally disappears with lying down or with compression of the jugular vein. Release of pressure may cause accentuation of the murmur for a few seconds. There is no thrill, systolic accentuation or increased peripheral pulsation.

Organic Murmurs

In contrast to the conditions described above, organic murmurs are the result of turbulent blood flow through abnormal cardiac structures or communications. Murmurs which are diastolic (other than a venous hum); right-sided; holosystolic; harsh in quality; associated with a thrill, ejection click, or fixed S_2 splitting; or accompanied by physical findings consistent with heart disease (cyanosis, clubbing, absent lower extremity pulses, signs of congestive heart failure) suggest that a murmur is organic.

ED Management

A murmur itself does not require acute management. Rather, intervention may be necessary for the underlying disease causing the murmur (such as endocarditis). Refer all patients with murmurs that do not meet the strict criteria of an innocent or functional murmur to a pediatric cardiologist.

Per the revised American Heart Association guidelines, very few patients with organic murmurs require SBE prophylaxis prior to procedures. Patients with murmurs secondary to rheumatic heart disease do require rheumatic fever prophylaxis (p. 699).

Indications for Admission

- Signs of congestive heart failure or acute rheumatic fever
- Suspected or confirmed infective endocarditis

Bibliography

Frank JE, Jacobe KM. Evaluation and management of heart murmurs in children. *Am Fam Physician.* 2011;**84**(7):793–800.

Mesropyan L, Sanil Y. Innocent heart murmurs from the perspective of the pediatrician. *Pediatr Ann.* 2016;**45**(8):e306–309.

Naik RJ, Shah NC. Teenage heart murmurs. *Pediatr Clin North Am.* 2014;**61**(1):1–16.

Infective Endocarditis

Infective endocarditis (IE) is an infection of the endothelium of the heart valves or great vessels. It is most commonly *subacute*, developing in patients with preexisting congenital heart disease, particularly valvular anomalies (aortic stenosis, prosthetic valve) and conditions associated with increased turbulence of blood flow (ventricular septal defect, aortic regurgitation). In this regard, conditions such as isolated secundum atrial septal defect are not likely to be related to IE.

A substantial percentage of IE cases occur in patients with no preexisting cardiac anomaly. These children have developed *acute* bacterial endocarditis and may suddenly become extremely ill.

For IE to occur, the endocardium must be exposed to potentially pathogenic bacteria. Dental treatments can result in bacteremia even without periodontal disease. Similarly, certain surgical procedures (tonsillectomy, urologic surgery) or the presence of a chronic indwelling parenteral catheter also place the patient at risk.

Clinical Presentation and Diagnosis

Diligence is required to suspect and treat IE and to refrain from other incorrect therapy. Inquire about any factors establishing a milieu for IE, particularly recent dental and surgical procedures, the presence of a venous catheter, and IV drug use.

Although fever in any patient with congenital heart disease raises the possibility of IE, certain situations are particularly worrisome. These are a protracted febrile illness, particularly without any obvious focus, even if thought to be of "viral" etiology; a documented change in the clinical picture, such as the development of a new heart murmur or congestive heart failure; the onset of hematuria; signs of either cutaneous emboli or embolic events to other organs; a new neurologic finding; or a focal infection such as pneumonia or meningitis.

Frequently, early signs and symptoms may be subtle. Classic findings such as change in a murmur, evidence of emboli, and splenomegaly may not be easily discernible. Nonetheless, carefully examine the conjunctivae, nail beds, palms, soles of the feet, and other skin surfaces to search for evidence of emboli, including tender nodules in the finger or toe pads (Osler nodes), small hemorrhages on the palms or soles (Janeway lesions), and linear subungual lesions (splinter hemorrhages). Perform a careful fundoscopic exam and serial auscultations, as murmurs may be transient and change may be rapid. Conversely, in fulminant acute IE, only the signs of severely compromised circulatory status may be present, without any heart murmur.

Obtain blood for a CBC, ESR, CRP, multiple blood cultures, as well as a urinalysis. The diagnosis is ultimately confirmed by obtaining positive blood cultures and/or positive findings on an echocardiogram. There may be a leukocytosis with a leftward shift, anemia, and elevation of the ESR and CRP. The urinalysis may reveal pyuria, hematuria, and proteinuria, as infective endocarditis is a cause of immune complex nephritis. Scrape any cutaneous emboli and examine after Gram's staining. If IE is being considered, consult a cardiologist to arrange for a two-dimensional echocardiogram. If a vegetation is identified, the study can indicate the diagnosis, even before the blood results have become available.

ED Management

While it may sometimes be crucial to initiate treatment rapidly, it is always imperative that an alternative diagnosis not be obscured. The treatment of IE involves protracted use of appropriate antibiotics, depending on culture and sensitivity results. Attempt to obtain at least two sets of blood cultures from any febrile child at risk for IE (congenital heart disease, normal heart but chronic indwelling catheter) *before antibiotics are administered*. Once the cultures have been obtained, give broad-spectrum IV antibiotics such as penicillin (200,000 units/kg/day div q 4h, 24 million units/day maximum) or ceftriaxone (100 mg/kg/day, 4 g/day maximum) combined with gentamicin (3 mg/kg/day div q 8h, 240 mg/day maximum). If there is particular suspicion for a Gram-negative organism, such as in an immunocompromised patient, use ampicillin (300 mg/kg/day div q 6h, 12 g/day maximum) or ceftriaxone combined with gentamicin.

These recommendations may not be adequate for patients with prosthetic heart valves or other special considerations. Consult with an infectious disease expert before initiation of therapy.

Endocarditis Prophylaxis

Children with congenital and acquired heart disease may require an urgent invasive procedure. In 2007, the American Heart Association, and others, published new guidelines for the consideration of appropriate antibiotics for IE prophylaxis. This statement dramatically changed the recommendations, so that prophylactic antibiotics are no longer indicated solely to prevent endocarditis for any genitourinary or gastrointestinal procedure. For respiratory tract procedures, if incision and/or biopsy of the respiratory mucosa is involved, give oral amoxicillin (50 mg/kg, 2 g maximum), parenteral ampicillin (50 mg/kg, 2 g maximum), or parenteral ceftriaxone (50 mg/kg, 1 g maximum). Recommendations for prophylaxis extend only to patients with prosthetic valves or conduits, previous IE, unrepaired cyanotic heart disease (even with a shunt in place), repaired congenital heart disease within the first six months of surgery or with a residual defect, and cardiac transplant recipients with a valvulopathy in the new heart.

Indications for Admission
- Suspected or confirmed infective endocarditis

Bibliography

Baltimore RS, Gewitz MH, Baddour LM, et al. Infective endocarditis in childhood: 2015 update. *Circulation.* 2015;**132**:1487–1515.

Elder RW, Baltimore RS. The changing epidemiology of pediatric endocarditis. *Infect Dis Clin North Am.* 2015;**29**(3):513–524.

Taib R. Infective endocarditis in children. *Southeast Asian J Trop Med Public Health.* 2014;**45**(Suppl .1):79–85.

Pericardial Disease

Three distinct disease processes can involve the pericardium: pericarditis, pericardial effusion, and pericardial tamponade. Infections are the most common etiology of pericardial diseases, but there are a variety of other causes in childhood (Table 3.4).

Pericarditis

Pericarditis is inflammation of the pericardium (infectious or noninfectious).

Pericardial Effusion

A pericardial effusion is the accumulation of fluid in the pericardial space.

Pericardial Tamponade

Pericardial tamponade is impaired cardiac output secondary to reduced ventricular filling. This is caused either by fluid accumulation in the pericardial space or by constriction of the

Table 3.4 Etiologies of pericarditis

Infections

Bacterial

    H. influenzae type B (extremely rare)

    Staphylococcus

    Streptococcus pneumoniae

    Pneumococcus

Other (tuberculosis, fungal)

Viral

Inflammatory

Collagen

Rheumatic

Traumatic

Chest wall injury

Postpericardiotomy syndrome

Oncologic

Leukemia

Lymphoma

Other

Blood dyscrasias

Drug induced (minoxidil)

heart from an abnormally thickened pericardium. The rapid accumulation of a small amount of fluid can produce tamponade, while chronic slow accumulation is more readily tolerated.

Clinical Presentation and Diagnosis

Pericarditis

Chest pain is the initial symptom in acute pericarditis. It is a constant, sharp sensation across the anterior precordium and is frequently associated with shoulder discomfort. The pain varies with position, being worse when supine and relieved when upright. Respiratory symptoms, particularly tachypnea, typically accompany the pain. There is often a history of a preceding URI. Fever is usually present and the patient may also complain of abdominal pain. There may be a history of open heart surgery in the past 10–14 days (post-pericardiotomy syndrome).

Pericardial Effusion

When a substantial pericardial effusion is present, the symptoms may mimic CHF. There may be tachypnea with chest retractions and nasal flaring. With impaired cardiac output, tachycardia and vasoconstriction occur, with pallor, low blood pressure, and cool extremities. Other findings secondary to systemic congestion are hepatosplenomegaly and neck vein distension.

Pericardial Tamponade

Cardiac tamponade is a true medical emergency. Classic findings include hypotension, distended neck veins, muffled heart sounds, and the presence of pulsus paradoxus, a ->10 mm Hg fall in systolic blood pressure associated with inspiration. A fall in the blood pressure of >20 mm Hg is serious. Pulsus paradoxus may also be found in respiratory disorders such as asthma and in congestive heart failure.

On auscultation, findings depend on the amount of fluid accumulation. When inflammation is present without fluid, as in acute pericarditis, there is often a loud friction rub audible. This is a scratchy, harsh sound heard throughout the cardiac cycle. The pericardial rub diminishes in proportion to the volume of fluid collection. The heart sounds in general decrease in intensity in direct proportion to pericardial fluid volume. Particularly ominous is the agitated child with signs of reduced cardiac output and a "quiet" auscultatory examination.

Obtain an ECG and chest x-ray. With pericarditis the ECG reveals elevated ST segments and, often, generalized T-wave inversions. Diminished precordial voltage usually indicates pericardial fluid accumulation. On x-ray, the heart size is increased with pericardial effusion but may be small with pericardial constriction without fluid (constrictive pericarditis). Other laboratory tests are nonspecific. With purulent pericarditis, there is leukocytosis and an elevated ESR and CRP. However, viral diseases will often be associated with normal values of both parameters, and the highest acute phase reactants can be seen with rheumatologic pericarditis.

ED Management

The approach to the child with pericardial disease varies depending on whether there is an effusion.

Pericarditis

For pericarditis without fluid accumulation, invasive treatment is not warranted. Admit the patient, give analgesics (aspirin, ibuprofen, or indomethacin) and observe for the development of complications (effusion, tamponade, myocarditis). Steroids are usually not indicated for initial management.

Pericardial Effusion

Closely follow the vital signs and degree of pulsus paradoxus, as pericardial fluid accumulation is usually a dynamic process. Rapidly changing circumstances may precipitate an acute crisis. Consult a cardiologist and admit the patient. Diagnostic pericardiocentesis may be required, especially if purulent pericarditis is suspected.

If purulent pericarditis is suspected, provide supplemental oxygen, establish IV access, and arrange for pericardiocentesis. Obtain blood and pericardial fluid specimens and begin broad-spectrum antibiotics (nafcillin 150 mg/kg/day div q 6h and cefotaxime 150–200 mg/kg/day div q 6h). Substitute vancomycin (40 mg/kg/day div q 6h) for nafcillin if MRSA is a possibility.

Pericardial Tamponade

When a substantial volume of pericardial fluid has accumulated, tamponade can develop rapidly. Arrange for immediate therapeutic drainage.

Indications for Admission

- Pericardial effusion (unless chronic)
- Pericarditis
- Pericardial tamponade

Bibliography

Adler Y, Charron P, Imazio M, et al. ESC Guidelines for the diagnosis and management of pericardial diseases: the Task Force for the Diagnosis and Management of Pericardial Diseases of the European Society of Cardiology (ESC). *Eur Heart J*. 2015;**36**:2921–2964.

Bergmann KR, Kharbanda A, Haveman L. Myocarditis and pericarditis in the pediatric patient: validated management strategies. *Pediatr Emerg Med Pract*. 2015;**12**(7):1–22.

Durani Y, Giordano K, Goudie BW. Myocarditis and pericarditis in children. *Pediatr Clin North Am*. 2010;**57**(6):1281–1303.

Johnson, JN, Cetta, F. Pericardial diseases. In Allen HD, Shaddy RE, Penny DJ, Feltes TF, Cetta F (eds.) *Moss and Adams' Heart Disease in Infants, Children, and Adolescents, Including the Fetus and Young Adult* (9th edn.). Philadelphia, PA: Lippincott Williams & Wilkins, 2016; 1427–1440.

Syncope

Syncope is a transient loss of consciousness, accompanied by loss of postural tone, resulting from decreased cerebral perfusion. Mechanisms of syncope can be classified into three broad groups: neurally mediated reflex syncope, orthostatic syncope, and cardiac syncope.

Clinical Presentation

The unconscious period may be preceded by a history of an inciting factor, such as a noxious stimulus, an excessively warm environment, emotional upset, or exercise. The patient may report a prodrome of dizziness, diaphoresis, headache, chest pain, palpitations, visual or auditory phenomena, respiratory distress, paresthesias, or a history of recurrent episodes. Findings on physical examination may include diaphoresis, hypotension (sometimes postural), tachycardia or bradycardia, lethargy, or dilated pupils.

Neurally Mediated Reflex Syncope (Including Vasovagal Syncope, Situational Syncope, Post-Micturition Syncope)

Vasodilation, with pooling of blood in capacitance vessels, causes decreased blood pressure with a resultant decrease in cerebral perfusion. Usually, an associated increase in vagal tone results in bradycardia and diaphoresis. Vasodepressor syncope is often precipitated by noxious stimuli, strong emotions, or fatigue, and is common in adolescents.

Orthostatic Hypotensive Syncope

This occurs on assuming an erect posture and is the result of abnormal vasomotor compensatory mechanisms in response to changes in position. It is rare in young children, but not uncommon in normal adolescents. It may also occur if the patient is dehydrated, chronically fatigued or malnourished, has suffered an acute blood loss, or is taking vasodilator drugs.

Cardiac

Although uncommon, cardiac causes of syncope can be life-threatening. The mechanism may involve hypoxemia due to cyanotic heart disease or decreased cardiac output secondary to myocardial dysfunction, arrhythmias, or obstructive lesions.

Structural Lesions

Syncope can occur in patients with obstructive lesions (severe valvar or subvalvar aortic stenosis, pulmonary hypertension) secondary to low cardiac output, cyanotic heart disease (tetralogy of Fallot) secondary to hypoxia, and congenital abnormalities of the coronary arteries. Most of these episodes occur during physical exertion; this history suggests a cardiac etiology and always requires a thorough work-up. Generally, there are auscultatory abnormalities, such as a murmur or abnormal second heart sound, or evidence of ventricular hypertrophy or strain on electrocardiogram.

Arrhythmias

Arrhythmias such as atrioventricular block (second or third degree) may cause syncope. Sick sinus syndrome is usually seen in the setting of repaired congenital heart disease. These patients may develop syncope secondary to severe bradycardia or sinus arrest. Syncope can also be associated with paroxysmal supraventricular tachycardia, atrial flutter and atrial fibrillation, especially in patients with WPW syndrome. Ventricular tachycardia or ventricular fibrillation may present with syncope in patients with repaired congenital heart disease, arrhythmogenic right ventricular cardiomyopathy (ARVC), or catecholaminergic polymorphic ventricular tachycardia (CPVT).

Syncope is also associated with long QT syndrome (LQTS), either congenital (the autosomal dominant Romano–Ward syndrome) or acquired, secondary to drugs (antibiotics [clarithromycin, erythromycin], anti-arrhythmics [sotalol, ibutilide, flecainide, quinidine, amiodarone], tricyclic antidepressants, antipsychotics), electrolyte imbalance, or starvation diets. Long QT syndrome can lead to a specific dysrhythmia, a polymorphic ventricular tachycardia called torsade de pointes. Consider LQTS in children with a history of syncope and a corrected QT interval >0.44 seconds.

Other Causes of Syncope (Rare)

Cerebral Hypoxemia

Hypoxia and anemia (rare) can cause syncope secondary to decreased cerebral oxygen delivery despite normal cardiac output. Respiratory causes include breath-holding spells in infants and toddlers (pp. 507–508) and hyperventilation in adolescents. The infant or child with a breath-holding spell becomes pallid or cyanotic before losing consciousness, while hyperventilating adolescents may have paresthesias or carpopedal spasm. In both, there is usually a history of emotional upset.

Hysterical Fainting

Hysterical fainting occurs primarily in patients with a histrionic (theatrical) personality style. These episodes can last for up to one hour and usually occur in front of others. The pulse and blood pressure are normal, and there is never any associated injury.

Fasting Hypoglycemia

Fasting hypoglycemia is the most common metabolic cause of syncope. Inquire about a history of diabetes or insulin use. Weakness, diaphoresis, confusion, and palpitations may occur prior to the actual syncopal episode, which is gradual in onset. Also, ethanol ingestions can be associated with hypoglycemia.

Consider seizures in the differential diagnosis. Frequent episodes of loss of consciousness suggest epilepsy. Migraine headaches involving the vertebral-basilar system can cause syncope, preceded by an aura and followed by the headache.

Diagnosis

A careful history usually suggests the diagnosis. Especially important is a description of the events leading up to the episode, particularly whether the syncope was abrupt and without warning, or preceded by lightheadedness, dizziness, sweating, palpitations, chest pain, or respiratory distress. Inquire about the setting of the syncopal event; consider exercise-induced syncope to be malignant until proven otherwise. Cardiac syncope can be sudden, without any warning. Inquire about the frequency of the attacks, any sequelae after the episode, possible drug ingestion, and family history of arrhythmia, syncope, sudden death, or deafness (which may be associated with the autosomal recessive form of LQTS).

On physical examination, check for orthostatic vital sign changes, odors on the breath (ethanol, ketones), and murmurs. Most cardiac etiologies can be ruled out by auscultation and a 12-lead ECG with a long rhythm strip. Causative arrhythmias such as supraventricular tachycardia, ventricular tachycardia, sick sinus syndrome, or heart block are usually not present on admission, but underlying predisposing conditions such as WPW and prolonged LQTS may be identified. If these are not found, 24-hour ambulatory monitoring is indicated when the history does not suggest another etiology for the syncope.

ED Management

Unless it is clear that the patient suffered a vasovagal episode, obtain an ECG with rhythm strip and blood for hematocrit, Dextrostix, and serum glucose. The diagnosis and management of hypoglycemia (pp. 194–197) and anemia (pp. 349–353) are discussed elsewhere.

Instruct patients with orthostatic syncope to get up slowly after lying or sitting and discontinue any implicated medications. Suggest increased fluid intake, and if the blood pressure is normal, recommend additional salt intake. Autonomic dysfunction and orthostatic hypotension can ultimately be documented by tilt table testing. Reassurance and primary care follow-up are all that are usually needed for hyperventilation or breath-holding. Consult with a pediatric cardiologist for LQTS, WPW, or other causes of cardiac syncope.

Follow-up

- Vasovagal, hyperventilation, or breath-holding episode: primary care follow-up in one week

Indications for Admission

- Recurrent syncope
- Cardiac syncope likely
- Significant injury caused by the syncopal episode

Bibliography

Friedman KG, Alexander ME. Chest pain and syncope in children: a practical approach to the diagnosis of cardiac disease. *J Pediatr*. 2013;**163**(3):896–901.

Pilcher TA, Saarel EV. A teenage fainter (dizziness, syncope, postural orthostatic tachycardia syndrome). *Pediatr Clin North Am*. 2014;**61**(1):29–43.

Stewart JM. Common syndromes of orthostatic intolerance. *Pediatrics*. 2013;**131**:968–980.

Dental Emergencies

Farhad Yeroshalmi

Children frequently present to the emergency department (ED) complaining of oral problems, primarily due to oral trauma or related to dental caries. Many of these can be diagnosed and treated by the ED physician, with subsequent referral to a dentist for consultation and/or definitive treatment.

Dental Anatomy

A basic knowledge of dental anatomy is necessary for evaluating and treating dental emergencies. The tooth itself is composed of four primary layers. The dental enamel, a mineralized, crystalline material, covers the coronal portion of the tooth. It is the hardest material found in the human body. A somewhat softer material, cementum, forms the outer surface of the root. Underneath the enamel and/or cementum is a less mineralized layer called dentin. The innermost portion of the tooth is the pulp chamber, which contains nerve tissue, as well as the vascular supply for nourishing the tooth structure. Periodontal ligament fibers attach the roots of the tooth to the surrounding alveolar bone. These structures are shown in Figure 4.1.

Complaints Associated With Dental Eruption

Clinical Presentation

Teething

Teething can be associated with irritable behavior (due to minor discomfort) and increased drooling. Teething infants often present to the ED with fever and diarrhea, although there is no conclusive evidence that tooth eruption is truly the cause. Therefore, evaluate the patient appropriately and consider teething a diagnosis of exclusion.

Treat teething pain with a frozen teething toy, but advise the parents to avoid using toys with multiple parts. For more significant pain, recommend acetaminophen (15 mg/kg q 4h), ibuprofen (10 mg/kg q 6h), or an over-the-counter non-irritating topical anesthetic. Be judicious when prescribing topical anesthetics for infants, as systemic absorption is rapid, so toxicity can occur if the product is misused.

Eruption Cyst or Hematoma

An eruption cyst is a fluctuant, fluid-filled sac overlying an erupting primary or permanent tooth. An eruption hematoma will have a bluish-purple appearance due to blood filling the

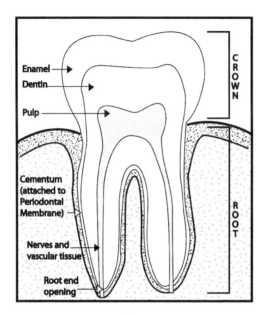

Figure 4.1 Tooth anatomy.

sac. Eruption cysts and hematomas are benign findings and will resolve spontaneously, either through biting pressure or upon eruption of the tooth.

Natal and Neonatal Teeth

Natal teeth are primary teeth that are present at birth. Neonatal teeth refer to teeth that erupt in the first 30 days of life. Both usually erupt in the mandibular incisor area and, in most cases, are part of the normal primary dentition and not supernumerary. Natal and neonatal teeth pose a theoretical aspiration risk, although no cases of aspiration have been reported in the literature.

Traumatic injury to the infant's tongue may be caused by the sharp incisal edges of these teeth, while trauma to a nursing mother's breast may interfere with feeding. Both of these conditions are indications for extraction and require referral to a dentist.

Bibliography

McDonald RE, Avery DR, Dean JA. Examination of the mouth and other relevant structures. In Dean JA, Avery DR, McDonald RE (eds.) *McDonald and Avery's Dentistry for the Child and Adolescent* (10th edn.). St. Louis, MO: Elsevier, 2016; 1–16.

Sarrell EM, Horev Z, Cohen Z, Cohen HA. Parents' and medical personnel's beliefs about infant teething. *Patient Educ Couns.* 2005;57(1):122–125.

Sood S, Sood M. Teething: myths and facts. *J Clin Pediatr Dent.* 2010;35(1):9–13.

Dental Caries and Odontogenic Infections

Dental caries is the most common chronic childhood disease in the United States and is frequently the cause of dental pain and oral infection. The caries process is initiated by the interaction of the bacteria *Streptococcus mutans* with fermentable carbohydrates, primarily sucrose. The acid that is produced as a byproduct of the bacteria's digestion of carbohydrates can dissolve the highly mineralized enamel that covers the tooth surface. Once the enamel is destroyed, further destruction of tooth structure can proceed fairly quickly until bacteria infect the innermost layer of pulp tissue. *Lactobacilli* may play a role in the progression of the lesions. Once organisms have reached the pulp, the infection can spread through the root into the adjacent periapical tissue, resulting in a dentoalveolar infection.

Most odontogenic infections are polymicrobial, with anaerobes predominating. Under healthy conditions, most of these organisms are not pathogenic. However, local (caries, trauma, foreign body, vascular insufficiency) and/or systemic factors (immune deficiencies) can facilitate the development of dental abscesses.

Clinical Presentation

Cavities

Dental caries commonly occur in the pits and fissures of the occlusal (chewing) surfaces of posterior teeth, interproximal surfaces of molars, and smooth tooth surfaces close to the gingiva. They initially appear as dull, opaque, white discolorations, which then cavitate and appear as brown holes. Although these lesions may be visible upon oral examination, they often remain asymptomatic until the infection spreads into the pulp tissue, and then present as pain upon eating sweet or cold foods. As the infection spreads, patients frequently report spontaneous pain, often interfering with sleep and eating.

Early Childhood Caries

Previously termed nursing bottle caries or baby bottle tooth decay, early childhood caries (ECC) is a form of rampant caries found in some young children. Typically, the labial and palatal surfaces of the primary maxillary incisors are the first teeth affected. If not treated, the caries can spread to the primary molars. The mandibular incisors are typically spared, except in the most severe cases. Children will often present with gross destruction of the maxillary incisors.

Dental Abscess

This is a localized, purulent infection caused by dental pulp necrosis, secondary to either dental caries or trauma to a non-carious tooth. An abscess can be chronic or acute. A chronic abscess is often asymptomatic, but can become an acute, symptomatic lesion. Some painful acute abscesses are not clinically evident and require a radiograph for diagnosis. Others may present with gingival erythema, tooth mobility, tenderness to tooth percussion, soft tissue swelling, and lymphadenopathy. Sometimes, a fistulous tract develops and opens onto the gingival mucosa, forming a parulis/abscess. This is more common in younger children, whose alveolar bone is relatively less dense.

Pericoronitis

Pericoronitis refers to inflammation or infection of the soft tissues adjacent to a partially erupted tooth. The teeth most commonly associated are the mandibular third molars (wisdom teeth). The condition is caused by food and bacteria becoming trapped under gingival tissue that partially covers the tooth. Symptoms can include localized swelling, pain, and a bad taste in the mouth due to suppuration. Frequently, there is localized lymphaden-opathy, and cellulitis and trismus can also develop.

Cellulitis

Localized infection from a carious or traumatized tooth can spread through soft tissues, causing cellulitis. This may be accompanied by fever, pain, trismus, and regional lymph-adenopathy. Include a thorough oral examination of any patient presenting with cellulitis of the face or neck, as the infection may be of odontogenic origin.

Deep Fascial Space Infections

Oral infections can also spread to the deep fascial spaces of the head and neck. Depending on the tooth and drainage area involved, varying degrees of pain, swelling, and trismus occur. In severe cases, involvement of the sublingual, pharyngeal, retro-pharyngeal, or pretracheal areas can occur, leading to dysphagia and/or respiratory compromise.

Ludwig's angina is a condition in which a mandibular dental abscess expands rapidly, causing diffuse swelling to the floor of the mouth, which then leads to airway compromise. This is usually associated with the permanent molars and is therefore uncommon in young children who have only primary teeth.

Diagnosis

A thorough intraoral evaluation is necessary for any patient with oral pain or face and neck swelling. In the absence of obvious dental caries, inquire about a history of dental trauma or past dental treatment. Inspect the oral cavity for obvious caries, gingival swelling and erythema, possibly from an infected tooth or an abscess. Palpate the gums for swelling and tenderness, and tap the molar occlusal surfaces of each tooth with a tongue blade to identify percussion sensitivity, and check for tooth mobility. Radiographs are indicated only if there is no obvious etiology for a swelling, or when numerous carious teeth are present.

ED Management

Caries

Refer asymptomatic children with dental caries and no evidence of acute infection to a dentist for comprehensive care. If the patient has dental-related pain, but no soft tissue inflammation or swelling, give analgesics and refer to a dentist as soon as possible, preferably the next day. Do not prescribe antibiotics for such patients.

Localized Dental Abscess

Consult with a dentist to perform incision and drainage of any fluctuant area. Prescribe analgesia with ibuprofen (10 mg/kg q 6h), or if severe, acetaminophen with codeine (0.5 mg/kg of codeine q 6h), although satisfactory pain relief is often achieved by the drainage procedure. Also prescribe oral antibiotics, either penicillin (25–50 mg/kg/day div q 6–8h) or clindamycin (20–30 mg/kg/day div q 6h). Treat localized pericoronitis in the same way as other localized dental abscesses. Additionally, irrigation with saline under the gingival flap that covers the affected tooth may help to alleviate discomfort.

Facial Cellulitis or Deep Fascial Space Infections

Admit the patient, consult an oral and maxillofacial surgeon, and start IV antibiotics. Use either penicillin 100,000–250,000 units/kg/day div q 4h or clindamycin 25–40 mg/kg/day div q 6h). Carefully assess the airway; any suggestion of compromise is an indication for early intubation. After initiation of antibiotic therapy, if there is a concern about the extent of a deep fascial space infection, obtain either a computerized tomography (CT) scan or magnetic resonance imaging (MRI).

Indications for Admission

- Facial cellulitis involving periorbital region
- Evidence of deep space infection (sublingual, submandibular, parapharyngeal) with potential for airway compromise
- Systemic involvement, including fever and/or dehydration due to inability or unwillingness to eat and drink
- Patients with immune compromise (HIV, diabetes, steroid therapy, cancer chemotherapy)
- Concern about outpatient adherence to the medical and/or follow-up recommendations

Bibliography

Chin JR, Kowolik JE, Stookey GK. Dental caries in the child and adolescent. In Dean JA, Avery DR, McDonald RE (eds.) *McDonald and Avery's Dentistry for the Child and Adolescent* (10th edn.). St. Louis, MO: Elsevier, 2016; 155–159.

Douglass AB, Douglass JM. Common dental emergencies. *Am Fam Phys.* 2003;**67**:511–516.

Kaban LB, Troulis MJ. *Pediatric Oral and Maxillofacial Surgery*, Philadelphia, PA: Saunders, 2004; 171–182.

Oral Trauma

Oral trauma is quite common in childhood, with injuries occurring in approximately 25% of school-age children. Causes include falls, seizures, sports injuries, motor vehicle accidents, fights, and inflicted injury. Lacerations, contusions and abrasion of facial soft tissues, gingiva, and intraoral mucosa are often associated with dental injuries. Fractures to facial bones and the bones that support the dentition can also occur. In a multiple-trauma victim, be sure to evaluate for dental injuries, which can easily be overlooked and potentially result in permanent damage.

Clinical Presentation

Dental Fractures

Treatment of dental fractures in the ED is rarely definitive, and any patient presenting with acute dental trauma requires referral to a dentist or oral surgeon within 24 hours. Appropriate intervention provided in a timely manner in the ED, however, is vital to prevent subsequent tooth loss and infection. See Table 4.1 for classification of dental fractures, along with appropriate management. Recommendations for treatment of fractured primary teeth do not differ markedly from those for permanent teeth. Depending on the age of the child at the time of trauma, and the expected longevity of the primary tooth, many dental practitioners will choose to be less aggressive in attempts to maintain a primary tooth.

Table 4.1 Classification of dental fractures

Fracture classification	Clinical findings	ED management
Enamel infraction	An incomplete fracture/crack No loss of tooth structure	No treatment needed
Enamel fracture	Fracture involves the enamel Loss of tooth structure	Elective dental referral X-ray any lip/cheek lacerations to search for tooth fragments or foreign material
Enamel–dentin fracture	Fracture involves enamel and dentin Loss of tooth structure No pulp exposure	Dental consult X-ray any lip/cheek lacerations to search for tooth fragments or foreign material
Enamel–dentin–pulp fracture	Fracture involves enamel and dentin Loss of tooth structure Exposure of the pulp	Immediate dental consult X-ray any lip/cheek lacerations to search for tooth fragments or foreign material
Crown–root fracture	Fracture involves enamel, dentin, and cementum Loss of tooth structure +/– Pulp exposure	Immediate dental consult Temporary stabilization of the loose segment to adjacent teeth until definitive treatment performed
Root fracture	Fracture involves cementum, dentin and pulp Coronal fragment may/may not be displaced	Immediate dental consult if coronal segment is mobile or displaced Reposition and stabilize the tooth with a flexible splint
Alveolar fracture	Fracture involves the alveolar bone +/– Involves the alveolar socket Mobility of the alveolar process Several teeth will move as a unit when mobility is checked	Immediate dental consult Reposition any displaced segment and splint

Tooth Displacement Injuries

Oral trauma frequently results in displacement of a tooth from its normal location, rather than fracture. As with fractures, the nature of the displacement and age of the patient will influence treatment decisions. Table 4.2 lists various displacement injuries and appropriate ED treatment.

Oral Soft Tissue Injuries

Lacerations

Lacerations of the lips, tongue, and oral mucosa are common in children of all ages. Lip lacerations which cross the vermilion border may present a cosmetic problem, since precise positioning of the wound margins is necessary for proper repair. Often, a child will present

Table 4.2 Dental displacement injuries

Injury	Clinical findings	ED management
Concussion	The tooth is tender to touch or tapping Tooth is not displaced No increased mobility	No treatment Soft diet for few days
Subluxation	The tooth is tender to touch or tapping Increased mobility Tooth is not displaced There may be bleeding from gingival crevice	Typically no treatment is needed A flexible splint to stabilize the tooth may provide patient comfort
Extrusive luxation	Tooth appears elongated Tooth is excessively mobile	Reposition the tooth by gently reinserting it into the tooth socket Stabilize using a flexible splint Primary tooth: extract if severely displaced/mobile
Lateral luxation	Tooth is displaced, usually in a palatal/lingual or labial direction Tooth will be immobile with fracture of the alveolar process	Reposition the tooth digitally or with forceps to disengage it from its bony socket and gently reposition it into its original location; stabilize using a flexible splint. Primary tooth: extract if severely displaced/mobile
Intrusive luxation	The tooth is displaced axially into the alveolar bone Tooth is immobile	Allow eruption without intervention, or reposition and stabilize using a flexible splint Primary tooth: Extract if there is a possibility of being displaced into the permanent successor
Avulsion	The tooth is completely displaced out of its socket and the dental arch	Permanent tooth: Prognosis related to the time tooth is out of the mouth Replant immediately and stabilize using a flexible splint If cannot reimplant, place tooth in Hanks Balanced Salt Solution (HBSS) or cold milk while awaiting immediate dental consultation Primary tooth: Do *not* replant

with lacerations of both the inner and outer surface of the lip. It is essential to identify whether these are two separate lacerations, or are in fact a communicating through-and-through laceration. Tongue lacerations occur frequently when children fall and accidentally bite a protruding tongue.

Punctures

Falling while running with an object in the mouth can cause soft tissue punctures. A puncture wound to the lateral palate may represent a significant trauma, with a risk of internal carotid injury, especially if the soft palate is involved. Of particular concern are deep or dirty wounds, foreign body contamination, and ongoing bleeding.

Bony Fractures

Alveolar Bone Fractures

The alveolar sockets are the bony processes in both the maxilla and mandible into which the teeth are embedded. The most common site for an alveolar fracture is in the area of the maxillary incisors. Clinical findings may include displacement and/or mobility of multiple teeth, along with mobility of the adjacent bone. Gingival bleeding is also commonly seen.

Mandibular Fractures

The mandible is a strong cortical bone with several weak areas that are susceptible to fracture. The necks of the condyles (below the temporomandibular joints) and the body of the mandible where the mental foramen are located are common sites for fracture. Frequently, the mandible will sustain multiple fractures resulting from one traumatic event. Clinical findings in mandibular fractures include painful jaw movement, malocclusion of the teeth, inability to close the mouth, and deviation of the mandible to one side during opening. Gingival bleeding, ecchymoses, intraoral edema, and paresthesias may also be present.

Diagnosis

Evaluation of airway, vital signs, mental status and cranial nerves are essential as part of the initial assessment. Obtain the history of the traumatic event, as well as the past medical history, including tetanus status and allergies. Treatment of life-threatening injuries obviously takes precedence. Once the patient is stabilized, use a systematic approach to physical evaluation of the face so that subtle injuries are not missed.

Extraoral Examination

- Inspect the face for asymmetry.
- Evaluate any abrasions, swelling, ecchymoses, and lacerations and check for the presence of foreign bodies.
- Palpate the facial bones (around each eye, each zygomatic arch, along the entire face from in front of the ears to the tip of the chin) for tenderness or discontinuities that may represent a fracture. To assess the mandibular condyles, place a gloved finger in each ear canal and have the patient open the mouth.
- Assess the integrity of the facial skeleton: place one hand on the anterior maxillary teeth and the other on the nasal bridge. Movement of the maxillary incisors and hard palate alone indicate a LeFort I fracture. Movement of the nasal bridge indicates a LeFort II fracture. Movement of the entire face indicates a LeFort III fracture.
- Ask a cooperative patient to bite down hard on a tongue blade using one side of the mouth. Twist the tongue blade medially. An intact mandible will preferentially break the

tongue blade. A patient with a mandibular fracture will not be able to break the tongue blade and will open the mouth due to pain. Repeat on the contralateral side.

- Note any deviations in mandibular opening and closing, and ask the patient if their bite feels normal.

Intraoral Examination

- Evaluate soft tissues for bleeding, swelling, lacerations, and abrasions.
- Thoroughly examine wounds for foreign bodies, including tooth fragments.
- Assess each tooth for mobility and fracture. Suspect an alveolar fracture if several adjacent teeth move as one unit.

Radiological Studies

Depending on the location and severity of the injuries, obtain the following radiographic studies:

- Upper face: axial and coronal CT scan; a skull series and Waters view radiographs are an alternative.
- Middle face: axial and coronal CT scan; as an alternative, obtain a Waters view, posteroanterior, submental vertex, and occlusal radiographs.
- Lower face: panoramic radiograph; posteroanterior, submental vertex, and occlusal are an alternative.
- If a condylar fracture is suspected, obtain a CT scan with cuts through bilateral condyles.

ED Management

Tables 4.1 and 4.2 outline treatment recommendations for dental fractures and displacement injuries. Advise the patient to see their dentist within 24–48 hours.

If a dentist is not immediately available and a primary tooth is so mobile as to be an aspiration risk, extract it. Grab the tooth firmly with gauze and twist it out. Immediately consult with an oral surgeon if there is a suspicion of alveolar, mandibular, or facial bone fracture.

Suturing of lacerations is not always indicated. Small intraoral wounds that do not pose an aesthetic problem heal quickly on their own. Similarly, tongue and lip lacerations that are small and have well approximated margins also do not require suturing. Suture lacerations that are deep or continue to bleed, lip lacerations that cross the vermilion border, and through-and-through lip and tongue lacerations. Prior to suturing, irrigate the wound thoroughly and inspect it carefully to rule-out the presence of foreign bodies, including fragments of any teeth that may have fractured during trauma. Do *not* inject local anesthetic directly into the wound area, as this could cause tissue swelling and hinder appropriate closure of the wound. Refer lacerations that require cosmetic repair to a plastic or oral surgeon.

Lateral puncture wounds to the palate may be complicated by vascular injury or foreign bodies. Carefully evaluate penetrating injuries for possible involvement of the carotid, palatine, and jugular blood vessels and perform a complete neurologic examination. A CT scan is indicated only if neurovascular involvement is suspected. Consult either an oral surgeon or otolaryngologist to determine the proper management for all puncture wounds to the palate. Sedation may be necessary when a wound requires extensive debridement and/or exploration to facilitate removal of foreign bodies.

Indications for Admission

- Mandibular or facial bone fractures
- Soft tissue swelling that may compromise the airway

Bibliography

Andreasen JO, Bakland LK, Flores MT, Andreasen FM, Andersson L. *Traumatic Dental Injuries: A Manual* (3rd edn.). Hoboken, NJ: Wiley-Blackwell, 2011.

Diangelis AJ, Andreasen JO, Ebeleseder, et al. International Association of Dental Traumatology guidelines for the management of traumatic dental injuries: 1. Fractures and luxations of permanent teeth. *Dent Traumatol.* 2012;**28**(1):2–12.

Olynik CR, Gray A, Sinada GG. Dentoalveolar trauma. *Otolaryngol Clin North Am.* 2013;**46** (5):807–823.

The Dental Trauma Guide. *Evidence Based Treatment Guide.* https://dentaltraumaguide.org (accessed May 11, 2017).

Oral Soft Tissue Lesions

Oral soft tissue lesions can result from a wide range of etiologies, including infection, inflammation, trauma, and developmental anomalies. Rarely are these of an emergent nature.

Clinical Presentation and Diagnosis

Infections

Herpes Simplex

Primary herpetic gingivostomatitis (HSV-1) is a common cause of gingivostomatitis in 1–3-year-olds. After a 1–2 day prodrome of fever, malaise, and vomiting, small vesicles appear anywhere on the oral mucosa, lips, tongue, perioral skin, or cheeks. These rapidly rupture, forming 2–10 mm lesions covered by a yellowish membrane. The membrane then sloughs, leaving a shallow, painful ulcer on an erythematous base. The patient may also present with erythematous, swollen gums that bleed easily. Fever up to 40.5 °C (105 °F), excessive salivation, diminished oral intake leading to dehydration, and marked local lymphadenopathy can also occur. Healing begins within 4–5 days and is usually completed within 1–2 weeks.

Recurrent Herpes

Recurrent herpes ("cold sores," herpes labialis) is thought to be secondary to stress (fever, menses, sunlight exposure). It presents with small vesicles, usually limited to the outer aspects of the lips and adjacent skin, although the hard palate and gingiva can also be involved. These rupture, coalesce, and become crusted. Healing takes 1–2 weeks.

Herpangina

Herpangina is typically a summertime infection caused by a number of enteroviruses, particularly type A Coxsackie viruses. The lesions are found only in the posterior oral cavity, which distinguishes them from herpes or aphthous ulcers. The soft palate, uvula, tonsils, and anterior tonsillar pillars are the sites of multiple, superficial, painful ulcers. A young child may be markedly irritable with fever and drooling, with severe dysphagia that can lead to dehydration. The lesions heal spontaneously over 1–2 weeks.

Hand–Foot–Mouth Disease

Hand–foot–mouth disease is caused primarily by type A16 Coxsackie viruses. Vesicles and ulcers occurring anywhere in the oral cavity are accompanied by fever, malaise, and abdominal pain. About 75% of patients also have a characteristic exanthem consisting of vesicles on an erythematous base located in one or more of the following sites: the palms and soles, dorsum of the hands and feet, dorsal aspects of the fingers and toes, buttocks, and genitalia. The lesions usually resolve within two weeks.

Necrotizing Ulcerative Gingivostomatitis

Necrotizing ulcerative gingivostomatitis (commonly referred to as NUG, Vincent's stomatitis, trench mouth) is a rare infectious disease of adolescents and young adults. *Prevotella intermedia, Fusobacterium, Treponema*, and *Selenomanos* species are among the microorganisms that have been found in the microflora of NUG lesions. It is associated with stress and smoking, although in rare cases there is underlying malnutrition or immune deficiency. Characteristic findings are painful gingiva that bleed easily, ulcerated interdental papillae covered by a grayish membrane, and foul-smelling breath, in addition to lymphadenopathy, malaise, and fever. In contrast to acute primary herpes gingivostomatitis, NUG occurs in older patients, the interdental papillae have a punched-out appearance, and there are no vesicles.

Acute Candidiasis (Thrush, Candidosis, Moniliasis)

Candida albicans (Monilia) is a common inhabitant of the oral cavity but may multiply rapidly and cause disease when host resistance is lowered. Thrush is most common in the first year of life. The complaint is diminished oral intake or white spots in the oral cavity. On inspection, the oral mucosa is beefy red with a curd-like white exudate on the tongue, gingiva, hard palate, or buccal mucosa. This can resemble milk, but it is not easily removed by scraping with a tongue depressor. On occasion, cracking or fissuring at the angle of the mouth, or cheilitis, is seen. Many infants simultaneously have a typical Candida diaper rash.

Thrush beyond the first year of life occurs in patients who have received broad-spectrum antibiotics, are using steroid inhalers, and those with autoimmune diseases and nutritional deficiencies. Persistent or recurrent thrush suggests possible HIV infection.

Papilloma

Papilloma (verruca vulgaris, condyloma acuminatum) can occur at any age. They present as single or multiple pedunculated or sessile nodules at any oral site. There may also be similar lesions on the skin.

Noninfectious Ulcers

Aphthous Ulcers

Aphthous ulcers, or canker sores, are solitary or multiple (five or fewer) very painful lesions on the non-keratinized mucosa (buccal, inner labial, ventral surface of tongue). They begin as erythematous papules that become well-circumscribed ulcers with a gray fibrinous exudate on an erythematous base. The etiology is unknown, although they are more common in families with allergies and their appearance is thought to be related to stress (infections, drugs, trauma, emotional upset). Fever is less common than with herpes. The ulcers usually last 7–14 days and recurrent episodes are the rule.

Traumatic Ulcer

Usually these are single ulcers, although the size, shape, and location all vary. Inquire as to recent ingestion of hot foods (pizza often causes burns to the anterior palate), dental treatment (children often bite the lip or tongue while it is numb, or the dental drill may have scratched the tongue or cheek), and oral habits (fingernail scratches of the gingival, chewing on the inside of the cheek). In the absence of repeated trauma, the lesion usually heals uneventfully within two weeks.

Mucocele

A mucocele is a fluid-filled nodule with translucent red or blue surface which may fluctuate in size. It occurs most commonly on the inner lower lip, secondary to the traumatic laceration of a minor salivary gland duct that permits accumulation and blockage of mucous.

Ranula

A ranula is a mucous retention cyst of a minor salivary gland. It presents as a large, soft swelling on the floor of the mouth. It may fluctuate in size and elevate the tongue.

Angular Cheilitis

Angular cheilitis presents with fissures at the corners of the mouth. These may bleed, ulcerate, and develop a crusted surface. Drooling, licking of the lips, and contact allergies may play a role and some patients may have frequent recurrences. The lesions can become infected with *Candida* and/or *Staphylococci*.

Irritation Fibroma

An irritation fibroma is a reactive hyperplastic lesion, usually secondary to chronic trauma. It can be located anywhere in the oral cavity, but the most common site is on the marginal gingiva. It appears as a painless, pedunculated or sessile nodule with a smooth pink surface.

Pyogenic Granuloma

A pyogenic granuloma is a reactive (irritation, trauma, poor oral hygiene) hyperplastic lesion that presents as a pedunculated or sessile nodule with a red surface. They frequently become ulcerated and bleed easily. They are more common in females and can be associated with pregnancy.

Fordyce Granules

Fordyce granules are oral sebaceous glands which often become evident at puberty. They appear as yellowish, multiple small papules, commonly on the vermilion border of the lip. These are asymptomatic and benign, but sometimes can be confused with candidiasis.

Gingival and Lingual Lesions

Geographic Tongue

Geographic tongue, or benign migratory glossitis, is a self-limited condition of unknown etiology. It presents as oval or irregular red patches in areas of desquamated papillae. While it is usually asymptomatic, some patients may complain of a burning sensation.

Coated Tongue

Coated tongue, or hairy tongue, represents elongation of the filiform papillae secondary to poor oral hygiene, dehydration, and medications (antibiotics, chlorhexidine). The presentation can range from whitish coating to brown/black "hairy" appearance.

Drug-Induced Gingival Overgrowth

Phenytoin, cyclosporin A, and calcium channel blockers can induce gingival hyperplasia. It presents with fibrous enlargement, primarily involving the interdental papillae in the anterior section of the mouth. In extreme cases, it may cover the crowns of teeth and interfere with eruption of teeth. Pain and difficulty with mastication can occur if the gingiva overgrow the occlusal surfaces of the teeth. In contrast, gingivitis presents with edematous and hemorrhagic gums.

Aggressive Periodontitis

Aggressive periodontitis presents with gingival inflammation and bleeding. In severe cases, teeth may become mobile. The etiology is unknown, although it is associated with diabetes, neutropenia, and hypophosphatasia.

ED Management

Ulcerative Lesions

For all oral ulcers, the major therapeutic goals are pain relief and maintenance of oral hygiene, so that adequate oral intake can continue. In patients who are not immuno-compromised, these conditions are self-limiting, and palliative treatment is all that is needed.

A number of options exist for pain management, but none is universally successful. Viscous lidocaine (2%) swabbed onto the lesions offers temporary relief, but caution the parents to not allow the child to swallow or rinse and spit the lidocaine (absorption of excessive amount). In addition, it is contraindicated for pharyngeal lesions (depression of the gag reflex). An alternative is to swab onto the lesions a 1:1 solution of Maalox/diphenhy-dramine or Kaopectate/diphenhydramine, but avoid using large quantities. Over-the-counter analgesic sprays offer only short-term relief, but they are safe and well-tolerated. Systemic analgesics, such as acetaminophen (15 mg/kg q 6h) and ibuprofen (10 mg/kg q 6h), can be helpful in the management of both pain and fever.

Emphasize the importance of encouraging oral intake. Ice cream, gelatin, milkshakes and pudding are often tolerated by children experiencing oral pain.

Necrotizing Ulcerative Gingivitis

Although NUG is an ulcerative disorder, its bacterial etiology requires specific treatment in addition to the palliative measures discussed previously. Give a seven-day course of penicillin VK (50 mg/kg/day div q 6h), metronidazole (30 mg/kg/day div q 6h), or clindamycin (20 mg/kg/day div q 6h). In addition, refer the patient to a dentist for treatment within 24–48 hours for debridement of necrotic gingival tissue.

Candidiasis

Treat with nystatin oral suspension (100,000 units/mL). Advise older patients to rinse with 4 mL for two minutes every six hours. If the patient is not old enough to rinse and spit, instruct the parent to place 1 mL along both sides of the buccal mucosa every six hours. In addition, keep the patient NPO for at least 30 minutes following administration of the nystatin. For patients who are immunocompromised, consult with the child's primary care physician or an infectious disease specialist, as more aggressive treatment may be needed.

Papillomas

Refer the patient to an oral surgeon for elective excisional biopsy and possible laser ablation of the lesions.

Mucocoele, Ranula

Refer the patient to an oral surgeon for excisional biopsy and removal.

Angular Cheilitis

Although the etiology of angular cheilitis is multifactorial, the lesions can often become infected with *Candida albicans* and/or *Staphylococci*. Treat with topical miconazole ointment, which has both antifungal and antibacterial properties, applied to the corners of the mouth every six hours. Refer the patient to a primary care provider to address any underlying conditions, such as drooling, frequent lip licking, and lip incompetence.

Irritation Fibroma, Pyogenic Granuloma

Refer the patient to an oral surgeon for excisional biopsy.

Fordyce Granules

These papules require no treatment other than reassuring the family that the finding is benign.

Geographic Tongue

No treatment is indicated if the condition is asymptomatic. If the patient complains of burning sensation, treat with a 1:1 mixture of diphenhydramine and Maalox, either used as a rinse or swabbed directly onto the painful area. Also advise the patient to avoid hot, spicy foods.

Coated Tongue, Hairy Tongue

No emergency treatment required, but treat any underlying systemic illnesses that can cause fever and dehydration. Encourage adequate hydration and recommend brushing of the tongue.

Gingival Hyperplasia (Drug Induced)

Refer the patient to a dentist for evaluation of hygiene and possible need for surgical resection of the tissue.

Periodontal Disease, Gingival Bleeding

Take a careful medical history, noting the duration and severity of the current complaint. Since local factors are the most common causes for gingival bleeding, look for poor oral hygiene, tooth eruption, foreign body entrapment, and self-injurious behaviors. If no local etiology can be identified, consider hormonal changes (puberty), thrombocytopenia, leukemia, clotting defects, and diabetes.

Follow-up

- Ulcerative lesions due to viral infection: immediately for severely diminished oral intake, otherwise 2–3 days
- NUG: dentist in 24–48 hours
- Candidiasis: 1–2 weeks
- Papillomas, mucocele, ranulas, fibromas, pyogenic granulomas: oral surgeon within several days
- Gingival hyperplasia: dentist within several days
- Periodontitis, gingival bleeding with known local etiology: dentist within several days

Indications for Admission

- Dehydration or inability to tolerate oral intake secondary to pain

Bibliography

Flaitz CM. Differential diagnosis of oral lesions and developmental abnormalities. In Casamassimo PS, Fields HW Jr, McTigue DJ, Nowak A (eds.) *Pediatric Dentistry: Infancy Through Adolescence* (5th edn.). St. Louis, MO: Elsevier Saunders, 2013; 11–53.

Hodgdon A. Dental and related infections. *Emerg Med Clin North Am.* 2013;**31**(2):465–480.

Le Doare K, Hullah E, Challacombe S, Menson E. Fifteen-minute consultation: a structured approach to the management of recurrent oral ulceration in a child. *Arch Dis Child Educ Pract Ed.* 2014;**99** (3):82–86.

Scully C, Welbury R, Flaitz C, de Almeida OP. *A Color Atlas of Orofacial Health & Disease in Children and Adolescents* (2nd edn.). London: Martin Dunitz, 2002.

Dermatologic Emergencies

Alexandra D. McCollum and Joshua M. Sherman

Dermatology is a visual specialty, and an accurate description of a "rash" makes it more likely that the practitioner will be able to classify a particular eruption and rapidly arrive at the right diagnosis. This chapter begins with definitions of dermatologic terms, which when used in conjunction with Table 5.1 can serve as a guide to the most common diagnoses.

Definition of Terms

Primary Lesions

Macule

A completely flat, nonpalpable lesion that is <1 cm in diameter.

Patch

A macule that is >1 cm in diameter.

Papule

A firm, palpable, elevated lesion that is <1 cm in diameter. A papule may be flat-topped, dome-shaped, or pointed.

Plaque

A papule that is >1 cm in diameter. It is a broad, elevated, flat-topped solid lesion often formed by a confluence of several papules.

Nodule

A palpable, solid papule >1 cm that is enlarged in all three dimensions: namely length, width, and depth.

Tumor

A large nodule.

Wheal

An evanescent, edematous, smooth, raised, pink to red papule or plaque. It is the characteristic lesion of urticaria, also known as hive(s).

Table 5.1 Dermatological diagnosis by type of eruption

Erythematous papules

Insect bite (papular urticaria)

Drug reaction

Viral exanthema

Scarlet fever

Papular acrodermatitis (Gianotti-Crosti)

Erythema toxicum neonatorum

Miliaria rubra

Candidiasis

Kawasaki disease

Erythematous nodules

Erythema nodosum

Pyogenic granuloma

Furuncle/carbuncle

Granuloma annulare^a

Erythematous plaques

Cellulitis

Tinea corporis

Psoriasis

Pityriasis rosea

Fixed drug eruption

Granuloma annulare

Contact dermatitis^b

Lupus erythematosus

Erythema chronicum migrans

Erythema marginatum

Eczematous lesions

Atopic dermatitis

Scabies

Seborrheic dermatitis

Contact dermatitis

Langerhans cell histiocytosis

Diaper dermatitis

Acrodermatitis enteropathica

Papulosquamous diseases

Psoriasis

Pityriasis rosea

Id reaction

Scabies

Secondary syphilis

Tinea

Lichen planus

Lupus erythematosus

Pustular eruptions

Acne

Candidiasis

Folliculitis

Staphylococcal pustulosis

Gonococcemia

Miliaria pustulosa

Infantile acropustulosis

Transient neonatal pustular melanosis

Erythema toxicum neonatorum

Impetigo

Skin-colored papules and nodules

Granuloma annulare^a

Molluscum contagiosum^c

Keloid

Verruca

Dermoid cyst

Reddish brown papules and nodules

Dermatofibroma

Pilomatricoma

Table 5.1 (cont.)

Neurofibroma	Mastocytoma

Vascular lesions

Nevus simplex	Port wine stain
Cutis marmorata	Pyogenic granuloma
Hemangioma of infancy	

Reactive erythematous eruptions

Drug eruptions	Erythema multiforme
Erythema marginatum	Urticaria
Erythema migrans	Viral exanthema
Photodermatitis	Contact dermatitis

Purpura or Petechiae

Idiopathic thrombocytopenic	Coagulopathy
Rocky Mountain spotted fever	Sepsis/DIC
Henoch–Schönlein purpura	Subacute bacterial endocarditis
Meningococcemia	TORCH infections

Vesicobullous

Vesicular

Dyshidrotic eczema	Miliaria crystallina
Scabies	Hand–foot–mouth disease
Herpes simplex	Varicella zoster
Eczema herpeticum	Allergic contact dermatitis

Bullous

Bullous impetigo	Staphylococcal scalded skin syndrome
Erythema multiforme major	Toxic epidermal necrolysis
Epidermolysis Bullosa	Pemphigus
Contact dermatitis – poison ivy	Photodermatitis

White lesions – patches and plaques

Pityriasis alba	Tinea versicolor
Postinflammatory hypopigmentation	Verrucae
Ash leaf macules	Vitiligo

White lesions – papules

Keratosis pilaris	Molluscum contagiosum[c]
Milia	

[a] Granuloma annulare can be either erythematous or skin-colored and presents as a papule which later develops into a nodule or plaque.
[b] Contact dermatitis can present as erythematous papules, vesicles, plaques, or mixed morphology in a well-demarcated distribution.
[c] Molluscum contagiosum can be skin-colored or have a white opalescent center, often with umbilication. They can also present swollen, erythematous, and tender.

Vesicle

A sharply circumscribed, elevated, fragile, clear fluid-filled lesion that is <1 cm in diameter and ruptures easily. Deroofed vesicles appear as small erosions.

Bulla

A vesicle that is >1 cm in diameter. A bulla may arise as a single large blister or through the coalescence of several vesicles.

Pustule

An elevated lesion containing purulent exudate. This lesion is usually filled with leukocytes, mostly neutrophils, but it can be sterile.

Secondary Lesions

Lesions that arise from alteration of a primary lesion, sometimes as a result of manipulation of the skin through scratching, picking, or rubbing.

Scale

An accumulation of layers of stratum corneum. Scales (or flakes) come in several types: adherent, nonadherent, coarse, shiny, smooth, lamellar, and polygonal. They may be greasy and yellowish, silvery and mica-like, fine and barely visible, or large, and sheet-like.

Crust

A crust (scab) results from dried serum (yellow), blood (dark red or brown), or purulent exudate (yellow to green) overlying areas of lost or damaged epidermis.

Erosion

A moist, shallow lesion in which part or all of the epidermis has been visibly lost or denuded. Erosions do not extend into the underlying dermis or subcutaneous tissue, so they heal without scarring.

Ulcer

An ulcer results from loss of both the epidermis and dermis, resulting in a punched-out lesion which may be filled with crust or necrotic skin. Alternatively, the base may be visible as a moist red surface. Ulcers heal with a scar.

Excoriation

A linear traumatic abrasion caused by scratching, rubbing, or scrubbing.

Scar

A permanent fibrotic skin change following damage to the dermis. Initially a scar is pink or violaceous, becoming hyper- or hypopigmented, sclerotic, or smooth over time. Scars may be atrophic (depressed and wrinkled) or hypertrophic (elevated and firm)

Acne

Acne vulgaris is the most common skin disease of the second decade, with an onset during puberty. It can be caused or exacerbated by medications, including phenytoin, isoniazid, iodides and bromides, and lithium. Acne can also be associated with polycystic ovarian syndrome (PCOS), androgen excess, or systemic steroid or adrenocorticotropic hormone therapy.

Clinical Presentation

Acne vulgaris primarily involves the face, chest, and upper back. Lesions include open (blackheads) and closed (whiteheads) comedones, papules, pustules, nodules, and cysts. Neonatal acne presents within the first few weeks of life on the forehead and cheeks and resolves usually by two months, requiring no treatment. The typical lesions of steroid acne are small erythematous papules and pustules, without comedones, primarily located on the back and chest.

Diagnosis

The diagnosis of acne vulgaris is usually straightforward, although a number of conditions may have a similar appearance. The differential diagnosis includes adenoma sebaceum, which appears as pink papules on the face of prepubertal patients with tuberous sclerosis (TS). Other cutaneous manifestations differentiate TS, including ash leaf spots, Shagreen patch, and periungual fibromas. In an infant, seborrheic dermatitis is often misdiagnosed as neonatal acne. Associated cradle cap and retro-auricular scaling distinguish seborrhea.

Although comedones can be found in children as young as 6–7 years of age, consider androgen excess (gonadal or adrenal tumors, congenital adrenal hyperplasia) if there is inflammatory acne (papules and pustules) in a prepubertal child.

ED Management

Acne vulgaris is a chronic disease. To help prevent permanent scarring, initiate treatment in the ED, but refer the patient to a primary care setting for ongoing care. Daily anti-acne medication, the use of very gentle cleansers, and the avoidance of sunburns are critical to therapy. Defer the initiation of medications such as isotretinoin and oral contraceptives to the primary care provider.

Topical retinoids and topical and oral antibiotics are the mainstays of treatment. For a patient ≥12 years of age, start with adapalene (0.1% gel; over-the-counter), applied in a thin layer nightly to the affected area. Add topical benzoyl peroxide and clindamycin gel combination, also applied in a thin layer to the affected area, but in the morning.

Add oral antibiotics, either doxycycline 50 to 100 mg bid or 100 mg q day. As an alternative, prescribe minocycline 50 mg q day, bid, or tid. An extended-release form of minocycline has very good compliance and is given as a single daily dose based on weight: 45–49 kg: 45 mg; 50–59 kg: 55 mg; 60–71 kg: 65 mg; 72–84 kg: 80 mg; 85–96 kg: 90 mg; 97–110 kg: 105 mg; 111–125 kg: 115 mg; 126–136 kg: 135 mg.

Treat steroid acne with topical benzoyl peroxide (2.5–10%), a topical antibiotic (as described above), and discontinuation of the steroids, if possible. The management of acne associated with PCOS includes either a combination oral contraceptive or progestin with topical therapies (described above). No therapy, other than reassurance, is required for neonatal acne.

Follow-up

- Primary care follow-up 2–3 days for patients requiring oral therapy, otherwise routine

Bibliography

Admani S, Barrio VR. Evaluation and treatment of acne from infancy to preadolescence. *Dermatol Ther.* 2013;**26**(6):462–466.

Eichenfield LF, Krakowski AC, Piggott C, et al. Evidence-based recommendations for the diagnosis and treatment of pediatric acne. *Pediatrics.* 2013;**131**(Suppl. 3):S163–S186.

Krakowski AC, Stendardo S, Eichenfield LF. Practical considerations in acne treatment and the clinical impact of topical combination therapy. *Ped Derm.* 2008;**25**(Suppl. 1):1–14.

Maronas-Jimenez L, Krakowski AC. Pediatric acne: clinical patterns and pearls. *Dermatol Clin.* 2016;**34**(2):195–202.

Alopecia

Alopecia is relatively common and, usually, a benign disorder in children. It is categorized as either localized or diffuse, and then further subcategorized as either scarring or non-scarring. The most common causes of localized alopecia include tinea capitis (pp. 137–139) and alopecia areata (presumed autoimmune disorder). Other causes of localized alopecia result from trauma or traction secondary to hair care techniques (braiding, straightening, blow drying) or trichotillomania, the purposeful removal of hair by the patient. These disorders are usually non-scarring and transient, but severe inflammatory forms of tinea capitis (kerion) can lead to permanent scarring.

The most common cause of diffuse alopecia in children is telogen effluvium. In most instances, the patient recently has suffered a significant stress (high fever, crash diet, parturition, convulsion, psychosocial event). Other etiologies include chemotherapeutic agents that cause anagen hair loss (cyclophosphamide, vincristine), drugs (ACE inhibitors, beta-blockers, antiepileptic drugs, lithium, cimetidine, oral contraceptives), radiation, toxins (lead, boric acid), endocrinopathies (hyper- and hypothyroidism, hypoparathyroidism), nutritional deficiencies (zinc, vitamin A), secondary syphilis, and systemic lupus erythematous. See Table 5.2 for the differential diagnosis of alopecia.

ED Management

Most cases of alopecia require no immediate treatment. Refer the patient to a dermatologist or primary care physician for follow-up, especially when the diagnosis is in doubt, or the alopecia is worsening or failing treatment, or there is chronic or scarring alopecia. See p. 139 for the treatment of a kerion.

Bibliography

DermNet New Zealand. Alopecia areata. www.dermnetnz.org (accessed June 26, 2017).

Alves R, Grimalt R. Hair loss in children. *Curr Probl Dermatol.* 2015;**47**:55–66.

Jackson AJ, Price VH. How to diagnose hair loss. *Dermatol Clin.* 2013;**31**(1):21–28.

Mubki T, Rudnicka L, Olszewska M, Shapiro J. Evaluation and diagnosis of the hair loss patient: part I. History and clinical examination. *J Am Acad Dermatol.* 2014;**71**(3):415.e1–415.

Table 5.2 Differential diagnosis of alopecia

Diagnosis	Differentiating features
Alopecia areata	Sudden onset; no scalp inflammation
	Sharply demarcated round or oval patches with total hair loss
	Exclamation point hairs at margins
Androgenetic	Bilateral frontoparietal recession and thinning over the vertex
	Begins in teenaged years
	No scalp inflammation
Telogen effluvium	History of emotional or physical stressors
	Physiologic; postpartum and newborn
	Diffuse thinning without scalp inflammation
	Positive hair pull test: >2–3 hairs removed at a time
Tinea capitis	Patchy/poorly demarcated with scalp inflammation and scaling
	Black dots within the patch
	KOH positive: chains of spores, positive fungal culture
Traction/trauma	Poorly demarcated areas of incomplete hair loss
	Occurs in scalp areas subjected to friction or pulling
	No scalp inflammation
Trichotillomania	Poorly demarcated, irregular-shaped areas of incomplete hair loss
	Eye lashes and eyebrows may also be involved
	History suggests psychopathology

Paller AS, Mancini AJ. Alopecia In Hurwitz S, Paller A, Mancini A (eds.) *Hurwitz's Textbook of Clinical Pediatric Dermatology* (4th edn.). Philadelphia, PA: WB Saunders, 2011; 130–154.

Atopic Dermatitis

Atopic dermatitis (AD) is a disease that predisposes the skin to excessive dryness and pruritus. It affects more than 10% of children, most of whom will also have or develop another atopic disorder, such as allergic rhinitis, asthma, or food allergy.

Clinical Presentation

Pruritic, dry, chronic, relapsing, eczematous lesions are major hallmarks of the disease. Infantile eczema occurs between birth and three years and is characterized by dry skin, erythema, papules, vesicles, oozing, and scales on the face, neck, chest, and extensor surfaces of the extremities. In older children subacute and chronic papular, scaly, and lichenified (thickened, leathery skin with accentuation of the normal skin markings) lesions occur, often in well-circumscribed plaques on the flexor aspects of the neck, arms, and legs. The antecubital and popliteal fossae are classically involved, and the periorbital and perioral regions may also be affected. The adolescent and adult forms demonstrate marked licheni-fication and flexural, hand, and foot involvement.

Other manifestations in children and adolescents may include nummular eczema (well-demarcated papular coin lesions) and pityriasis alba (discrete hypopigmented macules).

At any age the severe pruritus causes scratching which can lead to secondary bacterial infection. The superimposed pyoderma can confuse the clinical picture. Secondary herpes-virus infection (eczema herpeticum, pp. 125–126) can also occur and become generalized in atopic patients.

Atopic individuals can have a number of associated findings, including accentuated palmar creases, white dermatographism (blanching of the skin when stroked), and Dennie–Morgan folds or pleats (an extra groove of the lower eyelid). Keratosis pilaris (follicular hyperkeratosis) presents with scaly perifollicular papules on cheeks, upper arms, thighs, and buttocks.

Factors that can exacerbate symptoms in patients with AD include temperature, humid-ity, irritants, infections, foods, inhalant and contact allergens, and emotional stress.

Diagnosis

The diagnosis of atopic dermatitis is suggested by a family history of atopy, a personal history of allergies or asthma, dry and pruritic skin, and the typical location of the lesions that blend into the surrounding normal skin.

In infants, seborrheic dermatitis (pp. 132–133) causes a nonpruritic yellowish or sal-mon-colored, greasy eruption of the face, scalp, and intertriginous areas. The eruption of a contact dermatitis (pp. 111–113) has a sharp border with the uninvolved skin, and the history may suggest the offending agent. The lesions of tinea corporis (pp. 138–140) usually have central clearing and a raised scaly annular border. Bacterial infections (pp. 107–109) are not preceded by pruritus and are generally more localized than atopic rashes. Psoriatic lesions are usually well-demarcated with a silvery scale and are found on extensor surfaces, gluteal creases, scalp, and genital regions. The eruption of scabies (p. 130) does not follow the usual sites of predilection of AD, and the family or personal history of atopy may be negative. A secondary autoeczematization process may occur with scabies that makes differentiation between eczema and scabies difficult. To differentiate scabies, look for lesions in the interdigital spaces, on the areola, wrists, waist, and groin, and in infants on the palmo-plantar surfaces.

ED Management

Atopic dermatitis is a chronic condition that is best managed in the primary care setting, but therapy can be initiated in the ED. The goals are to hydrate the skin, prevent itching, and treat inflammation. Instruct the patient to avoid excessive bathing, harsh detergents, and fragrances, and to use moisturizers and emollients as first-line therapy (Cetaphil, Eucerin, Aquaphor, Vaseline). Use a low-potency corticosteroid for maintenance therapy, whereas intermediate- and high-potency corticosteroids are indicated for the treatment of clinical exacerbation over short periods of time (see Table 5.3).

Treat pruritus with diphenhydramine (5 mg/kg/day div qid) or hydroxyzine (2 mg/kg/day div qid).

Prescribe a mid-potency topical corticosteroid (0.1% triamcinolone ointment, 0.05% fluticasone cream, 0.1% mometasone cream) for the body and extremities and a low-

Table 5.3 Potency of topical corticosteroids

Class: potency	Generic name	Brand name	Strength/form
VII: Lowest	Hydrocortisone acetate	Cortifoam	0.1% lotion/ointment/ foam
	Hydrocortisone	Hytone, Cortaid	0.25–2.5% lotion/ ointment/solution
VI: Low	Desonide	Desowen	0.05% cream
	Flucinolone acetonide	Synalar	0.01% cream/solution
	Aclometasone	Aclovate	0.05% cream/ointment
V: Low/medium	Hydrocortisone butyrate	Locomid	0.1% ointment/ solution
	Prednicarbate	Dermatop	0.1% cream
IV to III: Medium/	Mometasone	Elocon	0.1% cream
high medium	Fluticasone proprionate	Cutivate	0.05% cream; 0.005% ointment
	Betamethasone valerate	Luxiq	0.1% cream/ointment/ lotion/foam
	Clocortolone pivalate	Cloderm	0.1% cream
II to I: High	Flucinonide	Lidex	0.05% cream/ ointment/gel/foam

Note: The duration of topical corticosteroid use varies by disease severity and location. Most patients will respond to 1–2 weeks of application daily bid. Longer courses require close follow-up. Do not use high-potency topical corticosteroids in the facial and intertriginous areas because it can lead to atrophy, striae, and telangiectasias. Extensive use of any potency topical steroids over large body surface areas for prolonged periods may lead to adrenal axis suppression, particularly in infants.

potency one (1–2.5% hydrocortisone ointment, 0.05% aclometasone, cream or ointment) for the face, neck, and other delicate areas. Limit the course to two weeks and do not use under occlusion in delicate areas.

Do not use oral steroids without consulting a dermatologist. Defer initiating topical nonsteroidal immunomodulator therapy (tacrolimus, opimecrolimus) to the primary care or dermatology office setting.

Reserve the use of wet wraps for severe flares and use only for a few days at a time, because they are time-consuming and children often are resistant to their application. Instruct the family to apply a mild- to moderate-potency topical steroid in a thin layer to the affected area, follow with emollient, cover with slightly damp Kerlix or cotton pajamas, and then place a dry Kerlix or dry pajamas over the treated sites, nightly for 3–5 nights.

If there is a secondary bacterial infection, use topical mupirocin tid on localized areas of involvement, but treat more extensive infections as a cellulitis (pp. 107–109) with oral antibiotics and arrange careful follow-up to document adequate response to treatment.

Follow-up
- Primary care follow-up in 1–2 weeks

Indications for Admission
- Severe involvement in a patient who cannot be adequately treated at home or shows signs of secondary infection that would be best treated with intravenous antibiotics
- Evidence of eczema herpeticum (pp. 125–126)

Bibliography

Eichenfield LF, Boguniewicz M, Simpson EL, et al. Translating atopic dermatitis management guidelines into practice for primary care providers. *Pediatrics*. 2015;**136**(3):554–565.

Krakowski AC, Eichenfield LF, Dohil MA: Management of atopic dermatitis in the pediatric population. *Pediatrics*. 2008;**122**:812–824.

National Eczema Association. Understanding your atopic dermatitis. https://nationaleczema.org/eczema/types-of-eczema/atopic-dermatitis (accessed June 26, 2017).

Rady Children's Hospital. Eczema diagnosis. www.rchsd.org/programs-services/dermatology/eczema-and-inflammatory-skin-disease-center/diagnosis (accessed June 26, 2017).

Tollefson MM, Bruckner AL. Atopic dermatitis: skin-directed management. *Pediatrics*. 2014;**134**(6): e1735–1744.

Bacterial Skin Infections

Bacterial skin infections, or pyodermas, are most commonly caused by group A Streptococcus and *Staphylococcus aureus*. Impetigo, folliculitis, furunculosis, and cellulitis are the usual forms of infection.

Clinical Presentation and Diagnosis

Impetigo

The most common type of bacterial skin infection is impetigo contagiosum (primary impetigo) caused by group A Streptococcus or *Staphylococcus aureus*. The eruption usually appears on the face and extremities as small erythematous macules which develop into vesicles that rupture. There is a typical honey-colored crust that is easily removed, but can recur. Fever and regional lymphadenopathy may also occur. Impetigo is extremely contagious, spreading by autoinoculation (satellite lesions), close contact, and fomites (towels). It is more common in 2–5-year-olds and in the warm, humid summer months.

Non-bullous impetigo is the most common form. Lesions often begin as papules that progress to vesicles surrounded by erythema. They eventually become pustules that break down to then form crusts.

Bullous impetigo is usually caused by phage group II staphylococci. Yellowish vesicles on the face, extremities, and trunk rupture, leaving well-demarcated, erythematous, circular macules with a "collarette of scale." There tends to be fewer lesions than in non-bullous impetigo, and the trunk is more frequently affected.

Folliculitis

Folliculitis is a pyoderma involving the hair follicles, particularly in areas subjected to sweating, friction, scratching, and shaving. Coagulase-positive *Staphylococcus* is the most frequent etiologic agent, although there are also viral and fungal etiologies. Folliculitis presents as pruritic, round-topped pustules most commonly seen on the scalp, face, thighs, and buttocks. The hallmark of a folliculitis is the presence of a hair shaft in most lesions.

Furunculosis

Furunculosis is an infection of the hair follicle in which purulent material extends through the dermis into the subcutaneous tissue, where a small abscess forms. Furuncles (boils) are tender, erythematous 1–5 cm nodules that become fluctuant, and then suppurate. They are seen in hair-bearing areas that are subject to perspiration and friction, including the face, thighs, buttocks, and scalp. In contrast, an abscess (pp. 762–763) is usually a solitary lesion that is not associated with hair follicles. Recurrent folliculitis is a risk factor for infection with community-acquired methicillin-resistant *Staphylococcus aureus*.

Cellulitis

Cellulitis, an infection involving the deeper dermis and subcutaneous tissues, causes a poorly demarcated, tender, erythematous swelling. It is often associated with fever, local lymphadenopathy, and proximal lymphangitic streaking. Sites of infection are often areas subjected to superficial trauma, such as the face and extremities. Common pathogens include methicillin-sensitive and -resistant *Staphylococcus aureus*, group A Streptococcus, and rarely *Streptococcus pneumoniae*.

Erysipelas

Erysipelas is an uncommon superficial infection caused by group A Streptococcus, involving the upper dermis and superficial lymphatics. It begins as a small area of redness that progresses to a tense, erythematous, tender, well-demarcated plaque.

Staphylococcal Scalded Skin Syndrome

Staphylococcal scalded skin syndrome (SSSS) is not a true cutaneous infection, but may be a manifestation of one. It is an acute exfoliative dermatosis caused by an epidermolytic toxin produced by phage group II strains of staphylococci, types 3A, 3B, 3C, 55, and 71. It must be distinguished from toxic epidermal necrolysis or TEN (pp. 116–119).

Staphylococcal scalded skin syndrome usually occurs in children <6 years of age. It begins abruptly, with a generalized macular erythema after a period of fever and irritability. There may be a pharyngitis, conjunctivitis, rhinorrhea, or discrete staphylococcal infection. The eruption becomes scarlatiniform (sandpaper-like) and tender, with wrinkling, bullae, sheet-like exfoliation, and a positive Nikolsky's sign (a peeling of normal-appearing skin with light pressure). Crusting around the mouth and sometimes nose and eyes is typical, but mucous membrane involvement is rare. Despite the marked skin tenderness and irritability, these patients do not appear toxic. If hydration is maintained, recovery occurs in 1–2 weeks.

Early in the course, SSSS may resemble scarlet fever (p. 409; nontender skin, pharyngitis, and strawberry tongue, negative Nikolsky), Kawasaki disease (pp. 414–417; erythema of the conjunctiva, lips, and oral mucosa, strawberry tongue, negative Nikolsky), and

Stevens–Johnson syndrome or TEN (target lesions, mucous membrane involvement, positive Nikolsky). The diagnosis of SSSS is confirmed by isolation of staphylococci from an orifice, or rarely the blood; it cannot be recovered from bullae or areas of exfoliation.

ED Management

Knowing the local community MRSA pattern is critical for choosing the most appropriate empiric treatment. If there is a significant concern, use either clindamycin *or* trimethoprim-sulfamethoxazole *plus* a first-generation cephalosporin.

Impetigo

Treat with mupirocin ointment (2%) tid for five days along with good local hygiene. For more extensive disease, or if mupirocin is unavailable or ineffective, treat for 7–10 days with cefadroxil (40 mg/kg/day div bid) or cephalexin (40 mg/kg/day div q 6h). If MRSA is a concern, either use clindamycin (20 mg/kg/day div q 6h) or add trimethoprim-sulfamethoxazole (8 mg/kg/day of TMP div bid) to the above regimen (cefadroxil or cephalexin).

Folliculitis

Folliculitis occasionally responds to 7–14 days of treatment with a topical antibiotic (mupirocin 2%, clindamycin 1%). If the response is inadequate, treat with the same oral antibiotics as for impetigo, for 7–10 days.

Cellulitis

Depending on the local community MRSA pattern, choose one of the regimens listed for impetigo. Admit for inpatient treatment with IV antibiotics if the child failed oral medications, or there are systemic symptoms such as fever, chills, vomiting, or with hemodynamic instability.

Erysipelas

Treat with penicillin (250 mg qid) for ten days. Admit for IV antibiotics (as for furunculosis and cellulitis) if there is an inadequate response.

Staphylococcal Scalded Skin Syndrome

If SSSS is suspected, obtain a CBC, blood culture, and polymerase chain reaction (PCR) for the toxin (if available). Obtain cultures and Gram's stains from the nose, throat, conjunctiva, and other potential foci of infection. The exfoliation is toxin-mediated so exfoliated sites will be sterile. Admit the patient and treat with IV anti-staphylococcal antibiotics, either nafcillin 150 mg/kg/day div q 6h or, if MRSA is a possibility, clindamycin (25–40 mg/kg/day div q 6h) or vancomycin (40 mg/kg/day div q 6h), if hemodynamically unstable.

Follow-up

- Impetigo: primary care follow-up in 2–3 days, if no improvement
- Folliculitis: primary care follow-up in 1–2 weeks
- Furunculosis, cellulitis, and erysipelas: primary care follow-up in 2–3 days

Indications for Admission

- Furunculosis or cellulitis in a patient with an immune deficiency

- Fever, proximal lymphadenopathy, and lymphangitic streaking in association with cellulitis or other deep skin infection
- Inadequate response to outpatient management
- Suspected staphylococcal scalded skin syndrome
- Hemodynamic instability

Bibliography

Fenster DB, Renny MH, Ng C, Roskind CG. Scratching the surface: a review of skin and soft tissue infections in children. *Curr Opin Pediatr.* 2015;**27**(3):303–307.

Mistry RD. Skin and soft tissue infections. *Pediatr Clin North Am.* 2013;**60**(5):1063–1082.

Raff AB, Kroshinsky D. Cellulitis: a review. *JAMA.* 2016;**316**:325.

Sanders JE, Garcia SE. Evidence-based management of skin and soft tissue infections in pediatric patients in the emergency department. Pediatr Emerg Med *Pract.* 2015;**12**(2):1–23.

Stevens DL, Bisno AL, Chambers HF, et al. Practice guidelines for the diagnosis and management of skin and soft tissue infections: 2014 update by the infectious diseases society of America. *Clin Infect Dis.* 2014; **59**:147.

Candida

Candidiasis is caused by the fungus *Candida albicans,* a normal cutaneous saprophyte that exists in the gastrointestinal tract, oral cavity, and vagina. Factors that predispose to candidiasis include local heat or moisture, long-term indwelling catheters, malignancy, chemotherapy, diabetes mellitus, and the use of systemic antibiotics, corticosteroids, or chemotherapy.

Clinical Presentation

Cutaneous Candidiasis

Cutaneous candidiasis is most frequently found in the intertriginous and diaper areas. It is characterized by moist, beefy red, well-demarcated, shallow plaques with raised, scaly edges. Satellite vesicles and pustules may be seen near the borders. In the anterior neck, axilla, and postauricular and inguinal folds, intertrigo will present as a weeping erythematous and macerated area, with or without satellite lesions. Intertrigo is often superinfected with *Staph* or group B *Strep.*

Oral Candidiasis

Oral candidiasis (thrush) presents in the first weeks of life with loosely adherent, cheesy white plaques on the tongue, soft and hard palates, and buccal mucosa. The mucosal surfaces are beefy red, and the lesions bleed when scraped lightly with a tongue blade. These lesions are often painful, and a marked decrease in oral intake can occur in young infants. Thrush in older patients is usually associated with some underlying condition (immunosuppression, broad-spectrum antibiotics), but it can occur in otherwise healthy infants. Recurrent thrush can be seen in HIV-infected children, and esophageal candidiasis occurs in up to 20% of these patients.

Diagnosis

The typical intense erythema, scaly border, and satellite lesions suggest the diagnosis of cutaneous candidiasis. See diaper dermatitis for differential diagnosis (pp. 113–115). When the diagnosis is in doubt, prepare a KOH prep from a skin scraping or send a fungal culture, but do not delay treatment.

Thrush is often confused with milk in the oral cavity, although milk can easily be scraped from the oral mucosa without causing any bleeding.

ED Management

Prescribe topical nystatin ointment, or miconazole, clotrimazole, or econazole cream. Apply bid or tid to cutaneous eruptions, such as intertrigo, for 2–3 weeks or two days past clearing. Avoid combination products containing neomycin, which can be irritating, as well as topical steroid combination preparations due to the risk of adverse effects from long-term use, especially in areas of occlusion. If the eruption is markedly inflamed, use a low-potency topical corticosteroid such as hydrocortisone 1–2.5% bid for 2–3 days, in addition to a topical antifungal. Instruct the parents to keep these areas clean and dry, if possible, and to use hypoallergenic, gentle cleansers. The additional use of a barrier product containing zinc oxide is often helpful.

For thrush, instill 1 mL of a nystatin oral suspension in each side of the mouth qid, after feedings, until at least two days past clearing. Advise the parent to rub persistent lesions with a gauze pad soaked with nystatin suspension and to discard any old pacifiers, nipples, or teething toys that may be contaminated. Sterilize nipples and pacifiers after use during the treatment phase and encourage treatment of *Candida* breast colonization and/or infection in lactating mothers. Suspect an underlying immunodeficiency or re-exposure to contaminated items as listed above in a patient with persistent or recurrent thrush in the absence of antibiotic use. For such a patient, or one who has failed to clear on nystatin, prescribe oral fluconazole (6 mg/kg once, then 3 mg/kg/day for 14 days) or clotrimazole troches for a patient >3 years of age (10 mg qid for 7–14 days, dissolve slowly in mouth, do not chew or swallow whole).

Follow-up

• Primary care follow-up in 1–2 weeks

Bibliography

Klunk C, Domingues E, Wiss K. An update on diaper dermatitis. *Clin Dermatol.* 2014;32(4):477–487.

Marty M, Bourrat E, Vaysse F, Bonner M, Bailleul-Forestier I. Direct microscopy: a useful tool to diagnose oral candidiasis in children and adolescents. *Mycopathologia.* 2015;180(5–6):373–377.

Pankhurst CL: Candidiasis (oropharyngeal). *BMJ Clin Evid.* 2013;2013:1304.

Warris A, European Paediatric Mycology Network (EPMyN). Towards a better understanding and management of fungal infections in children. *Curr Fungal Infect Rep.* 2016;10:7–9.

Contact Dermatitis

Contact dermatitis is an eczematous eruption due to local exposure to a skin irritant or sensitizing agent (allergen). The most common irritants are water (prolonged or repeated exposure), soaps, detergents, acids, alkalis, certain foods, saliva, urine, and feces.

Allergic contact dermatitis is a result of repeated exposures leading to a delayed type IV hypersensitivity. Common causes include urushiol from *Rhus* genus plants (poison ivy, oak, and sumac), latex, rubber, dyes, cosmetics, and additives to cleansers, lanolin, adhesives, neomycin, cobalt, chromate, and nickel.

Phytophotodermatitis is a non-immunologic, acute phototoxic reaction, which can occur after contact with plants containing psoralens upon subsequent exposure to UV light. Plants commonly associated with this response include lemon, lime, bergamot, celery, carrot, parsley, parsnip, fennel, dill, fig, mustard, and buttercup.

Clinical Presentation

Irritant contact dermatitis presents within minutes to hours of the contact as an acute eczematous reaction, with erythema, scaling, swelling, vesicles, and erosions of varying severity at the site of the contact. Lesions may be linear and have a sharp demarcation between the involved and uninvolved skin.

Allergic contact dermatitis presents within hours or days with erythema, edema, bullae, and vesicles, most commonly on the hands and face, but also seen on the feet, eyelids, ears, neck, axillae, and periumbilical area. Once again, the lesions may be linear and have a sharp demarcation between the involved and uninvolved skin. *Rhus* dermatitis presents within 1–3 days of exposure and persists for 1–3 weeks. If aerosolized, there may be severe facial edema presenting in a similar fashion as angioedema, but with fine vesiculation.

Phytophotodermatitis reactions may be eczematous and erythematous, with prominent vesicles and bullae, located in areas of psoralen contact. The cutaneous reaction may assume bizarre digitate, linear or drip patterns. The rash often resolves with subsequent hyperpigmentation. Photoxic reactions can easily be confused with child abuse, burns, or herpes simplex infection.

Diagnosis

The diagnosis is purely clinical, based on appearance and history of exposure. Inquire about exposure to possible offending agents (new soap, detergent, shoes, or foods, or playing in the woods) and whether there has been previous similar episodes or a known sensitivity to a substance. On examination, look for an eczematoid eruption either in nontypical locations or in a linear pattern, with sharp demarcations between involved and normal skin.

ED Management

Avoidance of the offending agent or allergen is critical. Treat an acute dermatitis with open wet dressings (tap water, normal saline, 5% Burrow's solution) PRN, calamine lotion, daily soothing baths (Aveeno, oatmeal), and antihistamines (hydroxyzine 2 mg/kg/day div tid or diphenhydramine 5 mg/kg/day div qid). For intense inflammation or pruritus, prescribe a low- to medium-potency topical corticosteroid (see Table 5.3) bid for two weeks.

Use a systemic corticosteroid for a dermatitis that is widespread or involves the mucous membranes or eye lids. Start with 0.5–1.5 mg/kg/day (40 mg/day maximum) of prednisone or prednisolone for 4–5 days, then taper over 4–6 days to prevent a rebound in the eruption.

For a chronic contact dermatitis the above modalities may be effective, but refer the patient to a dermatologist for definitive diagnosis and treatment.

Follow-up

- As needed based on severity; if on systemic steroids follow in two weeks

Indications for Admission

- Severe reactions with extensive involvement involving mucous membranes or threatening the eyes or upper respiratory tract

Bibliography

Bernstein DI. contact dermatitis for the practicing allergist. *J Allergy Clin Immunol Pract*. 2015;3(5): 652–628; quiz 659–660.

Goldenberg A, Silverberg N, Silverberg JI, Treat J, Jacob SE. Pediatric allergic contact dermatitis: lessons for better care. *J Allergy Clin Immunol Pract*. 2015;3(5):661–667.

Jacob SE, Goldenberg A, Pelletier JL, et al. Nickel allergy and our children's health: a review of indexed cases and a view of future prevention. *Pediatr Dermatol*. 2015;**32**(6):779–785.

Paller AS, Mancini AJ: Contact dermatitis. In Hurwitz S, Paller A, Mancini A (eds.) *Hurwitz's Textbook of Clinical Pediatric Dermatology* (4th edn.). Philadelphia, PA: WB Saunders, 2011; 61–70.

Pelletier JL, Perez C, Jacob SE. Contact dermatitis in pediatrics. *Pediatr Ann*. 2016;45(8):e287–292.

Diaper Dermatitis

Diaper rashes can begin as early as the first few weeks of life and may persist or wax and wane over the next 2–3 years. Diaper rash can be caused by friction and chaffing, irritant contact dermatitis, infection (bacterial, fungal), nutritional deficiencies (zinc, biotin, fatty acid, protein), dermatologic disorders (seborrhea, psoriasis, Langerhans cell histiocytosis), metabolic disorders (cystic fibrosis, maple syrup urine disease, methylmalonic acidemia, organic aciduria), or abuse/neglect. *Candida* superinfection commonly co-occurs with a diaper rash of any other etiology.

Clinical Presentation

Irritant Contact Dermatitis

Irritant contact dermatitis appears as a diffuse, shiny, erythematous, papular eruption on the convexities of the buttocks, genitalia, and lower abdomen, sparing the intertriginous folds.

Candida

Candida (see pp. 110–111) infections may be primary or secondary. *Candida* diaper dermatitis presents as widespread beefy red erythema, with or without a sharp white scaly margin, and satellite papules, pustules, and/or vesicles. Involvement of the inter-triginous creases and associated oral thrush are common, and the eruption can spread up the abdomen and down the thighs. The scrotum is often involved in males. Consider secondary candidiasis if a diaper rash does not respond to the usual therapeutic measures. Persistent or frequently recurring diaper candidiasis can occur in immunocompromised patients.

Seborrheic Dermatitis

Seborrheic dermatitis (see pp. 132–133) presents as salmon-colored, greasy scales on a well-demarcated erythematous base. Characteristically, a similar eruption is simultaneously seen on the face, along with scaling of the scalp and retroauricular areas. Involvement of the intertriginous creases is common, and secondary candidiasis can occur.

Langerhans Cell Histiocytosis (LCH or Histiocytosis X)

LCH may cause a diaper eruption which resembles seborrhea, but is more discretely papular. These papules may feel firm or slightly infiltrated or indurated and can appear hemorrhagic or purpuric. Furthermore, ulceration may occur, which is rare in seborrhea or psoriasis.

Acrodermatitis Enteropathica

Acrodermatitis enteropathica in the diaper area can mimic irritant contact dermatitis. It tends to be erosive and may involve the perioral region as well as the hands, feet, and intertriginous sites. The patient may also have failure to thrive, diarrhea, and alopecia.

Psoriasis

Psoriasis presents as persistent, well-demarcated red plaques with or without scaling (due to moisture in the diaper). New lesions are often small, 1–3 mm papules which subsequently enlarge and coalesce with adjacent lesions to form large plaques. Other psoriasiform lesions with micaceous scale may be found on the scalp, elbows, knees, lumbosacral, and anogenital regions.

Perianal Streptococcal Disease

Perianal group A streptococcal infection is characterized by a persistent, bright red, usually tender eruption which is sharply demarcated from the adjacent normal skin. There can be perianal tenderness and itching, and occasionally rectal pain, painful defecation, anal fissures, and secondary stool withholding.

Diagnosis

In general, the clinical presentations are sufficiently different, making the diagnosis apparent. When the picture is not typical, a secondary *Candida* infection of an irritant, contact, or seborrheic dermatitis has most likely occurred. Consider LCH if the eruption is recalcitrant, erosive, or purpuric. If the infant appears malnourished, with chronic diarrhea and alopecia, consider acrodermatitis. Psoriasis is suggested by the typical distribution and morphology of lesions elsewhere on the body. To confirm perianal streptococcal infection, obtain a bacterial culture or perform a rapid strep test.

ED Management

Meticulous diaper care is the cornerstone of management for all types of diaper rashes. Recommend frequent diaper changes, gentle cleansing, air drying when possible, liberal use of barrier products (zinc oxide- and petrolatum-based products) with every diaper change, and discontinuing all harsh soaps, powders, and perfumed products (including baby wipes).

Also, since *Candida* superinfection is common with diaper rashes of other etiologies, add antifungal therapy (see below), especially in refractory cases

Treat inflammation secondary to irritants, contact dermatitis, or seborrhea with a mild topical steroid (see Table 5.3) for a very short course – i.e., three times per day for three days. Caution the parents to not overuse steroids in this area due to high risk of side effects.

Many topical agents are available for the treatment of *Candida*, including nystatin, miconazole, and clotrimazole. Apply with every diaper change until two days past clearing. The "-azoles" are preferred in the diaper region or when it is difficult to distinguish tinea from *Candida*, as nystatin is only effective against *Candida* and other yeast fungi and not dermatophyte (tinea) infections. Add oral nystatin (1 mL each side of the mouth qid after feeding until two days past clearing) if there is concurrent oral thrush.

Treat perianal streptococcal infection with oral amoxicillin, 40 mg/kg/day, divided bid for ten days and topical mupirocin 2% tid for 7–10 days. Cephalexin 40 mg/kg/day PO divided bid for ten days (max. 500 mg/dose) and clindamycin (30 mg/kg per day div tid max. 900 mg/day for ten days) are acceptable alternatives.

A persistent diaper eruption may be the presenting sign of an underlying systemic disorder. Refer the patient to a dermatologist and for close primary care follow-up if the rash does not respond to these routine measures or the infant is not thriving or has recurrent infections.

Follow-up
• Routine primary care follow-up as needed depending on response to therapy

Indications for Admission
• Diaper dermatitis with suspicion of neglect, severe failure to thrive or LCH

Bibliography

Bonifaz A, Rojas R, Tirado-Sánchez A, et al. Superficial mycoses associated with diaper dermatitis. *Mycopathologia.* 2016;**181**(9–10):671–679.

Coughlin CC, Eichenfield LF, Frieden IJ. Diaper dermatitis: clinical characteristics and differential diagnosis. *Pediatr Dermatol.* 2014;**31**(Suppl. 1):19–24.

Klunk C, Domingues E, Wiss K. An update on diaper dermatitis. *Clin Dermatol.* 2014;**32**:477.

Shin HT. Diagnosis and management of diaper dermatitis. *Pediatr Clin North Am.* 2014;**61**:367.

Van Gysel D. Infections and skin diseases mimicking diaper dermatitis. *Int J Dermatol.* 2016;**55**(Suppl. 1):10–13.

Drug Eruptions and Severe Drug Reactions

Any drug can cause adverse reactions, which frequently involve the skin. The most common offending agents are the penicillins, sulfonamides, and anticonvulsants. Suspect that the eruption is drug-related when a medication has been newly prescribed within the past six weeks or has been used inconsistently in the recent past. The priority in the ED is expeditious diagnosis and treatment of serious drug reactions and anaphylaxis.

There are four common drug-related cutaneous eruption patterns: exanthematous, urticarial, fixed drug eruption, and phototoxic/allergic drug eruptions. Of particular concern are the more serious drug reactions with cutaneous manifestations. These include serum sickness-like reactions (SSLR), drug reaction with eosinophilia and systemic symptoms (DRESS), Stevens–Johnson syndrome (SJS), and toxic epidermal necrolysis (TEN).

Clinical Presentation and Diagnosis

Exanthematous Cutaneous Eruption

This is the most common (90% of cases) drug eruption. It is most frequently caused by amoxicillin and ampicillin ("amoxicillin rash"), developing in about 5–10% of patients taking either medication. The rash is an erythematous, nonpruritic, morbilliform, macular eruption primarily on the trunk, face, and extremities. The typical onset is between days 4 and 8, although the rash can occur after the first or last dose. This is not a true allergy and does not necessitate discontinuing the drug or avoiding penicillins in the future.

Stevens–Johnson Syndrome and Toxic Epidermal Necrolysis

Stevens–Johnson syndrome and toxic epidermal necrolysis are severe conditions involving blistering of two or more mucosal surfaces, widespread lesions and systemic involvement with fever and generalized malaise. One-third of children with SJS will have episcleritis and purulent conjunctivitis. The associated fever and pharyngitis frequently is misdiagnosed as an infection.

Serum Sickness

Serum sickness typically follows the administration of a drug, and is characterized by fever, lymphadenopathy, rash, arthritis, and/or arthralgias. Antigen–antibody complexes are deposited throughout the vascular system, leading to the intense inflammatory response.

See Table 5.4 for the diagnosis and management of the common types of drug eruptions. See Table 5.5 for the diagnosis of other types of drug eruptions. See Table 5.6 for the diagnosis and management of severe drug eruptions.

Table 5.4 Drug eruptions

Eruption type	Associated drugs	Presentation	Management
Exanthematous	Amoxicillin, ampicillin	Morbilliform or scarlatiniform	Discontinue medication
	Antiepileptics	Generalized, symmetric	Antihistamines
	Anti-Tb drugs	Centripetally progressive	Avoid sunlight
	NSAIDs		
Fixed drug	Sulfonamides, tetracyclines	Solitary or multiple	Discontinue medication
	Acetaminophen, NSAIDs	Erythematous or violaceous	

Table 5.4 (cont.)

Eruption type	Associated drugs	Presentation	Management
	Ciprofloxacin, metronidazole	Distinct patches or plaques	
	Penicillins, anti-Tb drugs	Face, trunk, genitalia	
Photosensitivity			
Phototoxic	Tetracyclines, griseofulvin	Sunburn	Discontinue medication
	Fluoroquinalones	May be edematous	Avoid sunlight
	NSAIDs, diuretics	Dose-dependent	Antihistamines
	Antipsychotics		Systemic steroids (if severe)
Photoallergic	Sunscreen, fragrance, latex	Eczematous and pruritic	Same as for phototoxic
	NSAIDs, thiazides		
	Sulfonamides		
Urticarial	Penicillins, cephalosporins	Evanescent, pruritic	Discontinue medication
	Sulfonamides	Edematous wheals, papules, plaques	Antihistamines
	NSAIDs, opiates	Angioedema may develop	Cool emollients
	Anti-Tb drugs	Dermatographism may be present	

Table 5.5 Other types of drug eruptions

Type of eruption	Most common causes
Acneiform	Corticosteroids, diphenylhydantoin, isoniazid, lithium, oral contraceptives
Erythema multiforme	Sulfonamides, penicillins, barbiturates, phenytoin, carbamazepine
Erythema nodosum	Sulfonamides, phenytoin, oral contraceptives
Lupus-like	Procainamide, hydralazine
Purpura	Penicillins, sulfonamides, oral contraceptives

Table 5.6 Serious drug reactions

Diagnosis	Drugs	Onset	Symptoms	Cutaneous findings	Treatment
DRESS	Antiepileptics Sulfonamides	1–6 wks	Fever Lymphadenopathy	Initially macular/erythematous Becomes papulovesicular, then exfoliative Facial edema Mucous membranes involved	Discontinue medication Systemic steroids (severe)
SJS/TEN	Antiepileptics Sulfonamides Beta-lactams Barbiturates Macrolides NSAIDs	1–8 wks	1–14 day prodrome: Fever, conjunctivitis, pharyngitis, rhinitis, arthralgia, myalgia, vomiting, diarrhea → mucous membrane erosion	Abrupt eruption of target lesions ≥2 sites mucous membrane involvement (+) Nikolsky's sign	Supportive care (PICU, burn unit) Meticulous wound care Maintain airway, hydration
SSLR	Cefaclor Beta-lactams Sulfonamides Macrolides	1–3 wks	Fever Arthralgia Lymphadenopathy	Erythema and urticaria Pruritus	Discontinue medication Antihistamines Topical steroids Systemic steroids (severe)

ED Management

Patients with DRESS, SJS, and TEN can deteriorate quickly from dehydration and internal organ involvement. Therefore, prompt recognition and intervention may be life-saving as these processes are associated with significant mortality.

Discontinue the offending agent. Treat pruritus with hydroxyzine (2 mg/kg/day divided every eight hours as needed) or diphenhydramine (5 mg/kg/day div qid) and a low-potency topical corticosteroid (see Table 5.6).

The treatment of anaphylaxis (pp. 37–41), acne (pp. 102–103), erythema multiforme (p. 120), erythema nodosum (p. 121), and urticaria (pp. 43–45) is discussed elsewhere.

Indications for Admission

- Suspicion for DRESS
- Suspicion for TEN
- Suspicion for SJS
- Anaphylaxis

Bibliography

Cleveland Clinic Center for Continuing Education. Drug eruptions. www.clevlandclinicmeded.com /medicalpubs/diseasemanagement/dermatology/drug-eruptions (accessed June 26, 2017).

Mockenhaupt M. Stevens–Johnson syndrome and toxic epidermal necrolysis: clinical patterns, diagnostic considerations, etiology, and therapeutic management. *Semin Cutan Med Surg.* 2014;**33** (1):10–16.

Smith R, Gargo E, Kirkham J, et al. Adverse drug reactions in children: a systematic review. *PloS One.* 2012;**7**(3):e24061.

Song JE, Sidbury R. An update on pediatric cutaneous drug eruptions. *Clin Dermatol.* 2014;**32** (4):516–523.

Stern RS. Clinical practice: exanthematous drug eruptions. *N Engl J Med.* 2012;**366**(26):2492–2501.

Erythema Annulare

Erythema annulare manifests as an erythematous annular lesion with a raised, non-indurated border and a clear center. The lesion enlarges centrifugally and there may be a fine collarette of scale left behind as the lesions progress. There can be single or multiple lesions on the trunk, buttocks, and thighs, but the hands and feet are usually spared. The etiology is unknown, but is thought to be a hypersensitivity reaction to an underlying condition such as dermatophyte, bacterial or viral infection, malignancy, or immunologic disorder. The lesions may be slightly pruritic but are often asymptomatic. The process is self-limiting but can last weeks to months with successive crops of lesions developing. Symptomatic treatment with antihistamines and a low-potency corticosteroid is variably effective.

Bibliography

Kumar P, Savant SS. Erythema annulare centrifugum. *Indian Pediatr.* 2015;**52**(4):356–357.

Erythema Multiforme

Erythema multiforme (EM) is a hypersensitivity reaction, most often to an infectious agent. In children, 50% of cases are associated with HSV type 1, but other viral infections (EBV, hepatitis, adenovirus), bacterial infections (tuberculosis, *Staph*, group A *Strep*, *Gonococcus*, *Mycoplasma*), and fungi (coccidiomycosis, histoplasmosis) are also implicated. EM is no longer divided into minor or major. If there is any mucous membrane involvement, the patient has SJS (see pp. 115–119).

Clinical Presentation

Erythema multiforme occurs in all age groups, although it is uncommon in children <3 years of age. A short prodromal phase, with symptoms of cough, coryza, sore throat, and myalgias can precede the eruption by 1–10 days. The classic lesions are dusky red, flat, round macules and target-shaped wheals, with a vesicle or bullae in the center, and occasionally with petechiae within the margins. The eruption can occur anywhere, but typically is on the palms and soles, dorsal surfaces of the hands and feet, and extensor surfaces of the arms and legs, while the mucus membranes are spared. The eruption is fixed for one week, then resolves over 2–3 weeks, but recurrences may occur. In contrast to urticaria, the rash is symmetric and fixed. Lesions appear in successive crops over 10–15 days, after which slow resolution occurs.

Diagnosis

When the characteristic target lesions are present, there is little difficulty in making the diagnosis. However, EM is most often confused with urticaria (pp. 43–45), in which the plaques are pruritic and individual lesions last less than 24 hours. A patient with SJS/TEN has the typical EM rash associated with oral mucous membrane involvement.

ED Management

If an etiology is not apparent (herpes, hepatitis, pharyngitis, etc.), but the patient appears well, a viral infection is the probable cause and work-up can be deferred. If the patient appears ill, obtain a heterophile antibody, cold agglutinins, and hepatitis surface antigen (HBsAg), and place a PPD. Also obtain a throat culture if there is a pharyngitis, and a chest x-ray if there are lower respiratory tract symptoms.

Appropriately treat any underlying illness (erythromycin for *Mycoplasma*, etc.). In mild cases, all that is needed is acetaminophen (15 mg/kg q 4h) and wet compresses (normal saline or 5% Burrow's solution) tid for localized bullae.

Follow-up

- Ill-appearing patient with EM: 2–3 days to check PPD and laboratory results

Indications for Admission

- Inability to take liquids adequately

Bibliography

DermNet New Zealand. Erythema multiforme. www.dermnetnz.org/topics/erythema-multiforme (accessed June 26, 2017).

Dinulos JG. What's new with common, uncommon and rare rashes in childhood. *Curr Opin Pediatr.* 2015;27(2):261–266.

Ferrandiz-Pulido C, Garcia-Patos V. A review of causes of Stevens–Johnson syndrome and toxic epidermal necrolysis in children. *Arch Dis Child.* 2013;98(12):998–1003.

Mathur AN, Mathes EF. Urticaria mimickers in children. *Dermatol Ther.* 2013;26(6):467–475.

Mockenhaupt M. Stevens–Johnson syndrome and toxic epidermal necrolysis: clinical patterns, diagnostic considerations, etiology, and therapeutic management. *Semin Cutan Med Surg.* 2014;33 (1):10–16.

Erythema Nodosum

Erythema nodosum (EN) is a hypersensitivity reaction that occurs most commonly in patients with respiratory infections, particularly group A streptococcal pharyngitis and primary tuberculosis. Other associations include fungal infections (coccidioidomycosis, histoplasmosis, dermatophytosis), Lyme disease, infectious mononucleosis, cat scratch disease, *Mycoplasma pneumoniae*, and drug reactions (bromides, sulfonamides, oral contraceptives). Erythema nodosum is more common in females, patients >10 years of age, and in the spring and fall.

Clinical Presentation

Erythema nodosum presents with multiple, 1–5 cm, oval, red, progressing to purple-colored, slightly elevated painful nodules symmetrically distributed over the pretibial area. Nodules can be warm and extremely tender and frequently are accompanied by arthralgias. Strep-induced erythema nodosum typically appears within three weeks of the infection. The eruption then usually disappears without scarring within six weeks. There may be recurrences over a period of weeks to months, but rarely thereafter.

Diagnosis

Usually the nodules are so characteristic that there is little difficulty in making the diagnosis.

Inquire about a history of upper respiratory infection, tick bites, trauma, recent travel, possible tuberculosis exposure, and medication use. Obtain a rapid strep test or a throat culture and place a 5 TU PPD. If tuberculosis, sarcoid, or a systemic fungal infection is suspected, also obtain a chest x-ray.

ED Management

The priority is treatment of the underlying disease or eliminating the offending drug. Bed rest, leg elevation, and ibuprofen (10 mg/kg q 6h) are helpful. Glucocorticoids are not necessary and antibiotics are indicated only in the setting of a streptococcal infection. Refer atypical, persistent, or recurrent cases to a dermatologist.

Follow-up

- Primary care in 2–3 days
- Rheumatology in 1–2 weeks if an underlying rheumatologic disease is suspected

Bibliography

Celebi S, Macimustafaoglu M, Berfu M, et al. Erythema nodosum in children. *J Pediatr Inf.* 2011; **5** (4):136–140.

DermNet New Zealand. Erythema nodosum. www.dermnetnz.org/topics/erythema-nodosum (accessed June 26, 2017).

Passarini B, Infusino SD. Erythema nodosum. *G Ital Dermatol Venereol.* 2013;**148**(4):413–417.

Starba A, Chowaniec M, Wiland P. Erythema nodosum: presentation of three cases. *Reumatologia.* 2016;**54**(2): 83–85.

Granuloma Annulare

Granuloma annulare (GA) is a relatively common cutaneous disorder of unknown etiology. Although GA may occur at any age, 40% of the cases appear in children <15 years of age.

Clinical Presentation

The classic lesion of GA is a nonscaling, erythematous to flesh-colored, annular plaque. Dome-shaped or slightly flattened papules, 3–6 mm in diameter may also be seen. These papules may be skin-colored, pink, or violaceous, and are typically arranged in the form of a ring. Ring size may vary from 1–10 cm in diameter and multiple rings are present in about 50% of patients. GA may occur on any part of the body, but it usually begins on the lateral or dorsal surfaces of the feet, hands, and fingers.

Diagnosis

Granuloma annulare must be distinguished from other annular eruptions, particularly tinea corporis, which is a scaling disease (GA has no scale). Erythema migrans (Lyme disease) can present as a single annular plaque with central clearing. To differentiate these, use low-power magnification (otoscope) to inspect the lesion. With GA there classically are individual papules that form the ring. In addition, on palpation the individual papules of GA can be appreciated, as opposed to the continuous ring of erythema migrans. See Table 5.7 for the differential diagnosis of annular lesions.

ED Management

The lesions of GA usually disappear spontaneously, often within several months to several years, with no residual scarring. If GA is severe or generalized, refer the patient to a dermatologist.

Follow-up

- 1–2 weeks

Bibliography

Keimig EL. Granuloma annulare. *Dermatol Clin.* 2015;**33**(3):315–329.

Patrizi A, Gurioli C, Neri I. Childhood granuloma annulare: a review. *G Ital Dermatol Venereol.* 2014;**149**(6):663–674.

Table 5.7 Differential diagnosis of annular lesions

Diagnosis	Morphology	Size	Location	Duration	Associated findings
Erythema migrans	Rapidly enlarging	>5 cm	Trunk	4–8 weeks	Fever, malaise, headache Arthralgia History of tick bite
	Round or oval plaques Annular or targetoid		Peripheral Extremities		
Erythema multiforme	Erythematous to violaceous	1–5 cm	Symmetrical	>7 days	Nonspecific viral URI Streptococcal pharyngitis Herpes infection Infectious mononucleosis
	Targetoid plaques		Acral Palms and soles		
Granuloma annulare	Pink to violaceous	1–5 cm	Distal extremities	Months to years	Asymptomatic
	Smooth papules and plaques				
Nummular eczema	Scaly plaques Excoriations	1–5 cm	Extremities	Weeks to months	Pruritus Follicular prominence
Tinea corporis	Scaly plaques Central clearing	Varies	Anywhere	Weeks to months	Cat or dog exposure
Urticaria	Erythematous and edematous Papules and plaques	Varies	Generalized	Usually <24 hours	Pruritus Angioneurotic edema

Adapted from Nopper A, Markus R, Esterly N. When it's not ringworm: annular lesions of childhood. *Pediatr Ann.* 1998;27:136–148.

Piette EW, Rosenbach M. Granuloma annulare: pathogenesis, disease associations and triggers, and therapeutic options. *J Am Acad Dermatol.* 2016;75(3):467–479.

Todd PS, Orlowski T, Schumacher-Kim W. A review of annular eruptions in children. *Pediatr Ann.* 2015;44(8):e199–204.

Herpes Simplex

Herpes simplex virus type 1 (HSV-1) is most commonly known as herpes labialis. It commonly affects the oral mucosa (cold sores). However, HSV-1 can cause disease in many other locations such as the genitalia, liver, lung, eye, and central nervous system.

Herpes simplex virus type 2 (HSV-2) classically involves the genitalia, although these infections can be caused by HSV-1 as well.

Clinical Presentation

The hallmark of herpes infection is a cluster of vesicles on an erythematous base.

The symptoms vary, based on whether the patient is experiencing a primary or non-primary infection.

Primary Infection

The onset of clinical illness is very sudden, with the appearance of multiple vesicular lesions superimposed on an erythematous base. Primary infection is often associated with systemic symptoms such as fever and malaise. The number and severity of lesions in a primary outbreak is usually greater than in recurrent infection. Lesions are usually painful and can last for up to 10–14 days.

Non-Primary Infection

This occurs when the virus, which has been dormant in sensory neurons, reactivates secondary to stress, ultraviolet light, local trauma, fever, or menstruation. These lesions are rarely associated with systemic symptoms, and they are fewer in number, less painful, and last a shorter duration than with primary herpes.

Neonatal Herpes

Neonatal disease occurs either as an ascending infection after premature rupture of the membranes or by direct spread to the neonate during passage through an infected birth canal. However, about 10% of neonatal herpes infections are acquired postnatally, likely from a close contact with active herpes labialis. Neonatal infection can be asymptomatic or present as a local infection or disseminated life-threatening disease. Generally, the infant becomes ill during the first 1–2 weeks of life when oral or cutaneous vesicles are noted, most commonly on the face or scalp. Fever, lethargy, and hepatosplenomegaly can occur, and with dissemination there may be ocular (keratoconjunctivitis), CNS (encephalitis), and pulmonary (pneumonia) involvement. Dissemination can also occur in the absence of cutaneous lesions. A similar spectrum of disease can occur in immunocompromised patients of any age.

Keratoconjunctivitis

Primary ocular disease presents as a purulent conjunctivitis with edema, vesicles, and corneal ulcers. In contrast to other etiologies of conjunctivitis, pain and photophobia are common because the cornea is involved. With recurrent disease, keratitis or corneal ulcers occur in association with a vesicular eruption of the conjunctiva, eyelids, periorbital skin, and tip of the nose.

Whitlow

Herpetic whitlow results from inoculation of the virus into the fingers, causing a painful, localized vesiculobullous eruption with swelling and erythema. It is usually found distally on the finger that the child habitually sucks. The course is 10–21 days and recurrences are common.

Eczema Herpeticum (Kaposi's Varicelliform Eruption)

This occurs in a patient with underlying atopic dermatitis. There are monomorphous (identical) ovoid, eroded, or vesicular lesions that may be associated with fever and toxicity. The lesions may be confused with a secondary bacterial infection.

Diagnosis

Always suspect herpes when there are grouped vesicles on an erythematous base. The presumptive diagnosis of a herpetic infection can be confirmed by performing a PCR from a scraping of the base of an open lesion. The diagnosis can be confirmed by culturing the virus from vesicle fluid; this requires at least 24–48 hours. In a neonate, have a high suspicion for disseminated herpes infection and obtain CSF for PCR detection.

ED Management

The mainstays of therapy for children with herpetic gingivostomatitis, labialis, and whitlow are analgesia (acetaminophen, ibuprofen), soaks (sitz baths, 5% Burrow's solution), and patience. Prescribe oral acyclovir (80 mg/kg/day div q 8h to a maximum of 1200 mg/24 hours) only when symptoms are severe. For a patient >12 years of age, start valacyclovir (2000 mg by mouth q 12h, for two doses) at the earliest signs of outbreak. Improvement is greatest if treatment is initiated within 48 hours of symptom onset. Use IV acyclovir (15 mg/kg/day div q 8h) if the patient cannot take oral medication. On occasion, an infant with severe oral disease can become dehydrated and require intravenous fluids. For a child with significant gingivostomatitis that interferes with adequate intake, swab the lesions with viscous lidocaine (2%). However, use it judiciously, as viscous lidocaine can cause seizures and has known cardiotoxic effects if large quantities are absorbed (when used as a rinse or for lesions in the posterior pharynx).

Genitalis

The management is summarized on p. 338. In general, treating primary or recurrent disease results in faster resolution of the pain and pruritus as well as decreased new lesion formation. Also, suppressive therapy can reduce the frequency of recurrences.

Eczema Herpeticum

Treat with PO or IV acyclovir, depending on the severity of the eruption and toxicity of the patient. Have a low threshold to start IV clindamycin (20–40 mg/kg/day div q 6h), as bacterial superinfection is common.

Keratoconjunctivitis

Refer any patient with suspected herpetic keratoconjunctivitis to an ophthalmologist for further evaluation and treatment (acyclovir ophthalmic ointment). *Never* prescribe ocular corticosteroids, which may facilitate spread of the infection.

Neonates and Immunocompromised Patients

Admit the patient and treat with IV acyclovir (60 mg/kg/day div q 8h) for 21 days. Attempt to culture the virus from mucocutaneous lesions, urine, saliva, and CSF.

Whitlow

Herpetic whitlow is a self-limiting condition. Use a dry dressing to cover the digit to prevent transmission and treat symptomatically (rest, elevation, anti-inflammatory agents). Acyclovir is indicated only for immunocompromised patients or those with severe infections.

Follow-up

- Gingivostomatitis and labialis: 1–2 days if no improvement
- Keratoconjunctivitis: as per the ophthalmologist
- Whitlow: primary care follow-up in 1–2 weeks

Indications for Admission

- Herpetic infection in a neonate or immunocompromised patient
- Poor oral intake and dehydration in an infant with gingivostomatitis
- Eczema herpeticum

Bibliography

Alter SJ, Bennett JS, Koranyi K, Kreppel A, Simon R. Common childhood viral infections. *Curr Probl Pediatr Adolesc Health Care*. 2015;**45**(2):21–53.

James SH, Kimberlin DW. Neonatal herpes simplex infection. *Infect Dis Clin North Am*. 2015;**19**(6):640–644

Ruderfer D, Krilov L. Herpes simplex viruses 1 and 2. *Pediatr Rev*. 2015;**36**(2):86–90.

Sanders JE, Garcia SE. Pediatric herpes simplex virus infections: an evidence-based approach to treatment. *Pediatr Emerg Med Pract*. 2014;**11**(1):1–19.

Whitley RJ. Herpes simplex virus infections of the central nervous system. *Continuum (Minneap Minn)*. 2015;**21**(6):1704–1713.

Hypopigmented Lesions

White or light patches of skin (depigmented or hypopigmented), are caused by either a decrease in the number of melanocytes or a decrease in the amount of melanin within the keratocytes. Table 5.8 describes the various presentations of disorders of hypopigmentation.

Table 5.8 Differential diagnosis of hypopigmented lesions

Diagnosis	Morphology	Distribution	Differentiating features
Pityriasis alba	Small, sharply demarcated	Cheeks	Pre-adolescents
	Minimal scale	Upper trunk	Worse in summer
	Accentuated in dark skin	Upper extremities	History of atopy
			Woods lamp and KOH (–)
Tinea versicolor	Well-demarcated	Upper trunk	Worse in summer
(pityriasis versicolor)	Oval macules and patches	Back, neck	Woods lamp (+): yellow-green
	Powdery scale	Upper arms	KOH (+): "spaghetti and meatballs"
Tuberous sclerosis	"Ash leaf" spots	Trunk	Other stigmata:
	Well-demarcated patches		Adenoma sebaceum
			Shagreen patches
			Periungual fibromas
			Woods lamp and KOH (–)
Vitiligo	Oval or irregular	Anywhere	Positive family history
	Macules or patches	Axillae	Other autoimmune disorders
	Coalesce →larger patches	Genitalia	Woods lamp and KOH (–)
		Periorbital	Ivory white, hyperpigmented border
		Acral	Can be segmental

ED Management

Pityriasis Alba

There is no effective treatment, although most children outgrow the disease by early to mid-adolescence. Occasionally, therapy with a very mild topical steroid (1% hydro-cortisone cream, bid) and moisturizers may diminish the demarcation between normal and whiter skin. Stress to the family that sun protection is imperative because the affected areas cannot tan normally and may be more susceptible to sunburn, while tanning of the surrounding skin accentuates the difference between the normal and hypopigmented skin.

Tinea Versicolor

The treatment is discussed on p. 140.

Tuberous Sclerosis

There is no treatment. Rather, refer the patient to a primary care provider to investigate for other stigmata of the disease.

Vitiligo

The single most important piece of advice is for the patient to use appropriate sun protection, as areas of vitiligo are unable to tan normally and therefore are not protected from the sun.

Follow-up

- Primary care follow-up in 2–4 weeks

Bibliography

Gupta AK, Lyons DC. Pityriasis versicolor: an update on pharmacological treatment options. *Expert Opin Pharmacother.* 2014;**15**(12):1707–1713.

Iannella G, Greco A, Didona D, et al. Vitiligo: pathogenesis, clinical variants and treatment approaches. *Autoimmun Rev.* 2016;**15**(4):335–343.

Lio PA. Little white spots: an approach to hypopigmented macules. *Arch Dis Child Educ Pract Ed.* 2008;**93**:98–102.

Miazek N, Michalek I, Pawlowska-Kisiel M, Olszewska M, Rudnicka L. Pityriasis Alba: common disease, enigmatic entity – up-to-date review of the literature. *Pediatr Dermatol.* 2015;**32**(6):786–791.

Phiske MM. Vitiligo in children: a birds eye view. *Curr Pediatr Rev.* 2016;**12**(1):55–66.

Infestations: Lice

Three varieties of lice, the head louse, the body louse, and the pubic louse, parasitize humans. The head louse is transmitted by direct personal contact, by contact with infected upholstery, and by sharing hats, combs, brushes, and towels. Body and pubic lice are acquired via bedding, clothing, and person-to-person (sexual) contact. The body louse can carry rickettsial disease (typhus and trench fever) and spirochetal disease (relapsing fever).

Clinical Presentation

Pediculosis Capitis (Head Lice)

The patient usually presents with pruritus of the scalp, ears, and back of the neck at the hairline. They may also exhibit an eczematous eruption on the scalp and neck. Nits (eggs) are oval and yellow-white, measuring 0.3–0.8 mm in size. They are found close to the scalp, firmly cemented to the hair around the ears and the occiput. They project from the side of the hair shaft and do not surround it. Nits more than 1.25 cm (0.5 in) from the scalp are probably no longer viable. Adult lice are usually not seen. Secondary impetigo, folliculitis, or furunculosis is common and may mask the primary disease.

Pediculosis Corporis (Body Lice)

These lice live in the lining and seams of clothing and occasionally emerge to bite the host. Erythematous macules become intensely pruritic papules and urticarial wheals, with secondary eczematization and impetiginization.

Pediculosis Pubis (Pubic Lice; "Crabs")

Itching is frequently the initial symptom, but secondary infection is common. Pubic and axillary hair and the eyelashes can be affected. The organisms can be identified as brownish crawling "flecks" and nits may be seen attached to the hair shafts. Lice bites can cause nonblanching gray–blue macules (maculae cerulae) on the lower abdomen and thighs.

Diagnosis

The diagnosis of lice infestation is based on the history of possible contact, itching, and visualization of the lice or nits. Nits fluoresce under Wood's lamp examination, and microscopic identification of a nit confirms the diagnosis. Body and pubic lice infestation may resemble eczema or folliculitis. Body lice can also simulate scabies.

ED Management

Treat pruritus associated with any infestation with hydroxyzine (2 mg/kg/day div qid) or diphenhydramine (5 mg/kg/day div qid).

Pediculosis Capitis

Treat with either a permethrin or pyrethrin-based shampoo. Instruct the parents to apply a single ten-minute application of a permethrin (Nix), after first shampooing and towel-drying the scalp. An equally effective alternative is two ten-minute applications of a pyrethrin-based product (A200, Rid), one week apart. Treat all contacts at the same time. Recommend that the parents use a fine-toothed comb to remove nits. Instruct the family to wash the clothing and bedding in very hot water (>52 °C [125 °F]) for ten minutes followed by high-heat drying, and to place all hats, combs, and headgear in a plastic bag until after the second shampoo.

As a result of increasing resistance in many urban areas, a variety of other topical agents are now being used. Malathion is the most effective of these, but it is flammable and malodorous. Elimite (5% permethrin) applied overnight is also effective.

Pubic Lice

Apply a pyrethrin-based product for ten minutes, and then repeat in one week. Advise the patient to have all sexual contacts treated.

Body Lice

Frequent bathing and laundering (>52 °C [125 °F] for at least ten minutes) of clothing and bedding followed by high-heat drying are all that is usually necessary. If lice are noted, treat with a pyrethrin: apply to the entire body from the jawline down, leave on overnight, and then wash off in the morning.

Eyelash Lice

Treat with petrolatum, applied bid for eight days. Mechanically remove any nits.

Follow-up
- Primary care follow-up in 1–2 weeks

Bibliography

Devore CD, Schutze GE. Head lice. *Pediatrics*. 2015;**135**(5):e1355–1365

Feldmeier H. Treatment of pediculosis capitis: a critical appraisal of the current literature. *Am J Clin Dermatol*. 2014;**15**(5):401–412.

Gunning K, Pippitt K, Kiraly B, Sayler M. Pediculosis and scabies: treatment update. *Am Fam Physician*. 2012;**86**(6):535–541.

Yetman RJ. The child with pediculosis capitis. *J Pediatr Health Care*. 2015;**29**(1):118–120.

Infestations: Scabies

Scabies is caused by *S. scabiei* and is a common infestation, with the highest prevalence in children <2 years old. It is acquired by close personal contact, although spread via fomites (clothing, linen, and towels) is possible, as the mite can survive for 2–5 days away from humans. Pruritus begins about three weeks after the primary infestation, or sooner if the individual has been previously sensitized. Nocturnal pruritus and subsequent sleep disturbance is a common cause of late-night ED visits.

Clinical Presentation

The usual complaint is generalized pruritus, especially interfering with sleep at night. The most common sites of involvement are the interdigital webs, flexor aspects of the wrists, extensor surfaces of the elbows, and nipples, axillae, perineum, and abdomen. The head, neck, palms, and soles can be infected in infants and young children. Papules, pustules, vesicles, and burrows (elevated, white serpiginous tracts), excoriations, and eczematization may be seen. Other family members may complain of itching and there may be a history of contact with an infected person.

Diagnosis

Scabies is a "great imitator" of other pruritic eruptions. The diagnosis is suggested by a history of contact with an infected person, the intense pruritus, and the variable nature of the lesions. Atopic dermatitis most commonly occurs on the flexor surfaces, while involvement of the interdigital webs is uncommon.

ED Management

Start treatment if the clinical suspicion is high. Prescribe permethrin 5% (Elimite cream), which is the drug of choice for scabies in patients >2 months of age. Instruct the parent to massage the cream into the skin from head to toe, and leave it on for 8–14 hours (preferably at night before bed). Treat the scalp of infants. Treat all close contacts, including babysitters, simultaneously. Advise the family to launder bedclothes and linens (hot water wash and high-heat dry), or store them away for at least one week. Repeat the treatment 7–10 days later. Treat the pruritus with hydroxyzine (2 mg/kg/day div tid) or diphenhydramine (5 mg/kg/day div qid).

Bibliography

Banerji A. Scabies. *Pediatr Child Health*. 2015;20(7):395–402.

Boralevi F, Diallo A, Miquel J, et al. Clinical phenotype of scabies by age. *Pediatrics*. 2014;133(4): e910–916.

Gunning K, Pippitt K, Kiraly B, Sayler M. Pediculosis and scabies: treatment update. *Am Fam Physician*. 2012;86(6):535–541.

Rezaee E, Goldust M, Alipour H. Treatment of scabies: comparison of lindane 1% vs permethrin 5. *Skinmed*. 2015;13(4):283–286.

Rosamilia LL. Scabies. *Semin Cutan Med Surg*. 2014;33(3):106–109.

Neonatal Rashes

Compared to a child or adult, the skin of a newborn is thinner, does not sweat as much, and has less hair and fewer melanocytes. As a result, newborn skin appears dry and scaly, and is more likely to develop blisters or erosions in response to minor traumas. In addition, infants have an increased body surface area, which places them at increased risk for the absorption of, and potential toxicities from, any topically applied agent. Fortunately, most neonatal eruptions are transient and harmless

Clinical Presentation and Diagnosis

Cutis Marmorata

Cutis marmorata is a reticulated, bluish-red mottling or vascular network that is seen when the infant is exposed to cold or in distress, and then improves when warm. This is a normal physiologic condition that requires no treatment. Extreme, persistent, and/or deeply violaceous forms may be associated with Down's syndrome, Cornelia de Lange syndrome, Trisomy 18, or cutis marmorata telangiectatica congenita.

Erythema Toxicum Neonatorum

Erythema toxicum is a self-limited erythematous eruption that is very common in full-term newborns within the first week of life. It is characterized by a combination of small (<3 mm) papules and pustules on an erythematous base. The lesions can be anywhere on the body, except the palms and soles. Despite the appearance, the infant is asymptomatic and well-appearing. If confirmation is necessary, unroof a pustule and obtain a Gram or Wright stain of the contents. Eosinophils are characteristic of erythema toxicum, in contrast to the neutrophils, seen with a bacterial infection

Milia

Milia are tiny (<2 mm), white pearly micropapules seen on the cheeks, nose, chin, and forehead of about 50% of newborns. They are asymptomatic and typically disappear, without treatment, within the first few months of life.

Miliaria

Miliaria rubra (heat rash or prickly heat) is an erythematous pinpoint papular eruption that appears on occluded areas, such as the back, that are subject to overheating and bundling. Miliaria crystallina (sudamina) is a more superficial form of miliaria and is characterized by pinpoint, clear, thin-walled vesicles on otherwise normal skin (no erythema). The rash is asymptomatic and occurs primarily in the intertriginous areas. Sunburn can cause this type of miliaria.

Mongolian Spots (Dermal Melanocytosis of Infancy)

Mongolian spots are poorly circumscribed, dark brown to blue/black patches that are usually found over the lumbosacral area and buttocks, and occasionally on the dorsal surface of the hands or the ankles. They are very common in newborns, occurring in more than 90% of African-Americans and Native Americans, 80% of Asians, and 70% of Hispanics. Mongolian spots are present at birth and most fade over the first few years of life, while others persist into adulthood. They may be single or multiple, and can vary greatly in size. Although they can be confused with bruises, Mongolian spots do not undergo the color changes seen with bruising or a coagulopathy. Extensive, persistent Mongolian spots have been reported in association with lysosomal storage diseases, such as GM1 gangliosidosis and Hurler syndrome.

Neonatal Acne

Neonatal acne is thought to be secondary to maternal and infantile androgens stimulating sebaceous glands. It presents in the first few weeks of life with erythematous papules and pustules and comedones, almost exclusively on the face. The course is usually self-limited over the first three months of life and washing with mild soap and water is all that is required. A more extensive evaluation is necessary if there are other signs of hyperandrogenism (pubic or axillary hair).

Neonatal Herpes

Herpes occurs by either an ascending infection after premature rupture of the membranes or direct spread to the neonate during passage through an infected birth canal. Neonatal infection can be asymptomatic or present as a local infection or disseminated life-threatening disease. Generally, the infant becomes ill during the first week of life when oral or cutaneous vesicles are noted, most commonly on the face or scalp. Fever, lethargy, and hepatosplenomegaly can occur, and with dissemination there may be ocular (keratoconjunctivitis), CNS (encephalitis), and pulmonary (pneumonia) involvement. Postnatal acquisition in the neonatal period has a high risk for dissemination, which can occur in the absence of cutaneous lesions.

Seborrhea

Seborrheic dermatitis (cradle cap) presents at 2–10 weeks of life with erythematous to salmon-colored plaques with yellowish scaling on the scalp, face (eyebrows and postauricular areas) neck, axilla, and diaper region. The disease usually starts at the scalp and may spread downward. In the diaper area, the eruption has a similar appearance to candidiasis, with involvement of intertriginous areas.

Transient Neonatal Pustular Melanosis

Transient pustular melanosis is a self-limited neonatal eruption of unknown etiology. In contrast to erythema toxicum, it is present at birth, occurring more commonly in African-American infants. It is characterized by clusters of vesicles and papulopustules, found primarily on the chin, forehead, back, and lower legs. The lesions easily rupture within 24–48 hours, leaving a collarette of scale with resultant hyperpigmentation, which fades over subsequent months. As with erythema toxicum, the contents are sterile, but neutrophils are seen on Gram or Wright stain.

ED Management

Reassurance is all that is needed for erythema toxicum, milia, Mongolian spots, neonatal acne, and transient neonatal pustular melanosis.

Miliaria

Management consists of cool baths, gentle cleansers and avoidance of occlusive skin barriers and overheating.

Seborrhea

Seborrhea may resolve spontaneously within 3–4 weeks, although treating the infant's scalp usually clears the remainder of the eruption. Remove adherent scale by gently massaging with mineral oil and scrubbing. Shampoo with ketoconazole 1% shampoo (not tear-free, must rinse well) 1–2 times per week, alternating with gentle tear-free shampoo. Treat severe facial eruptions with a 3–5-day course of 1% hydrocortisone cream bid. Use a topical antifungal cream (ketoconazole 2% cream bid for two weeks) in the intertriginous areas.

Neonatal Herpes

Since neonatal herpes can resemble any of the transplacental TORCH infections or bacterial sepsis, especially when there are no cutaneous lesions, perform a complete sepsis work-up including lumbar puncture (with HSV PCR on the CSF), blood HSV PCR, surface HSV culture and TORCH titers. Do not dismiss the possibility of neonatal herpes if the mother denies ever having herpes or having active disease at the time of delivery. Start intravenous (IV) acyclovir (two weeks to three months of age: 20 mg/kg/dose q 8h: infants under two weeks of age: q 12h) if diagnosis of neonatal HSV is suspected (pp. 124–126).

Follow-up

- Primary care follow-up in 1–2 weeks

Indications for Admission

- Neonatal herpes

Bibliography

American Academy of Pediatrics. Herpes Simplex. In Kimberlin DW, Brady MT, Jackson MA, Long SA (eds.) *Red Book: 2015 Report of the Committee on Infections Diseases* (30th edn). Elk Grove Village, IL: American Academy of Pediatrics, 2015: 432.

Clark GW, Pope SM, Jaboori KA. Diagnosis and treatment of seborrheic dermatitis. *Am Fam Physician.* 2015;**91**(3):185–190.

Newborn Nursery at Lucile Packard Children's Hospital. Skin. https://med.stanford.edu/newborns/professional-education/photo-gallery/skin.html (accessed June 26, 2017).

Tüzün Y, Wolf R, Bağlam S, Engin B. Diaper (napkin) dermatitis: a fold (intertriginous) dermatosis. *Clin Dermatol.* 2015;**33**(4):477–482.

Palpable Purpura

Vascular reactions are categorized as blanching (nonpurpuric) and nonblanching (purpuric). Palpable purpura are nonblanching, slightly elevated lesions.

The distinction between palpable and nonpalpable purpura is of critical importance, as nonpalpable purpura often represents bruises or ecchymoses, caused by trauma or a clotting abnormality. However, severe fulminant infectious disorders, such as meningococcemia, can present with purpuric lesions that may not be palpable. In contrast, palpable purpura almost always signifies some type of vasculitis, secondary to a serious disease. Possible etiologies include meningococcemia with coagulopathy, SBE, SLE, Rocky Mountain spotted fever, HSP, and drug reactions.

Clinical Presentation

Palpable purpura presents as elevated, nonblanching, erythematous to violaceous plaques and nodules. Dependent areas, such as the legs, feet, and buttocks, are the most common sites.

Henoch–Schönlein purpura (HSP) is the most common vasculitis of childhood and classically presents with nonthrombocytopenic purpura, along with some combination of abdominal pain, arthritis, and glomerulonephritis. Purpuric lesions are most concentrated on the buttocks and extensor surfaces of the lower extremities. The majority of cases of HSP are preceded by a URI and there are reports of familial HSP.

Diagnosis

Rapidly obtain a complete history, including medication use, previous illnesses, travel, tick bite, and whether there has been fever, other rashes, headache, or arthralgias. Maintain a high suspicion for sepsis (high fever, lethargy, or toxicity in association with petechiae and palpable purpura), especially meningococcemia.

In general, the purpura is not palpable in cases of physical abuse. Also, the history, distribution of the lesions (face, back, arms), and different types of injuries (burns, linear marks, fractures) suggest the diagnosis.

See the appropriate sections for the evaluation of patients with possible SLE (pp. 709–711), SBE (pp. 74–75), and Rocky Mountain spotted fever (pp. 433–435).

ED Management

The priority in evaluating a nonblanching vascular process is to expeditiously rule-out or treat sepsis or other serious vasculitic disorders. Evaluate any child with purpuric lesions in an extensive distribution or of a long-standing nature for an underlying infection, auto-immune disorder, or child abuse.

If the patient is febrile or appears toxic, treat palpable purpura as *bacterial sepsis* until proven otherwise. Immediately obtain a CBC, blood culture, and urine cultures, and begin treatment with broad-spectrum antibiotics. If meningitis cannot be ruled out clinically, also perform a lumbar puncture.

If HSP is suspected, assess renal function by measuring the blood pressure and obtaining a basic serum chemistry and urinalysis. Treat a drug eruption (pp. 115–119) by discontinuing the offending agent. If there is any suspicion for child abuse, contact the child protection team and social services, and document diligently (pp. 597–603).

Indications for Admission

- Possible sepsis
- Acute abdomen or renal compromise
- Suspected child abuse
- Severe arthralgia affecting ambulation

Bibliography

Kummerle-Deschner JB, Thomas J, Benseler SM. Childhood vasculitis. *Rheumatol.* 2015;**74** (10):863–866.

Mayo Clinic. Henoch-Schönlein purpura. www.mayoclinic.org/diseases-conditions/henoch-schonlein-purpura/home/ovc-20209932 (accessed June 26, 2017).

Park SJ, Suh JS, Lee JH, et al. Advances in our understanding of the pathogenesis of Henoch–Schönlein purpura and the implications for improving its diagnosis. *Expert Rev Clin Immunol.* 2013;**9** (12):1233–1238

Reid-Adam, J. Henoch–Schönlein purpura. *Pediatr Rev.* 2014;35(10):447–449

Yang YH, Yu HH, Chiang BL. The diagnosis and classification of Henoch-Schönlein purpura: an updated review. *Autoimmun Rev.* 2014;**13**(4–5):355–358.

Pityriasis Rosea

Pityriasis rosea is an acute, benign, self-limited eruption of unknown etiology. It is presumed to be viral in origin because of the frequent prodromal symptoms, seasonal clustering, and lifelong immunity that develops in 98% of patients. However, person-to-person transmission has not been confirmed.

Clinical Presentation

Pityriasis rosea occurs predominantly in adolescents and young adults, and less commonly in children <5 years of age. After a variable prodrome of malaise, about 75% of cases present with an initial lesion called a herald patch. This is a 2–5 cm scaling erythematous plaque with a "collarette of scale" (the scaling forms a circle within the borders of the plaque), seen most commonly on the chest, neck, or back. The generalized eruption that follows 2–21 days later characteristically consists of small, ovoid papules also with a collarette of scale. The long axes of these lesions follow the cleavage lines on the back and trunk in a so-called Christmas tree pattern. This can be more easily appreciated by having the patient twist his or her spine at the waist and by examining the axillae. Lesions continue to occur for up to two weeks, with clearing in 6–10 weeks. Postinflammatory hypo- or hyperpigmentation can result.

Diagnosis

The history of the herald patch and the characteristic nature of the lesions of the generalized eruption usually suffice to confirm the diagnosis of pityriasis rosea. However, the herald patch may resemble a tinea corporis infection, although these grow slowly and are not followed by a generalized eruption. The lesions of erythema migrans are not scaly, expand more rapidly, and grow to larger dimensions than a herald patch. See Table 5.7 for the differential diagnosis of annular lesions.

The eruption of secondary syphilis can look very similar, but may involve the palms and soles. Obtain a VDRL if the patient is sexually active.

ED Management

For most patients no treatment is necessary. Topical antipruritics or oral antihistamines (hydroxyzine 2 mg/kg/day div tid; diphenhydramine 5 mg/kg/day div qid) alleviate the pruritus. Topical corticosteroids may be useful in very inflammatory cases, but they do not shorten the course of the disease.

Follow-up

- Primary care follow-up in 2–4 weeks
- Dermatologist if lesions persisting for longer than 12 weeks

Bibliography

American Academy of Dermatology. Pityriasis rosea. www.aad.org/public/diseases/rashes/pityriasis-rosea (accessed June 26, 2017).

Drago F, Ciccarese G, Broccolo F, et al. Pityriasis rosea in children: clinical features and laboratory investigations. *Dermatology*. 2015;**231**(1):9–14.

Drago F, Ciccarese G Rebora A, Broccolo F, Parodi A. Pityriasis rosea: a comprehensive classification. *Dermatology*. 2016;**232**(4):431–437.

Eisman S, Sinclair R. Pityriasis rosea. *BMJ*. 2015;**351**:h5233.

Psoriasis

Psoriasis is an inherited disorder of unknown etiology. About 25% of patients develop the disease before age 15, 10% before age 10, and 6.5% before age 5. Patients with active lesions present at birth (congenital psoriasis) have also been reported.

Clinical Presentation

Psoriasis is characterized by well-demarcated red plaques which are often covered with copious amounts of white or silver (micaceous) scales. New lesions present as small, 1–3 mm papules that subsequently enlarge and coalesce with adjacent lesions to form large plaques. Partial coalescence can result in gyrate or serpiginous plaques. Linear psoriatic plaques induced by local cutaneous trauma lesions may also occur, reflecting the Koebner phenomenon. The most common sites for psoriasis are the elbows, scalp, knees, genitalia, lumbosacral region, and extensor surfaces of the arms and legs. In infants, psoriasis may also present in the diaper area. Nail changes are also often present, including nail plate pitting, onycholysis, and yellowish discoloration of the nail plate ("oil drop").

Guttate psoriasis presents with a sudden outbreak of hundreds of small, red, drop-like (guttate), nonconfluent papules. The lesions are generally symmetrical and are distributed on the trunk and proximal aspects of the extremities. Guttate psoriasis is often triggered by group A streptococcal infection.

Diagnosis

Classic lesions of psoriasis are not difficult to diagnose, especially when there is a positive family history. The only other similar common disease which exhibits the Koebner phenomenon is lichen planus, in which the papules are usually pruritic and limited to a few areas of the body, including the flexor surfaces and oral mucosa. Pityriasis rosea can be differentiated on the basis of the herald patch and the "Christmas tree" distribution on the torso. If the diagnosis remains in doubt, consult a dermatologist who can perform a skin biopsy.

ED Management

If the psoriasis is mild and limited to only a few sites, therapy may be initiated in the ED. Recommend mild soaps or cleansers (Dove or Cetaphil), moisturizers, and mild- to moderate-potency topical steroids. Treat scalp psoriasis with thick adherent plaques with P&S liquid or Derma-Smoothe oil, applied overnight, followed 6–8 hours later by an anti-seborrheic tar or steroid shampoo. It is important to explain to the patient that psoriasis is a chronic condition that is treated but not cured and that there are often alternating periods of exacerbation and remission. Refer patients with psoriasis to a dermatologist.

Follow-up

- Dermatology follow-up in 2–4 weeks

Bibliography

Bronckers IM, Paller AS, van Geel MJ, van de Kerkhof PC, Seyger MM. Psoriasis in children and adolescents: diagnosis, management and comorbidities. *Paediatr Drugs.* 2015;**17**(5):373–384.

Fotiadou C, Lazaridou E, Ioannides D. Management of psoriasis in adolescence. *Adolesc Health Med Ther.* 2014;**5**:25–34.

Mahe E. Childhood psoriasis. *Eur J Dermatol.* 2016;**26**(6):537–548.

Megna M, Napolitano M, Balato A, et al. Psoriasis in children: a review. *Curr Pediatr Rev.* 2015;**11**(1):10–26.

Michalek IM, Loring B, John SM. A systematic review of worldwide epidemiology of psoriasis. *J Eur Acad Dermatol Venereol.* 2017;**31**(2):205–212.

Tinea

Superficial dermatophytoses are called tinea. The name of any particular tinea infection is based on the clinical location and the species of infecting organism (e.g., *Trichophyton tonsurans* tinea capitis).

Clinical Presentation

Tinea Capitis

Tinea capitis is caused by infection of the hair shaft, causing patchy alopecia with scaling, erythema, and infected hairs that are broken off at scalp level (black dots). Suboccipital lymphadenopathy is often present. Patients may also present with a nonspecific, "seborrheic dermatitis-like" picture, with minimal diffuse hair loss and scale. An acute hypersensitivity reaction with a boggy, inflammatory mass (kerion) can develop.

Tinea Corporis

Tinea corporis, or ringworm, is a superficial infection of the skin. Infection occurs via contact with an infected individual, infected animal (kitten or puppy), and fomites. The lesions are well-circumscribed annular plaques, with central clearing, and a raised, scaly, papular, or vesicular border.

Tinea Cruris

Tinea cruris, or "jock itch," is an infection of the groin and upper thighs that is rare before puberty. More frequent in hot, humid environments and in obese or very athletic individuals, tinea cruris is exacerbated by tight-fitting and chafing clothing. Sharply demarcated, bilaterally symmetric, scaly, erythematous plaques that spare the scrotum and labia are typical.

Tinea Pedis

Tinea pedis, or "athlete's foot," is a pruritic eruption that is more common in postpubertal patients. Findings range from mild scaling to marked erythema, maceration, fissuring, and vesiculation involving the toes and interdigital webs. The infection may spread to the soles and sides of the feet, but the dorsal aspects of the toes are usually spared. An allergic response to the fungus (id reaction) occasionally causes an erythematous vesicular eruption on the trunk, upper extremities, and palms.

Tinea Unguium

Tinea unguium (onychomycosis) is a fungal infection of the nail plate that can be a primary infection or occur in association with dermatophytosis elsewhere (hands, feet). The infection usually begins at the distal/lateral edges of the nail, which become discolored, lusterless, and friable, with subungual hyperkeratosis and separation of the distal nail from the nail bed (onycholysis).

Tinea Versicolor

Tinea versicolor (pityriasis versicolor) is an infection of the upper trunk and back, proximal arms, and neck that is particularly common in warm climates. The causative organism is *Pityrosporum orbiculare*, a dimorphous yeast which is part of the normal skin flora. It presents as hypo- or hyperpigmented, well-demarcated, oval macules and patches with fine scale and little or no erythema or pruritus. It is diagnosed more commonly in the summertime, as the involved areas will not tan while the surrounding uninfected skin does.

Tinea Incognito

Tinea incognito is any tinea (corporis, cruris, pedis) infection that has been modified by treatment with topical corticosteroids. This temporarily decreases the inflammatory response to the cutaneous fungal infection while the infection slowly progresses. As a result, there is often less pruritus, decreased scaling, and the lesions tend to be more macular with increased erythema. The eruption may be extensive and sometimes pustular.

Diagnosis

Diagnosis is clinical based on lesion type and location. If the diagnosis is in doubt, culture the fungus (Sabouraud's agar or dermatophyte test medium [DTM]) or submit a sample for

KOH prep. A minority of tinea capitis and all tinea versicolor infections will fluoresce under Wood's lamp examination.

Tinea capitis is the only common etiology of childhood alopecia that causes scalp inflammation. The eruption may fluoresce under a Wood's lamp and black dots may be seen. The scalp is normal in alopecia areata, and trichotillomania, while seborrheic dermatitis causes scaling without hair loss. Bacterial infections of the scalp are uncommon and usually there is no hair loss, as with a kerion. Bacterial folliculitis of the scalp will show discrete perifollicular erythema and purulence.

Tinea corporis can resemble contact dermatitis, the herald patch of pityriasis rosea, erythema migrans, and nummular eczema. The characteristic central clearing and raised, well-demarcated scaly border usually suggest the diagnosis.

Tinea cruris can be confused with contact dermatitis, intertrigo, and erythrasma, a *Corynebacterium* infection that fluoresces coral-red under Wood's lamp examination. In addition, secondary candidal infection can occur and confuse the picture, but a broad-spectrum topical antifungal, such as miconazole, will treat both dermatophytes and *Candida*.

Before the diagnosis of tinea pedis is made in a prepubertal patient, consider dyshidrotic eczema, atopic dermatitis, and contact dermatitis, which can involve the dorsum of the foot. The id reaction is characterized by the absence of fungus in the area of the reaction, an identifiable focus of fungal infection (usually on the feet), and spontaneous clearing when the primary fungal infection is eradicated.

Tinea unguium must be confirmed with a positive culture of nail clippings, as psoriasis, eczema, trauma, and congenital ectodermal syndromes all have a similar appearance.

Tinea versicolor resembles pityriasis alba, postinflammatory hypopigmentation, and vitiligo, although none of these conditions fluoresce under Wood's lamp examination.

The diagnosis of tinea incognito is suggested by the history of steroid use, as well as the appearance of the lesions. To confirm, send skin scrapings for microscopy or culture.

ED Management

Tinea Capitis

Tinea capitis cannot be treated topically. Obtain a culture prior to treating the patient with oral griseofulvin (20–25 mg/kg/day microsize; 10–15 mg/kg/day ultramicrosize) for 6–8 weeks. Leukopenia, neutropenia, and hepatotoxicity are uncommon side effects. If therapy extends longer than eight weeks, obtain a CBC and LFTs. Oral terbinafine is also an option, but refer the patient to a dermatologist first. Use selenium (Selsun) or ketoconazole shampoo twice a week to decrease the period of infectivity. Inform the family that regrowth of hair may take several months. Inquire about other symptomatic contacts as they may serve as an infectious focus in the house.

Tinea Corporis, Tinea Cruris, Tinea Pedis

Treat with clotrimazole or miconazole, bid or tid, for four weeks. Refer a recalcitrant case to a dermatologist for oral terbinafine treatment. In addition, soak inflammatory lesions with normal saline or 5% Burrow's solution compresses. Keep affected areas dry; this is particularly important for tinea pedis and tinea cruris, where antifungal powders are helpful. Instruct the patient to wear cotton (instead of synthetic) underwear and socks to help dissipate moisture.

Tinea Unguium
Refer the patient to a dermatologist to determine if oral terbinafine is necessary.

Tinea Versicolor
Treat for two weeks with either 2.25% selenium sulfide shampoo or 2% ketoconazole shampoo, daily for one week, then once monthly. Advise the patient to apply the shampoo to the affected skin daily, for five minutes, prior to rinsing. Topical antifungals are also effective. Inform the patient that the normal skin pigment will not return until after the treated lesions are exposed to ultraviolet light.

Tinea Incognito
Discontinue the use of topical corticosteroids and treat the eruption with a topical antifungal such as econazole 1% cream (apply to affected area daily for 2–4 weeks). Topical terbinafine (1% cream) can be used in patients over 12 years of age (apply to affected area bid for 1–4 weeks). If topical treatment is not effective, refer the patient to a dermatologist for possible systemic antifungal therapy.

Follow-up
- Primary care follow-up in two weeks
- Tinea unguium: dermatologist within two weeks

Bibliography

Bell-Syer SE, Khan SM, Torgerson DJ. Oral treatments for fungal infections of the skin of the foot. *Cochrane Database Syst Rev.* 2012;**10**:CD003584.

DermNet New Zealand. Kerion. www.dermnetnz.org/topics/kerion (accessed June 26, 2017).

Hawkins DM, Smidt AC. Superficial fungal infections in children. *Pediatr Clin North Am.* 2014;**61** (2):443–455.

John AM, Schwartz RA, Janniger CK. The kerion: an angry tinea capitis. *Int J Dermatol.* 2016. DOI: 10.1111/ijd.13423

Paloni G, Valerio E, Berti I, Cutrone M. Tinea incognito. *J Pediatr.* 2015;**167**(6):e1450–1452.

Verrucae and Molluscum
Verrucae, or common warts, occur in about 10% of children and young adults. They are benign, self-limited, superficial intra-epidermal tumors caused by human papillomavirus and spread via autoinoculation, person-to-person, and fomite contact. Lesions are most common on the fingers, hands, elbows, and plantar surfaces. The incubation period is 1–6 months and two-thirds of all lesions spontaneously resolve within two years. A patient can have from one to several hundred warts.

Molluscum contagiosum is caused by a pox virus. It occurs most commonly at 3–15 years of age and spreads by direct person-to-person contact and autoinoculation.

Clinical Presentation

Common Warts

Common warts (verruca vulgaris) occur predominantly on the dorsal surfaces of the hands and the periungual regions. They usually begin as pinpoint, flesh-colored papules that grow larger (1–10 mm), with roughened surfaces, grayish color, and sharply demarcated borders. Often these lesions are studded with black dots (thrombosed capillaries).

Flat Warts

Flat warts (verruca plana) are tan to flesh-colored, soft, flat, small (2–6 mm) papules that occur primarily on the face, neck, arms, and hands. These are particularly common in shaved areas. Contiguous lesions can become confluent and plaque-like.

Plantar Warts

Plantar warts (verruca plantaris) usually occur in weight-bearing areas of the sole of the foot. They are flat, with sharp margins, and black dots are seen within the lesions. Pressure forces them into the tissues of the foot and this leads to marked tenderness when walking. They often coalesce into a single large plaque called a mosaic wart.

Venereal Warts

Venereal warts (condylomata acuminata) are soft, reddish pink, filiform lesions that may coalesce into larger, cauliflower-like clusters. They are located primarily on the genitalia and around the anus, and the rectal mucosa may also be involved. Condylomata acuminata are usually sexually transmitted, although they can spread from a caretaker diapering or by autoinoculation from warts elsewhere on the body. Sexual abuse is a concern when venereal warts are found on a young child. While the vast majority of anogenital warts found in children <2 years of age are the result of maternal perinatal transmission, the initial onset of lesions in older patients are of more concern for sexual abuse. In general, the older the prepubertal child is at first presentation of genital warts, the greater is the likelihood of sexual transmission.

Molluscum

The lesions start as small papules that typically grow to 3–6 mm in diameter, but they can be as large as 2–3 cm. They usually are flesh-colored or opalescent and dome-shaped, with a central umbilication. Papules are found on the face, trunk, extremities, and pubic region, either alone or in clusters, and number from one to several hundred. Most lesions resolve within 9–12 months; some may persist for 2–3 years. Chronic conjunctivitis or keratitis may occur with eyelid lesions. Particularly severe eruptions with thousands of lesions can occur in patients with atopic dermatitis or depressed cellular immunity.

Diagnosis

The diagnosis of common or flat warts can be confirmed by the absence of skin markings over the lesions and the presence of black dots (thrombosed dermal capillaries) beneath the surface. Gentle paring with a scalpel causes small bleeding points which represent intact capillaries.

Periungual warts can be confused with the periungual fibromas of tuberous sclerosis, but usually other cutaneous manifestations of tuberous sclerosis are present (adenoma sebaceum, ash leaf spots, Shagreen patches).

Plantar warts may resemble calluses, corns, and black heel (talon noir). Calluses do not have sharp, well-demarcated margins and no black dots are seen. Corns typically occur at the metatarsophalangeal joints. There are no black dots, but they have sharp margins and a characteristic translucent particle at the core. Skin markings over the lesion remain intact. Black heel occurs in athletes who make frequent sudden stops, causing blackish pinpoint hemorrhages. The margin is not well-demarcated, and paring does not reveal bleeding points.

Condylomata acuminata must be differentiated from the condylomata lata of secondary syphilis. The latter are 1–3 cm grayish pink nodules occurring in the same regions. Dark field microscopy or serology (VDRL and FTA) is necessary to confirm the diagnosis.

The diagnosis of molluscum is usually easily established by the distinctive appearance of the flesh-colored papules with central umbilication. To verify the diagnosis, opening a papule will reveal a small central core, which resembles a cluster of grapes when visualized under magnification.

ED Management

Since untreated warts often spontaneously resolve within several months to years, watchful waiting is often the best approach. If treatment is desired, recommend an over-the-counter liquid salicylic acid preparation with duct tape for occlusion. Apply nightly after bathing, and repeat the procedure after paring the wart or rubbing with a washcloth, emery board, or pumice stone.

Refer a patient with lesions on the face, multiple hand warts, periungual and subungual warts, large plantar warts, or venereal warts to a dermatologist for other available therapies, which include liquid nitrogen, cantharidin, electrodessication and curettage, and podophyllin. See pp. 608–611 for the evaluation and management of possible sexual abuse.

Reassure a patient with molluscum that the disorder is benign, and refer to their pediatrician or dermatologist for treatment if desired.

Follow-up

• Primary care or dermatology follow-up in 1–2 weeks

Bibliography

Brotherton JM. Human papillomavirus vaccination: where are we now? *J Paediatr Child Health.* 2014;**50**(12):959–965.

Butala N, Siegfried E, Weissler A. Molluscum BOTE sign: a predictor of imminent resolution. *Pediatrics.* 2013;**131**(5):e1650–1653.

Oranje AP, de Waard-van der Spek FB. Recent developments in the management of common childhood skin infections. *J Infect.* 2015;**71**(Suppl. 1):S76–79.

Paller AS, Mancini AJ: Viral diseases of the skin. In Hurwitz S, Paller A, Mancini A (eds.) *Hurwitz's Textbook of Clinical Pediatric Dermatology* (4th edn.). Philadelphia, PA: WB Saunders, 2011; 355–365.

Rush J, Dinulos JG. Childhood skin and soft tissue infections: new discoveries and guidelines regarding the management of bacterial soft tissue infections, molluscum contagiosum, and warts. *Curr Opin Pediatr.* 2016;**28**(2):250–257.

Ear, Nose, and Throat Emergencies

Daran Kaufman and Jeffrey Keller

Acute Otitis Media

Acute otitis media (AOM) is a suppurative infection of the middle ear caused by bacteria and viruses. It accounts for up to one-third of pediatric acute health care visits. The incidence is highest during the winter months, secondary to the greater frequency of viral upper respiratory infections (URIs). Children with normal immunity may have multiple episodes in a year. Risk factors for AOM include daycare attendance, second-hand smoke exposure, use of a pacifier, bottle feeding, and a family history of ear infections. Children with Down syndrome or craniofacial abnormalities are at increased risk of otitis media.

The most common bacterial etiology identified is *Streptococcus pneumoniae* (30–40%), which is now decreasing in frequency secondary to vaccination, followed by nontypable *Haemophilus influenzae* (20–30%), *Moraxella catarrhalis* (10–20%), and *Streptococcus pyogenes*. Gram-negative enteric organisms (*Escherichia coli*, *Klebsiella*, *Proteus*, *Pseudomonas*) and *Staphylococcus aureus* are responsible for about 15% of cases in the first few months of life, but are exceedingly rare afterward. Viruses, including parainfluenza, respiratory syncytial virus, influenza, adenovirus, and enterovirus are common pathogens (up to 50% of cases).

Clinical Presentation

Acute otitis media is usually preceded by a URI with cough and rhinorrhea. Additional symptoms begin 2–3 days later and may include fever, pain, dizziness, buzzing in the ear, or decreased hearing. In infants, there are nonspecific symptoms, such as irritability, increased crying, decreased feeding, sleep disturbance, vomiting, or diarrhea. In younger patients there may only be fever, a persistent URI, or behavioral changes (cranky, not feeding or sleeping well). Ear tugging is an unreliable sign of AOM. Occasionally, there is a history of severe ear pain that improved abruptly when a bloody or yellowish discharge began to drain from the external canal (tympanic membrane perforation). In summary, clinical history alone is an inaccurate predictor of AOM; therefore, examine the ears of a patient with any of the symptoms mentioned above, even if otoscopy in the previous 24–36 hours did not reveal an otitis media.

Diagnosis

The American Academy of Pediatrics and the American Academy of Family Physicians practice guidelines state that the diagnosis of AOM must meet the following three criteria: rapid onset, the presence of middle ear effusion (MEE), and signs and symptoms of middle ear inflammation.

Table 6.1 Differential diagnosis of otalgia

Diagnosis	Differentiating features
Acute myringitis	Inflammation of tympanic membrane
	Bullae possible
Dental abscess	Edema, erythema, or tenderness of gingiva
Otitis externa	Pain on traction of pinna, tenderness over tragus
Parotitis	Edema, tenderness over angle of mandible
	Inflammation of Stensen's duct
Pharyngitis	Erythema, exudate, or herpangina on oropharyngeal examination
Serous otitis media	Dark, retracted tympanic membrane
	Air-fluid level or bubbles behind tympanic membrane
TMJ disease	Pain with palpation of TMJ, especially with mouth opening/closing

Examine the tympanic membrane (TM) for shape (concave, retracted, bulging), color (pearly gray, injected, erythematous, yellow), the presence of landmarks (light reflex, malleus), and mobility. Redness alone is not sufficient to make the diagnosis, since crying can cause erythema of the drum. Perform pneumatic otoscopy, focusing on the light reflex. Decreased mobility of the tympanic membrane, which can be confirmed by tympanometry (flat tympanogram), is the most sensitive indicator of a middle ear effusion. A combination of erythema, bulging with or without a purulent effusion, loss of normal anatomic landmarks and decreased mobility are characteristic of an acute otitis media. Tympanic membrane perforation with recent onset of bloody or purulent ear discharge is also diagnostic. The history of a recent URI, complaints of ear pain, and constitutional symptoms such as listlessness and fever are insufficient to make the diagnosis without the typical otoscopic findings. See Table 6.1 for the differential diagnosis of otalgia.

The optimal position for examination varies with the age of the patient. Examine infants and young children supine on the table, restrained by an adult. Place an older child on the parent's lap, seated face-to-face with the examiner. One of the parent's arms can tightly embrace the child, while the other holds the patient's head.

In some cases, there may be impacted cerumen in the ear canal obstructing the view of the tympanic membrane. Remove cerumen by curetting or irrigating with warm water 20 minutes after instilling several drops of hydrogen peroxide (if no tympanic membrane perforation is suspected).

ED Management

Despite the presence of an otitis media, perform a thorough physical examination to be certain that the patient does not have a more serious infection, such as meningitis. If the patient is toxic-appearing, admit for aggressive inpatient parenteral management.

Table 6.2 Treatment guidelines for AOM by age[a]

Age	With otorrhea[a]	Uni/bilateral[a] with severe symptoms[b]	Bilateral without otorrhea[a]	Unilateral without otorrhea[a]
6 months – 2 years	Antibiotics	Antibiotics	Antibiotics	Antibiotics or additional observation[c]
≥2 years	Antibiotics	Antibiotics	Antibiotics or additional observation[c]	Antibiotics or additional observation[c]

[a] Applies only to patients with well-documented acute AOM.
[b] A toxic-appearing patient, otalgia for >48 hours, temperature >102 °F (38.9 °C) in the past 48 hours, or if follow-up is uncertain.
[c] If observation is offered a mechanism must be in place to ensure follow-up and begin antibiotics if the patient worsens or fails to improve within 48–72 hours.
Adapted from Lieberthal AS, Carroll AE, et al. The diagnosis and management of acute otitis media. *Pediatrics*. 2013 Mar;131(3):e964–999.

The American Academy of Pediatrics practice guideline recommends a 48–72 hour period of observation, without antimicrobial treatment, for selected patients in whom follow-up can be assured if symptoms worsen (Table 6.2). See Table 6.3 for antibiotic choices and doses.

Regardless of the treatment option, pain management is critical. Use analgesics such as acetaminophen (15 mg/kg q 4h) or ibuprofen (10 mg/kg q 6h). In the ED, instilling a single dose of one to two drops of 2% viscous lidocaine may ameliorate extreme discomfort. Do not recommend antihistamine–decongestant combinations, which are of no benefit. Instruct the parents to return in 2–3 days if the child remains symptomatic (fever, ear pain, decreased hearing). If AOM is confirmed on re-examination, initiate antibiotic treatment. Patients whose symptoms are worsening at any time or who have continued symptoms at the completion of treatment require re-examination.

Under Two Months of age

Treat an afebrile, well-appearing infant <2 months of age with amoxicillin. However, if there is fever (>38.1 °C; 100.6 °F), toxicity, irritability, evidence of a systemic infection, a complicated neonatal course, or a previous hospitalization with antibiotic treatment, perform an evaluation for sepsis, treat with IV antibiotics, and admit the patient (see Evaluation of the Febrile Child, pp. 390–394).

A sterile effusion occurs in more than 40% of children following an AOM. This usually resolves without intervention, although a temporary conductive hearing loss can persist until the effusion resolves.

Tympanocentesis with culture is indicated for systemic toxicity, severe unremitting pain, inadequate response to conventional therapy, or a suppurative complication (facial nerve paralysis, mastoiditis, meningitis, brain abscess), and may be necessary in some immunocompromised patients. Obtain an otolaryngology consult.

Table 6.3 Antibiotic doses for otitis media and sinusitis

Antibiotic	Dose	Notes
Amoxicillin	80–90 mg/kg/day div bid or tid	First choice if not penicillin-allergic
Amoxicillin-clavulanate ES[a]	90 mg/kg of amoxicillin div q 12h	Use for treatment failure after 3 days
Azithromycin: first day days 2–5 or or	10 mg/kg q day 5 mg/kg q day 12 mg/kg × 5 days 20 mg/kg/day × 3 days	Use for type 1 penicillin hypersensitivity[b]
Cefdinir	14 mg/kg/day div q day or bid	Use for non-type 1 penicillin hypersensitivity
Cefpodoxime	10 mg/kg/day div q day or bid	Use for non-type 1 penicillin hypersensitivity
Ceftriaxone IM	Unable to take PO: 50 mg/kg × 1 Treatment failure: 50 mg/kg/day × 3	
Cefuroxime	30 mg/kg/day div q 12h	Non-type 1 penicillin hypersensitivity
Clarithromycin	15 mg/kg/day div q 12h	Use for type 1 penicillin hypersensitivity[b]
Clindamycin	20 mg/kg/day div tid or qid	Use for type 1 penicillin hypersensitivity[b]
Erythromycin-sulfisoxazole	50 mg/kg/day of erythro div qid	Use for type 1 penicillin hypersensitivity[b]
Trimethoprim/sulfamethoxazole	8–10 mg/kg of TMP div bid	Use for type 1 penicillin hypersensitivity[b]

[a] Consider as first choice for otitis-conjunctivitis syndrome because of high prevalence of penicillinase resistance among non-typable *H. flu* (most common etiologic agent).
[b] Urticaria or anaphylaxis.

Follow-up

- Patient not treated with antibiotics: 2–3 days
- Patient treated with antibiotics: 2–3 days if still febrile or with persistent otalgia

Indications for Admission

- Infant <1 month of age, with temperature over 38.1 °C (100.6 °F)
- Toxic appearance
- Immunocompromised patient with fever
- Suppurative complication (mastoiditis, meningitis, brain abscess) or seventh nerve palsy

Bibliography

Ngo CC, Massa HM, Thornton RB, Cripps AW. Predominant bacteria detected from the middle ear fluid of children experiencing otitis media: a systematic review. *PLoS One.* 2016;**11**(3): e0150949.

Principi N, Marchisio P, Esposito S. Otitis media with effusion: benefits and harms of strategies in use for treatment and prevention. *Expert Rev Anti Infect Ther.* 2016;**14**(4):415–423.

Schilder AG, Chonmaitree T, Cripps AW, et al. Otitis media. *Nat Rev Dis Primers.* 2016;**2**:16063.

Sjoukes A, Venekamp RP, van de Pol AC, et al. Paracetamol (acetaminophen) or non-steroidal anti-inflammatory drugs, alone or combined, for pain relief in acute otitis media in children. *Cochrane Database Syst Rev.* 2016;**12**:CD011534.

Venekamp RP, Burton MJ, van Dongen TM, et al. Antibiotics for otitis media with effusion in children. *Cochrane Database Syst Rev.* 2016;**6**:CD009163.

Cervical Lymphadenopathy

Palpable cervical lymph nodes >1 cm in diameter are present in approximately 80–90% of preschool and young, school-age children, especially if they have had a recent upper respiratory tract infection. Nonetheless, consider cervical lymphadenopathy in three broad etiologic categories: reactive, adenitis, or associated with systemic illness.

Clinical Presentation

Reactive

Most enlarged cervical lymph nodes are reactive, found in conjunction with a viral or bacterial infection of the head or neck. These nodes are generally benign and no work-up or specific treatment is necessary.

Most often the presentation reflects the primary illness (URI, pharyngitis, etc.). Other complaints include pain, a neck mass, stiff neck (unwillingness to move the neck side to side), or torticollis. Reactive nodes are usually multiple, discrete, firm, smaller than 1–2 cm in diameter, nontender, and mobile. The overlying skin is neither erythematous nor adherent. In general, reactive adenopathy subsides in 2–3 weeks, but it can persist.

Adenitis

An adenitis is an infection of the lymph node itself, most commonly (60–85%) caused by *Staphylococcus aureus* or group A Streptococcus, although viral and anaerobic infections have been implicated. Atypical *Mycobacterium* and *Mycobacterium tuberculosis* can result in a node with all the signs of acute infection. Cat scratch disease (Bartonellosis) may cause cervical, axillary, or inguinal adenitis.

With an adenitis, the node becomes enlarged, tender, and fluctuant. The overlying skin can be warm, erythematous, and occasionally adherent. The hallmarks of an atypical *Mycobacterium* infection are the presence of skin erythema overlying a nontender lymph node in an afebrile, otherwise well-appearing child. The node often suppurates. Cat scratch disease is characterized by a papule at the site of the scratch, followed in 5–60 days by regional lymphadenitis. Despite the impressive lymphadenopathy, the patient usually appears well, although 30% may have fever.

Systemic Disease

Systemic diseases, especially infectious mononucleosis and mono-like syndromes (cytomegalovirus, toxoplasmosis, leptospirosis, brucellosis, and tularemia), sarcoidosis, Kawasaki syndrome, and HIV can cause cervical as well as generalized lymphadenopathy. Some medications, such as phenytoin and isoniazid, can cause generalized lymphadenopathy. Always consider the possibility of a malignancy (leukemia, Hodgkin's disease, non-Hodgkin's lymphoma, neuroblastoma).

Mononucleosis and mono-like illnesses (pp. 425–427) can present with generalized tender lymphadenopathy, sometimes in association with an exudative pharyngitis, macular rash, and hepatosplenomegaly. These nodes are firm and mobile. Kawasaki disease (pp. 414–417) and HIV (pp. 396–399) are discussed elsewhere.

A malignant node is fixed, nontender, hard, and matted. It is frequently supraclavicular in location and may be described as persistent or continuously growing. Weight loss, weakness, pallor, night sweats, fever, petechiae, and ecchymoses are other possible findings.

Table 6.4 Differential diagnosis of cervical lymphadenopathy and neck masses

Diagnosis	Differentiating features
Branchial cleft cyst	Smooth and fluctuant along the lower anterior border of SCM muscle
Cervical ribs	Bilateral, hard, immobile masses
Cystic hygroma	Soft, compressible
	Usually transilluminates
Dermoid cyst	Midline mass with calcifications on x-ray
Hemangioma	Present at birth
	Red or bluish color
Kawasaki	Nonpurulent conjunctivitis and mucous membrane changes
	Polymorphic rash
	Edema of dorsum of extremities
Malignancy	May have: weight loss, pallor, bleeding, fever, hepatosplenomegaly
	Node is fixed, hard, matted, and persistent or growing
Meningitis	Nuchal rigidity, photophobia, toxicity
Parotitis	Swelling obscures the angle of the jaw
	Intraoral exam: edema, erythema, or drainage from Stensen's duct
Thyroglossal duct cyst	Midline mass between thyroid bone and suprasternal notch
	Moves up when patient sticks out tongue

Diagnosis

Perform a thorough examination of the head, neck, teeth, and gums to find a source of infection draining into the affected node(s). Weakness, fever, rash, hepatosplenomegaly, and generalized lymphadenopathy are all indicative of a systemic disease. See Table 6.4 for the differential diagnosis of cervical adenitis.

There are seven features of the affected node(s) to consider.

Single or Multiple (Unilateral or Bilateral)

Enlargement of a single node generally occurs in an adenitis, although tuberculous adenitis causes bilateral involvement. Reactive adenopathy and systemic diseases most often result in multiple, bilateral involvement.

Location(s)

The location of a reactive node can suggest the site of the primary infection (preauricular–conjunctiva or external ear canal; occipital–scalp; submental and submandibular–intraoral). Supraclavicular adenopathy is suspicious for a malignancy, while occipital adenopathy suggests a viral illness (particularly roseola and rubella). Generalized lymphadenopathy most commonly occurs during mononucleosis or a mono-like infection, although leukemia is a possible etiology.

Size

Reactive nodes are typically small (<2 cm). Massive enlargement can occur with an atypical *Mycobacterium* infection.

Rate of Growth

Nodes that slowly enlarge suggest a malignancy, while rapid enlargement occurs in an infected or reactive node.

Mobility

In general, a freely movable node is benign. A node that is fixed to adjacent structures or matted to other nodes suggests a malignancy, mycobacterial infection, or cat scratch disease.

Consistency

Soft or firm nodes are benign, while fluctuance occurs in adenitis. A rubbery consistency is noted in sarcoidosis, and malignant nodes are usually rock hard.

Overlying Skin

Bacterial adenitis causes erythema and warmth of the overlying skin. However, adherence occurs in cat scratch disease and atypical *Mycobacterium* infection. A reactive node does not affect the overlying skin.

ED Management

Reactive

"Benign" reactive nodes found in conjunction with a head or neck infection require treatment of the primary illness only. If the pharynx is erythematous, obtain a rapid strep test or a throat culture. Benign nodes can be followed without intervention, although persistence for more than 4–6 weeks may indicate the need for further testing. Reassure the family and arrange for primary care follow-up.

Adenitis

When bacterial adenitis is diagnosed, obtain a throat culture or rapid strep test and give an oral antibiotic with staphylococcal and streptococcal coverage, such as amoxicillin-clavulanate (875/125 formulation; 90 mg/kg/day of amoxicillin div bid) or clindamycin (20 mg/kg/day div q 6h). Warm compresses, applied for 15–30 minutes every 3–4 hours, are a useful adjunct. Have the patient return in 2–3 days. If there is clinical improvement, or a positive strep test or culture, continue the antibiotics for a total of ten days. If the node has not responded to antibiotics and warm compresses, obtain an ultrasound and admit the patient for IV antibiotics. If, instead, the node has become fluctuant, also obtain an ultrasound and consult with an otolaryngologist or surgeon to arrange for an incision and drainage. Obtain *Bartonella* titers if the patient has had contact with a kitten.

Admit patients who are toxic or have nodes unresponsive to oral antibiotic therapy for parenteral treatment: nafcillin 150 mg/kg/day div q 6h, ampicillin-sulbactam (150 mg/kg/day div q 6h), or cefazolin 75 mg/kg/day div q 8h. Use clindamycin (40 mg/kg/day div q 6h) if MRSA is a concern. Obtain a CBC with differential, heterophile antibody, and a blood culture prior to starting intravenous therapy. Indications for a node biopsy include age greater than ten years, persistent and unexplained weight loss or fever, skin ulceration or fixation to the node, supraclavicular location, or continuously increasing size. If atypical mycobacterial infection is suspected, surgical curettage/excision is required as the infection is frequently resistant to antitubercular medication (pp. 428–429), but avoid incision and drainage, which can result in a chronic fistula. If tuberculosis is suspected because of possible exposure or travel, place a 5 TU PPD. If the PPD is positive, consider *Mycobacterium* as the cause of the infection. Obtain a chest x-ray and admit the patient for surgical consultation, collection of culture specimens, and institution of antituberculous therapy (pp. 435–439).

Systemic Disease

When a mononucleosis syndrome is suspected, obtain a heterophile antibody (≥5 years of age) or EBV titers (<5 years of age). Treatment is supportive. Note that the heterophile antibody may be negative early in the disease and in young or immunocompromised patients. If a malignancy is suspected, the initial evaluation includes a chest x-ray and CBC with differential and reticulocyte count prior to hematology consultation. See pp. 159–160 for the treatment of parotitis.

Follow-up

- Bacterial adenitis: 2–3 days

Indications for Admission

- Cervical adenitis associated with toxicity or inadequate oral intake
- Cervical adenitis unresponsive to outpatient treatment
- Evaluation of a suspected malignancy
- Institution of antituberculous therapy

Bibliography

Locke R, Comfort R, Kubba H. When does an enlarged cervical lymph node in a child need excision? A systematic review. *Int J Pediatr Otorhinolaryngol.* 2014;**78**(3):393–401.

Meier JD, Grimmer JF. Evaluation and management of neck masses in children. *Am Fam Physician.* 2014;**89**(5):353–358.

Rajasekaran K, Krakovitz P. Enlarged neck lymph nodes in children. *Pediatr Clin North Am.* 2013;**60** (4):923–936.

Rosenberg TL, Nolder AR. Pediatric cervical lymphadenopathy. *Otolaryngol Clin North Am.* 2014;**47** (5):721–731.

Epistaxis

Epistaxis usually originates from the anterior nasal septum (Kiesselbach's area). Trauma (nose picking, punch, fall), URIs, environmental allergies, excessive use of decongestants or topical nasal steroids, an overly dry environment, and foreign bodies are predisposing factors. Rarely, structural abnormalities (hemangioma, telangiectasia, or angiofibroma), a bleeding diathesis (usually thrombocytopenia), or hypertension is involved. While children are often rushed into the ED because of "massive" blood loss, clinically significant bleeding is unusual.

Clinical Presentation

Usually an anterior septal source is evident. It is rare for the bleeding to be bilateral, but blood crossing behind the nasal septum can mimic a bilateral bleed. Sometimes, if the site is posterior or if the child is sleeping, the blood may present as hematemesis.

Diagnosis

Examine the nasal cavity with the child sitting on the parent's lap, using a bright light (otoscope). If a bleeding source is found, the examination may be terminated, as multiple sites are unusual, except in the case of a fractured nasal septum. If the patient has suffered nasal trauma, look for a septal hematoma, which appears as a bluish-black mass on the anterior septum, filling the nasal cavity. Occasionally, a mucosal hemangioma or telangiectasia is seen. If no cause is found, but blood is noted trickling down the throat, assume that there is a posterior source.

Examine the skin for hemangiomata or telangiectasias, which may also be present in the nasal cavity. Pallor, tachycardia, gallop rhythm, or orthostatic vital sign changes suggest significant blood loss. Jaundice, petechiae, purpura, lymphadenopathy, and hepatospleno-megaly may reflect a bleeding diathesis.

In general, no work-up is required for a nosebleed in an otherwise well child with an anterior septal source. Obtain a hematocrit if anemia is suspected, but evaluate for a bleeding diathesis (pp. 353–357) if the patient has any of the physical findings enumerated above, a long history of recurrent nosebleeds, easy bruising, hemarthrosis, multiple sub-conjunctival hemorrhages, or a family history of excessive bleeding.

ED Management

Most anterior bleeds respond to pressure. Pinch the nares together for a full five minutes with the child sitting upright leaning forward (to prevent swallowing of blood). If this is unsuccessful, soak gauze with 1:1000 aqueous epinephrine or 0.05% oxymetazoline solution and place it in the nasal cavity. Alternatively, if the bleeding remains brisk, pack the nose with petrolatum-impregnated gauze, merocel nasal packing, or Gelfoam. If the patient has recurrent bleeds, after hemostasis is obtained, apply topical anesthesia with 4% lidocaine or benzocaine and cauterize the site, if visible, for three seconds with a silver nitrate stick. Treat hemangiomata or telangiectasias in the same way, but do not use cautery if a bleeding diathesis is suspected (possible tissue slough). Humidification, saline nose drops during the day, and the application of petrolatum (Vaseline) to the septum at bedtime help reduce the recurrence of nose bleeds. If a nasal septal hematoma is suspected, consult an otolaryngologist for immediate drainage to prevent a septal abscess and subsequent nasal deformities.

If routine measures are ineffective or the source is posterior, either consult an otolaryngologist or place a posterior pack. Anesthetize the nose with a topical anesthetic (as above), insert a posterior nasal balloon pack (Epistat or Rapid Rhino, blow up the posterior balloon, pull anterior until it fits snugly in the nasopharynx, and then inflate the anterior balloon until the bleeding stops. Fill both balloons with saline solution. If nasal balloon packs are not available, pass an uninflated Foley catheter through the nose into the pharynx, inflate the balloon, and then pull the catheter back until it fits snugly posteriorly in the nose. Fill the nose with petrolatum-impregnated gauze up to the balloon and place a clamp across the catheter where it exits the nose. If an anterior or posterior nasal pack is placed, give the patient broad-spectrum antibiotics to prevent an acute sinusitis (see Table 6.3). Otolaryngology consultation is indicated.

Follow-up

- Unilateral anterior pack: 48 hours for pack removal

Indications for Admission

- Bilateral anterior pack
- Posterior pack
- Bleeding diathesis or significant blood loss

Bibliography

Béquignon E, Teissier N, Gauthier A, et al. Emergency Department care of childhood epistaxis. *Emerg Med J*. 2016. pii: emermed-2015-205528.

McGarry GW. Recurrent epistaxis in children. *BMJ Clin Evid*. 2013;**2013**:0311.

Qureishi A, Burton MJ. Interventions for recurrent idiopathic epistaxis (nosebleeds) in children. *Cochrane Database Syst Rev*. 2012;**9**:CD004461.

Siddiq S, Grainger J. Fifteen-minute consultation: investigation and management of childhood epistaxis. *Arch Dis Child Educ Pract Ed*. 2015;**100**(1):2–5.

Stoner MJ, Dulaurier M. Pediatric ENT emergencies. *Emerg Med Clin North Am*. 2013;**31**(3):795–808.

Foreign Bodies

Foreign bodies found in the nose or ear commonly include inanimate objects (toys, earrings, etc.), vegetable material, and insects. The nose is the most common site of foreign body impaction in children <3 years of age, and the ear is the most frequent site in patients 3–8 years of age. However, the signs and symptoms of a foreign body may be subtle, and there may be no clear history of insertion. Button batteries require immediate removal to prevent alkaline burns, necrosis, or perforation secondary to chemical leakage or electrical current.

Clinical Presentation and Diagnosis

Aural

A foreign body in the ear can cause pain, tinnitus, and in the case of a live insect, extreme discomfort. Recurrent otitis externa raises the possibility of an aural foreign body. Although usually a benign condition, inexpert attempts at removal can push the object further into the canal, perforate the eardrum, and cause bleeding and swelling of the canal.

Nasal

A nasal foreign body presents with a unilateral foul-smelling discharge with unilateral obstruction. Usually the object can be seen anteriorly in the nose, but swelling of the mucosa can obscure visualization.

Esophageal

An esophageal foreign body (pp. 478–479) is an unusual but potentially serious problem. Most objects pass into the stomach. However, possible sites for lodging include the esophageal inlet due to cricopharyngeus muscle spasm, the inferior margin of the cricoid cartilage, the level of the aortic arch, and just superior to the diaphragm. Symptoms may include pain, dysphagia, vomiting, and dyspnea (secondary to laryngeal compression), although a patient may be asymptomatic. Subsequent edema can cause esophageal obstruction (dysphagia and drooling), upper airway obstruction, and possible perforation leading to mediastinitis.

ED Management

Aural

Usually, a foreign body in the external auditory canal is easily removed with suction, a wire loop, curette, right angle hook, Katz extractor, or small alligator forceps, while irrigation can be used for nonvegetable objects. Prior to attempting to remove a live insect, drown it with mineral oil, 1% lidocaine with 1:1000 epinephrine solution, or 95% alcohol. Do not instill any solution if a tympanic membrane perforation is suspected (blood in the canal in association with ear pain). Arrange for outpatient otolaryngology consultation if the object cannot be removed.

Nasal

Most nasal foreign bodies become impacted between the anterior nasal septum and the inferior turbinate. Prior to attempting to remove the foreign body, anesthetize the nasal mucosa with 4% lidocaine spray and suction any nasal discharge with a Frazier-tip catheter to enhance visualization. Use a nasal speculum with either a curette, Katz extractor, or an alligator forceps to remove the object. As an alternative, a large foreign body can be removed by the caregiver by applying positive pressure via a mouth-to-mouth forced breath to a supine patient, while occluding the opposite (unobstructed) nostril. Consult with an otolaryngologist if removal is unsuccessful or if the object is in the posterior nasal cavity. Do not use topical decongestants routinely, as it may allow the object to migrate further posteriorly and result in aspiration. Antibiotics are not required after successful removal of the foreign body.

Esophageal

Most esophageal foreign bodies, whether round, irregular, or sharp, will pass without difficulty. However, drooling, dysphagia, stridor, or substernal pain or fullness suggests that the object may be lodged in the esophagus. In such cases obtain antero-posterior and lateral neck and chest radiographs, to determine the presence and number of radio-opaque foreign bodies and whether the object(s) is in the esophagus or trachea. An esophageal foreign body typically aligns in a coronal orientation while a laryngeal or tracheal foreign body lies in the sagittal plain. If it is not clear if the foreign body is radiopaque, obtain a searching image x-ray by placing an identical object in a cup of water next to the patient. If foreign body aspiration is likely, but no object is identified on the neck and chest radiographs, obtain abdominal film(s).

A patient with a foreign body, but minimal symptoms, can be monitored for 12–24 hours to see if the object passes spontaneously. However, if the patient is symptomatic arrange for removal under general anesthesia through rigid esophagoscopy. If a disk battery (pp. 478–479) is identified in the esophagus or a sharp object is noted in the esophagus or stomach, consult an otolaryngologist to arrange emergent removal under general anesthesia.

Follow-up

- Blunt foreign body (including button battery) that has passed into the stomach: return at once if vomiting or abdominal pain occur

Indication for Admission

- Esophageal foreign body which has been present >12–24 hours
- Symptomatic patient

Bibliography

Craig SS, Cheek JA, Seith RW, West A. Removal of ENT foreign bodies in children. *Emerg Med Australas.* 2015;**27**(2):145–147.

Friedman EM. Videos in clinical medicine: removal of foreign bodies from the ear and nose. *N Engl J Med.* 2016;**374**(7):e7.

Gupta R, Nyakunu RP, Kippax JR. Is the emergency department management of ENT foreign bodies successful? A tertiary care hospital experience in Australia. *Ear Nose Throat J.* 2016;**95**(3):113–116.

Stoner MJ, Dulaurier M. Pediatric ENT emergencies. *Emerg Med Clin North Am.* 2013;**31**(3):795–808.

Mastoiditis

Mastoiditis is a bacterial infection of the mastoid bone and air cells, usually caused by an untreated AOM. Although the incidence of mastoiditis has decreased significantly with introduction of antibiotics, it remains the most common complication of otitis media, with an incidence of about six cases per 100,000 non-immunocompromised children <14 years of age. It most often occurs in children <2 years of age.

Streptococcus pneumoniae remains the most common cause of mastoiditis. However, universal vaccination is causing a decrease in the number of cases while increasing the cases secondary to multidrug-resistant *S. pneumoniae*. Other etiologies are *Pseudomonas aeruginosa, S. aureus, S.* pyogenes, and nontypable *Haemophilus influenzae*.

Clinical Presentation

Mastoiditis often takes a few weeks to develop and typically follows an untreated or incompletely treated otitis media. The physical findings include swelling, erythema, and tenderness over the mastoid process behind the ear. The auricle is typically displaced antero-inferiorly because of mastoid swelling, and in some cases a fluctuant collection of purulent material can be palpated on the lateral surface of the mastoid process (e.g., subperiosteal abscess). The ipsilateral tympanic membrane is frequently, but not always, erythematous and bulging. Edema and sagging of the posterior external auditory canal wall may be seen upon careful examination of the external auditory canal. Fever >38.3 °C (101 ° F) is common.

Since the advent of pneumococcal vaccination, patients present with more complicated and severe disease, including subperiosteal abscesses. This usually requires surgical intervention in addition to antibiotics.

Diagnosis and ED Management

If mastoiditis is suspected based on clinical findings, obtain an axial/coronal CT scan of the temporal bones to rule-out possible extension of infection beyond the mastoid. Clouding of the mastoid air cells and loss of the intermastoid cell septa secondary to the osteomyelitic process are seen in coalescent mastoiditis. The radiographic findings of fluid in the middle ear and mastoid without the loss of bony septa may be the result of a recent otitis media and do not necessarily indicate acute mastoiditis, in the absence of the typical clinical findings. Plain mastoid radiographs are not useful.

Admit all children with acute mastoiditis, consult an otolaryngologist, and treat with IV ceftriaxone (100 mg/kg/day div q 12h) *and* clindamycin (40 mg/kg/day div q 6h). Tympanocentesis can be helpful in obtaining fluid for Gram's stain and culture. Surgical drainage is indicated if a subperiosteal or intracranial abscess is seen on CT scan or if the patient does not improve clinically with 24–48 hours of intravenous antibiotics.

Indication for Admission

- Mastoiditis

Bibliography

Blumfield E, Misra M. Pott's puffy tumor, intracranial, and orbital complications as the initial presentation of sinusitis in healthy adolescents, a case series. *Emerg Radiol.* 2011;18:203–210.

DeMuri GP, Wald ER. Complications of acute bacterial sinusitis in children. *Pediatr Infect Dis J.* 2011;30(8):701–702.

Marom T, Roth Y, Boaz M, et al. Acute mastoiditis in children: necessity and timing of imaging. *Pediatr Infect Dis J.* 2016;35(1):30–34.

Psarommatis IM, Voudouris C, Douros K, et al. Algorithmic management of pediatric acute mastoiditis. *Int J Pediatr Otorhinolaryngol.* 2012; **76**:791–796.

Tamir So, Roth Y, Dalal L, Goldfarb A, Marom T. Acute mastoiditis in the pneumococcal conjugate vaccine era. *Clin Vaccine Immunol.* 2014; **21**: 1189

Neck Masses

Although the majority of neck masses in children are benign enlarged lymph nodes, the possibility of a malignancy is often a concern. In general, neck masses can be considered in four categories: lymph nodes (pp. 147–150), congenital masses, benign tumors, and malignancies.

Clinical Presentation and Diagnosis

Congenital Masses

Branchial Cleft Cyst

A branchial cleft cyst is often not diagnosed until late childhood or early adulthood (average age, 13 years), when it becomes infected. It presents as a discrete, erythematous, tender, fluctuant mass in the lateral neck, typically anterior to the sternocleidomastoid muscle. On occasion, there is a fistula anterior to the muscle with an orifice that drains mucus and retracts with swallowing. If the acute infection is properly treated with antibiotics, the cyst shrinks, but may re-expand during subsequent upper respiratory infections.

Thyroglossal Duct Cyst

A thyroglossal duct cyst usually presents as an asymptomatic midline neck mass at or below the level of the hyoid bone. The sexes are affected equally, and 50% of cases present prior to age ten years. These frequently become infected and respond to antibiotics, only to reemerge during the next URI. In between, the mass is cystic or solid, nontender, and mobile. The pathognomonic feature is elevation of the mass when the tongue is protruded. Occasionally, it contains ectopic thyroid tissue.

Congenital Muscular Torticollis

Congenital muscular torticollis, or fibromatosis colli, presents at 1–2 weeks of age as a hard, nontender mass within the body of the sternocleidomastoid. Characteristically, the head is tilted to the affected side, the baby faces away from the lesion, and there can be flattening of the unaffected side of the head. The family may report that the baby looks in one direction only.

Benign Tumors

Cystic Hygroma

A cystic hygroma usually presents as an irregular, soft, painless, compressible lateral neck mass that transilluminates and can increase in size during straining. Fifty percent are present at birth and 90% are noted during the first two years of life. Massive enlargement can cause obstruction of the airway or the esophagus. Typical locations are the submental, preauricular, and submandibular areas.

Hemangioma

Hemangiomas are more frequently present at birth, and all present during the first year of life. Unlike cystic hygromas, there is a 3:1 female preponderance. Most are of the cavernous type, often located within the parotid gland, in the preauricular area. Infection or hemorrhage can cause acute enlargement, and the mass becomes bluish in color when the infant is crying or straining.

Dermoid Cyst

A dermoid cyst typically is an asymptomatic, cystic midline mass located in the submental region. A teratoma has a similar presentation, but calcifications or teeth are often seen on x-ray.

Malignant Tumors

About one-quarter of all the malignancies of childhood occur in the neck and more than half of these are either Hodgkin's disease (pp. 360–361) or lymphosarcoma. Hodgkin's disease usually (80%) presents in the upper neck as a painless, hard or firm, fixed, slowly enlarging unilateral node. Most patients are more than five years old. Forty percent of non-Hodgkin's lymphomas present extranodally in the neck throughout the pediatric age range, and the disease is often (40%) bilateral. A slowly growing, hard or rubbery, fixed mass is seen. Weight loss and hepatosplenomegaly are features of both diseases.

A rhabdomyosarcoma can originate in the nasopharynx or ear; symptoms are determined by the site. A nasopharyngeal mass presents as chronic adenoidal hypertrophy, with adenoidal facies, snoring, mouth breathing, serous otitis, and a serosanguinous nasal discharge. There may also be extension to the base of the skull with cranial nerve deficits. A mass in the ear causes chronic otitis, ear discharge, and mastoiditis. Weight loss can occur with a mass in either location. Other rare neck malignancies include fibrosarcoma (mandible most common site), thyroid cancer (history of neck irradiation), and both primary (causing Horner's syndrome) or metastatic (located in orbit or nasopharynx) neuroblastoma.

ED Management

Congenital Masses

Treat an infected branchial cleft cyst or thyroglossal duct cyst with cephalexin (40 mg/kg/day div q 12h), cefadroxil (40 mg/kg/day div bid), or amoxicillin-clavulanate (90 mg/kg/day of amoxicillin div bid), and warm soaks every two hours. If MRSA is a concern, either use clindamycin (20 mg/kg/day div q 6h) or give trimethoprim-sulfamethoxazole (8 mg/kg/day of TMP div bid) along with either cephalexin or cefadroxil. Since these lesions have a tendency to become re-infected, refer the patient to an otolaryngologist so that elective excision can be performed.

A neck ultrasound or thyroid scan is a prerequisite for thyroglossal duct excision, as the cyst may contain all of the patient's thyroid tissue. Instruct the parents of a child with a sterno-cleidomastoid tumor and torticollis to perform stretching exercises, four times a day: Straighten the head into a midline position, then rotate the head to the affected side and hold for ten seconds.

Benign Tumors

If there are no signs or symptoms of airway compromise, referral to an otolaryngologist is indicated for patients with massive enlargement of a cystic hygroma or hemangioma or extreme disfigurement. On occasion, a dermatologist or plastic surgeon should see the child so that cosmetic reconstruction can be planned. Dermoid cysts and teratomas require elective excision.

Malignant Tumors

If a malignancy is suspected (hard, nontender, slowly growing mass; systemic signs and symptoms; a clinical picture consistent with a mass in the ear or nasopharynx), obtain a CBC, reticulocyte count, and a chest x-ray to rule-out mediastinal or hilar node enlargement. Admit the patient, and consult an oncologist. Do not give the patient corticosteroids.

Follow-up

• Infected branchial cleft cyst or thyroglossal duct cyst: 48–72 hours

Indications for Admission

• Airway or esophageal obstruction
• Suspected malignancy

Bibliography

Brigger MR, Cunningham MJ. Malignant cervical masses in children. *Otolaryngol Clin North Am.* 2015;48(1):59–77.

Geddes G, Butterfly MM, Patel SM, Marra S. Pediatric neck masses. *Pediatr Rev.* 2013;34(3): 115–125.

Goins, MR, Beasley MD. Pediatric neck masses. *Oral Maxillofac Surg Clin North Am.* 2012;24 (3):457–468.

Meier JD, Grimmer JF. Evaluation and management of neck masses in children. *Am Fam Physician.* 2014;89(5):353–358.

Prosser JD, Myer CM. Branchial cleft anomalies and thymic cysts. *Otolaryngol Clin North Am.* 2015;48 (1):1–14.

Otitis Externa

Otitis externa (AOE), also known as swimmer's ear, is an inflammation of the external auditory canal. It generally occurs in the summertime, when swimming leads to the trapping of excess moisture in the external auditory canal. Excessive cerumen, local trauma, eczema, foreign bodies, and immunocompromise are additional risk factors. This results in a mixed infection of fungi (*Aspergillus* and *Candida*) and bacteria (*Pseudomonas*, *Klebsiella*, *S. aureus*, and *Enterobacter*).

Clinical Presentation and Diagnosis

Generally there is a history of recent swimming or of manipulation of the external canal with a pointed object or q-tip. The patient is usually afebrile, but complaining of ear pain and itching, with a thick white, yellow, or green discharge from the external canal. Extreme discomfort when pulling the pinna or tragus distinguishes the discharge of otitis externa from that caused by a perforated tympanic membrane. Otoscopy is significant for an erythematous external canal, which can be so swollen that it prevents visualization of the tympanic membrane. In the absence of a history of swimming or ear canal manipulation, consider a foreign body impaction.

ED Management

Treat otitis externa with topical, broad-spectrum antibiotic ear drops. Preparations which contain hydrocortisone often reduce swelling more effectively. Use acetic acid with or without hydrocortisone (3–5 drops tid × 7 days), ciprofloxacin-hydrocortisone (3 drops bid × 7 days), ofloxacin (5 drops bid <12 years, 10 drops bid ≥12 years, × 10 days), or polymyxin B-neomycin-hydrocortisone (3–5 drops tid × 7 days). If a perforated tympanic membrane cannot be ruled out, use a preparation that is less caustic to the middle ear structures, such as ofloxacin or ciprofloxacin/dexamethasone. Instill the drops either directly into the canal or onto a cotton earwick, which ensures delivery of the drug throughout the external canal. In addition, keep the canal dry; further swimming is not permitted unless the child wears earplugs. Complete resolution takes 5–7 days. If there is no improvement in two days, refer the patient to an otolaryngologist for cleaning of the ear canal and possible ear wick placement. If the child is prone to recurrences and no tympanic membrane perforation is present, use two drops of a prophylactic mixture of half rubbing (isopropyl) alcohol and half water after every swim.

Severe otitis externa with associated cellulitis of the pinna requires admission for systemic antibiotics. Consult an otolaryngologist.

Follow-up

- 48 hours, if the symptoms do not begin to improve.

Bibliography

Block SL. Mastoiditis mimicry: retro-auricular cellulitis related to otitis externa. *Pediatr Ann.* 2014;**43** (9):342–347.

Lorente J, Sabater F, Rivas MP, et al. Ciprofloxacin plus fluocinolone acetonide versus ciprofloxacin alone in the treatment of diffuse otitis externa. *J Laryngol Otol.* 2014;**128**(7):591–598.

Prentice P. American Academy of Otolaryngology: head and neck surgery foundation clinical practice guideline on acute otitis externa 2014. *Arch Dis Child Educ Pract Ed.* 2015;**100**(4):197.

Rosenfeld RM, Schwartz SR, Cannon CR, et al. Clinical practice guideline: acute otitis externa. *Otolaryngol Head Neck Surg.* 2014;**150**(1 Suppl.):S1–S24.

Parotitis

Sialoadenitis is an acute inflammatory process of one or more of the salivary glands, with the most frequently affected being the parotid gland. Parotitis results from salivary stasis, secondary to viruses (mumps, Coxsackieviruses), bacteria (*Staphylococcus aureus, Streptococcus viridans, Streptococcus pneumonia*), salivary duct stone (sialolith), or dehydration in chronically ill or debilitated patients.

Recurrent parotitis of childhood (RPC) is a separate clinical entity in which periodic acute episodes of parotid swelling occur in one or both parotid glands. Although the etiology is unknown, it is thought to be secondary to poor dental hygiene.

Clinical Presentation

Acute parotitis presents with swelling and pain overlying the affected parotid gland, obscuring the angle of the mandible. Infectious parotitis may cause unilateral or bilateral swelling with severe tenderness. The swelling can develop rapidly and often presents during or after a meal, when salivary flow is stimulated. Intraoral examination may reveal swelling, erythema, or a discharge from the opening of Stensen's duct, which is on the buccal mucosa opposite the second upper molar. With a bacterial parotitis, purulent material can be expressed from Stenson's duct by gently massaging the affected gland.

Diagnosis

In general, an enlarged parotid is the only mass that obscures the angle of the mandible. See Table 6.4 for the differential diagnosis of neck masses.

ED Management

The treatment of parotitis is aimed at increasing salivary flow in order to flush infected material from within the salivary duct and gland. Encourage hydration and recommend the use of sialogogues, such as lemon swabs or sucking candies. In addition, provide analgesia (acetaminophen 15 mg/kg q 4h, ibuprofen 10 mg/kg q 6h) and warm compresses.

If there is evidence of duct obstruction, overlying erythema and tenderness, or purulent drainage from Stenson's duct, give anti-staphylococcal antibiotics such as cephalexin (40 mg/kg/day div q 12h), cefadroxil (40 mg/kg/day div bid), or amoxicillin-clavulanate (90 mg/kg/day of amoxicillin div bid). If MRSA is a concern, either use clindamycin (20 mg/kg/day div q 6h) or add trimethoprim-sulfamethoxazole (8 mg/kg/day of TMP div bid) to the above regimens. Obtain a CT scan of the neck if the patient has persistent or recurrent parotitis, an abscess, or if an anatomic obstruction (e.g., stone) is suspected.

Recurrent parotitis of childhood responds well to medical treatment and the episodes often disappear after puberty.

Follow-up

*   Parotitis: 48–72 hours

Indications for Admission

*   Patient toxic or unable to manage PO hydration
*   Parotid abscess

Bibliography

Barskey AE, Juieng P, Whitaker BL, et al. Viruses detected among sporadic cases of parotitis, United States, 2009–2011. *J Infect Dis.* 2013; **208**(12):1979–1986

Campbell JR. Parotitis. In Feigin RD, Cherry JD, Demmler-Harrison GJ, Kaplan SL (eds.) *Textbook of Pediatric Infectious Diseases* (7th edn.). Philadelphia, PA, Saunders; 2014; 189–193.

Ellies M, Laskawi R. Diseases of the salivary glands in infants and adolescents. *Head Face Med.* 2010;**6**:1

Francis CL, Larsen CG. Pediatric sialadenitis. *Otolaryngol Clin North Am.* 2014;**47**(5):763–778

Michaels MG, Nowalk AJ. Infectious disease. In Zitelli BJ, McIntire SC, Norwalk AJ (eds.) *Atlas of Pediatric Physical Diagnosis* (6th edn.) Philadelphia, PA: Saunders/Elsevier, 2012; 469–529.

Periorbital and Orbital Cellulitis

The orbital septum is a fibrous membrane running from the periosteum of the orbital bones to the tarsal plates. It separates the skin and subcutaneous tissues from intraorbital structures. Although the clinical pictures are similar, differentiation of periorbital (preseptal) cellulitis from orbital (postseptal) cellulitis is critical.

Clinical Presentation

Both periorbital and orbital cellulitis present with warm, tender, erythematous lid swelling, usually associated with fever and regional adenopathy.

Periorbital Cellulitis

Periorbital cellulitis can be divided into two types. The infection may be preceded by an obvious break in the skin (insect bite, laceration, impetigo), with the causative agents being *S. aureus* or group A *Streptococcus*. More commonly, the infection occurs as a result of local spread from an ethmoid sinusitis with a *Moraxella catarrhalis* or *pneumococcus* infection. In a sinusitis-related case, the patient may have a history of a persistent nasal discharge, and the upper eyelid may be affected first, with subsequent spread to the lower lid. With either type of periorbital cellulitis, mild to moderate conjunctival swelling and hyperemia with a mucoid to purulent discharge may be present.

Orbital Cellulitis

The hallmarks of a postseptal infection are proptosis, chemosis, and decreased painful extraocular mobility, in association with fever and toxicity. Decreased visual acuity may also occur late in the course.

Diagnosis

Distinguishing periorbital from orbital cellulitis is critical because more aggressive medical and surgical intervention may be required with the latter. Passively open the eyelids and examine the eyes for conjunctival injection, discharge, proptosis, chemosis, and decreased extraocular mobility, and check the visual acuity. In addition, a patient with orbital cellulitis may have limited or painful extraocular movements in the unaffected eye. If the distinction between periorbital and orbital infection is not clear on clinical grounds, obtain a noncontrast axial/coronal CT scan of the orbit and sinuses. If orbital cellulitis is suspected, promptly consult both an otolaryngologist and an ophthalmologist.

Lid erythema and swelling may be caused by a viral or bacterial conjunctivitis (marked palpebral conjunctival injection), an insect bite (a painless punctum may be identified), or infectious mononucleosis (bilateral swelling with fever and pharyngitis). An allergic reaction or nephrotic syndrome can cause lid swelling (generally bilateral) in the absence of erythema, tenderness, or fever. Proptosis can be secondary to an orbital tumor although the signs of infection are usually absent, while hyperthyroid exophthalmos can be confused with proptosis. Ecchymosis can be due to trauma (consider child abuse) but can also be seen with orbital tumors (neuroblastoma).

ED Management

As mentioned above, when the distinction between a periorbital and orbital infection is not clear, radiologic studies can be helpful. Since an orbital cellulitis can be a life-threatening illness, always err on the side of overdiagnosing a postseptal infection.

Periorbital Cellulitis

A child with mild preseptal cellulitis secondary to a break in the skin may be treated as an outpatient with cefadroxil (40 mg/kg/day), cephalexin (40 mg/kg/day div qid), amoxicillin-clavulanate (875/125 formulation, 90 mg/kg/day of amoxicillin div bid), or cefuroxime (30 mg/kg/day div bid). If MRSA is a concern, either use clindamycin (20 mg/kg/day div q 6h) or add trimethoprim-sulfamethoxazole (8 mg/kg/day of TMP div bid) to one of the above regimens. If the infection is sinusitis-related, give a topical nasal decongestant (oxymetazoline bid) and amoxicillin-clavulanate or cefuroxime (as above). Also recommend warm compresses qid.

Admit the patient if there is a significant fever >39.4 °C (103.0 °F), significant eyelid edema, decreased extraocular mobility, inability to tolerate oral antibiotics, or signs of systemic toxicity. Obtain a CBC and blood culture, and treat with IV antibiotics (ampicillin-sulbactam 150 mg/kg/day div q 6h, cefuroxime 100 mg/kg/day div q 8h, or vancomycin 40 mg/kg/day div q 6h for possible MRSA) and a topical nasal decongestant.

Orbital Cellulitis

The IV antibiotic treatment is the same as for a preseptal cellulitis (see above), but include vancomycin in the regimen if there is any possibility of MRSA. As mentioned above, obtain an axial/coronal CT scan of the paranasal sinuses and orbits and both otolaryngology and ophthalmology consultations early in the evaluation of the patient. Abscess drainage is indicated if there is extreme toxicity, evidence of intracranial spread (focal neurologic findings), decreased visual acuity, or no response to 24 hours of antibiotics. However, treat small subperiosteal abscesses with 24–48 hours of IV antibiotics prior to surgical intervention.

Follow-up

- Preseptal cellulitis: 24–48 hours. Instruct the family to return immediately for IV therapy if symptoms worsen

Indications for Admission

- Preseptal cellulitis associated with fever or toxicity, or unresponsive to 24–48 hours of oral antibiotics
- Orbital cellulitis

Bibliography

Bedwell J, Bauman NM. Management of pediatric orbital cellulitis and abscess. *Curr Opin Otolaryngol Head Neck Surg.* 2011;**19**(6):467–473.

Blumfield E, Misra M. Pott's puffy tumor, intracranial, and orbital complications as the initial presentation of sinusitis in healthy adolescents, a case series. *Emerg Radiol.* 2011;**18**:203–210.

Mathew AV, Craig E, Al-Mahmoud R, et al. Paediatric post-septal and pre-septal cellulitis: 10 years' experience at a tertiary-level children's hospital. *Br J Radiol.* 2014;**87**(1033):20130503.

Meara DJ. Sinonasal disease and orbital cellulitis in children. *Oral Maxillofac Surg Clin North Am.* 2012;**24**(3):487–496.

Peritonsillar Abscess

Occasionally, a bacterial pharyngitis can evolve into a peritonsillar abscess, which is a collection of purulent material in the peritonsillar space between the tonsil's capsule and the surrounding pharyngeal muscles. The infection may then spread into the surrounding soft tissues. This usually occurs in an adolescent who has not been treated with antibiotics, although adequate antimicrobial coverage does not always prevent this complication. Virtually all cases of peritonsillar abscess are caused by group A beta-hemolytic *Streptococci*, although uncommonly *S. aureus* and anaerobes are implicated.

Clinical Presentation

A peritonsillar abscess causes severe sore throat and toxicity, with difficulty opening the mouth (trismus), drooling, and a "hot potato" muffled voice. The tonsil may be markedly erythematous and covered with a whitish exudate, while the uvula is swollen and deviated to the contralateral side. Anterior and superior to the tonsil there is soft palate swelling which is sometimes fluctuant. The head may be tilted to the unaffected side, and tender cervical adenopathy is usually prominent on the same side as the abscess. In severe cases, signs of upper airway obstruction may also be present.

Diagnosis and ED Management

If a peritonsillar abscess is suspected, either perform an incision and drainage, or obtain ENT consultation to determine whether incision and drainage or needle aspiration is the most appropriate course of action. In general, imaging is not necessary.

After the drainage procedure, in a mild case, in which adequate oral intake is possible, treat with antibiotics and analgesia (ibuprofen, 10 mg/kg q 6h; acetaminophen with codeine 1 mg/kg q 6h, 30 mg maximum). Cultures taken from the aspirates of acute peritonsillar abscess frequently yield multiple organisms, some of which are beta-lactamase producers. Therefore, give a 7–10-day course of amoxicillin-clavulanate (875/125 formulation, 90 mg/kg/day of amoxicillin div bid) or, if penicillin-allergic, clindamycin (30 mg/kg/day div qid). If adequate oral intake is not possible, admit the patient and treat with intravenous penicillin G (50,000–100,000 units/kg/day div q 6h) or clindamycin (40 mg/kg/day div q 6h) and IV hydration. A single dose of dexamethasone (0.6 mg/kg, 10 mg maximum) may be helpful in reducing pain and discomfort during the first 24 hours after the procedure.

Follow-up

- Peritonsillar abscess (drained): next day

Indications for Admission

- Severe dysphagia preventing oral intake
- Patient not taking adequate oral fluids, status-post incision and drainage of a peritonsillar abscess

Bibliography

Baldassari C, Shah RK. Pediatric peritonsillar abscess: an overview. *Infect Disord Drug Targets*. 2012;**12**(4):277–280.

Goldstein NA, Hammerschlag MR. Peritonsillar, retropharyngeal, and parapharyngeal abscesses. In Cherry JD, Harrison GJ, Kaplan SL, Steinbach WJ, Hotez PJ (eds.) *Feigin and Cherry's Textbook of Pediatric Infectious Diseases* (7th edn.). Philadelphia, PA: Saunders, 2014; 167–175.

Kim DK, Lee JW, Na YS, et al. Clinical factor for successful nonsurgical treatment of pediatric peritonsillar abscess. *Laryngoscope*. 2015;**125**(11):2608–2611.

Nguyen T, Haberland CA, Hernandez-Boussard T. Pediatric patient and hospital characteristics associated with treatment of peritonsillar abscess and peritonsillar cellulitis. *Clin Pediatr (Phila)*. 2015;**54**(13):1240–1246.

Qureshi H, Ference E, Novis S, et al. Trends in the management of pediatric peritonsillar abscess infections in the U.S., 2000–2009. *Int J Pediatr Otorhinolaryngol*. 2015;**79**(4):527–531.

Pharyngotonsillitis

Pharyngitis is most often caused by viral infections (adenovirus, parainfluenza, rhinovirus, coronavirus, CMV, EBV, Coxsackie A virus). Approximately 20–30% of cases are caused by group A beta-hemolytic *Streptococci* ("strep throat"). Other rare etiologies include *Mycoplasma*, group C and G *Streptococcus*, toxoplasmosis, *Chlamydia*, *Neisseria gonorrhea*, tularemia, and diphtheria (very rare).

Clinical Presentation and Diagnosis

The older child usually complains of pain or difficulty with swallowing. The toddler may act cranky or irritable, refuse food or fluids, and have sleep disturbances. Other findings may include drooling or difficulty handling secretions, fever, otalgia, and tender anterior cervical lymphadenopathy. Infection of the pharynx causes erythema of the tonsils and tonsillar pillars with or without tonsillar enlargement. In older patients, epiglottitis (pp. 641–643) may present with severe dysphagia.

Viral Infections

Low-grade fever (<38.3 °C; 101 °F) associated with conjunctivitis, rhinitis, or cough suggests a viral etiology. Tonsillar exudate, toxicity, and severe difficulty swallowing are unusual findings in the common viral infections. However, adenovirus can cause a severe pharyngitis with exudate and ulceration. Thick, gray mucus covering the tonsils can be seen in infectious mononucleosis and mono-like syndromes (CMV, toxoplasmosis, tularemia). Generalized lymphadenopathy, hepatosplenomegaly, an erythematous maculopapular rash, fever (>38.3 °C; 101°F), periorbital edema, urticaria, upper airway obstruction secondary to lymphoid hyperplasia, and severe, prolonged lethargy are other manifestations of infectious mononucleosis, especially in the adolescent (pp. 425–427). Herpangina (coxsackieviruses) causes a vesicular eruption in the posterior pharynx.

Sreptococcal Infection

Streptococcal infection is suggested by whitish yellow exudate on the tonsillar surface, palatal petechiae, a red uvula, tender anterior cervical lymphadenopathy, halitosis, headache, and fever >38.3 °C (101°F). On occasion, associated severe abdominal pain can mimic acute appendicitis. Marked dysphagia, with drooling and difficulty breathing, occurs less frequently. An erythematous sandpaper-like scarlatiniform rash with perioral pallor may develop. Other findings are a "strawberry" tongue, accentuation of the rash in the flexion creases (Pastia's lines), and, late in the course, periungual desquamation.

ED Management

Clinical evaluation alone is an inaccurate method for diagnosing strep throat. Streptococcal infection may be diagnosed either by a throat culture on 5% sheep blood agar or by a rapid agglutination test, which is useful for early diagnosis. False-negative results, although rare, are possible with all the rapid *Streptococcus* tests, so a throat culture is indicated if the rapid test is negative.

Treat pharyngitis symptomatically, with gargles, lozenges, cold liquids, soft foods, and acetaminophen (15 mg/kg q 4h) or ibuprofen (10 mg/kg q 6h). Avoid salty foods and acidic drinks (orange juice). If a rapid strep test or throat culture is positive for beta-hemolytic *Streptococci*, treat with antibiotics to prevent rheumatic fever as well as to shorten the course of the acute pharyngitis. Therapy consists of ten days of oral antibiotics: penicillin VK (25 mg/kg/day div tid), amoxicillin (50 mg/kg once daily), cefadroxil (20 mg/kg once daily), or, for penicillin-allergic patients, azithromycin (12 mg/kg once daily for five days or 20 mg/kg once daily for three days), erythromycin ethyl succinate (40 mg/kg/day div bid or tid), or clindamycin (25 mg/kg/d div qid). However, there is a 10–20% rate of strep resistance to macrolides. If compliance is not assured, give one dose of intramuscular benzathine penicillin G mixed with procaine penicillin (600,000 units of benzathine <27 kg [60 lb]; 1,200,000 units of benzathine >27 kg [60 lb]). At least 20% of group A beta-hemolytic *Streptococci* are resistant to tetracycline, while sulfonamides (including trimethoprim-sulfamethoxazole) do not reliably eradicate acute streptococcal infections and therefore are not appropriate therapy. Patients with *severe* pharyngeal discomfort may benefit by a dose of dexamethasone (0.6 mg/kg PO or IM, 10 mg maximum).

When the clinical picture is suggestive of infectious mononucleosis or the patient has been suffering an unusually prolonged or severe sore throat, an evaluation for mononucleosis is indicated. Obtain a CBC with differential to look for atypical lymphocytosis and a monospot test or heterophile antibody.

Follow-up

- Strep throat: 1–3 days if symptoms worsen, otherwise as per routine care
- Mononucleosis: primary care follow-up in two weeks, to assess for splenomegaly

Indications for Admission

- Severe dysphagia preventing oral intake
- Patient not taking adequate oral fluids, status-post incision and drainage of a peritonsillar abscess

Bibliography

Cohen JF, Bertille N, Cohen R, Chalumeau M. Rapid antigen detection test for group A streptococcus in children with pharyngitis. *Cochrane Database Syst Rev.* 2016;7:CD010502.

Fierro JL, Prasad PA, Localio AR, et al. Variability in the diagnosis and treatment of group A streptococcal pharyngitis by primary care pediatricians. *Infect Control Hosp Epidemiol.* 2014;**35**(Suppl. 3):S79–S85.

Russo ME, Kline J, Jaggi P, Leber AL, Cohen DM. The challenge of patient notification and the work of follow-up generated by a 2-step testing protocol for group A streptococcal pharyngitis in the pediatric emergency department. *Pediatr Emerg Care.* 2017; DOI: 10.1097/PEC.0000000000001144.

Shapiro DJ, Lindgren CE, Neuman MI, Fine AM. Viral features and testing for streptococcal pharyngitis. *Pediatrics.* 2017;**139**(5).

Van Driel ML, De Sutter AI, Keber N, Habraken H, Christiaens T. Different antibiotic treatments for group A streptococcal pharyngitis. *Cochrane Database Syst Rev.* 2013;**4**:CD004406.

Retropharyngeal Abscess (RPA)

A retropharyngeal abscess is a complication of viral upper respiratory tract infections, streptococcal pharyngitis, trauma, or an extension of a vertebral osteomyelitis. Retrophayngeal lymph nodes become infected in young children and develop into an abscess. These nodes involute as the child gets older, making infection less likely in adolescents. Adolescents who develop RPA, do so most often as a result of local trauma (endoscopy, etc.). Most infections are polymicrobial with *S. aureus*, group A strep and anaerobes such as *Bacteroides* and *Peptostreptococcus* being the most common.

Clinical Presentation

The patient presents with fever, drooling, respiratory distress, and hyperextension of the neck. Torticollis or limited neck movement (side to side or up and down) may also be present. On examination, there may be anterior bulging of the posterior pharyngeal wall, although the throat exam is often normal. In severe cases upper airway obstruction with stridor or stertor (harsh crackling sounds over the larynx or trachea) may also be present. Chest pain is an ominous sign in this setting and suggests mediastinitis.

Diagnosis

If a retropharyngeal abscess is suspected, obtain a soft tissue lateral neck x-ray. Findings include widening of the retropharyngeal space and loss of the normal cervical lordosis. A crying child with his neck flexed can produce a false-positive x-ray. If the radiograph is positive or you have a high suspicion for an RPA, obtain a neck CT scan with IV contrast, which will confirm the diagnosis and delineate the extent and location of an abscess relative to the airway and blood vessels.

ED Management

Request an ENT consultation to help confirm the diagnosis, assess for airway compromise, and determine if surgical drainage is required. Treat with beta-lactamase resistant antibiotics, such as IV ampicillin-sulbactam (150 mg/kg/day div q 6h) or IV clindamycin (40 mg/kg/day div q 6–8h) if the patient is allergic to penicillin. However, if MRSA is a concern, use vancomycin (40 mg/kg/day div q 6h). Respiratory distress or failure to respond to medical treatment within 24–48 hours is an indication for incision and drainage in the operating room.

Indications for Admission

- Retropharyngeal abscess

Bibliography

Elsherif AM, Park AH, Alder SC, et al. Indicators of a more complicated clinical course for pediatric patients with retropharyngeal abscess. *Int J Pediatr Otorhinolaryngol.* 2010;74:198–201.

Goldstein NA, Hammerschlag MR. Peritonsillar, retropharyngeal, and parapharyngeal abscesses. In Cherry JD, Harrison GJ, Kaplan SL, Steinbach WJ, Hotez PJ (eds.) *Feigin and Cherry's Textbook of Pediatric Infectious Diseases* (7th edn.). Philadelphia, PA: Saunders, 2014; 167–175.

Grisaru-Soen G, Komisar O, Aizenstein O, et al. Retropharyngeal and parapharyngeal abscess in children: epidemiology, clinical features and treatment. *Int J Pediatr –Otorhinolaryngol.* 2010;74:1016–1020

Stoner MJ, Dulaurier M. Pediatric ENT emergencies. *Emerg Med Clin North Am.* 2013;31(3):795–808.

Serous Otitis Media

Serous otitis media (SOM), also known as otitis media with effusion (OME), is the presence of nonsuppurative fluid in the middle ear. Although no overt signs of infection are seen in SOM, bacteria have been found in 30–70% of cultures of the fluid.

Clinical Presentation and Diagnosis

Despite adequate treatment, serous otitis frequently follows an episode of acute otitis media. Usually, there are no complaints of pain or fever, although an infant may be fussy when recumbent, while an older child may note decreased hearing or mild balance disturbances.

On pneumatic otoscopy, the tympanic membrane appears darkened and retracted, with decreased mobility, but without evidence of acute infection (i.e., no erythema). There may be an air-fluid level with bubbles visible behind the drum. The limited mobility can be confirmed by impedance testing (retracted tympanic membrane with negative middle ear pressure).

ED Management

The best management of SOM is watchful waiting for a three-month period. The empirical use of antihistamine–decongestant combinations is of no value, while antibiotics and corticosteroids offer only a temporary benefit and therefore are not indicated.

Refer the patient to a primary care provider to assess the frequency of acute infections. Arrange for a hearing evaluation if fluid has been present for >3 months. Myringotomy and pressure equalizing tubes may be indicated for unresponsive, recurrent otitis media or significant conductive hearing loss (hearing threshold >20 dB), especially in a child with speech delay.

Bibliography

Atkinson H, Wallis S, Coatesworth AP. Otitis media with effusion. *Postgrad Med.* 2015;**127** (4):381–385.

Daniel M. Antibiotics for otitis media with effusion in children. *Clin Otolaryngol.* 2013;**38**(1):56–57.

Griffin G, Flynn CA. Antihistamines and/or decongestants for otitis media with effusion (OME) in children. *Cochrane Database Syst Rev.* 2011;9:CD003423.

Venekamp RP, Burton MJ, van Dongen TM, et al. Antibiotics for otitis media with effusion in children. *Cochrane Database Syst Rev.* 2016;(**6**):CD009163.

Sinusitis

Sinusitis (also known as rhinosinusitis) is defined as inflammation of one or more of the paranasal sinuses, which develop as outpouchings of the nasal chamber. They enlarge as the child grows, so that the importance of a particular sinus varies with the age of the patient. The maxillary and ethmoid cells are present at birth while the sphenoid and frontal sinuses are not aerated until approximately five and seven years of age, respectively.

The organisms responsible for most cases of acute sinusitis are similar to those implicated in acute otitis media and include *S. pneumoniae*, nontypable *H. influenzae, M. catarrhalis*, and *S. aureus*. In contrast, anaerobes, *S. aureus*, alpha *Streptococcus*, and nontypable *H. influenzae* are the predominant infectious etiologies of chronic sinusitis, which is also frequently caused by a noninfectious etiology, chronic hyperplastic eosinophilic sinusitis.

Clinical Presentation

The most common signs and symptoms of acute sinusitis are dry cough (typically occurs at night or during naps), persistent (>7–10 days) nasal discharge, and fever. Children ≥5 years of age may complain of a headache that is accentuated by leaning forward. Younger patients (<5 years) may have malodorous breath in the absence of a pharyngeal or dental infection. Facial pain and swelling occur, but are not as common as in adults.

Diagnosis

Acute sinusitis is a common complication of viral URIs and can usually be diagnosed on clinical grounds alone. Suspect sinusitis if a patient has nasal discharge/congestion and/or daytime cough which persists longer than expected for the typical URI (>10 days), and is not improving, or worsens after five days. Complaints of fever, headache, and cough are variable, and children may not exhibit the classic signs and symptoms of facial tenderness or dental pain. However, observed or reported periorbital swelling or medial infraorbital discoloration of the skin suggests ethmoid sinusitis.

Radiographs are of limited value. Axial/coronal CT scans of the paranasal sinuses are indicated only for patients who have not responded to medical management, or in whom there is concern for intracranial or orbital extension, and may require aspiration or surgical intervention. Transillumination and ultrasound are not helpful.

Various combinations of headache, cough, fever, and nasal discharge can occur with viral URIs, influenza, or pneumonia. Malodorous breath may be secondary to a dental abscess, pharyngitis, or nasal foreign body. Cough-variant asthma usually presents with a nocturnal cough.

ED Management

If the patient has mild persistent symptoms, an additional three days of observation is an appropriate course of action. Otherwise, the antibiotic treatment of acute sinusitis is summarized in Table 6.3; prescribe a 14–21-day course. Amoxicillin is the first-line choice. In addition, prescribe a topical nasal vasoconstrictor (oxymetazoline bid) for 48 hours, but do not use decongestants or H_1 antihistamines. Treat a patient who has recurrent sinusitis (>3–4 episodes/year) with a topical nasal steroid, such as budesonide, fluticasone, or mometasone, one spray in each nostril daily for 4–6 weeks. Adenoidectomy may be indicated for some patients with recurrent sinusitis refractory to treatment.

Drainage, irrigation, and culture of the paranasal sinuses are indicated for patients who are immunocompromised, unresponsive to medical therapy, toxic, or suffering from one of the rare intracranial complications (brain abscess, subdural empyema, cavernous sinus thrombosis) or an orbital cellulitis. Nasal cultures are of limited value, as they do not accurately predict the pathogen responsible for acute sinusitis.

Admit a patient with acute frontal sinusitis if there is an air-fluid level and moderate to severe pain, and treat with IV antibiotics because of increased risk of intracranial spread. Also admit a patient with sphenoid sinusitis.

Follow-up

- Acute sinusitis: 48–72 hours. If symptoms persist, change to an alternative medication or consult an otolaryngologist for possible parenteral antibiotics and sinus drainage

Indications for Admission

- Acute frontal sinusitis with air-fluid level and moderate to severe pain
- Sphenoid sinusitis
- Systemic toxicity
- Unremitting headache or incapacitating symptoms
- Orbital cellulitis or intracranial complication

Bibliography

Hicks CW, Weber JG, Reid JR, Moodley M. Identifying and managing intracranial complications of sinusitis in children: a retrospective series. *Pediatr Infect Dis J.* 2011;**30**:222–226

Magit A. Pediatric rhinosinusitis. *Otolaryngol Clin North Am.* 2014;**47**(5):733–746.

Shaikh N, Wald ER. Decongestants, antihistamines and nasal irrigation for acute sinusitis in children. *Cochrane Database Syst Rev.* 2014;**10**:CD007909.

Wald ER. Applegate KE, Bordley C, et al. Clinical practice guideline for the diagnosis and management of acute bacterial sinusitis in children aged 1 to 18 years. *Pediatrics.* 2013;**132**(1):e262–280.

Upper Respiratory Infections

Upper respiratory infections are generally mild illnesses caused by numerous organisms. However, if a URI does not resolve within 3–4 days, consider the possibility of other illnesses, such as allergies, otitis media, or sinusitis.

Clinical Presentation

Most often, the patient is afebrile, or has a low-grade temperature, with watery or mucoid rhinorrhea. Sneezing, coughing, and conjunctival injection are other features. Infants may have noisy breathing or decreased ability to feed.

Adrenal Insufficiency — Life threatening defy of Cortisol & Aldosterone. Dental

Diagnosis

Cause — ① Infn - Viral, Bacterial ② Procedure ← surgical

Inquire about fever, cough, appetite, vomiting, diarrhea, treatments given at home, and whether anyone else at home is ill. Perform a complete examination, looking for evidence of bacterial infection such as nasal discharge (sinusitis, allergic rhinitis), otitis media, pharyngitis, and nuchal rigidity (meningitis). Auscultate the lungs for decreased breath sounds or rales (pneumonia) or wheezing (asthma or bronchiolitis).

ED Management

Although there are a myriad of over-the-counter cold remedies, there are few data supporting efficacy. Antihistamine–decongestant combinations available over the counter have been shown to have little effect on the common cold. Recommend rest, fluids, and acetaminophen (15 mg/kg q 4h) or ibuprofen (10 mg/kg q 6h) for fever. For infants, give normal saline nose drops (two drops in one nostril at a time), followed by gentle aspiration with a bulb syringe. A vaporizer may be helpful for all age groups.

Follow-up

- Return to primary care provider if symptoms worsen (toxicity, fever >39.4 °C or 103 °F, ear pain) or do not resolve within 3–4 days.

Bibliography

Hyper aldosteronism — Loss of Na & water retention of K — Hyperkalemia.

Fan Y, Ji P, Leonard-Segal A, Sahajwalla CG. An overview of the pediatric medications for the symptomatic treatment of allergic rhinitis, cough, and cold. *J Pharm Sci.* 2013;**102**(12):4213–4229.

Fashner J, Ericson K, Werner S. Treatment of the common cold in children and adults. *Am Fam Physician.* 2012;**86**(2):153–159.

Isbister GK, Prior F, Kilham HA. Restricting cough and cold medicines in children. *J Paediatr Child Health.* 2012;**48**(2):91–98.

Lowry JA, Leeder JS. Over-the-counter medications: update on cough and cold preparations. *Pediatr Rev.* 2015;**36**(7):286–297.

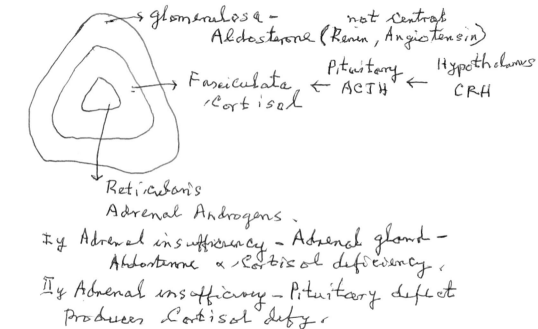

→ glomerulosa — not central
Aldosterone (Renin, Angiotensin)
→ Fasciculata ← ACTH ← CRH
Pituitary   Hypothalamus
Cortisol
Reticularis
Adrenal Androgens.
I y Adrenal insufficiency — Adrenal gland — Aldosterone & Cortisol deficiency.
II y Adrenal insufficiency — Pituitary defect Produces Cortisol defy.

Endocrine Emergencies

Aviva Sopher, Tamar G. Baer, Morri Markowitz, and
Sandra J. Cunningham

Adrenal Insufficiency

The adrenal cortex is divided into three zones: the outermost glomerulosa, which produces aldosterone (mineralocorticoid), the middle fasciculata, which produces cortisol (glucocorticoid), and the innermost reticularis, which produces dehydroepiandrosterone (DHEA) and androstenedione (adrenal androgens). Cortisol production is regulated primarily by pituitary adrenocorticotropic hormone (ACTH) secretion, which in turn is regulated by the hypothalamic release of corticotrophin releasing hormone (CRH).

Lesions of the hypothalamus, pituitary, or adrenal cortex may cause adrenal insufficiency. In general, primary adrenal insufficiency (originating from the adrenal gland) results in inadequate production of both aldosterone and cortisol. Secondary adrenal insufficiency (originating from the pituitary) results in inadequate production of cortisol. Congenital adrenal hyperplasia (CAH), an inherited defect in steroid biosynthesis (most often 21-hydroxylase deficiency), is a relatively common cause. Other etiologies include autoimmune adrenalitis, adrenal hemorrhage in meningococcemia, trauma, HIV infection, tumor, infiltrative disease, tuberculosis, and bilateral adrenalectomy.

Central (hypothalamic or pituitary) adrenal insufficiency may be idiopathic, or secondary to CNS tumors, congenital abnormalities, or trauma. Exogenous steroid therapy is a frequent cause of adrenal insufficiency. Glucocorticoid treatment for more than 7–10 days places the patient at risk. *steroid Rx > 7-10 days can ppte deficiency*

Adrenal insufficiency can result in a life-threatening emergency caused by relative or absolute deficiencies of cortisol and aldosterone. Crisis occurs when the adrenal gland fails to adequately respond to stress with an up to tenfold increase in cortisol secretion. This rise in cortisol secretion is dependent on increased ACTH release. Crisis may be precipitated by bacterial or viral infections, or dental or surgical procedures. Prompt recognition of the presenting symptoms and immediate treatment is imperative. *Cortisol & Aldosterone↓*

Adrenal Insuff'y - Life threatening - due to Infections or Surgical procedures

Clinical Presentation

The initial complaints are often nonspecific. The presentation may be gradual, with subtle complaints such as weakness, fatigue, malaise, anorexia, poor growth, and weight loss. With aldosterone deficiency (as occurs in primary adrenal insufficiency), salt craving may be reported and the blood pressure may be normal or low. Alternatively, there may be an acute presentation, with fever, weakness, lethargy, abdominal pain, nausea, vomiting (possibly

Szes – Hypoglycemia, or Hyponatremia.

bilious), guarding and rebound tenderness, dehydration, hypotension, and/or shock. Seizures, secondary to hypoglycemia or hyponatremia, may also occur. The presentation may also be fulminant, and sudden death can occur.

With primary adrenal insufficiency a subtle physical examination finding is skin hyperpigmentation, most often found on the lips and buccal mucosa, nipples, groin, palmar or axillary creases, and areas of old scars or friction (knees, elbows, knuckles). Skin hyperpigmentation is a sign of increased ACTH secretion, so it does not occur with secondary or tertiary adrenal insufficiency (due to pituitary or hypothalamic disease). Other possible signs include petechiae and purpura (overwhelming sepsis, usually meningococcemia), hypoglycemic seizures (glucocorticoid insufficiency), midline craniofacial malformations (e.g., septo-optic dysplasia, cleft lip/palate, holoprosencephaly), and micropenis (hypopituitarism). Central adrenal insufficiency is often associated with other hypothalamic/pituitary hormone deficiencies, which may manifest as growth failure, delayed pubertal progression, micropenis (secondary to growth hormone deficiency), and, in the case of CNS lesions, diabetes insipidus.

Primary adrenal insufficiency is usually associated with deficient aldosterone production with resultant significant losses of sodium and water and retention of potassium. These patients present with more severe hyponatremia, hyperkalemia, and volume depletion. As aldosterone production is primarily regulated by the renin-angiotensin enzyme system; central secondary or tertiary adrenal insufficiency are not associated with aldosterone deficiency. Autoimmune Addison's disease (a type of primary adrenal insufficiency) may also be associated with mucocutaneous candidiasis, hypothyroidism, hypokalemia, hepatitis, vitiligo, alopecia, and pernicious anemia.

The use of steroids for more than 7–10 days can cause suppression of the patient's endogenous hypothalamic–pituitary–adrenal axis. The abrupt withdrawal of steroids can then result in clinical adrenal insufficiency or acute adrenal crisis, as the patient is unable to mount an ACTH response or respond to ACTH. Acute insufficiency can also occur when there is a physiologic stress (surgery, infection, trauma) without an appropriate increase in the exogenous dose of glucocorticoids.

A female infant with CAH is usually diagnosed soon after birth because of ambiguous genitalia, ranging from mild clitoromegaly to a completely penile urethra with labioscrotal folds. A male infant with CAH typically has normal external genitalia and is therefore not often diagnosed in the immediate newborn period, unless a positive screen is reported. The patient may present at 1–3 weeks of life (or later infancy) with fatigue, poor feeding, and vomiting, resembling the clinical picture of sepsis. Alternatively, there may be a fulminant presentation with dehydration, shock, or sudden death. There may be a family history of consanguinity, CAH, or neonatal deaths. On physical examination, hyperpigmentation (as described above) may be noted, while a completely virilized girl will not have testes detected.

Diagnosis

The key to diagnosing acute adrenal crisis is to maintain a high degree of suspicion, especially in a previously well infant who has mild to moderate illness but deteriorates quickly. The prominent gastrointestinal symptoms of adrenal crisis can resemble gastroenteritis (diarrhea is frequent), an acute abdomen (involuntary guarding and rebound tenderness), and intestinal obstruction (bilious vomiting). An elevated 17-OH progesterone confirms the diagnosis.

If impending or acute adrenal crisis is suspected, do not delay treatment while waiting for confirmatory laboratory tests. Initiate diagnostic testing and treatment simultaneously.

Cortisol deficiency –

Hypoglycemia & (Neutropenia < 5000 WBS)

Obtain blood for CBC, electrolytes, glucose, and serum cortisol, plasma renin activity, ACTH, and aldosterone while establishing IV access.

Acute primary adrenal insufficiency may cause hyponatremia, hypochloremia, and hyperkalemia with peaked T-waves on ECG. Hypoglycemia and neutropenia (WBC $<5000/mm^3$) can occur, although these can also be signs of sepsis. In addition, there is increased plasma renin, increased urinary excretion of sodium if the patient is aldosterone-deficient (i.e., salt-wasters), and decreased urinary excretion of potassium.

Normally, patients in shock have an elevated serum cortisol level (> 15 mcg/dL), but with adrenal insufficiency, the serum cortisol is inappropriately low.

Normally i stress, Serum Cortisol is high > 15 µg/dl. ✶

ED Management   *in Adr. crisis it will be low.*

Once the diagnosis is suspected, therapy includes immediate, aggressive fluid management and steroid replacement. Obtain a fingerstick glucose measurement and assess possible hyperkalemia (aldosterone deficiency or resistance) by looking for peaked T-waves on EKG. Infants with CAH may tolerate hyperkalemia better than older children. If needed, definitive assessment of adrenal function can be performed after the acute emergency has passed. *STRESS dose - HC (Solu-Cortef) IM/IV*

Acute Crisis   *✶) < 3yrs - 25mg, 3-12yrs - 50mg, >12yrs 100mg*

Glucocorticoid Stress Dose   *then Same dose ÷ Q 4H or Q 6H - over 24hrs*

Give a stat dose of hydrocortisone (Solu-Cortef), IV push/IM (0–3 years of age: 25 mg; ≥3–12 years of age: 50 mg; ≥12 years of age: 100 mg), followed by the same dose as a 24-hour IV infusion or div q 4–6h. The response is usually rapid.

Fluid Management   *repeat boluses untill Normotensive. ✶*

Clinical assessment tends to underestimate the severity of the hypovolemia. Consider the patient to be at least 10% dehydrated. Start an IV and give 20 mL/kg of normal saline over 30 minutes. Repeat the boluses until the patient becomes normotensive. Once the blood pressure is normal, continue with D_5 NS for patients with salt-losing adrenal insufficiency. Change non-salt-losers to D_5 ½ NS, if the electrolytes are normal.

Total fluid requirements are in the range of 1.5–2 times maintenance; reassess as therapy continues. Add potassium (10–20 mEq/L) once the patient voids, as the administration of cortisol will rapidly induce kaliuresis and a fall in the serum potassium. If the patient is hypoglycemic (blood glucose <70 mg/dL), give 2–4 mL/kg of D_{10} (maximum dose 25 g), infused slowly at a rate of 2–3 mL/min, and recheck the glucose in 15 minutes. Repeat the D_{10} if the hypoglycemia persists (blood glucose <70 mg/dL).

Shock

If shock persists despite the crystalloid boluses, give a plasma expander, such as plasmanate (20–40 mL/kg) or a vasopressor, such as dopamine (see Shock, pp. 28–36). Vasopressors may be ineffective unless preceded by adequate cortisol replacement.

Mineralocorticoid Replacement

Mineralocorticoid replacement is not necessary during the acute ED treatment because high-dose glucocorticoids interact with mineralocorticoid receptors and normal saline is

Hypoglycemia - < 70 mg%.
Rx D10 W, 2-4 ml/kg at 2-4ml/mte, check glucose in 15 mtes & repeat PRN.

Cortisol induces kaliuresis → Hypokalemia

given (steps 1 and 2). Once the patient is stable and can take oral fluids, give 9α-fluor-ocortisol (Florinef) 0.1–0.3 mg PO to salt-wasters. Supplemental oral sodium may also be necessary.

Underlying Pathology

Identify and treat any underlying cause of the stress. Infections are the most common precipitating factor. *MC*

Complications

ICU monitoring may be necessary, especially if the patient remains comatose or hypotensive, or the underlying pathology takes a fulminant course (sepsis). Complications of excessive fluid, salt, or steroid replacement include hypernatremia, hypokalemia, pulmonary edema, congestive heart failure, and hypervolemia. *PO, IM, IV.*

Stress Dosing in Adrenal Insufficiency *HC 25–50 mg/m^2/day div q6H*

Patient Taking Maintenance Corticosteroids (e.g., Patient With CAH or Addison's Disease)

For a minor illness, such as low-grade fever (<38.8 °C; 102 °F), give 25 mg/m^2 div q 6h of hydrocortisone. A stress dose is not necessary for afebrile patients. For a moderate illness, such as fever ≥102 °F (>38.8 °C), vomiting, anesthesia, or a bacterial infection, give 50 mg/m^2 div q 6h. If the patient cannot tolerate oral medications, give the same dose IM or IV. Admission will be necessary if the patient cannot subsequently tolerate oral steroids.

Patient Taking Pharmacologic Doses of Steroids (for Asthma, Nephrotic Syndrome, ITP, Leukemia, Collagen Vascular Diseases, etc.)   *etc*

Most pharmacologic doses are greater than physiologic doses. However, if the current steroid dose is less than the recommended stress dose (see below), a stress dose is still necessary. If the stress is a serious infection, with an etiology that may be adversely affected by high-dose steroids (such as fungal infection in a patient with cystic fibrosis), consult with pediatric infectious disease and endocrine specialists. If a patient receiving a tapering dose of corticosteroids develops symptoms of adrenal insufficiency, increase the dose to the most recent dose at which he or she was asymptomatic, then initiate a more gradual taper after consulting with a pediatric endocrinologist. *7–10 days or longer*

* Patient Who Has Recently Completed a Steroid Course *in the previous 6 months*

Prev 6 mths A history of completing a 7–10-day, or longer, course of corticosteroids in the previous six months places a patient at risk for developing adrenal insufficiency. If the patient is symptomatic for an acute adrenal crisis, treat as above. If the adrenal status is uncertain, treat for presumed adrenal insufficiency, as noted above.

For all of the above scenarios, continue the oral stress dose, 25–50 mg/m^2 of hydrocortisone for the duration of the stress, and then taper quickly, over 4–7 days, to the previous or maintenance dose. If the patient has symptoms of adrenal insufficiency during a taper, the tapering schedule may be too rapid. Increase the dose to the most recent dose at which the patient was asymptomatic. Then, initiate a more gradual taper after consulting with a pediatric endocrinologist.

Oral stress dose – Hydrocortisone
? 25–50 mg/m^2
? Per day – duration of stress   HC
then taper over 4–8 days.

Infant - 25 mg, child 50 mg, Adult 100 mg

Advise the family of a steroid-dependent child to obtain and wear a MedicAlert bracelet or carry a card that indicates the presence of adrenal insufficiency, the current steroid dose (as well as the indication and the steroid doses that should be used for stress), and the prescribing physician's name and contact numbers. In addition, instruct the family members and/or caretakers to administer emergency intramuscular hydrocortisone (infant 25 mg, child 50 mg, adult 100 mg) in the event the patient has persistent vomiting or altered mental status. Remind the caretakers to check expiration dates, new prescriptions, and to have the hydrocortisone easily available in the event of an emergency.

Follow-up

- Stress doses of hydrocortisone required: daily, until the stress has resolved

Indications for Admission

- Addisonian or adrenal crisis
- Vomiting, inadequate oral intake, or postural vital sign changes in a patient known to be at risk for adrenal insufficiency
- Medication compliance at home is uncertain
- Electrolyte abnormalities

Bibliography

Auron M, Raissouni N. Adrenal insufficiency. *Pediatr Rev.* 2015;**36**(3):92–102

Bornstein Sr, Allolio B, Arlt W, et al. Diagnosis and treatment of primary adrenal insufficiency: an Endocrine Society Clinical Practice Guideline. *J Clin Endocrinol Metab* 2016;**101**(2):364–389.

Levy-Shraga Y, Pinhas-Hamiel O. Critical illness-related corticosteroid insufficiency in children. *Horm Res Paediatr.* 2013;**80**(5):309–317.

Levy-Shraga Y, Pinhas-Hamiel O. Novel insights into adrenal insufficiency in childhood. *Minerva Pediatr.* 2014;**66**(6):517–532.

Diabetes Insipidus

ADH helps reabsorb water from urine (kidney)

Diabetes insipidus (DI) is characterized by an inability to concentrate urine in the presence of hyperosmolality/hypernatremia. DI can be caused by either vasopressin (ADH) deficiency (central DI) or resistance of the ADH receptor (nephrogenic DI). ADH controls water homeostasis by activating reabsorption of water from urine.

A variety of acquired hypothalamic and pituitary lesions are associated with central DI, including tumors (craniopharyngioma, optic glioma, germinoma), infiltrative disorders (Langerhans cell histiocytosis, sarcoidosis, granulomatous disease), operative trauma to the posterior pituitary gland, autoimmune lymphocytic hypophysitis, drugs (ethanol, phenytoin, opioids, alpha-adrenergics), infections (meningitis/encephalitis), trauma (basilar skull fractures), and vascular lesions (aneurysm). The etiology of central DI may also be genetic, congenital, or idiopathic.

Nephrogenic DI is caused by renal unresponsiveness to ADH. The defect may be congenital or secondary to hypercalcemia, hypokalemia, drugs (lithium, amphotericin, cisplatin, rifampin, methicillin), or chronic renal disease (ureteral obstruction, polycystic kidney disease, renal medullary cystic disease, sickle cell disease).

Nephrogenic - Lyte anomalies
Drugs
, Chr. renal disease.

N-pla -Osm 275-295

ADH Secretion ① ↑plasma Osm ② Dehydration

Normal plasma osmolality ranges between 275 and 295 mOsm/kg. Normally, at a serum osmolality of <280 mOsm/kg, the plasma vasopressin level is ≤1 pg/mL. Above 280 mOsm/kg, the normal threshold for vasopressin release, the plasma vasopressin level rises in proportion to the plasma osmolality, up to a maximum concentration of 20 pg/mL (at a blood osmolality of 320 mOsm/kg). Peak antidiuretic effect is achieved at a vasopressin concentration of 5 pg/mL. *8% loss of blood Volume*

Vasopressin secretion is also induced by hypovolemia, but in contrast to the increases in vasopressin secretion with minor changes in plasma osmolality, no change in vasopressin secretion occurs until the blood volume decreases by approximately 8%. Vasopressin secretion is inhibited by glucocorticoids, so that enhanced vasopressin activity occurs in primary or secondary glucocorticoid insufficiency and contributes to the hyponatremia in these conditions.

Clinical Presentation

Diabetes insipidus causes renal loss of free water, which leads to excessive urine output and thirst. Water loss is compensated for by increasing water intake, so that dehydration is unusual in an awake patient who has free access to water and whose sensation of thirst is intact. Infants, children with developmental delay or altered mental status, and patients whose thirst centers are affected by the primary process (hydrocephalus, postconcussive syndrome) are at an increased risk for hypernatremic dehydration.

An infant with DI is usually irritable but eager to suck, often exhibiting a distinct preference for water over milk and presenting with failure to thrive. An older child commonly presents with polyuria and polydipsia. Nocturia, secondary enuresis, constipation, and a preference for ice water are common. Recurrent episodes of dehydration and hypernatremia can result in poor growth and mental retardation, while polyuria and large volumes of urine can cause dilation of the urinary tract, impaired bladder function, and chronic renal failure.

Central nervous system symptoms, such as irritability, altered consciousness, increased muscle tone, convulsions, and coma can occur secondary to hypernatremia. These findings correlate with the degree and rapidity of the rise in serum sodium.

Na > 145, pl Osm > 300, Urine Osm < 300

Diagnosis
Urine SG < 1010

The cardinal diagnostic features of diabetes insipidus are:

- a high rate of dilute urine flow (urine output >4 mL/kg/h) over at least two hours;
- clinical signs of dehydration (weight loss, hypotension), which may not be as apparent because of the hypernatremia;
- mild to marked degree of serum hypernatremia (>145 mEq/L);
- hyperosmolality (>300 mOsm/kg);
- low urine osmolality (<300 mOsm/kg) and low specific gravity (<1.010), despite a normal or elevated serum osmolality.

If there is severe dehydration or a low glomerular filtration rate, urine output decreases and urine osmolality increases above the serum; this may temporarily obscure the diagnosis.

Other causes of polyuria include psychogenic polydipsia (nocturia unusual), organic polydipsia (hypothalamic lesion), osmotic diuresis (diabetes, IV contrast administration,

Insensible fluid loss = 400-600 mL/m²/day (D_5 ½ NS)

chronic renal insufficiency), hyperglycemia associated with diabetes mellitus, diuretic use, and postoperative diuresis, as well as ADH unresponsiveness due to hypercalcemia or hypokalemia. With a urinary tract infection (pp. 692–696), there will be symptoms such as urgency, frequency, and dysuria. Diabetes insipidus may be distinguished from these other diagnoses by the history, serum and urine electrolytes and osmolality, BUN, and creatinine.

A large urinary volume can lead to bladder distention, which can then mimic obstructive uropathy.

Serum Osm > 300, Urine Osm < 300 suggests DI,

ED Management   *(300)*

If DI is suspected, obtain a basic metabolic panel, serum osmolality, urinalysis and urine culture, urine electrolytes, and urine osmolality. A serum osmolality >300 mOsm/kg with a urine osmolality <300 mOsm/kg are highly suggestive of the diagnosis of DI. Perform a complete neurologic examination, with visual field assessment, if possible. Admit the patient and consult with a pediatric endocrinologist who will initiate vasopressin treatment if the serum sodium is >145 mmol/L and the osmolality is >295 mOsm/kg.

Arrange for an MRI of the pituitary gland with and without gadolinium. Normally, the posterior pituitary is seen as an area of enhanced brightness on T1-weighted images following the administration of gadolinium. This "bright spot" is absent in both central and nephrogenic diabetes insipidus, due to vasopressin deficiency in the former and enhanced vasopressin release in the latter. In primary/psychogenic polydipsia, the posterior bright spot is normal.

Fluid Therapy

DI can be treated with meticulous fluid management, initiated immediately in the ED, once the diagnosis is established. Use a flow sheet to document fluid intake and output, replacement of urine output and insensible losses, vital signs, urine specific gravity, and serum electrolytes. The components of fluid management include:

- insensible fluid loss replacement (400 – 600 mL/m²/day) with D_5 ½ NS;
- urine output replacement, mL per mL, with D_5W or $D_{2.5}$ ¼ NS IV or free water orally;
- correction fluid to lower the serum sodium to the normal range; Use the following equation (over 8–24 h):

$$\text{Volume required(mL)} = 4 \times \text{patient's weight(kg)} \times \left(Na_{current} - Na_{goal}\right).$$

Treatment of DI in Infants

Since the primary source of nutrition in infants is in liquid form, there is a risk of hyponatremia in infants with DI treated with vasopressin or DDAVP. Instead, use a low-solute formula (PM 60/40) or breast milk to reduce urine output by reducing renal solute load.

Treatment of Nephrogenic DI

The goals of therapy are to maintain normal growth and development by providing adequate calories, to decrease urine volume, and to avoid severe dehydration and hyponatremia. Medications used to decrease the polyuria include:

Thiazide Diuretics

Thiazides promote sodium excretion by interfering with sodium reabsorption in the distal tubule of the nephron and by altering inner medullary osmolality. A thiazide plus an amiloride diuretic is the most commonly used combination for the treatment of congenital X-linked nephrogenic diabetes insipidus. Give hydrochlorothiazide (2 mg/kg/day divided bid; 100 mg/day maximum for children, 200 mg/day maximum for adults).

Amiloride Diuretics

Amiloride counteracts the thiazide-induced hypokalemia. The dose is 0.625 mg/kg/day in patients weighing 6–20 kg; in adolescents, give 5–20 mg/day, up to a maximum of 40 mg/24 hours.

Indomethacin

Indomethacin (2 mg/kg/day) enhances proximal tubular sodium and water reabsorption.

Indications for Admission

- New-onset or symptomatic DI
- Hypernatremia
- Inability to drink oral fluids or to keep up with losses
- Titration of dosing

Bibliography

Jain V, Ravindranath A. Diabetes insipidus in children. *J Pediatr Endocrinol Metab*. 2016;**29**(1):39–45.

Leroy C, Karrouz W, Douillard C, et al. Diabetes insipidus. *Ann Endocrinol (Paris)*. 2013;**74**(5–6):496–507.

Ooi HL, Maguire AM, Ambler GR. Desmopressin administration in children with central diabetes insipidus: a retrospective review. *J Pediatr Endocrinol Metab*. 2013;**26**(11–12):1047–1052.

Qureshi S, Galiveeti S, Bichet DG, Roth J. Diabetes insipidus: celebrating a century of vasopressin therapy. *Endocrinology*. 2014;**155**(12):4605–4621.

Diabetic Ketoacidosis

Diabetic ketoacidosis (DKA) is defined as hyperglycemia (glucose >200 mg/dL), the presence of ketones in the urine or blood, and metabolic acidosis (pH <7.3 or serum bicarbonate <15 mEq/L). DKA may be the initial presentation of new-onset type 1 diabetes mellitus (DM) or a complication in a previously diagnosed patient. DKA occurs less frequently in patients with type 2 DM. Infection is the most common precipitating factor, but trauma, pregnancy, emotional stress, and noncompliance are other causes. An absolute or relative insulin deficiency is present, along with increased levels of counterregulatory hormones (glucagon, cortisol, growth hormone, and catecholamines), leading to deranged metabolism, hyperglycemia, osmotic diuresis, hypertonic dehydration, and finally, ketoacidosis. In ketoacidosis, the acidosis is secondary to ketonemia with β-hydroxybutyrate and its redox partner, acetoacetate.

Table 7.1 Differential diagnosis of DKA

Coma	Ketonuria (without hyperglycemia)
CNS trauma, infection, bleeding	Anorexia of any etiology
Hypoglycemia	Fasting states
Lactic acidosis	Gastroenteritis with vomiting
Nonketotic hyperosmolar coma	Salicylate poisoning
Sedative-hypnotic or narcotic overdose	
Hyperglycemia	**Metabolic acidosis**
Hypernatremia	Salicylate poisoning
Iron toxicity	Severe gastroenteritis with hypovolemia
Salicylate poisoning (glucose <300 mg/dL)	Other ingestions: ethanol, ethylene glycol, iron, isoniazid, methanol
Sepsis	
Stress	

Clinical Presentation

The patient usually presents with abdominal pain, nausea, vomiting, dehydration, fatigue, and hyperpnea. Isolated vomiting can also be a presentation of DKA. The history often reveals polydypsia, polyuria, nocturia, enuresis, and, with new-onset diabetes, recent weight loss or lack of weight gain in a growing child. Characteristic Kussmaul breathing (deep sighing breathing) can be present, but the respirations may be depressed if the patient is severely acidotic (pH ≤6.9). Neurologic findings range from drowsiness to coma and are related to the level of hyperosmolality and the degree of volume depletion and acidosis.

DKA is categorized as mild (pH 7.2–7.3), moderate (pH 7.1–7.2), or severe (pH <7.1)

Diagnosis

In the known diabetic, consider DKA when the patient complains of abdominal pain, vomiting, or malaise. The diagnosis may be more difficult to make in a patient presenting for the first time (Table 7.1). In addition to acidosis and ketonemia, significant hyperglycemia (>500 mg/dL) is common, although DKA can occur with a glucose of 200–300 mg/dL.

In DKA, sodium stores are depleted but serum sodium may be low, normal, or high, depending on the water balance. The measured sodium is lower than the true value because of the shift of water into the extracellular space (sodium decreases 1.6 mEq/L per each 100 mg/dL rise in glucose over 100 mg/dL) and the increase in serum lipid and protein levels (pseudohyponatremia). In addition, the low sodium level may reflect water retention secondary to increased secretion of antidiuretic hormone.

While there is usually a total body potassium deficit, the initial serum potassium concentration may be normal or elevated because of hyperosmolality, insulin deficiency, and the shifting of potassium into the extracellular space. A low initial potassium level (<3.5 mEq/L) is an unusual and ominous finding.

Finally, in the absence of infection, the WBC count may be elevated (18,000–20,000/mm^3), secondary to the increase in circulating catecholamines and hemoconcentration.

ED Management

After a rapid evaluation of the patient's status, initiate therapy to correct fluid deficits, electrolyte imbalances, acidosis, and hyperglycemia. Avoid overly vigorous management, which can cause excessively rapid changes in glucose, osmolality, and pH, and therefore contribute to the development of complications, such as cerebral edema. Treat any concomitant pathology or complications (sepsis, increased ICP, or coma).

History

Determine the duration of the current illness and any precipitating factors such as infection, trauma, or stress. If the patient is a known diabetic, document the current insulin regimen (and adherence) and the time of the last injection.

Physical Examination

Focus the examination on the vital signs (including the presence of Kussmaul respirations), degree of dehydration, level of consciousness, fundoscopic examination, and possible sites of infection. Document the vital signs and neurologic status at least hourly.

Initial Laboratory Evaluation

Obtain blood for STAT glucose, electrolytes, BUN, creatinine, lactate, calcium, phosphorous, osmolality, beta-hydroxybutyrate, pH (venous or arterial), CBC, HgbA1c, and a bedside fingerstick glucose measurement. Also obtain a urinalysis and an ECG (check for peaked T-waves). Prior to beginning insulin therapy for a patient with new-onset diabetes, send additional blood for insulin, C-peptide, thyroid autoantibody titers and relevant autoantibodies (insulin autoantibodies [IAA], islet cell antibodies [ICA], and glutamic decarboxylase antibodies [GAD]). Also obtain blood cultures if infection is suspected.

Initial Management

Place the patient on a cardiorespiratory monitor and start and maintain a flow sheet. Perform a rapid assessment of level of consciousness and evaluate for signs of cerebral edema; repeat at least hourly. In general, the goals are slow, steady rehydration over 48 hours, a decrease in the serum glucose of 80–100 mg/dL/h, and a stable corrected sodium while the measured sodium increases.

Fluid Resuscitation

A patient with DKA has some degree of dehydration. However, significant dehydration can exist and the patient will continue to urinate until intravascular volume depletion affects the glomerular filtration rate. If available, the difference between a premorbid weight and present weight provides the best assessment of volume depletion. In general, a child with moderate to severe DKA is at least 7–10% dehydrated.

Insert two IV catheters so that maintenance and replacement fluids and the insulin drip can be managed separately. Initially, administer an isotonic saline fluid bolus (20 mL/kg) over approximately 60 minutes. Reassess the patient after the initial bolus (peripheral pulses, capillary refill) and repeat, if necessary, in order to maintain adequate peripheral perfusion.

Deficit Fluids

Calculate deficit fluids using recent weight loss or an estimation of percentage dehydration. Replace the total deficit with normal saline, divided evenly over 24–48 hours. Use a slower rate (over 48 hours) of fluid replacement for children under two years, or if there is severe acidosis, an elevated corrected sodium, significant hyperosmolality (>350 mOsm/kg), or a long prodromal illness. Subtract the amount of fluid given as a fluid bolus from the total deficit.

Maintenance Fluids

Calculate the daily maintenance fluid requirements and administer as normal saline. Replacement of ongoing losses may be necessary, especially if there is polyuria (>5 mL/kg/h). For a polyuric patient, measure the urinary losses every 4–8 hours, and then replace half of this volume over the next 4–8 hours with ½ NS in a separate "piggy-back" line. Also replace the volume of vomitus with ½ NS in this line.

Potassium

Correction of the acidosis will exacerbate the hypokalemia. If the serum potassium is <5.0 mEq/L, add 20 mEq K acetate/L and 20 mEq K phosphate/L, *once urine output is documented*. If a serum potassium level is unavailable, obtain an ECG to look for evidence of hyperkalemia (peaked T-waves, shortened QT interval) or hypokalemia (flattened T-waves, widened QT interval). If the patient is hypocalcemic, use KCL instead of K phosphate. Measure the phosphorus and calcium every 4–6 hours and repeat the ECG every 2–4 hours.

Insulin and Glucose

After the initial fluid resuscitation, begin an insulin drip with the goal of decreasing the blood sugar by 80–100 mg/dL/h. Start the insulin drip at 0.1 units/kg/h. Do not give an insulin bolus. Add 100 units of regular insulin to 100 mL of normal saline (resultant concentration = 1 unit/mL), and infuse at 0.1 mL/kg/h. Prior to running the drip, allow 50 mL of the mixture to flow through the IV in order to saturate insulin binding sites in the tubing. Start the insulin drip at 0.05 units/kg/h if the patient is markedly hyperglycemic (glucose >1000 mg/dL), is under two years of age, or has recently received a subcutaneous dose of insulin.

Add D_5 to the fluids when the glucose reaches 250–300 mg/dL, but continue the insulin infusion. Adjust the rate of the drip to maintain a blood glucose of 120–180 mg/dL. Lower the rate by one-half (0.5 units/kg/h) if the glucose is falling below this level. If the patient is becoming hypoglycemic at this rate, increase the dextrose in the IV solution to $D_{7.5}$–$D_{12.5}$. Calculate the glucose requirement per unit of insulin; most patients require 3–5 g of glucose/unit of insulin. Once the acidosis is resolved (pH >7.30, bicarbonate >15 mEq/L) and the patient can tolerate a PO diet, begin subcutaneous insulin. Stop the insulin drip one hour after the subcutaneous insulin dose.

Bicarbonate

Do not use sodium bicarbonate unless the venous pH is <6.9 with associated hemodynamic compromise. The dose is 0.5–1 mEq/kg by IV infusion over one hour, *not as an IV push*. Mix a 50 mL ampule of sodium bicarbonate with 250 mL sterile water to create a concentration of 44 mEq/300 mL.

Example Calculation

Patient with DKA who weighs 40 kg and has 10% dehydration:

Initial Fluid Bolus

$$20 \text{ mL/kg} = 800 \text{ mL}$$

Fluid Deficit

$$10\% \text{ of } 40 \text{ kg} = 4 \text{ kg}(= 4L \text{ or} 4000 \text{ mL of fluid loss})$$
$$4000 \text{ mL(fluid deficit)} - 800 \text{ mL(initial fluid bolus)} = 3200 \text{ mL}$$
$$3200 \text{ mL divided over 48 hours} = 66 \text{ mL/h}$$

Maintenance Fluids

$$40 \text{ kg patient maintenance} = 1900 \text{ mL/day}$$
$$1900 \text{ mL divided over 24 hours} = 79 \text{ mL/h}$$

Insulin

$$0.1 \text{ units/kg/h} = 4 \text{ mL/h}$$

Initial Fluids

$$(\text{Deficit} - \text{bolus}) + (\text{maintenance}) = 145 \text{ mL/h normal saline} + 20 \text{ mEqK}$$
$$\text{phosphate/L} + 20 \text{ mEqK acetate/L}$$

Continue normal saline until the osmolality is <310 mOsm/kg and the sodium rises to approximately 140 mEq/L as the blood sugar falls, then change to ½ NS. However, if the corrected sodium is >160 mEq/L, consult with a pediatric endocrinologist and use a lower sodium concentration in the IV fluid.

Laboratory Assessments

Repeat the glucose and venous pH hourly. Obtain electrolytes, osmolality, BUN, and creatinine every two hours until the trend is normalizing, then every four hours until normal. Calculate the corrected sodium with each set of laboratory values:

Corrected sodium = measured sodium + 1.6 × [(measured glucos e − 100)/100]

Obtain calcium and phosphorus levels every 4–6 hours until the DKA is resolving. Obtain an ECG every 2–4 hours, looking for peaked T-waves (hyperkalemia).

Even with meticulous care, a patient with DKA is at risk for developing cerebral edema. Risk factors include age under three years, an elevated BUN, severe acidosis, and failure of the serum sodium to rise as expected as the glucose falls. Signs and symptoms of increased ICP (pp. 527–529) classically occur 6–18 hours into treatment and include headache, vomiting, lethargy, disorientation, fundoscopic changes (absent venous pulsations, blurring of optic disk margins), and decorticate or decerebrate posturing. Any neurologic signs at presentation, *prior* to treatment, reflect the patient's hyperosmolality.

If the patient complains of headache and becomes lethargic *during* treatment, but has a normal fundoscopic examination, obtain a stat CT scan of the head. If the patient is unresponsive, posturing, has pupillary changes, or has milder symptoms with fundoscopic abnormalities, immediately treat for increased intracranial pressure (pp. 527–529) with mannitol 1 g/kg IV over ten minutes, endotracheal intubation if airway protection is compromised because of the patient's mental status, and elevation of the head to 30°. Alternatively, use 3% saline, 5 mL/kg over 30 minutes.

Also observe the patient for other problems associated with therapy for DKA, such as fluid overload with edema or CHF.

Management of Mild DKA (pH >7.2)

Administer a normal saline bolus (20 mL/kg), if needed (as above). If the patient is not dehydrated, give ½ NS at a maintenance rate plus deficit (based on clinical examination and recent weight loss). Give a known diabetic subcutaneous regular insulin (usually 0.1 unit/kg). In the case of a new-onset diabetic not in DKA, treat with appropriate hydration and consult with a pediatric endocrinologist. Do not treat with insulin until after consultation, as such a patient is particularly sensitive to exogenous insulin. Obtain baseline measurements of serum insulin, C-peptide, HbA_{1c}, IAA, ICA, GAD antibodies, and thyroid function tests.

Hyperglycemia During Stress

Hyperglycemia may occur in response to stress, such as sepsis or corticosteroid administration, although most patients with stress do not become hyperglycemic. Diabetes cannot be definitively diagnosed during another illness, but the patient requires close follow-up. Obtain IAA, ICA, and GAD antibodies to evaluate the risk of type 1 diabetes, which is greater in a child with positive antibodies, with or without known relatives with diabetes. Refer a patient with any positive antibody test to a pediatric endocrinologist, in about six weeks, for evaluation of glucose tolerance.

Type 2 Diabetes

Type 2 diabetes is increasing in frequency among children, though it is more commonly an incidental finding than the cause for an ED visit. It is characterized by insulin resistance and relative insulin hyposecretion. Patients can present with polydipsia, polyuria, and polyphagia, and infrequently weight loss. However, ketosis and/or acidosis are rare, unless the patient presents with a significant infection. Alternatively, glucosuria or hyperglycemia may be noted as incidental findings.

A patient with type 2 diabetes is usually obese and frequently has acanthosis nigricans, most commonly on the posterior neck, but lesions may also be found on the anterior neck, the axillae, and in the groin. The blood sugar is >200 mg/dL and the fasting glucose is >125 mg/dL. Management depends on the severity of presentation; a dehydrated patient requires IV fluid and a ketotic patient needs insulin. Also give insulin to a patient who remains hyperglycemic after a bolus of normal saline. Consult with a pediatric endocrinologist to determine whether treatment with an oral agent is indicated.

Hyperosmolar hyperglycemic state (HHS) is a serious complication of type 2 DM, with a mortality rate of 10–20%. It is characterized by hyperosmolarity, hyperglycemia, dehydration, and minimal ketoacidosis. Hyperosmolar hyperglycemic state can be the initial presentation of type 2 DM or can occur in patients with a known history of type 2 DM during an intercurrent illness. Unlike DKA, the onset is more insidious and patients may initially present with nonspecific flu-like symptoms. Plasma glucose levels (>600 mg/dL), as well as serum osmolality (>320 mOsm/kg) are significantly elevated. The bicarbonate level is generally >15 mEq/L, the venous pH >7.30, and urine and serum ketones are small or absent. Neurologic features are prominent, including stupor and coma. Volume depletion in HHS is greater than in DKA, requiring aggressive fluid resuscitation with normal saline. Although many patients with HHS will respond to fluids alone, administer IV insulin as in DKA to facilitate correction of the hyperglycemia. Do not give insulin without adequate fluid resuscitation. Correct electrolyte imbalances as in DKA, and assess the patient for an underlying infection.

Follow-up
- Mild DKA in a known diabetic when compliance and follow-up can be assured: 1–2 days
- Stress hyperglycemia with positive antibody test: endocrinology follow-up in six weeks

Indications for Admission
- Newly diagnosed diabetes
- Moderate or severe DKA
- Known diabetic with an intercurrent illness which limits oral rehydration or therapy (nausea and vomiting)
- HHS

Bibliography

Decourcey DD, Steil GM, Wypij D, Agus MS. Increasing use of hypertonic saline over mannitol in the treatment of symptomatic cerebral edema in pediatric diabetic ketoacidosis: an 11-year retrospective analysis of mortality. *Pediatr Crit Care Med.* 2013;**14**:694–700.

Nallasamy K, Jayashree M, Singhi S, Bansal A. Low-dose vs standard-dose insulin in pediatric diabetic ketoacidosis: a randomized clinical trial. *JAMA Pediatr.* 2014;**168**(11): 999–1005.

Olivieri L, Chasm R. Diabetic ketoacidosis in the pediatric emergency department. *Emerg Med Clin North Am.* 2013;**31**(3):755–773.

Wolfsdorf JI, Allgrove J, Craig ME, et al. ISPAD Clinical Practice Consensus Guidelines 2014: diabetic ketoacidosis and hyperglycemic hyperosmolar state. *Pediatric Diabetes.* 2014;**15**(Suppl. 20):154–179.

Hypercalcemia

Although serum calcium levels vary somewhat by patient age and laboratory, hypercalcemia is generally accepted to be a serum calcium >11 mg/dL or a blood ionized calcium >5.5 mg/dL (1.4 mmol/L). In contrast to hypocalcemia, hypercalcemia is uncommon in children.

Clinical Presentation

Patients with serum calcium levels <12 mg/dL are often asymptomatic. The hallmark symptoms of hypercalcemia are pain, weakness, and cognitive impairment. The pain may be gastrointestinal in origin, accompanied by nausea, vomiting, and constipation. In addition, there may be renal colic caused by genitourinary stone formation, with or without hematuria. Finally, the patient may have osteolytic bone lesions.

Neurologic symptoms can range from confusion or agitation to stupor and coma, with weakness eventually including the respiratory muscles. Since calcium acts as an antidiuretic hormone (ADH) antagonist, the patient may have polyuria, polydypsia, and dehydration. Long-standing hypercalcemia may lead to band keratopathy. An uncommon sign of hypercalcemia in children is hypertension.

In Williams Syndrome, hypercalcemia may be associated with elfin facies (upturned nose, long philtrum, hypotelorism, receding chin), full lips, stellate pattern of the iris with blue eyes, strabismus, medial flare of the eyebrows, supravalvular aortic stenosis, and mental retardation. In these patients the hypercalcemia usually resolves a year or two after birth.

Diagnosis

The diagnosis of hypercalcemia is confirmed by documenting either a high ionized calcium concentration or an elevated serum calcium level in the absence of a high serum protein level. Associated serum laboratory abnormalities may include any of the following: decreased phosphorus or bicarbonate; increased BUN, alkaline phosphatase, PTH, 25-hydroxyvitamin D, 1,25-dihydroxyvitamin D, PTHrP, thyroid hormones, or vitamin A level. Urine findings may include an elevated pH (≥ 7.0), calciuria, phosphaturia, and aminoaciduria. Radiographs may reveal generalized bone demineralization, bone tumors, resorption of subperiosteal bone in distal phalanges, nephrocalcinosis, or renal stones.

ED Management

If the serum calcium is >12.0 mg/dL or the patient is symptomatic with a calcium between 11–12 mg/dL, consult a pediatric endocrinologist and begin treatment after obtaining the blood tests noted above. Many hypercalcemic patients are dehydrated at presentation, so that calcium levels may decline solely with rehydration. If the patient remains hypercalcemic, increase calciuresis by giving IV normal saline at 2–3 times maintenance rates. Adding furosemide (1 mg/kg IV q 6h) may be effective, but first ensure adequate hydration, otherwise the hypercalcemia can worsen. Check the serum electrolytes at least every six hours during this aggressive stage of therapy. Dialysis is indicated for renal failure.

For patients that are being hospitalized for treatment of hypercalcemia, other treatment modalities an endocrinologist might prescribe include corticosteroids, which are particularly efficacious in malignancies and hypervitaminosis D; calcitonin, which is most effective in cases of immobilization or other causes of bone resorption; and bisphosphonates, which are the most effective agents at reducing bone resorption and calcium levels.

Indications for Admission

- Treatment required for hypercalcemia

Bibliography

Davies JH. Approach to the child with hypercalcaemia. *Endocr Dev.* 2015;**28**:101–118.

McNeilly JD, Boal R, Shaikh MG, Ahmed SF. Frequency and aetiology of hypercalcaemia. *Arch Dis Child.* 2016;**101**(4):344–347.

Minisola S, Pepe J, Piemonte S, Cipriani C. The diagnosis and management of hypercalcaemia. *BMJ.* 2015;**350**:h2723.

Reynolds BC, Cheetham TD. Bones, stones, moans and groans: hypercalcaemia revisited. *ArchDis Child Educ Pract Ed*. 2015;**100**(1):44–51.

Hyperkalemia

Hyperkalemia is defined as a serum potassium ≥5.5 mEq/L, although in infants up to 6.0 mEq/L is normal. In general, elevated potassium occurs secondary to increased potassium intake, transcellular shifts of potassium and/or decreased potassium excretion. Prompt recognition and management of hyperkalemia is critical in order to prevent lethal cardiac arrhythmias.

The most common causes of hyperkalemia are metabolic acidosis with insulin deficiency as seen in DKA, and acute kidney injury, such as acute glomerulonephritis and acute tubular necrosis. Other etiologies of hyperkalemia include adrenal insufficiency, hypoaldosteronism, chronic renal failure, hypovolemia, ingestions (beta-blocker, digoxin), cytotoxic chemotherapy, tumor lysis syndrome, medication side effects (succinylcholine, ACE inhibitors), trauma, rhabdomyolysis, and familial periodic paralysis. Most often an elevated potassium level reflects pseudohyperkalemia caused by hemolysis or in association with thrombocytosis or leukocytosis.

Clinical Presentation

A patient with a serum potassium <6.0 mEq/L is usually asymptomatic. At higher levels there may be muscle weakness, paresthesias, and flaccid paralysis, associated with asymptomatic ECG changes (see below). At a serum potassium >7.0 mEq/L there is a risk of ventricular arrhythmias, which are more likely if there is associated hyponatremia, hypocalcemia, or acidosis.

Diagnosis

If the potassium is ≥6.0 mEq/L, immediately obtain an ECG to identify cardiac conduction abnormalities such as peaked T-waves (T-wave > one-half the R- or S-wave) and a shortened QT interval. Later changes (K^+ >6.5–7.0 mEq/L) may include flattening of the P-wave, lengthening of the PR interval, and widening of the QRS complex.

ED Management

The treatment of hyperkalemia involves increasing cellular uptake of potassium and enhancing potassium excretion through either the gastrointestinal tract or kidneys. Aggressive intravenous therapy is necessary for patients who are symptomatic (muscle weakness, cramps, etc.) or have ECG changes (>7.0 mEq/L). Prompt treatment is crucial to protect the myocardium, as the potassium-lowering effects of the other therapies are not immediately effectively. Give 10% calcium gluconate (60 mg/kg = 0.6 mL/kg, 20 mL maximum) by slow IV infusion over 3–5 minutes.

Increasing Cellular Uptake of Potassium

Glucose and Insulin

Give both 0.5–1 g/kg of glucose (2–4 mL/kg of a 25% dextrose solution) over 30 minutes *and* regular insulin (1 unit per 5 g of glucose given) in separate intravenous lines. The potassium-lowering effect of insulin occurs within 10–20 minutes. Serum glucose must be monitored closely for hyper- or hypoglycemia.

Nebulized β-Agonists

Beta-agonists, such as albuterol, are effective at shifting potassium into cells with a peak in about 40–80 minutes, but they are less predictable than other therapies. Treat with 10–20 mg in 4 mL normal saline (4–8 times the dose used for the treatment of asthma). This treatment can be administered simultaneously with the glucose and insulin.

Sodium Bicarbonate

Sodium bicarbonate is indicated if there is acute hypovolemia and metabolic acidosis. Give 1 mEq/kg (50 mEq maximum dose) IV over 10–15 minutes. Use 1 mL/kg of an 8.4% solution, except for patients <6 months of age (2 mL/kg of a 4.2% solution).

Enhancing Potassium Excretion

Kayexalate

In the absence of peaked T-waves, treat with polystyrene sulfonate (Kayexalate), 1 g/kg dissolved in 4 mL of water, with sorbitol (PO or PR). This dose lowers the serum potassium by 0.5–1 mEq/L by enhancing gastrointestinal excretion, but the onset is slow and duration is variable.

Furosemide

If the patient is not anuric, treat with furosemide (1–2 mg/kg q 6h). The onset of action is within one hour.

Special Considerations

Acute Kidney Injury

Dialysis is indicated if the patient has life-threatening hyperkalemia (serum potassium >7 mEq/L).

Diabetic Ketoacidosis (DKA)

Although patients in DKA may have normal or elevated potassium levels, they are almost always total body potassium depleted. In addition, administering insulin and correction of acidosis will drive potassium into cells and cause hypokalemia if potassium is not added to fluids. Therefore, if the serum potassium is <5.0 mEq/L, add 20 mEq K acetate/L and 20 mEq K phosphate/L, once urine output is documented.

Adrenal Insufficiency

Mild hyperkalemia (and hyponatremia) will generally correct with initiation of stress dose hydrocortisone treatment, although in more severe cases of hyperkalemia the treatments mentioned earlier in this section may be necessary.

Indications for Admission

- Hyperkalemia with clinical symptoms and/or ECG changes
- Diabetic ketoacidosis

Hypertonicity stimulates (1) ADH (2) Thirst.

- Hyperkalemia requiring dialysis
- Severe hyperkalemia (K^+ >7.0 mEq/L)

Bibliography

Auron M, Raissouni N. Adrenal insufficiency. *Pediatr Rev.* 2015;36(3):92–102.

Chime NO, Luo X, McNamara L, Nishisaki A, Hunt EA. A survey demonstrating lack of consensus on the sequence of medications for treatment of hyperkalemia among pediatric critical care providers. *Pediatr Crit Care Med.* 2015;**16**(5):404–409.

Clausen T. Hormonal and pharmacological modification of plasma potassium homeostasis. *Fundam Clin Pharmacol.* 2010;**24**(5):595–605.

Daly K, Farrington E. Hypokalemia and hyperkalemia in infants and children: pathophysiology and treatment. *J Pediatr Health Care.* 2013;**27**(6):486–496

Hypernatremia   *Na ≥ 145.*

Hypernatremia is defined as a serum sodium level ≥145 mmol/L, and occurs when there is a relative excess of sodium compared to water in the body. Hypernatremia is generally caused by dehydration when water loss exceeds salt loss but can also be caused by excessive intake of sodium. Normally, hypertonicity stimulates both the secretion of ADH and an extremely powerful compensatory thirst, which can keep up with as much as 15–20 L of pure water loss.

Patients with adipsic hypernatremia do not feel the urge to drink fluids even in the presence of hyperosmolar dehydration due to a disruption in the regulation of thirst by the osmosensor. The hypernatremia in these patients is accelerated by events such as gastroenteritis, fever, or excessive sweating. A disordered thirst mechanism can occur in approximately 10% of patients with central diabetes insipidus. Adipsic hypernatremia can occur with malformations of the brain (holoprosencephaly, hypoplasia of the corpus callosum), vascular lesions, neoplasms, AIDS, cytomegalovirus encephalitis, pseudotumor cerebri, and empty sella turcica.

Regardless of the etiology, acute hypernatremia has a mortality of 10–70%. CNS morbidity has been reported in up to two-thirds of patients, although it is unclear whether this is a result of the primary disease or the treatment.

Classification of Hypernatremia

Classification of hypernatremia is generally based on the balance between total body sodium and total body water.

Low Na, Lower Water,

Low Total Body Sodium (TBNa); Lower Total Body Water (TBW)

Most often, this form of hypernatremia occurs in the setting of hypernatremic dehydration in infants, usually secondary to gastrointestinal losses. Osmotic diuretics (glucose, mannitol, urea) can also cause water loss in excess of salt loss.

Normal TBNa; Low TBW   *DI, ↓Thirst, ↑ Insensible Loss, Tachypnea, Restricted access*

Central and nephrogenic DI cause excessive renal water loss. In central DI caused by trauma, hydrocephalus, or neoplasia there may be a concomitant derangement in the thirst mechanism, further predisposing to hypernatremia. Increased insensible losses (hypermetabolic states with fever) and tachypnea can also result in hypernatremia, while restricted access to water (infants, developmentally impaired children, bedridden patients) is another risk factor.

Increased TBNa; Normal TBW (Uncommon)

Primary hyperaldosteronism, Cushing's syndrome, and salt poisoning (inappropriately mixed infant formula, salt tablet ingestion, iatrogenic sodium bicarbonate administration) result in excess body sodium. Except in the case of salt poisoning, very high serum sodium levels are unusual.

Clinical Presentation

The clinical signs and symptoms of hypernatremia result from the physiologic response to serum hypertonicity. Most conscious patients will experience voracious thirst, and will drink water as long as they have free access to it. If ADH action and oral water intake do not adequately compensate, serum hypertonicity ensues. Brain cells shrink in a hypertonic environment, leading to CNS signs and symptoms. Lethargy, alternating with irritability, and a high-pitched cry (infants) occur early and are followed by tremors, ataxia, muscle twitching, tonic spasms, seizures (both focal and generalized), and ultimately coma.

Physical signs may include hypertonia, hyperreflexia, and nuchal rigidity (secondary to hypertonia). Since intracellular fluid shifts extracellularly, the intravascular volume is maintained, so that signs of intravascular volume depletion are late findings. Chvostek's sign may occasionally be elicited, and a smooth, velvety, or doughy feel to the skin may be noted. Focal neurologic findings suggest the possibility of CNS hemorrhage as a sequela of brain shrinkage.

A patient with hypernatremia associated with DI may not have signs of intravascular depletion and dehydration if the thirst mechanism and access to water are preserved.

Salt poisoning may cause pulmonary edema (tachypnea, hepatomegaly, rales) and acute CNS pathology without signs of intravascular depletion. Primary hyperaldosteronism is associated with weakness, headaches, and hypokalemia.

An infant exposed to extreme heat and humidity is at risk for hypernatremic dehydration due to limited access to water. Always consider child abuse or neglect in such cases.

Diagnosis

Hypernatremia is usually discovered incidentally when electrolytes are obtained because of gastroenteritis, fever, altered mental status, seizures, polyuria, or polydipsia. In general, since the presentation of hypernatremia is nonspecific, early diagnosis requires a high index of suspicion. Consider hypernatremia if the skin has a velvety, doughy feel, or if the clinical history fits the common etiologies.

If increased total body sodium from improper feeding technique is suspected, obtain some of the infant formula from the home and send it to the company and/or laboratory for evaluation. Also, watch how the caregiver prepares powdered formula and/or dilutes concentrated formula.

Once hypernatremia is documented, use the urine osmolality and urine sodium to categorize the patient (Table 7.2).

ED Management

Be judicious in the fluid management of any patient with an electrolyte abnormality, as rapid correction carries its own risks, such as cerebral edema. If there are signs of intravascular depletion (resting tachycardia, orthostatic vital sign changes, weak peripheral pulses,

Table 7.2 Diagnosis of hypernatremia

TNBA[a]	TBW[b]	Urine osmolality	Urine sodium
Low	Lower		
	GI losses (>800 mOsm/kg)	Hypertonic	<10 mEq/L (low)
	Osmotic diuresis	Hypertonic	>20 mEq/L (high)
Normal	Low		
	Diabetes insipidus	Isotonic/hypotonic	Variable
	Insensible losses	Hypertonic	Variable
Increased	Low/high		
	Salt poisoning	Isotonic/hypertonic	>20 mEq/L (high)

[a] TBNa: total body sodium.
[b] TBW: total body water.

Hyperglycemia & Hypocalcemia accompany - Hypernatremia.

poor capillary refill), give repeated boluses of 20 mL/kg of isotonic crystalloid (normal saline, Ringer's lactate) until perfusion is normalized. Hypernatremia is not a contraindication to using isotonic fluids, as these are hypotonic relative to the patient's serum, so the hypernatremia will not be exacerbated.

Hyperglycemia and hypocalcemia often accompany hypernatremia. Once the intravascular volume has been restored, obtain a CBC, electrolytes, glucose, calcium, creatinine, urinalysis, urine sodium and osmolality, and any other laboratory tests pertinent to the patient's presentation.

TBNa and TBW Depletion

In hypernatremic dehydration, the key to therapy is restoration of isotonicity gradually in order to avoid a rapid fluid shift into brain cells. Otherwise, cerebral edema can ensue. First, give normal saline boluses until perfusion is normalized (as above). Estimate the free water deficit using the formula:

Free H_2O deficit (L) = [(Serum sodium level − 140)/140] × Weight (kg) × 0.6.

An alternative method of calculation is:

$$4 \times \text{weight (kg)} \times [(\text{Sodium current}) - (\text{Sodium goal})]$$

Replace the water deficit over 48 hours, using D_5 ½ NS with one ampule of 10% calcium gluconate added per 500 mL of replacement fluid. Also add 40 mEq/L of potassium acetate after adequate urinary output is established. Replace ongoing losses simultaneously while closely monitoring the clinical status and serum electrolytes. The goal is a slow fall in the serum sodium of 0.5–1.0 mEq/h. Measure the sodium and glucose hourly to document the rate of sodium correction, and follow the calcium and potassium every 2–4 hours until normal levels are documented or the replacement is nearly complete.

D_5 ½ NS
1 Ampule Ca gluconate/500 ml fluid
+ K-acetate 40 mEq/L after urination

Replace H_2O deficit over 48 hrs.
also replace ongoing loss
Na Correction 0.5-1.0 mEq/hour

TBNa Normal; TBW Depleted

Give insensible fluid loss of 400–600 mL/m^2/day as ½ NS. Additionally, give mL for mL urine output replacement as D_5 ¼ NS IV or free water PO deficit correction (as calculated above) with D_5 ¼ NS over 24 hours. Treat central DI with vasopressin (pp. 177–178).

Increased TBNa/Salt Poisoning

Treat with peritoneal dialysis if the serum sodium is >200 mEq/L or the patient has seizures or is comatose. Otherwise, give NS at a maintenance rate with furosemide (1 mg/kg) to achieve a net loss of sodium in excess of water.

Hypertension may be the presenting sign of a patient with hyperaldosteronism, although malignant hypertension is rare. Consult a pediatric endocrinologist.

Indications for Admission

- Symptomatic hypernatremia
- New-onset DI
- Severe dehydration

Bibliography

Braun MM, Barstow CH, Pyzocha NJ. Diagnosis and management of sodium disorders: hyponatremia and hypernatremia. *Am Fam Physician*. 2015;**91**(5):299–307.

Chisti MJ, Ahmed T, Ahmed AM, et al. Hypernatremia in children with diarrhea: presenting features, management, outcome, and risk factors for death. *Clin Pediatr (Phila)*. 2016;**55**(7):654–663.

Majumdar I, Black TA, Nair J. Hypernatremia management. *Clin Pediatr (Phila)*. 2017. DOI: https://doi.org/10.1177/0009922816685819.

Powers KS. Dehydration: isonatremic, hyponatremic, and hypernatremic recognition and management. *Pediatr Rev*. 2015;**36**(7):274–283.

Hypocalcemia

Hypocalcemia is generally accepted to be a blood ionized calcium <4.0 mg/dL (1.0 mmol/L), or a total serum calcium <8.5 mg/dL in the absence of hypoalbuminemia or acidosis. In the neonate these numbers are shifted down 0.5 and 1.0 mg/dL respectively. Alkalosis, which causes increased calcium binding to protein, can decrease the ionized calcium fraction without a significant change in the serum total calcium level. Severely ill children are at risk for concomitant hypocalcemia, while chronic hypocalcemia is associated with hypoparathyroid conditions and vitamin D disorders.

Clinical Presentation

Clinical manifestations of hypocalcemia primarily involve the neuromuscular system. Muscle cramps and paresthesias are the hallmark symptoms. These can be sustained, producing tetany, or intermittent, as in a seizure. Contractions of the larynx can produce stridor or complete airway occlusion. Newborns may present with nonspecific symptoms of poor feeding, vomiting, and lethargy.

Characteristic signs include the Chvostek (facial muscle twitching elicited by tapping the facial nerve at the inferior maxillary edge just anterior to the ear) and Trousseau (carpal spasm elicited by maintaining a blood pressure cuff at just above systolic pressure for <5 minutes).

Typically, the hyperventilating adolescent presents with hypocalcemic symptoms in addition to anxiety, tachypnea, and labored breathing. There may be a history of recent emotional upset or past psychiatric disorders.

Findings in patients with long-standing hypocalcemia may include cataracts and basal ganglia calcifications, along with radiographic evidence of rickets.

Diagnosis

Hyperventilation

Suspect hyperventilation-induced hypocalcemia in an older child or adolescent who presents with tachypnea, anxiety, and carpopedal spasm. If the presentation is not typical for anxiety-related hyperventilation, obtain an ABG. An increased pH, decreased pCO_2, and normal pO_2 confirm the diagnosis and rule-out other causes of hyperventilation, such as hypoxia or a metabolic acidosis. See Table 7.3 for the differential diagnosis of hypocalcemia.

Table 7.3 Differential diagnosis of hypocalcemia

Diagnosis	Differentiating features
Cardiac bypass surgery	Positive history
End-organ vitamin D resistance	↑ serum calcitriol
Hypernatremic dehydration	↑ serum sodium
Hypoparathyroidism	↑ phosphate; normal alkaline phosphatase
	↓ PTH
Inadequate hepatic 25-hydroxylation	↑ serum LFTs
Inadequate vitamin D intake,	↓ serum 25-hydroxy vitamin D absorption or production
Lack of renal 1-hydroxylation	Normal renal function and 25-hydroxyvitamin D
Overwhelming sepsis	Premorbid finding
Pancreatitis	↑ serum amylase and lipase
	Abdominal pain and vomiting
Phosphate overload (renal failure, tumor lysis, enemas)	Positive history
Pseudohypoparathyroidism	↑ phosphorous and PTH
	Mental retardation
	Short fourth and fifth metacarpals/metatarsals
	↓ serum calcitriol
Rhabdomyolysis	Acute phase
Severe acute illnesses	Positive history
Vitamin D disorders	↓ serum phosphate; ↑ alkaline phosphatase, PTH

Other Etiologies

Immediately obtain an ECG to determine the corrected QT (QTc) interval, which is prolonged with hypocalcemia. In addition, obtain blood for total and/or ionized calcium, electrolytes, BUN, creatinine, phosphorus, magnesium, PTH, 25-hydroxyvitamin D, and liver function tests, including albumin and alkaline phosphatase.

ED Management

Hyperventilation

Instruct the patient to breathe slowly in and out of a paper bag or a face mask with a reservoir attached and the side ports taped shut. This causes rebreathing of CO_2, leading to a decreased plasma pH and, thus, an increased ionized calcium. Occasionally sedation is required. Use either hydroxyzine (1 mg/kg, 20 mg maximum), diphenhydramine (1–2 mg/kg, 50 mg maximum), or a more rapid-acting anxiolytic, such as IV lorazepam (0.03 mg/kg, 1 mg maximum) or diazepam (0.05–0.2 mg/kg, 5 mg maximum). Once the hyperventilation has stopped, try to discover the precipitating cause and reassure the patient and the family as to the benign nature of the episode.

Other Etiologies

Give a symptomatic patient (seizures, laryngospasm, tetany) 0.5 mL/kg of 10% calcium gluconate (10 mL maximum) *slowly* IV over 10–15 minutes, while continuously monitoring the ECG. The bolus may be repeated once. If symptoms persist consider other diagnostic possibilities, such as hypokalemia, hypomagnesemia, or a seizure disorder. After the bolus (es) are completed, give a continuous calcium IV infusion, starting with 200 mg/kg/day of calcium gluconate, which is equivalent to about 20 mg/kg/day of elemental calcium. Increase the dose to 500 mg/kg/day for neonates.

Oral calcium administration will be ineffective in hypoparathyroidism and vitamin D disorders unless calcitriol (or other appropriate forms of vitamin D) is also given. Consult a pediatric endocrinologist.

Follow-up

- Hyperventilation that seems to be a manifestation of anxiety: primary care follow-up within one week for evaluation and possible psychiatric referral

Indications for Admission

- Hypocalcemia requiring IV treatment

Bibliography

De Sanctis V, Soliman A, Fiscina B. Hypoparathyroidism: from diagnosis to treatment. *Curr Opin Endocrinol Diabetes Obes.* 2012;**19**(6):435–442.

Hasan ZU, Absamara R, Ahmed M. Chvostek's sign in paediatric practice. *Curr Pediatr Rev.* 2014;**10** (3):194–197.

Shaw NJ. A practical approach to hypocalcaemia in children. *Endocr Dev.* 2015;**28**:84–100.

Hypoglycemia

Hypoglycemia occurs when there is failure to maintain glucose homeostasis secondary to defects in substrate, enzymes, or hormones. Clinical hypoglycemia is defined as a plasma glucose concentration low enough to cause symptoms and/or signs of impaired brain function (typically at a plasma glucose level <50–60 mg/dL). However, the laboratory definition of hypoglycemia depends upon the method by which the specimen was obtained: consider hypoglycemia to be a whole blood glucose level <50 mg/dL in a full-term newborn infant, child or adult. Recurrent hypoglycemia during the period of rapid brain growth in infancy can result in long-term neurological sequelae, psychomotor retardation, and seizures. Therefore, prevention, rapid diagnosis, and aggressive therapy are essential to prevent these severe consequences of hypoglycemia.

Although there are many etiologies of hypoglycemia, it is most commonly seen in diabetics having an "insulin reaction" secondary to insulin overdose, skipped or late meals, or exercise without an adjustment in food intake or insulin dosage. In a nondiabetic under eight years of age, ketotic hypoglycemia is the most frequent cause. Inadequate intake (prolonged fasting, malnutrition), gastroenteritis, ingestions (alcohol, oral hypoglycemic agents, propranolol, salicylates), hyperinsulinemia, hormone deficiencies (panhypopituitarism, growth hormone, ACTH, cortisol), liver disease, or a ketogenic diet may lead to hypoglycemia.

Clinical Presentation

The presentation is nonspecific but can be age-dependent. Autonomic symptoms arise from both sympathetic and parasympathetic divisions and include sweating, hunger, paresthesias, tremors, pallor, anxiety, nausea, and palpitations. CNS glucose deprivation causes warmth, fatigue, weakness, dizziness, headache, inability to concentrate, drowsiness, blurred vision, difficulty speaking, confusion, bizarre behavior, loss of coordination, difficulty walking, coma, and seizures. A neonate can present with jitteriness, irritability, poor feeding, apnea, perioral cyanosis, irregular respirations or tachypnea, hypothermia, hypotonia, seizures, and an abnormal cry. An infant or older child can have gastrointestinal symptoms (hunger, nausea, abdominal pain) or neurologic complaints (headache, speech and vision disturbances, weakness, anxiety, behavior changes, short attention span, ataxia, seizures, coma). These symptoms may occur with or without the signs of catecholamine excess (sweating, pallor, tachycardia). In general, vomiting associated with hypoglycemia suggests acidosis, gastroenteritis, food poisoning, or acute liver disease.

A patient with hypoglycemia secondary to hormone deficiencies, such as growth hormone deficiency or panhypopituitarism, can present at birth with microphallus or undescended testes. An infant or child with a metabolic defect may present with metabolic acidosis, hepatosplenomegaly, increased uric acid and lactic acid levels, and positive urine or serum ketones. This hypoglycemia typically occurs when feeding is interrupted, as can occur when the overnight feeding is held or an infection interrupts the normal feeding pattern.

Ketotic Hypoglycemia

Ketotic hypoglycemia, low blood glucose levels accompanied by ketosis, presents most commonly between 18 months and 5 years of age and remits spontaneously by 8–9 years. It may be due to multiple factors that contribute to substrate limitation, such as defects in protein catabolism or amino acid synthesis. Hypoglycemia typically occurs in a lean child with decreased muscle mass, when food intake is limited by anorexia or vomiting caused by an intercurrent illness. It usually presents in the morning, before breakfast or when breakfast is skipped, and in many cases the child has either skipped the evening meal or eaten poorly. Hypoglycemia occurs after 2–24 hours of fasting, and, at the time of hypoglycemia, insulin and plasma alanine levels are low, serum ketones are elevated with ketonuria, blood lactate and pyruvate levels are normal, and the concentrations of counterregulatory hormones (growth hormone and cortisol) are increased.

Hyperinsulinism

Hyperinsulinism caused by generalized β-cell dysfunction is the most common cause of persistent hypoglycemia in infants and young children. Insulin concentrations are inappropriately elevated (>5–10 microunits/mL) during the episode of hypoglycemia. There are several distinct genetic forms of congenital hyperinsulinism, although transient cases of hyperinsulinism have been associated with various risk factors, including maternal diabetes, intrauterine growth restriction, and perinatal asphyxia. It generally presents in infants <1 year of age, and there may be a history of constant hunger and frequent nighttime feeds. Hypoglycemia occurs soon (usually 30 minutes to 2 hours) after feeding and is associated with negative or small urinary ketones (insulin prevents ketosis) with inappropriately low plasma ketones concentrations (β-OH-butyrate and acetoacetate) and high insulin levels. In milder, autosomal dominant forms of hyperinsulinism, patients may not present with hypoglycemia until later in childhood or in adulthood.

Hereditary Fructose Intolerance

Hereditary fructose intolerance is caused by an inability to break down fructose, leading to an accumulation of fructose 1 phosphate, which inhibits glycogen breakdown and gluconeogenesis. Typically, a nursing infant is asymptomatic until fruits and juices are added to the diet. It can also present following the consumption of a commercial formula containing sucrose (soy-based formulas). Fructose causes vomiting, diarrhea, and hypoglycemia acutely. Chronic exposure to fructose results in hepatomegaly, jaundice, failure to thrive, and renal tubular dysfunction.

Diagnosis

If hypoglycemia is suspected or the patient has altered mental status or seizures, obtain a fingerstick glucose determination. Confirm any measurement <60 mg/dL with a laboratory measurement of the plasma glucose from a "gray top" tube.

Perform a thorough history regarding the timing of the episode of hypoglycemia in relation to food and exercise. Birth weight, gestational age and family history are also critical pieces of information. If there is suspicion of ingestion, obtain a full list of medications present in the household. Insulin, sulfonylureas, beta-blockers, salicylates and alcohol are most commonly associated with hypoglycemia.

Physical findings of short stature, microphallus, and midline defects (cleft palate, single maxillary central incisor) suggest hypopituitarism, along with low cortisol and growth hormone levels. Increased skin pigmentation may indicate compensatory ACTH release (primary adrenal insufficiency). Hepatomegaly occurs in glycogen storage diseases, galactosemia, liver disease, and disorders of gluconeogenesis, fatty acid oxidation, and carnitine metabolism, but not in ketotic hypoglycemia. Among syndromes associated with hypoglycemia, suspect Beckwith–Wiedemann if the patient has an omphalocele, hemihypertrophy, and macroglossia.

If ketotic hypoglycemia is suspected, obtain insulin and plasma alanine levels (which will be low), while serum ketones are elevated with ketonuria, and blood lactate and pyruvate levels are normal. Otherwise, if the patient is not a known diabetic, obtain whole blood glucose, cortisol, growth hormone, insulin, uric acid, electrolytes, liver function tests, plasma ammonia, lactate, pyruvate, alanine, and C-peptide levels (for suspicion of exogenous insulin administration). At the time of hypoglycemia, also send urine for ketones, reducing substances, and save an aliquot for analysis of amino acids, organic acids, and acylglycines. It is important to draw these specimens *prior* to treatment.

The absence of ketones or their presence in only trace or small amounts is characteristic of hyperinsulinism, as well as disorders of carnitine metabolism, fatty acid oxidation, and ketogenesis. An elevated lactate suggests an inborn error of metabolism, while positive urine reducing substances occurs in disorders of galactose, fructose, and tyrosine metabolism. If the symptoms followed a meal, determine whether fructose or galactose was the sole sugar consumed. An elevated insulin level with a low C-peptide suggests exogenous insulin administration.

ED Management

Regardless of the etiology, the treatment of hypoglycemia is glucose. The goal of therapy is to prevent hypoglycemia in order to protect the brain from damage. Maintain the plasma glucose concentration >70 mg/dL.

Encourage an alert child to drink a carbohydrate-containing solution initially (orange juice, apple juice, soft drink with sugar), followed within an hour by a carbohydrate- and protein-containing meal or snack. If the patient is unconscious, vomiting, or unable to take fluids orally, give a bolus of 0.5 g/kg of dextrose (5 mL/kg of D10) over 1 minute. Follow bolus therapy with a continuous infusion of 10% glucose, with maintenance electrolytes, at a maintenance rate. Sodium chloride must be in the maintenance fluid to prevent hyponatremia as the hypoglycemia improves. Recheck glucose 15 minutes after bolus while receiving maintenance glucose infusion. If hypoglycemia recurs, give another bolus of 0.5 g/kg (5 mL/kg). Adjust the infusion rate and concentration to maintain a glucose level of about 80 mg/dL. Note that 5 mL/kg/h of D10 is equal to a glucose infusion rate of 8 mg/kg/min. D10 is preferred over higher concentrations of dextrose in neonates and infants.

Hyperinsulinism

If the hypoglycemia persists with inappropriately elevated insulin levels, consult an endocrinologist and give glucagon (30–50 mcg/kg, up to 1 mg IV, IM, or SQ) while continuing the glucose infusion, as a glycemic response requires adequate amounts of substrates. Patients without hyperinsulinism typically require glucose infusion rates of 6–8 mg/kg/min to maintain euglycemia, while children with hyperinsulinism may require glucose infusion rates that are 2–4 times greater because of their increased glucose utilization. Insertion of a central line may be needed to deliver adequate glucose concentrations. In severe cases of hyperinsulinemic hypoglycemia, a glucagon infusion can be administered at 5–10 mcg/kg/h, but avoid a rate >10 mcg/kg/h, which can stimulate paradoxical insulin secretion.

To treat hyperinsulinism, give a trial of diazoxide to suppress insulin secretion (5 mg/kg/day in three divided doses, gradually increasing to 20 mg/kg/day maximum). Other possible treatments include a long-acting somatostatin analog (octreotide) given IV, SC or as a continuous IV infusion and nifedipine. Glucagon can be used to stabilize the hypoglycemia in patients prior to surgery.

Ketotic Hypoglycemia

Instruct the family of a child with ketotic hypoglycemia that the child must avoid prolonged periods of fasting. Recommend a bedtime snack consisting of both carbohydrate and protein to prevent further episodes of hypoglycemia. During intercurrent illness, instruct the parents to provide carbohydrate-rich drinks at frequent intervals during both the day and night. Also, have the family test the urine for ketones during an intercurrent illness, as ketonuria may precede the onset of hypoglycemia by several hours. An ED visit for IV glucose may be necessary if carbohydrate-containing drinks are not tolerated. Discharge the patient when the glucose normalizes, oral intake is adequate, and close follow-up is arranged.

Follow-up
- Ketotic hypoglycemia: primary care follow-up in one week

Indications for Admission
- Hypoglycemic episode in a nondiabetic, unless patient is known to have ketotic hypoglycemia and the glucose normalizes
- Hypoglycemia in a diabetic if the cause is unclear or self-destructive behavior is likely

Bibliography

Langdon DR, Stanley CA, Sperling MA. Hypoglycemia in the toddler and child. In Sperling M (ed.). *Pediatric Endocrinology* (4th edn.). Philadelphia, PA: Elsevier Saunders, 2014; 920–955.

Royal Children's Hospital Melbourne. Hypoglycemia. www.rch.org.au/clinicalguide/guideline_index/hypoglycaemia_guideline (accessed May 23, 2017).

Rozenkova K, Guemes M, Shah P, Hussain K. The diagnosis and management of hyperinsulinemic hypoglycemia. *J Clin Res Pediatr Endocrinol.* 2015;7(2):86–97.

Thornton S, Stanley CA, De Leon DD, et al. Recommendations from the Pediatric Endocrine Society for evaluation and management of persistent hypoglycemia in neonates, infants, and children. *J Pediatr.* 2015;167(2):238–245.

Hyponatremia

Hyponatremia is defined as a serum sodium (Na) concentration <135 mEq/L. Hyponatremia may be associated with hypovolemia, euvolemia, or hypervolemia.

Hypovolemia (low Total Body Water; Lower Total Body Na)

Most often, hypovolemic hyponatremia is caused by loss of sodium in excess of water secondary to extrarenal losses (vomiting, diarrhea, sweat, third-spacing). Renal salt-wasting occurs with diuretics, osmotic diuresis, salt-wasting nephropathy, adrenal insufficiency, proximal renal tubular acidosis, metallic alkalosis, and pseudohypoaldosteronism. Severe salt-wasting can also be secondary to cerebral insults.

Euvolemia (High Total Body Water; Normal Total Body Na)

The most common cause of euvolemic hyponatremia is the syndrome of inappropriate secretion of antidiuretic hormone (SIADH), secondary to CNS pathology (meningitis, trauma) or pulmonary disease (pneumonia, tuberculosis). Additionally, drugs, such as nicotine, morphine, barbiturates, isoproterenol, antineoplastic agents, carbamazepine, and acetaminophen have all been implicated as "antidiuretic" agents. Other etiologies of euvolemic hyponatremia are hypothyroidism, nephrotic syndrome, and water intoxication. Glucocorticoid deficiency can cause either euvolemic or hypovolemic hyponatremia.

Hypervolemia (Higher Total Body Water; Relatively High Total Body Na)

Hypervolemic hyponatremia is characterized by edema, as in congestive heart failure, cirrhosis, nephrotic syndrome, and renal failure.

Clinical Presentation

The clinical presentation of hyponatremia is determined by the intravascular volume and the absolute concentration and rate of fall of serum sodium.

Hypovolemia

With depletion of the intravascular space, signs of hypovolemia predominate. There may be tachycardia, orthostatic vital sign changes, poor capillary refill, weight loss, and decreased skin turgor. Laboratory abnormalities include elevations of the BUN, renin, aldosterone, and uric acid. Urinary sodium excretion is low (<20 mEq/L) with extrarenal etiologies and high (>20 mEq/L) with renal causes.

Euvolemia

The clinical findings are related to the serum sodium level. A rapid decrease to the 120–125 mEq/L range may cause gastrointestinal symptoms such as anorexia, nausea, and vomiting associated with agitation, headache, muscle cramps, seizures, and coma. Other neurologic signs (decreased deep tendon reflexes, pathologic reflexes, Cheyne–Stokes respiration, and pseudobulbar palsy) can be present, especially when the level is <120 mEq/L. The patient may be asymptomatic, however, with a sodium <120 mEq/L if the fall in the serum sodium occurred slowly, over days to weeks.

Hypervolemia

In hypervolemic hyponatremia, there may be signs of fluid excess, including edema, tachycardia, hypertension, headache, pulmonary rales, and hepatomegaly.

Diagnosis

Most often mild hyponatremia (≥130 mEq/L) is discovered incidentally, when electrolytes are obtained because of vomiting, diarrhea, or dehydration. In such cases, no further work-up is needed. For patients with more significant hyponatremia (<130 mEq/L), a history of diabetes or renal disease, or neurologic symptoms (altered mental status, seizures), obtain blood for repeat electrolytes, glucose, and CBC, and urine for sodium, creatinine, and osmolality *prior* to correcting hyponatremia. It is also necessary to rule-out pseudohyponatremia as seen in hypertriglyceridemia:

$$\text{Triglycerides}(\text{mg}/\text{dL}) \times 0.002 = \text{decrease in plasma Na level}(\text{mEq}/\text{L})$$

and hyperproteinemia:

$$(\text{Protein}[\text{g}/\text{dL}] - 8) \times 0.25 = \text{decrease in plasma Na}(\text{mEq}/\text{L})$$

Also, check for distributive hyponatremia, secondary to the presence of excess solutes, such as glucose or mannitol. In a hyperglycemic patient, most typically seen in diabetes mellitus, for every 100 mg/dL increase in glucose over 100 mg/dL, the serum sodium is lowered by 1.6 mEq/L

If a euvolemic or hypervolemic state is likely, contact a pediatric endocrinologist. The work-up may include vasopressin, renin, aldosterone, uric acid, and cortisol levels, thyroid function tests, and a lipid panel, as well as urinary osmolality and creatinine.

The urinary sodium level can help distinguish among the various etiologies of hyponatremia. With dehydration and volume depletion, the proximal tubular reabsorption of sodium and water will be high, leading to a urinary sodium <10 mEq/L. It will also be low in most hypervolemic states; a urine sodium >20 mEq/L suggests renal salt-wasting, SIADH, and other euvolemic conditions. With renal failure the urine sodium may be >40 mEq/L, except in acute glomerulonephritis (when it is typically low).

Patients with decreased effective intravascular volume due to CHF, cirrhosis, nephritic syndrome, or lung disease will present with signs of their underlying disease, which often includes peripheral edema. Patients with primary salt loss will also appear volume-depleted. If the salt loss is from the kidney (e.g., diuretic therapy or polycystic kidney disease), urinary sodium will be elevated, as may be the urine volume. Salt loss from other sites (e.g., the gut in gastroenteritis or the skin in cystic fibrosis) will cause urine sodium to be low, as in other forms of systemic dehydration.

SIADH is characterized by the hyponatremia, along with an inappropriately increased urine osmolality (>100 mOsm/kg), normal or slightly elevated plasma volume, and a normal to high urine sodium level. Serum uric acid is low in patients with SIADH, whereas it is high in those with hyponatremia due to systemic dehydration from other causes of decreased intravascular volume.

Consider drug-induced hyponatremia in patients taking potentially contributory medications. A careful search for a tumor (thymoma, glioma, bronchial carcinoid) causing SIADH is necessary if there is not an obvious cause. Patients will present with nonspecific symptoms of hyponatremia, such as anorexia, lethargy, weakness, and in severe cases, obtundation and convulsions. Signs of diminished intravascular volume, edema, hypothyroidism, adrenal insufficiency, and renal disease are absent by definition.

ED Management

Immediately treat symptomatic hypovolemia (poor peripheral pulses, delayed capillary refill, orthostatic changes) without waiting for the laboratory confirmation of hyponatremia. Give 20 mL/kg boluses of isotonic crystalloid (normal saline, Ringer's lactate) until adequate perfusion is established. Obtain blood for serum electrolytes, BUN, and creatinine and urine for urinalysis, sodium, creatinine, and osmolality. Begin definitive therapy once the initial serum and urine studies confirm the diagnosis.

If the hyponatremia is acute and there are severe neurological symptoms secondary to a serum sodium level <125 mEq/L (lethargy, psychosis, coma, or generalized seizures, especially in younger children), give hypertonic saline (3% [513 mEq/L] or 5% 9855 mEq/L]) to raise the sodium above 125 mEq/L. Replace this deficit over four hours, using the following formula:

$$\text{Sodium needed(mEq)} = (125 - \text{patient's sodium}) \times (0.6) \times (\text{body weight in kg})$$

As a general guide, 12 mL/kg of 3% sodium chloride will increase the serum sodium approximately 10 mEq/L. Raise the serum sodium to 135 mEq/L over the subsequent 24 hours. Do not exceed a rate of correction of >0.5 mEq/L/h or 12 mEq/day. Measure the serum sodium every two hours until it is >135 mEq/L and all symptoms have resolved. Subsequent treatment then depends on the initial assessment of the intravascular volume status.

Use a slower rate of correction for chronic hyponatremia, as the hypertonic saline may result in both cell shrinkage and central pontine myelinolysis. This is characterized by somnolence, disorientation, and aphasia, which may progress over a few weeks to quadriplegia, which becomes evident 24–48 hours after a rapid correction of hyponatremia. It has a characteristic appearance on CT and MRI, and often causes irreversible brain damage.

Hypovolemia

Replace volume with NS or D_5 NS. In adrenal insufficiency, sodium deficits are difficult to replace without corticosteroid replacement.

Euvolemia

Limiting the water intake to two-thirds maintenance, including all fluids (e.g., IV medications), may be all that is required. Immediately begin treatment if the cause of SIADH is identified, but acute treatment of the hyponatremia due to SIADH is indicated only if there is cerebral dysfunction. Because patients with SIADH have volume expansion, salt administration is not very effective in raising the serum sodium level, as it is rapidly excreted in the urine due to suppressed aldosterone levels and elevated atrial natriuretic peptide concentration.

Hypervolemia

If the patient is edematous, restrict fluids to two-thirds maintenance. Give furosemide (1 mg/kg/dose IV) if there is pulmonary edema and respiratory compromise.

Indications for Admission

- Symptomatic hyponatremia
- Hyponatremia of undetermined etiology
- Factitious hyponatremia (psychiatric admission)

Bibliography

Braun MM, Barstow CH, Pyzocha NJ. Diagnosis and management of sodium disorders: hyponatremia and hypernatremia. *Am Fam Physician.* 2015;**91**(5):299–307.

Powers KS. Dehydration: isonatremic, hyponatremic, and hypernatremic recognition and management. *Pediatr Rev.* 2015;**36**(7):274–283.

Reid-Adam J. Hyponatremia. *Pediatr Rev.* 2013;**34**(9):417–419.

Srivatsa A, Majzoub JA. Disorders of water homeostasis. In Lifshitz F (ed.) *Pediatric Endocrinology.* New York: Informa Healthcare USA, 2007; 651–692.

Zieg J. Evaluation and management of hyponatraemia in children. *Acta Paediatr.* 2014;**103**(10):1027–1034.

Thyroid Disorders

Normal thyroid gland function is critical for normal growth and neurocognitive development. Thyroid disorders are common and can present in subtle or dramatic fashion.

Hyperthyroidism, or thyrotoxicosis, is characterized by increased production of triiodothyronine (T3) and thyroxine (T4), a suppressed TSH level and characteristic clinical symptoms. Hyperthyroidism primarily affects children over six years of age and is more common in females. Pathogenesis may be due to the inappropriate production of thyroid hormone, such as in Graves' disease (diffuse toxic goiter, most common), autonomously functioning thyroid nodules, or thyroid adenomas. Hyperthyroidism may also be due to release of supraphysiologic levels of thyroid hormones from destruction of thyroid follicles, such as in subacute viral thyroiditis, amiodarone-induced thyroiditis, and Hashitoxicosis. Exogenous overdosage can also occur.

Thyroid storm is a rare, life-threatening complication of hyperthyroidism with severe cardiovascular, thermoregulatory, gastrointestinal, and neurobehavioral symptoms. In 50% of episodes there is an identifiable precipitating factor (stress, infection, surgery, childbirth). The syndrome complex may occur either in a previously undiagnosed patient or someone with poorly controlled hyperthyroidism. Untreated thyroid storm has a mortality of up to 90%.

Euthyroid hyperthyroxinemia is the term used to describe the various conditions in which the serum T4 level, either total or free, is elevated in the absence of thyrotoxicosis. This may be caused by increased T4-binding by serum proteins, increased concentration of thyroid binding globulin (TBG), or a generalized (pituitary and peripheral tissues) resistance to thyroid hormone.

Hyperthyroidism can also present in the neonatal period. A newborn can develop neonatal Graves' disease, which occurs when the thyroid-stimulating immunoglobulins (TSI) of maternal Graves' disease cross the placenta and can cause transient or permanent thyroid disease in the infant. Previous maternal therapy with radioactive iodine or surgery does not eliminate the presence of thyroid antibodies.

Hypothyroidism is defined as low to absent levels of thyroid hormones. It may be present at birth (congenital) or develop later in life (acquired). Chronic autoimmune thyroiditis (Hashimoto's) is the most common cause of acquired hypothyroidism. Congenital hypothyroidism occurs in 1 in 1500–3000 newborns, and is most commonly due to thyroid gland dysgenesis. Early diagnosis and treatment is crucial to ensure normal development and cognition, and a delay in therapy is associated with intellectual disability. Thyroid screening, with either thyroid-stimulating hormone (TSH) or T4, is part of the newborn screen in every state. Patients with the highest percentile of TSH or the lowest percentile of T4 from each day are recalled. Therefore, false-positives occur, but this is necessary to ensure that all truly hypothyroid newborns are identified. Hypothyroidism beyond the newborn period is most commonly caused by chronic autoimmune thyroiditis.

Clinical Presentation

Hyperthyroidism

The onset of hyperthyroidism is gradual, with complaints of palpitations, sweating, heat intolerance, weight loss despite increased appetite, tremor, nervousness, increased frequency of bowel movements, and emotional lability. Short attention span, inability to concentrate, deteriorating school performance, attacks of dyspnea, and easy fatigability may occur. Insomnia, restless sleep, and nocturia are common and are often associated with fatigue and lethargy during the day. Newborns may exhibit irritability, inability to feed (breast or bottle), low birth weight, and inadequate weight gain. There is usually a history of maternal thyroid disease, thyroid surgery, or radioactive iodine treatment.

Children who develop Graves' disease before the age of three years can experience transitory speech and language delays, intellectual disability, and craniosynostosis. Children may have accelerated growth velocities and delayed puberty. In female adolescents, oligomenorrhea and irregular menses are common. Other diseases have been observed in association with Graves' disease and include Hashimoto's thyroiditis, vitiligo, systemic lupus erythematosus, rheumatoid arthritis, Addison's disease, insulin-dependent diabetes mellitus, myasthenia gravis, and pernicious anemia.

On examination, almost all hyperthyroid patients (except in the case of exogenous overdose) have a goiter, and a characteristic bruit may be heard over the thyroid. The skin is warm and moist, and tachycardia (particularly increased resting pulse rate), increased systolic blood pressure, and widened pulse pressure are common. Eye findings, when present, include lid retraction, staring, lid lag, and exophthalmos. There may be proximal muscle weakness, brisk deep tendon reflexes, and fine tremors of the eyelids, fingers, or tongue, but pretibial myxedema is very rare.

Graves' Ophthalmopathy

In most children and adolescents with Graves' disease, the signs and symptoms are relatively mild and include lid lag, lid retraction, stare, proptosis, conjunctival injection, chemosis, and periorbital and eyelid edema. Less commonly, patients may complain of eye discomfort, pain, or diplopia. Severe ophthalmopathy, associated with marked chemosis, severe proptosis, periorbital ecchymosis, corneal ulceration, eye muscle paralysis, and optic atrophy, is very unusual. Ophthalmoplegia may be secondary to severe exophthalmos, nerve entrapment, or myasthenia gravis, which is a rare coexisting disease.

Thyroid Storm

Thyroid storm is a life-threatening manifestation of hyperthyroidism that is very rare in childhood. It often starts abruptly, with the sudden onset of severe thyrotoxic symptoms and fever (usually >38.5 °C [101.3 °F], often up to 41.1 °C [106 °F]), cardiovascular symptoms (tachycardia out of proportion to the fever, high-output cardiac failure, arrhythmias, shock), gastrointestinal dysfunction (vomiting, diarrhea, hepatomegaly, jaundice), and neurological changes (agitation, tremor, seizures, psychosis, stupor, coma). Thyroid storm can be precipitated by infection, trauma, surgery, concomitant ingestion of sympathomimetic agents (e.g., pseudoephedrine), withdrawal of antithyroid medication, and radioactive iodine therapy.

Hypothyroidism

Hypothyroidism presents with a combination of poor appetite, slowing growth velocity, cold intolerance, constipation, hypotonia, poor school performance, delayed puberty, and delayed dentition. On physical examination there may be bradycardia and delayed deep tendon reflexes, and a goiter may be appreciated. An infant with untreated congenital hypothyroidism will present with poor feeding, prolonged jaundice, constipation, hoarse cry, and lethargy. An umbilical hernia, macroglossia, a wide posterior fontanelle, and mottled skin may be seen on physical examination.

Diagnosis

Hyperthyroidism

The typical gradual onset makes the early diagnosis of hyperthyroidism difficult, although the presence of a goiter or bruit, along with other symptoms of hyperthyroidism, usually suggest the diagnosis. The differential diagnosis of hyperthyroidism includes anxiety attack, sepsis, pheochromocytoma, gastroenteritis, and congestive heart failure. Other possible midline neck masses include thyroglossal duct cyst, dermoid cyst, cystic hygroma, and neuroblastoma (with Horner's syndrome). Exophthalmos or ophthalmoplegia can be confused with a neuroblastoma, intraorbital tumor, and orbital cellulitis.

If hyperthyroidism is suspected, obtain a CBC, electrolytes, and liver function tests (thioamides can affect liver function), in addition to thyroid function tests, including T3, T4, free T4, TSH, thyroid antibodies (antithyroglobulin, thyroid peroxidase), TSI, and TSH receptor Ab (TSHRAb). Typical findings are elevated free T4, total T4 or T3, with a suppressed (low) TSH, although early in the course of thyrotoxicosis, a patient may present with an elevated T3 level and a normal T4 level. A neonate born to mothers with Graves' disease is at high risk for thyrotoxicosis. If there is any concern for hyperthyroidism in an infant more than three days of age, obtain FT4 and TSH levels.

If hypothyroidism is suspected, obtain TFTs (T3, T4, free T4, TSH), as well as antithyroglobulin and thyroid peroxidase antibodies. The free T4 and total T4 will be low while the TSH is elevated. Primary T4 testing is the mainstay of newborn screening with heel-stick samples obtained between two and five days of life. If a newborn is brought to the ED with documentation of a failed thyroid screen, consult a pediatric endocrinologist and obtain blood for TSH, free and total T4, and TBG.

ED Management

Hyperthyroidism (Thioamides)

Methimazole (MMI) is now the drug of choice to control hyperthyroidism, as propylthiouracil (PTU) has been implicated in drug-induced fulminant hepatic necrosis. Consult with a pediatric endocrinologist to initiate MMI treatment, typically with 0.1–1 mg/kg/day (30 mg/day maximum), usually divided q 8–12h (see Table 7.4). Side effects include nausea, rash, mild leukopenia, liver toxicity, and bone marrow suppression. Obtain a CBC if a patient taking MMI complains of a sore throat, fever, mouth ulcers, arthralgias or malaise. If leukopenia is confirmed, discuss changing the treatment regimen with the endocrinologist.

Table 7.4 Dosing of thionamides in hyperthyroidism and thyroid storm

Age	Thionamide dose
Infant	1.25 mg/day MMI
1–5 years	2.5–5 mg/day MMI
5–10 years	5–10 mg/day MMI
10–18 years	10–20 mg/day MMI
Thyroid storm	PTU: 5–10 mg/kg/day divided q 6–8h (1200 mg/day maximum) *or* MMI: 0.6–0.7 mg/kg/day divided q 6–8h (30 mg/day maximum)

In addition to the antithyroid medication, give oral atenolol (25–50 mg once or twice a day, 100 mg/day maximum) to treat the adrenergic symptoms.

Thyroid Storm

Thyroid storm requires *immediate treatment*, including respiratory and cardiovascular support, body temperature control, management of precipitating factors, and limiting the amount of thyroid hormone available to peripheral tissues. The goals are to decrease the thyroid hormone levels acutely and block their peripheral effects. Call for an immediate pediatric endocrinology consult, obtain blood for T3, T4, FT4, TSH, cortisol, CBC, electrolytes, and liver function tests, and initiate therapy using the following modalities.

Propranolol

Perform an EKG and consult a cardiologist if the patient is not in sinus rhythm. Treat the symptoms of hyperthyroidism with propranolol, although it has no effect on the cause. Give a child 1–3 mg/kg/day divided q 6h (60 mg/day maximum) and an older adolescent 20–40 mg q 6h. If gastrointestinal symptoms preclude oral treatment, give IV at a starting dose of 0.01 mg/kg to a maximum dose of 5 mg over 10–15 minutes. The dose may be repeated three or four times, but consult a pediatric cardiologist. Possible side effects include hypotension, hypoglycemia, bronchospasm, and heart block. Atenolol, a cardioselective beta-blocker, is a second-line choice. Give 1–2 mg/kg/day (100 mg/day maximum).

PTU and MMI

Despite the potential toxicity, PTU is preferred over MMI for the acute treatment of thyroid storm. PTU inhibits production of thyroid hormone and blocks peripheral conversion of T4 to T3. Give 5–10 mg/kg/day div q 6–8h or 100–200 mg every 4–6 hours (1200 mg/day maximum) orally, rectally, or via nasogastric tube. Alternatively, use MMI, 0.6–0.7 mg/kg/day divided q 6–8h, maximum 30 mg/day.

Oral Iodide (Lugol's Solution)

Lugol's solution is 5% iodine and 10% potassium iodide; it contains 126 mg iodine/mL, or 8 mg iodine/drop. Give children and adolescents 4–8 drops (32–64 mg iodine) PO q 6–8h, starting at least one hour after the MMI to avoid a potential increase in thyroid hormone production. Alternatively, use potassium iodide (1 g/mL), 150–200 mg PO tid for infants <1 year of age; 300–500 mg PO tid for children and adolescents. Propranolol is so effective in blocking the β-adrenergic effects that iodides are often unnecessary. If the patient cannot take PO, give sodium iodide 125–250 mg IV, up to 1–2 g/day.

Dexamethasone

In extreme cases, such as a patient with heart failure, arrhythmias, severe adrenergic symptoms, or shock give dexamethasone (0.2 mg/kg IV q 6–12h) or hydrocortisone (2 mg/kg IV bolus, followed by 36–45 mg/m^2/day IV div q 6h [100 mg/dose maximum]). Both block T4 to T3 conversion.

Temperature Regulation

Use antipyretics (acetaminophen 15 mg/kg; ibuprofen 10 mg/kg), cooling blankets, and muscle relaxants, as needed. Do not give aspirin, which may elevate the T4 level.

Ophthalmopathy

In general, eye findings improve in association with control of the hyperthyroidism (MMI treatment), so that specific treatment is usually not necessary. Occasionally, local measures may be necessary to treat symptoms. For example, eye drops or ointment preparations containing methylcellulose may be necessary to prevent corneal drying. Sleeping with the head elevated may help to reduce chemosis and periorbital edema. If there are severe symptoms, consult an ophthalmologist.

Hypothyroidism

In a neonate with confirmed hypothyroidism, start treatment with thyroxine, 10–15 mcg/kg/day as a single daily dose (the majority of patients receive 37.5 mcg). Use a brand-name drug, as there may be unacceptable variations with generics. Instruct the parents to crush the tablets, add a few drops of water, formula, or breast milk to make a paste, and then smear on the inner cheek. Do not prescribe an oral suspension, as the concentration is unreliable. The goal is to maintain both the T4 (10–13 mg/dL) and TSH 1–2 milliunits/mL in the high range of normal for newborns. For a patient beyond the newborn period, defer treatment and promptly refer the patient to a pediatric endocrinologist.

Follow-up
- Hyperthyroidism without thyroid storm: 2–3 days
- Neonatal hypothyroidism: pediatric endocrinology follow-up 1–3 days
- Acquired hypothyroidism: pediatric endocrinology follow-up within one week

Indications for Admission
- Thyroid storm or thyrotoxic periodic paralysis
- Hyperthyroidism with heart failure, arrhythmias, shock, or psychosis

Bibliography

Hanley P, Lord K, Bauer AJ. Thyroid disorders in children and adolescence: a review. *JAMA Pediatrics.* 2016;**170**(10):1008–1019.

Pediatric EM Morsels. Thyroid storm. http://pedemmorsels.com/thyroid-storm/. (accessed May 23, 2017).

Ross DS, Burch HB, Cooper DS, et al. 2016 American Thyroid Association guidelines for diagnosis and management of hyperthyroidism and other causes of thyrotoxicosis. *Thyroid*. 2016;**26**(10):1343–1421.

Styne, DM. Disorders of the thyroid gland. In *Pediatric Endocrinology*. New York: Springer 2016; 91–122.

van der Kaay, DCM, Wasserman JD, Palmert MR. Management of neonates born to mothers with Graves' disease. *Pediatrics*. 2016;**137**(4):e20151878.

Environmental Emergencies

Anthony J. Ciorciari, Haamid Chamdawala,
and Katherine J. Chou

Burns

Each year, approximately 250,000 children in the United States are burned seriously enough to require medical attention, and burns are the third-most frequent cause of pediatric injury-related mortality.

Common types of burn injuries are thermal (scald and flame), chemical (acids and alkalis), electrical, and radiation (sunburn). Scald burns are the most frequent type in children under five years of age, while flame burns are most common in those 5–13 years of age. In teenagers, burn injury most often results from accidents involving flammable liquids.

Up to one-third of child abuse cases involve burns, accounting for 10–25% of all childhood burns. The most common mechanism is scalding. Other causes include burns from appliances, matches, and tobacco products.

Clinical Presentation

The presentation and severity of a thermal injury is determined by the type and temperature of the agent causing the burn and the duration of exposure to the agent.

Determining the surface area and depth of tissue involved are priorities in evaluating the extent of a burn injury. The "rule of nines" used in older children and adolescents requires modification for infants and young children, because the percentage of the total body surface area (BSA) represented by the various body parts changes with age. To estimate the BSA involved, use the patient's own hand, which, including the fingers, is approximately 0.8–1% of the BSA. Depth can be difficult to estimate, since the injury is usually not uniform in all affected areas, and the depth may progress over time. Scald burns, other than those caused by immersion, tend to be superficial, while chemical burns are typically deeper. Electrical burns (pp. 214–217) can cause tissue damage that is much deeper than suspected during the initial examination.

First-Degree Burns

First-degree burns involve only the superficial epidermis. Sunburn is the most common example of a first-degree burn. The area appears pink or light red and blanches with pressure. The burn is dry, without blister formation and is hypersensitive. Healing generally takes place within seven days, without scarring.

Second-Degree Burns

Second-degree burns are also known as partial-thickness burns. They are subdivided into superficial and deep partial-thickness burns. Superficial partial-thickness burns involve the epidermis and the papillary layer of the dermis. They present with blisters and bullae and are typically bright red or mottled in color. They have a moist surface, and the superficial skin can be wiped away. These burns are extremely painful. With proper care, they heal within 14–21 days with a small risk of hypertrophic scarring.

Deep partial-thickness burns involve the epidermis and both the papillary and reticular layers of the dermis. Most are caused by flame, oil grease, and very hot liquids. The skin may appear yellow-white or dark red (nonblanching), with a dry or mildly moist surface. There is sensation to pressure only, secondary to nerve destruction. These injuries may be difficult to distinguish from third-degree burns and may require >21 days (up to two months) for healing with residual scar formation.

Third-Degree Burns

Third-degree, or full-thickness, burns are usually caused by flame, hot grease or oil, chemicals, or prolonged immersion. All skin elements are lost, with coagulation of blood vessels. The skin is dry or leathery, grayish-white, and waxy. Thrombosed superficial veins may be visible. The patient has sensation to deep pressure only. Wound closure requires resurfacing and grafting, because the burned surface will not support the migration of normal epithelium from the unburned periphery.

Fourth-Degree Burns

Fourth-degree burns have the same etiologies as third-degree burns. They involve the subcutaneous layer, fascia, tendon, muscle, and/or bone. The extensive amount of necrotic tissue can produce systemic toxicity from tissue breakdown products and deep infection.

Diagnosis

The evaluation of any burn injury includes determination of the cause, location, and depth of the burn. Look for evidence of inhalation injury or other associated injuries, and note any preexisting illness. Always consider child abuse when the patient presents with burns to the buttocks or burns with a sharp delineation from immersion or the application of a hot object to the skin.

Burns can be classified as minor, moderate, or major, based on the severity of the burn and the involved BSA. Minor burns are first-degree, as well as second-degree injuries encompassing <10% total BSA. Moderate burns include partial-thickness burns that cover 10–20% total BSA. Full-thickness injuries covering <10% total BSA are also considered moderate. Major burns include partial-thickness burns >20% BSA and third-degree burns >10% BSA, as well as burns of the hands, face, eyes, ears, feet, and perineum.

Burns can also be classified as minor, moderate, and major based upon the severity of the burn as well as risk group. Minor burns include partial- or full-thickness burns <5% BSA in a child under ten years of age, partial- or full-thickness burns <10% BSA in a child ten years of age or older, and full-thickness burns <2% BSA. Moderate burns include partial- or full-thickness burn involving 5–10% BSA in a child younger than ten years of age, partial- or full-thickness burns involving 10–20% BSA in a child ten years of age or older, full-thickness burns involving 2–5% BSA, suspected inhalation injury, and circumferential burns. Major burns include any burn in an infant, any burn involving the face, eyes, ears, genitalia, or joints, burns complicated by fractures or other trauma, high-voltage burns, burns complicated by inhalation injury, partial- or full-thickness burns of >10% BSA in a child under ten years of age, partial- or full-thickness burns >20% BSA in a child ten years of age or older, and full-thickness burn >5% BSA.

ED Management

First-Degree Burns

Treat pain with acetaminophen (10–15 mg/kg q 4h) or ibuprofen (10 mg/kg q 6h). Hydrocortisone ointment (1%) may help reduce the pain and swelling of severe sunburn, especially if the eyelids and face are involved, but do not apply steroids to higher-degree burns. Cool showers and oatmeal baths are also helpful. Severe itching can occur after a few days and persist for more than one week; treat with hydroxyzine (2 mg/kg/day div tid, 50 mg/dose maximum) or diphenhydramine (5 mg/kg/day div qid, 50 mg/dose maximum).

Second-Degree Burns

Immediately remove any clothing that is hot or soaked with chemical. Use mineral oil mixed with cool water to remove substances like tar. Decrease the burning process by applying sterile gauze pads soaked with slightly cooled (12 °C; 53.6 °F) or room-temperature saline. To be effective in preventing microvascular changes, the cooling must occur within 30 minutes after the burn occurred.

Before the burn is cleaned, parenteral analgesia, such as IM or IV morphine sulfate (0.05–0.15 mg/kg q 4–6h, as needed), may be required. Do not attempt IV access in a burned area. Gently clean the burned surface with chlorhexidine solution and rinse thoroughly. Debride devitalized tissues using aseptic technique.

To promote restoration of mobility, open and debride blisters over joints. Also open and debride large blisters over immobile areas, but leave small blisters on immobile areas intact. If there is a concern about follow-up, debride all blisters as intact or spontaneously collapsed blisters can serve as a focus for wound infection.

Silver sulfadiazine has both Gram-positive and Gram-negative activity and provides good prophylactic antibiotic coverage. It also facilitates debridement. However, do not use silver sulfadiazine on the face, for children with hypersensitivity to sulfonamides, or for infants under two months of age (bacitracin ointment is an acceptable alternative). Use a sterile tongue depressor to apply a 2 mm layer, and cover with either a nonadherent or petrolatum-impregnated dressing, then wrap with gauze.

If the hand and fingers are involved, dress each finger individually and splint the hand with the wrist extended to 15–30 degrees, metacarpophalangeal joints at 60–90 degrees of flexion, the interphalangeal joints fully extended, and the thumb fully abducted. Use a sling to elevate the extremity above the level of the heart.

Clean and dress the burn daily. At each dressing change, remove the silver sulfadiazine completely, as it loses its antibacterial activity.

Biobrane (Woodruff Laboratories, Santa Ana, CA), a biosynthetic dressing coated with collagen peptides, is indicated for superficial second-degree burns (those with no chance of becoming third-degree burns). Apply it directly to a cleaned burn area, then cover with an absorbent dressing that should be changed every 24 hours. The Biobrane will separate on its own in 1–2 weeks. Apply it to flat surfaces only.

Third-Degree Burns

If the burn encompasses <2% total BSA, with no involvement of the face, hands, feet, or perineum, the care is the same as for second-degree burns. If >2% total BSA is involved, admit the patient to a burn unit.

General Approach to the Burned Child

1. Stop the burning process by removing burned clothing and copiously lavage all chemical burns. Apply cool or room-temperature soaks to reverse the thermal gradient and relieve pain (second-degree burns), but avoid hypothermia.
2. Assess and maintain ventilation. Check for signs of inhalation injury (pp. 226–229); if any are present, measure the oxygen saturation and immediately perform fiberoptic laryngoscopy to rule-out involvement of the upper airway. Obtain a carboxyhemoglobin level if the patient was in a closed-space fire. If there is a marked metabolic acidosis or hyperlactatemia, treat the patient for possible cyanide toxicity (see p. 229).
3. Initiate IV fluid therapy for patients with >20% partial- or full-thickness burns. Immediately place a large-bore IV catheter in either a central or peripheral vein found in an unburned area. Treat signs of hypovolemia with a 20 mL/kg bolus of normal saline or lactated Ringer's solution. Use dopamine (5–20 mcg/kg/min) if poor perfusion persists. For patients not in shock, administer 2–4 mL/kg/%BSA burned of normal saline or lactated Ringer's solution over the first 24 hours. Give one-half of the calculated total over the first 8 hours (starting from the time of the burn incident) and the remainder over the next 16 hours. For a child weighing <30 kg add the estimated daily maintenance fluid requirement. A larger patient >30 kg does not need the maintenance fluids added as part of the fluid replacement. The goal is a urine output from 1 mL/kg/h in a young child to 0.5 mL/kg/h in an adolescent.

   Insert an indwelling urinary catheter using aseptic technique in any burn victim needing IV fluids. Discard any urine obtained when the catheter is inserted, as this may have been in the bladder before the burn injury. Check the urine (with a dipstick) for hemoglobin or myoglobin; if positive, obtain a microscopic urinalysis to differentiate hematuria from rhabdomyolysis. If myoglobin is present, increase the fluid rate to maintain a brisk urine output (2 mL/kg/h).
4. Take a careful history. Inquire about the cause of the burn, preexisting illnesses, chronic medications, and allergies. Suspect child abuse (pp. 604–608) if the accident occurred when the child was reportedly alone, the injury is attributed to a sibling, the history varies from one interview to another, there is a previous history of accidental trauma, the history is incompatible with the observed injury, or there is delay in seeking medical attention.
5. Check the tetanus immunization status and give 0.5 mL of tetanus toxoid booster (Tdap) if the last immunization was more than five years ago. If the patient has received fewer than three tetanus toxoid boosters, give 0.5 mL of tetanus immune globulin as well as 0.5 mL of tetanus toxoid booster.
6. Perform a careful physical examination. Check for corneal injury with fluorescein staining if the lids are burned, the eyelashes have been singed, or eye damage is suspected. Evaluate the patient for associated injuries, especially fractures and head

trauma, and signs of child abuse. Non-accidental burn injuries include pattern burns, sharply demarcated burns of the hands, feet, buttocks, and perineum, and stocking-glove burn injuries.

7. Insert a nasogastric tube and attach it to suction if the burn exceeds 20% of total BSA or if there is nausea, vomiting, or abdominal distention. An ileus is common as a result of splanchnic vasoconstriction.

8. Give pain medication as needed (IV morphine sulfate, 0.1–0.15 mg/kg q 15–60 min).

9. Perform the initial burn wound care as described above.

10. Examine the patient for circumferential injuries. Remove all rings, bracelets, and restrictive clothing. Look carefully for signs of impaired circulation, including cyanosis, impaired capillary refill, changes in sensation, deep tissue pain, or paresthesias.
    If circulatory impairment is a possibility, call a burn surgeon or a plastic surgeon as an escharotomy may be necessary.

Follow-up (Minor Burns)

- First-degree burns: return at once if blisters form.
- Second- and third-degree burns: return at once if there are any signs or symptoms of impaired circulation (numbness, tingling, or color change distal to the bandage) or infection (fever, vomiting, poor feeding, or change in mental status). Otherwise, follow-up with a primary care provider in 3–4 days

Indications for Admission

- Moderate burn
- Major burn: transfer to a burn center
- Patient with any size burn whose family seems unable to cope with recommendations for care and follow-up

Guidelines for Transferring the Burn Victim

In addition to the usual considerations when transferring any patient to another institution, there are several special concerns when transferring a burn victim:

1. The patient's airway must be securely protected. An accidental extubation in a burn victim with a swollen airway can prove fatal. A physician who is able to perform an emergency intubation and/or emergency cricothyroidotomy must accompany the patient.

2. Just prior to transport, remove all saline-soaked dressing and replace them with sterile dry gauze dressings to prevent hypothermia.

3. Treat the patient with adequate sedation and analgesia to minimize pain and agitation.

Bibliography

Bodger O, Theron A, Williams D. Comparison of three techniques for calculation of the Parkland formula to aid fluid resuscitation in paediatric burns. *Eur J Anaesthesiol*. 2013;**30**(8):483–491.

Gonzalez R, Shanti CM. Overview of current pediatric burn care. *Semin Pediatr Surg*. 2015;**24**(1):47–49.

Haines E, Fairbrother H. Optimizing emergency management to reduce morbidity and mortality in pediatric burn patients. *Pediatr Emerg Med Pract.* 2015;**12**(5):1–23.

Krishnamoorthy V, Ramaiah R, Bhananker SM. Pediatric burn injuries. *Int J Crit Illn Inj Sci.* 2012;**2**(3):128–134.

Schiestl C, Meuli M, Trop M, Neuhaus K. Management of burn wounds. *Eur J Pediatr Surg.* 2013;**23**(5):341–348.

World Health Organization. Management of burns. www.who.int/surgery/publications/Burns_management.pdf (accessed June 20, 2017).

Drowning

Drowning is a process resulting in primary respiratory impairment from submersion or immersion in a liquid medium. This results in a liquid–air interface in the child's airway. Therefore, do not use the terms wet drowning, dry drowning, secondary drowning, and near-drowning. Approximately one-third of deaths from unintentional drowning occur in patients <19 years of age, while drowning is the second most common cause of injury and death in children aged 1 month to 14 years of age. Among toddlers, most incidents occur in bathtubs and swimming pools. Risk factors include inadequate supervision, developmental disorders, use of alcohol and/or illicit drugs, and associated trauma.

Death may be caused directly by laryngospasm, or by cerebral hypoxia, carbon dioxide narcosis, or cardiac arrest.

Aspiration of either saltwater or freshwater results in hypoxemia. There is no longer a distinction made between the two. As little as 1–3 mL/kg of water can cause pulmonary vasoconstriction and impaired gas exchange, as surfactant is either destroyed or washed out. Compliance is reduced and ventilation/perfusion mismatch develops. These pulmonary complications can develop slowly or rapidly.

Hypothermia is the double-edged sword of drowning. Cold water (< 20 °C; 68 °F) decreases metabolic demands and shunting blood from nonvital to vital organs, but adverse effects such as dysrhythmias (sinus bradycardia, atrial and ventricular fibrillation, asystole) often occur.

Clinical Presentation and Diagnosis

Inquire about the site and duration of submersion, water temperature, possibility of trauma or physical abuse, drug or alcohol use, and past medical history.

A drowning victim's mental status may range from fully alert to comatose. The patient may have no signs of respiratory distress or may present with tachypnea, nasal flaring, and/or retractions. Auscultation of the lungs may reveal adventitious sounds (crackles and/or wheezes), and any type of dysrhythmia may be seen on ECG. Among adolescents, inquire about drinking or drug use prior to the event. The chest radiograph can be normal or show evidence of air space disease either localized or diffuse.

Trauma is often involved in near-drowning. Pay particular attention to the possibility of head or cervical spine injuries. Consider internal injuries to the chest or abdomen, especially if the patient does not respond appropriately to resuscitation interventions. Arterial blood gases may show a metabolic and/or respiratory acidosis.

ED Management

Handle the patient carefully because of the possibility of cervical spine injury (pp. 741–743). Place a rectal temperature probe to confirm the core temperature, rapidly assess the airway and breathing, and provide 100% oxygen. Consult with a pediatric pulmonologist about the possibility of noninvasive ventilation (NIV) for a patient who is alert and maintaining their airway, but remains hypoxic. Indications for assisted ventilation via bag-mask apparatus and endotracheal intubation are apnea, an oxygen saturation <85% while inspiring 100% oxygen, or signs of neurologic deterioration. If intubation is needed, place an orogastric tube to relieve gastric distention. The patient may require positive end expiratory pressure (PEEP) if there is an inadequate response to the initial ventilator settings. Treat bronchospasm with nebulized albuterol (0.03 mL/kg in 3 mL of normal saline) and repeat as needed. There is no evidence that steroids are beneficial in aspiration-induced bronchospasm.

Assess the cardiac status and continuously monitor the ECG. If the patient is pulseless, start basic life support, then advanced life support as warranted by the ECG rhythm and the clinical status. However, most resuscitation drugs are not effective in a severely hypothermic patient and are therefore contraindicated during rewarming (see Hypothermia, pp. 224–226). One exception is glucose. Give 0.5–1 g/kg (1–2 mL/kg D_{50}; 0.25–0.5 mL/kg D_{25}) to any patient with altered mental status. Also give naloxone (0.4–2.0 mg IV or 4.0 mg ET) to an adolescent if the history suggests a narcotic overdose.

Start at least one large-bore IV with normal saline or lactated Ringer's solution. However, give fluids cautiously since these patients are at risk for pulmonary and cerebral edema, and warm the fluids if the patient is hypothermic. Initial laboratory studies include CBC, electrolytes, BUN, creatinine, glucose, CPK, ABG, serum pregnancy test (for a female of childbearing age), serum osmolality, and type and cross (if there is any suspicion of trauma). If the history or physical examination suggests an intoxication, obtain a blood alcohol level and urine for toxicology. Also obtain an ECG and a chest radiograph. The need for other tests, such as additional x-rays or CT scans, are determined by the history of the event and serial assessments.

An initially well-appearing child may rapidly develop both pulmonary and neurologic complications any time within the first 24 hours. However, most asymptomatic children may be discharged after eight hours' observation if the physical examination, the initial chest x-ray, and all tests are normal; the physician is assured that the family is reliable; and adequate follow-up is arranged. Poor prognostic signs include a submersion duration of >9 minutes, prolonged apnea, or coma.

Follow-up

- At once if pulmonary (cough, tachypnea, dyspnea) or neurologic (altered mental status) symptoms develop, otherwise primary care follow-up in 2–3 days

Indications for Admission

- History of prolonged submersion
- Respiratory or neurologic symptoms
- A patient with an abnormal chest x-ray, for at least 24 hours

Bibliography

Engel SC. Drowning episodes: prevention and resuscitation tips. *J Fam Pract*. 2015;**64**(2):E1–E6.

Schilling UM, Bortolin M. Drowning. *Minerva Anestesiol*. 2012;**78**(1):69–77.

Szpilman D, Bierens JJ, Handley AJ, Orlowski JP. Drowning. *N Engl J Med*. 2012;**366**(22):2102–2110.

Vanden Hock TL, Morrison LJ, Shuster M, et al. Part 12: cardiac arrest in special situations: 2010 American Heart Association guidelines for cardiopulmonary resuscitation and emergency cardiovascular care. *Circulation*. 2010;**122**:S829.

Electrical Injuries

Small children, especially toddlers, frequently sustain low-voltage electrical injuries when they insert objects (pins, keys, etc.) into household sockets or chew on electrical cords. Older children are more likely to sustain high-voltage electrical injuries by contacting live third rails or power lines when climbing.

Most of the harmful effects from electrical injuries are due to the heat generated, which is directly related to current strength, tissue resistance, pathway, type of current (i.e., direct or alternating), and duration of contact. Serious electrical injuries are uncommon, but carry a mortality risk of approximately 40%.

Electrical injuries are usually categorized in terms of high (>1000 V) or low (<500–1000 V) voltage. In the United States, household current is low-voltage (110 V). Because voltage is directly related to current, high-voltage injuries are usually more serious than low-voltage, although a low-voltage contact applied to areas of low resistance can also cause serious injury. Exposure to an electrical socket with a wet hand can result in a current of 50–100 mA, which is enough to cause ventricular fibrillation. Low-voltage injuries account for more than one-half of all deaths from electrical injuries.

Clinical Presentation and Diagnosis

Electrical injuries can cause multiorgan dysfunction and a variety of burns and traumatic injuries. A child who has had contact with electric current can present with first-, second-, or third-degree burns of the skin, as well as entrance and exit burns (which are usually third-degree burns). There may also be burns at flexor creases and at the oral commissure, which may be associated with delayed labial artery bleeding of 2–21 days after the burn.

If the electrical current takes a vertical path, or if there is extensive skin damage, cardiac involvement is more likely. Cardiac complications include all forms of dys-rhythmias, ranging from occasional ectopic atrial and/or ventricular premature contractions (VPCs), supraventricular tachycardia, first-, second-, and third-degree AV blocks, ventricular tachycardia, and ventricular fibrillation. ECG abnormalities are usually evident upon initial ED evaluation and commonly include accelerated sinus rhythm and nonspecific ST–T-wave changes, although damage to the myocardium is uncommon. Pulmonary involvement can include pulmonary contusion, hemothorax, pneumothorax, and/or ventilatory arrest.

Central nervous system involvement may be due to the electrical injury itself or the subsequent fall after the event. The patient can present with any type of mental status change. Other neurologic symptoms, such as paralysis, can occur immediately or can be delayed for up to several days. Electric current can cause tetany of skeletal muscle and both upper and lower motor neuron findings may be noted. This can lead to all types of musculoskeletal injury, from strains to fractures and/or dislocations.

Vascular injuries directly from the electric current can include hemorrhage, either immediate or delayed, in addition to thrombosis. Renal complications can include renal failure, which may be due to either third-spacing of fluid or rhabdomyolysis.

Gastrointestinal injuries can occur in up to 25% of high-voltage injuries. The most common complication is adynamic ileus. Other conditions that may be seen include hepatic, gallbladder, and pancreatic necrosis as well as stress ulcers.

High-Voltage Injuries

The patient may present with a variety of complications involving a number of organ systems. Asystole, respiratory arrest, and hypoxia-induced ventricular fibrillation are the most common causes of immediate death. Other complications include hemolysis, rhabdomyolysis, direct burns of the lung or viscera, neurologic injuries, renal failure, and musculoskeletal injuries such as fractures and dislocations. Burns are usually characteristic of high-voltage injuries. The types of burns that may be seen include the following.

Flash Burns

Flash burns are caused by electrical arcs on the skin. They resemble thermal burns and require the same treatment.

Arc Burns

The temperature of an electrical arc can reach 2500–5000 °C. These high-voltage burns have a dry center (up to 3 cm) with a surrounding area of congestion. There may be internal injury along the arc pathway.

Contact Burns

These may look like flash burns early in the course of care and may also suggest internal injury.

Low-Voltage Injuries

Most low-voltage injuries initially present with a small, localized, painless, white parchment-like patch of skin. However, if a child has bitten on an electrical wire, there can be considerable edema of the lips, tongue, and gums. Rarely, severe intraoral edema may result in airway obstruction. If the child conducts electricity, muscle paralysis and ventricular dysrhythmias may occur. Fortunately, conduction with low voltage is rare, so these are usually limited injuries.

ED Management

High-Voltage Injuries

Rapidly assess the adequacy of the airway. Use the chin-lift maneuver without hyperextension to maintain patency if there is the possibility of a cervical spine injury, either directly from the electrical injury or from resulting trauma (e.g., fall from a tree or ladder). If the patient is not breathing, ventilate with a bag-mask resuscitator and prepare for intubation. If respirations are adequate, administer 100% oxygen via a nonrebreather mask.

Assess the cardiovascular status, obtain an ECG, and secure a large-bore IV. If the patient is pulseless and the ECG monitor reveals ventricular fibrillation or pulseless ventricular tachycardia, defibrillate with an energy level of 2 J/kg (monophasic or biphasic; see Ventricular Fibrillation, pp. 58–64).

If the patient presents with signs of inadequate tissue perfusion, give an IV fluid bolus of 20 mL/kg of NS and repeat as needed. If the patient remains hemodynamically unstable, continue rapid IV hydration and start a dopamine drip at 5–20 mcg/kg/min (see Shock, pp. 28–36). However, inadequate tissue perfusion may be due to an associated thoracic, abdominal, or long-bone injury sustained after the electrical insult. Always consider major trauma in patients presenting in shock after an electrical injury.

If the patient has a normal pulse rate and blood pressure, give IV hydration with D5 ½ NS at a rate of 1.5–2 times maintenance. Aim for a urine output of at least 2–3 mL/kg/h, but do not add potassium for the first 24 hours (unless the patient has documented hypokalemia). The presence of rhabdomyolysis (hemoglobin or myoglobin on urine dipstick and/or an elevated creatine phosphokinase [CPK]) indicates significant deep tissue injury and predicts renal failure unless a brisk urine output is quickly established.

Initial laboratory tests include blood for an ABG, CBC, electrolytes, glucose, BUN, creatinine, PT and PTT, serum osmolality, pregnancy test (for adolescent females of childbearing age), a urinalysis, and a 12-lead ECG. Obtain radiographic studies of any region you suspect may have been injured. Do rely on CPK-MB as a single criterion for myocardial infarction as an elevation in the absence of other evidence of myocardial injury (chest pain and/or EKG changes) is not specific for myocardial damage. The role of troponin in electrical injuries has not been studied extensively.

Perform a secondary survey to check for surface thermal burns, orthopedic injuries, or evidence of compartment syndrome. If the patient presents with an altered mental status, evidence or suspicion of an intoxicant, or a distracting injury, clear the cervical spine radiographically. However, a head CT is also indicated for continued altered mental status after electrical injury.

Categorize and treat surface thermal burns in the usual fashion (see Burns, pp. 207–211).

Low-Voltage Injuries

Quickly assess the patency of the airway, especially if there are burns of the mouth. Perform a careful physical examination, looking for evidence of both an entrance and an exit wound. For the common electrical burn of the mouth, provide local wound care with topical bacitracin. If localized tissue charring is present and there is any suggestion of injury to underlying structures, immediately consult with a surgeon. When significant portions of the lips are involved (especially the oral commissure), consult a plastic surgeon or oral surgeon. Warn the parents that 2–21 days after the injury, as the burned tissue begins to separate, bleeding from the labial artery may occur. This bleeding can be controlled by local pressure but occasionally requires suture ligation in the ED.

Burns that are sustained by placing a metal object into a wall socket can usually be managed with routine local burn care only. Cardiovascular and neurologic complications are rare. Therefore, if the vital signs (particularly the pulse) and mental status are normal, in the absence of a history of loss of consciousness, tetany, wet skin, or evidence of current flow across the heart, an ECG and cardiac monitoring are not necessary.

Follow-up

- Immediate, for any signs or symptoms of impaired circulation (numbness, tingling, color change distal to the bandage) or infection (fever, vomiting, poor feeding, change in mental status). Otherwise, primary care follow-up in 3–4 days

Indications for Admission

- The presence of both an entrance and an exit wound
- Any neurologic or cardiovascular instability
- Patient with mouth burns unwilling or unable to take adequate fluids by mouth
- High-voltage electrical burns

Bibliography

Alemayehu H, Tarkowski A, Dehmer JJ, et al. Management of electrical and chemical burns in children. *J Surg Res.* 2014;**190**(1):210–213.

Dokov W. Assessment of risk factors for death in electrical injury. *Burns.* 2009;**35**:114–117.

Glatstein MM, Ayalon I, Miller E, Scolnik D. Pediatric electrical burn injuries: experience of a large tertiary care hospital and a review of electrical injury. *Pediatr Emerg Care.* 2013;**29**(6):737–740.

Roberts S, Meltzer JA. An evidence-based approach to electrical injuries in children. *Pediatr Emerg Med Pract.* 2013;**10**:1–16.

Frostbite

Frostbite occurs when ice crystals form within the soft tissues as a consequence of prolonged exposure to cold. For this to occur, the soft tissues have to be cooled to –4 to –2.2 °C (24.8–28 °F). Low ambient temperatures and high wind velocity quicken the freezing process. The tissue temperature is influenced by the circulation in the extremity and the cold stress, which in turn depends on the environmental temperature, wind chill, moisture, and protective insulation. Circulation in the extremity, which influences the tissue's internal heat flow, is affected by constrictive garments, the position of the extremity, local pressure, and vasospasm. The most severe damage occurs to tissues that freeze, thaw, and then refreeze. Factors that predispose to cold injury include inadequate nutrition, smoking, alcohol and drug use, fatigue, and tight clothing.

Superficial frostbite involves the skin only. Deep frostbite involves the underlying tissues, such as muscles and tendons.

Clinical Presentation and Diagnosis

Frostbite most commonly involves distal, relatively poorly perfused regions of the body, such as fingertips, toes, earlobes, and the nose. In children, areas that have poor heat-generating ability and insulation, including the cheeks and chin, are also at high risk for frostbite. However, any area of skin that has prolonged exposure to cold can be affected.

Initially, frostbite presents with a painful cold feeling and skin blanching. This is followed by numbness, while the involved area becomes waxy, white, and firm. Deeply frostbitten skin feels hard and appears white with a yellow to blue tint. Superficial frostbitten skin also feels firm, but will be soft and indent when pressure is applied. All patients experience a sensory deficit (touch, pain, temperature) in the involved region that may extend just proximal to the line of demarcation of the frostbite.

Upon thawing an area of superficial frostbite, there is a throbbing pain followed by a tingling sensation. Deeper injuries become mottled-blue, swollen, and extremely painful upon warming. Edema occurs within three hours after thawing, with vesicles and bullae forming in more severe cases after 6–48 hours. Immediately following thawing, findings such as sensation to pinprick, good color, warm tissue, and large, clear non-hemorrhagic blebs which, if the digits are involved extend completely to the tips, suggest a relatively favorable prognosis for tissue viability. Poor prognostic signs include the late occurrence of small, dark hemorrhagic blebs that do not extend to the tips of the extremities, cyanosis, and the absence of edema.

ED Management

The goal of therapy, which is prevention of further soft tissue destruction, is accomplished via rapid rewarming. Thaw the frozen part by immersion in water heated to 37.8–42 °C (100–108 °F), but do not use warmer water, which may cause burns. If possible, have the child move the frostbitten body part during rewarming. A whirlpool is ideal for an extremity, as thawing time is decreased when water is circulated. Carefully monitor the temperature. As the bath cools (check with a thermometer), add hotter water to maintain the desired temperature range. Avoid rubbing or massaging the frostbitten area.

The warming usually takes 15–30 minutes; remove the extremity after thawing has occurred. The endpoint is when the affected area becomes soft, develops a purple-red color, and sensation starts to return. While in the last stages of rewarming, the patient may experience severe pain and require analgesia (morphine sulfate 0.10–0.15 mg/kg IV).

After thawing, inspect the wound. Debride any ruptured blebs, apply an antibiotic ointment (such as bacitracin) or aloe vera, and apply bulky sterile dressings. Place cotton between affected fingers or toes. Again, the use of a potent analgesic such as morphine may be necessary, but prophylactic antibiotics are not indicated. Obtain plastic surgery consultation early in the course of treatment. An escharotomy is indicated if the digits are not freely mobile. Give tetanus toxoid (Tdap 0.5 mL) if the last immunization was more than five years ago.

Follow-up

- Daily follow-up, until injured areas are healing well

Indications for Admission

- Frostbite of hands and feet

Bibliography

Fudge JR, Bennett BL, Simanis JP, Roberts WO. Medical evaluation for exposure extremes: cold. *Clin J Sport Med*. 2015;**25**(5):432–436.

Handford C, Buxton P, Russell K, et al. Frostbite: a practical approach to hospital management. *Extrem Physiol Med*. 2014 22;3:7.

Hutchison RL. Frostbite of the hand. *J Hand Surg Am*. 2014;**39**(9):1863–1868.

McIntosh SE, Opacic M, Freer L, Grissom CK, et al. Wilderness Medical Society practice guidelines for the prevention and treatment of frostbite: 2014 update. *Wilderness Environ Med*. 2014;**25**(4 Suppl.): S43–S54.

Petrone P, Asensio JA, Marini CP. Management of accidental hypothermia and cold injury. *Curr Probl Surg*. 2014;**51**(10):417–431.

Heat-Excess Syndromes

Most cases of heat illnesses occur during the summer months. Environmental conditions that increase the risk include the lack of air-conditioning and enclosure in a small, unventilated space such as an automobile. Extreme physical activity, underlying illness, alcohol abuse, inadequate fluid intake, and drugs such as cocaine, salicylates, amphetamines, phenothiazines, antihistamines, or anticholinergics, coupled with any of the predisposing environmental factors, place a person at a high risk for developing hyperthermic injury.

Children are less efficient thermoregulators compared to adults. They exhibit a slower speed of acclimatization, have a lower sweating rate, and produce more metabolic heat per kilogram of body weight, placing a greater strain on thermoregulatory mechanisms. Children also have a higher set point (the change in core temperature when sweating starts) than adults.

Clinical Presentation and Diagnosis

Heat Cramps

Heat cramps are painful muscle cramps that are probably caused by electrolyte depletion in association with insufficient blood supply to an exercising muscle. Large muscle groups, such as the hamstrings and the gastrocnemius, are most likely to be involved. Clinically, the affected muscles are contracted. However, the onset may be delayed, occurring when the patient is showering after exercise or resting. The patient has a normal mental status and normal vital signs, but the core temperature may be slightly elevated. There may or may not be sweating.

Heat Exhaustion

Heat exhaustion is caused by excessive sweating associated with inadequate intake of water and salt in a hot environment. Symptoms include headache, dizziness, fatigue, anxiety syncope, visual disturbances, nausea, vomiting, diarrhea, malaise, myalgias, and muscle cramps. The patient is usually tachycardic and tachypneic, and may have orthostatic vital sign changes. At the time of presentation, however, sweating may not be present. The rectal temperature is typically 38–40 °C (100.4–104.0 °F).

Heat Stroke

Heat stroke is a life-threatening emergency that occurs when the core body temperature exceeds 40.0 °C (104.0 °F). The estimated mortality is >50%. It is associated with acute neurologic changes, including irritability, aggression, or emotional instability, along with any of the symptoms of heat exhaustion. Heat stroke has been classified as either classic or exertional. Classic heat stroke occurs in an infant secondary to poor water intake. It has a relatively slow onset, with the insidious development of anorexia, nausea, vomiting, headaches, dry skin, and progressive deterioration of mental function. Sweating is usually absent (however, there are cases where sweating is present) and rhabdomyolysis and hypoglycemia are uncommon. Exertional heat stroke usually occurs in a patient who engages in prolonged physical activity. It presents with the rapid onset of severe prostration, headache, syncope, tachycardia, tachypnea, and hypotension. Lactic acidosis is common and rhabdomyolysis, hypoglycemia, and hypocalcemia are often present. The most important prognostic sign is the duration, not the degree, of the hyperthermic state.

ED Management

Heat Cramps

Treat heat cramps by placing the patient at rest in a cool environment. In mild cases, replace salt with a salt-containing oral rehydration solution. For severe cases, start an IV and give the patient 20 mL/kg of normal saline. Obtain blood for CBC and electrolytes (including calcium and magnesium). The patient may be discharged after clinical improvement (well-hydrated, no cramps).

Heat Exhaustion

Immediately place the patient in a cool environment, remove any excess clothing, and sponge with lukewarm tap water. Then increase the heat dissipation by placing fans directed to blow air across the patient. Assess the airway and breathing and administer 100% oxygen. Start a large-bore IV, give 20 mL/kg of normal saline, then reassess the patient's hydration status and response to fluids. Obtain a CBC, electrolytes, and urinalysis. Discharge the patient after cooling and volume replacement, if vital signs are normal and symptoms have resolved.

Heat Stroke

Rapidly assess airway and breathing and intubate a patient who is comatose, having seizures, or has an oxygen saturation <85% while breathing 100% oxygen. Obtain vital signs including a rectal temperature (use a rectal probe), and monitor the cardiac rhythm. Undress the patient completely and start the cooling process by spraying with lukewarm tap water, then position fans to blow air across the body. It is estimated that the evaporation of 1 g of water transfers seven times as much heat as melting 1 g of ice. However, use ice packs to the axillae, neck, and groin as supplemental treatment. Continue this aggressive cooling, at a rate of approximately 0.2 °C (0.4 °F) per minute until the core temperature reaches 38 °C (100.4 °F), to prevent overshoot hypothermia. Do not use cold water immersion, as it may cause overshoot hypothermia and bradycardia. Prevent shivering, which generates body heat, with IV lorazepam (0.1 mg/kg IV). Alcohol baths are contraindicated due to the potential of alcohol intoxication. Acetaminophen and ibuprofen have no role in the treatment of heat stroke.

Start two large-bore IVs, immediately give 0.5–1 g/kg dextrose (1–2 mL/kg D_{50}; 2–4 mL/kg D_{25}) and two 20 mL/kg boluses of normal saline, then reassess the circulatory status. If the patient remains in shock after the second bolus of crystalloid, severe vasodilation is likely. Use central venous pressure (CVP) monitoring to guide further fluid therapy, since continued boluses may cause pulmonary edema. If the CVP is low, give repeated fluid boluses. If the CVP is normal, and the patient is still hypotensive, start dopamine at a rate of 2–5 mcg/kg/min. Insert a Foley catheter, and carefully monitor intake and output.

Initial laboratory studies include CBC, PT/PTT, electrolytes, BUN, creatinine, glucose, CPK, LFTs, serum osmolality, salicylate level, pregnancy test (for females of childbearing age), fibrinogen, lactate, urinalysis, and an ECG. Reassess the patient frequently to identify complications such as neurologic deterioration, liver and pulmonary injury, rhabdomyolysis, and disseminated intravascular coagulation.

Follow-up

- Heat cramps: primary care follow-up in 1–2 weeks
- Heat exhaustion: next day

Indications for Admission

- Heat stroke

Bibliography

Atha WF. Heat-related illness. *Emerg Med Clin North Am.* 2013;**31**(4):1097–1108.

Casa DJ, DeMartini JK, Bergeron MF, et al. National Athletic Trainers' Association position statement: exertional heat illnesses. *J Athl Train.* 2015;**50**(9):986–1000.

Lipman GS, Eifling KP, Ellis MA, et al. Wilderness Medical Society practice guidelines for the prevention and treatment of heat-related illness: 2014 update. *Wilderness Environ Med.* 2014;**25**(4 Suppl.):S55–S65.

Santelli J, Sullivan JM, Czarnik A, Bedolla J. Heat illness in the emergency department: keeping your cool. *Emerg Med Pract.* 2014;**16**(8):1–21.

Seeyave DM, Brown KM. Environmental emergencies, radiological emergencies, bites and stings. In Shaw KN, Bachur RG (eds.) *Fleisher & Ludwig's Textbook of Pediatric Emergency Medicine* (7th edn.). Philadelphia, PA: Wolters Kluwer, 2016; 718–760.

Hyperbaric Oxygen Therapy

Hyperbaric oxygen therapy (HBOT) involves the administration of oxygen under increased ambient pressure. While the indications for HBOT are controversial, the most common emergency conditions which appear to benefit from HBOT are decompression sickness, air embolism, and carbon monoxide (CO) poisoning. Table 8.1 lists conditions that are approved for treatment with HBOT, either primarily or adjunctively.

Decompression Sickness and Air Emboli

Decompression sickness occurs most commonly on ascension in free or assisted diving when nitrogen in the blood comes quickly out of solution, resulting in bubble formation in the circulation and tissues. Type I decompression sickness can present with a dull deep pain (usually in a joint or tendon area) which usually resolves in 5–10 minutes, pruritus, or a rash that may be mottling or papular. The upper extremities are usually affected more than the lower extremities. Type II decompression sickness presents with pulmonary symptoms (cough, respiratory distress, chest discomfort), neurologic symptoms (headaches, vertigo, nystagmus, paresis, paralysis, and mental status changes), visual disturbances (scotomata), and circulatory symptoms (shock or thrombus formation).

Table 8.1 Indications for HBOT

Traditional indications	Current indications
Carbon monoxide poisoning	Acute air embolism
Decompression sickness	Acute traumatic ischemia
Gas gangrene	Compromised skin grafts and flaps
Wound healing	Necrotizing soft tissue infections
	Osteoradionecrosis
	Soft tissue radionecrosis
	Thermal burns

Adapted from Weiss LD, Van Meter KW. The applications of hyperbaric oxygen therapy in emergency medicine. *Am J Emerg Med* 1992;10:558–567.

Arterial gas emboli result from leakage of air bubbles into the circulation and may cause circulatory obstruction. They may be iatrogenic (cardiovascular procedures, central line placement, lung biopsies, hemodialysis) or may be a complication of uncontrolled ascents in scuba diving.

When treating both of these disorders, HBOT relies upon two basic laws of physics: Boyle's law (the pressure of a gas is inversely proportional to its volume), and Henry's law (the amount of gas dissolved in solution is directly proportional to its partial pressure). HBOT causes a reduction in the size of the trapped bubbles and forces them back into solution from the circulatory system and tissues.

Carbon Monoxide Poisoning

Carbon monoxide competes with oxygen for hemoglobin and cytochrome binding sites. Toxicity results from several mechanisms, including direct hypoxic damage to tissues, inhibition of cellular respiration by disruption of the cytochrome system and mitochondrial enzymes leading to production of oxygen free radicals, and lipid peroxidation in the central nervous system. Signs and symptoms of carbon monoxide poisoning include fatigue, nausea, vomiting and neurologic abnormalities ranging from headache to personality deficit to frank coma.

The half-life of carboxyhemoglobin (COHb) is approximately 240–320 minutes (range of 128–409 minutes) at sea level (1 atmosphere) in 21% oxygen. It is decreased to approximately 40–80 minutes while receiving 100% oxygen, to approximately 15–30 minutes at 2.5–3.0 atmospheres in 100% oxygen.

Since the serum (either venous or arterial) COHb level may not reflect COHb tissue levels and often does not correlate with the degree of toxicity, the signs and symptoms of toxicity are equally important in determining the need for therapy for CO poisoning. HBOT is recommended for a patient with a history of unconsciousness after exposure to CO regardless of COHb level, a history of or continued mental status change or other neurologic deficit, cardiac dysfunction or ischemia, persistent metabolic acidosis, a COHb level >25% regardless of symptoms, or for any pregnant woman with a history of CO exposure (regardless of COHb level). The only absolute contraindication to HBOT is an untreated pneumothorax.

If the indications for HBOT are nonurgent (burns or wounds; CO exposure presenting with a mild headache that has resolved with 100% O_2 therapy), defer treating patients with significant upper respiratory infections, asthma, fever, seizure disorder, diabetes, or a history of chest surgery or pneumothorax. Also, unstable patients who have had a cardiac arrest and/or require pressors for support may experience little improvement in clinical symptoms after HBOT because of other ongoing medical problems, and they are difficult to resuscitate inside the hyperbaric chamber. A patient who has suffered a cardiac arrest has a very poor prognosis and may not experience enough benefit from HBOT to warrant the risks.

Initial ED Management and Preparation for HBOT

Initial priorities include addressing the ABCs, providing 100% oxygen via a tight-fitting nonrebreather mask or endotracheal tube, and obtaining a COHb level from venous or arterial blood using a heparinized 1 mL syringe. If the patient is in respiratory distress or requires ventilatory support, secure an IV and obtain an ABG, ECG, and chest x-ray. Other tests may be indicated, including serum electrolytes, liver function tests, and creatinine. In addition, assess the patient for other traumatic injuries, smoke inhalation, or cyanide poisoning. These conditions must be fully addressed before the patient is taken into the hyperbaric chamber.

Once it is determined that HBOT is indicated, prepare the patient for the chamber. If the patient is intubated with a cuffed endotracheal tube, replace the air in the cuff with saline or water, since fluids do not compress under pressure. Change glass IV bottles, which may implode under pressure, to flexible plastic IV bags. Adjust IV drip rates manually with pressure bags. Open the nasogastric tube (if inserted) to gravity to allow for equalization of pressure between the stomach and the atmosphere. Make sure that the patient's clothing is made of cotton or flame-retardant material, and remove any fire hazards, including matches, lighters, jewelry, watches, alcohol, cosmetics, lubricants, hairsprays, cell phones, and newspapers from the patient before going into the chamber.

Sedate and paralyze (pp. 14–19) intubated patients to minimize the risk of extubation, and consider restraints for patients with altered mental status who may improve and awaken during treatment and injure themselves or chamber personnel. Optional considerations include prophylactic administration of a decongestant (pseudoephedrine 1 mg/kg, 30 mg maximum) to an awake patient to help prevent middle ear and sinus barotrauma.

While practices vary among institutions, one current acceptable treatment protocol for CO poisoning involves administering 100% O_2, via tight-fitting mask or endotracheal tube, at 2.8 ATA for two 23-minute periods interrupted by a 5-minute interval on 21% oxygen (an "air break").

HBOT may result in barotrauma to any air-filled cavity which cannot equilibrate with ambient pressure. The middle ear and/or sinuses are most commonly affected. Rarely, barotrauma may cause a pneumothorax or air embolus.

Oxygen toxicity to the CNS may occur with prolonged exposure to 100% oxygen. Additionally, the seizure threshold may be lowered, and autonomic regulation of respiration may be affected. However, neurotoxicity is unusual with the low-pressure, short-duration treatments used in most clinical situations.

Pulmonary toxicity may occur after six continuous hours of exposure to 100% O_2 at 2 ATA. However, no HBOT protocol requires this length of treatment.

Other side effects include accelerated cataract growth, temporary worsening of myopia or improved presbyopia, claustrophobia, and fatigue. Technical complications of HBOT include a fire risk within the chamber where oxygen is being used, and the inadequacy of equipment and personnel to perform prolonged resuscitation on a patient while pressurized within the chamber.

Follow-up

- Asymptomatic patient: next day

Indications for Admission

- Any patient treated with HBOT who has continued significant respiratory, cardiovascular, or neurologic compromise
- Other medical conditions that necessitate admission (e.g., severe burns or significant smoke inhalation)

Bibliography

Bleecker ML. Carbon monoxide intoxication. *Handb Clin Neurol.* 2015;**131**:191–203.

Camporesi EM. Side effects of hyperbaric oxygen therapy. *Undersea Hyperb Med.* 2014;**41**(3):253–257.

Hampson NB, Plantadosi CA, Thom SR, Weaver LK. Practice recommendation in the diagnosis, management, and prevention of carbon monoxide poisoning. *Am J Resp Crit Care Med.* 2012;**186**:1095–1101.

Moon RE. Hyperbaric oxygen treatment for decompression sickness. *Undersea Hyperb Med.* 2014;**41** (2):151–157.

Thom SR. Hyperbaric oxygen: its mechanisms and safety. *Plast Reconst Surg.* 2011;**127** (Suppl. 1):131S–141S.

Hypothermia

Hypothermia, a core temperature ≤35 °C (95 °F), is usually caused by accidental exposure. At <35 °C (95 °F) the human body loses its ability to generate sufficient heat to maintain bodily functions. Below 30 °C (86 °F) the body assumes the temperature of the surrounding environment.

Children are at particular risk, because of their large body surface area (BSA), lack of fat insulation, inadequate shivering, and inability to escape a cold environment. Prolonged out-of-hospital resuscitation and cold water immersion are common causes of hypothermia. Predisposing factors include malnutrition, hypoglycemia, major trauma, hypothyroidism, Addison's disease, and drug use or abuse (alcohol, antipsychotics, gamma-hydroxybutyrate, opiates, and sedative-hypnotics). Although most cases of accidental exposure are seen in winter, hypothermia may occur in the spring and fall during wet, windy weather. Hypothermia may develop acutely within minutes in a cold water immersion victim, or insidiously over days in a neonate in a poorly heated home.

Clinical Presentation

Mild Hypothermia (32 °C [89.6 °F] to 35 °C [95 °F])

The patient may present with tachypnea, tachycardia, ataxia, dysarthria, and shivering. There may be loss of coordination, but the patient is hemodynamically stable.

Moderate Hypothermia (32 °C [89.6 °F] to 28 °C [82.4 °F])

There may be a slowing of the heart rate or dysrhythmias, as well as a loss of shivering. The mental status may also be altered.

Severe Hypothermia (<28 °C [82.4 °F])

There is a change in the mental status, vascular collapse, loss of reflexes, and malignant dysrhythmias.

Diagnosis

Consider a patient with cold skin, altered mental status, and bradycardia to be hypothermic until proved otherwise. In addition, any severe injury or illness can be associated with hypothermia. Since the diagnosis of hypothermia rests on measuring the core temperature, use a thermocouple probe inserted 3–5 cm into the rectum. Do not use a tympanic thermometer, which is unreliable

A "J," or Osborne wave, may be observed on the ECG of upto 80% of patients with moderate or severe hypothermia. This is a secondary wave, following the S-wave, seen in aVL, aVF, and throughout the chest leads. It is sometimes confused with a right bundle branch block. Other ECG findings include prolonged PR, QRS, and/or QT intervals.

Investigate for precipitating and complicating factors such as alcohol or drug intoxication, near-drowning, head trauma, sepsis, or hypoglycemia. Consider other causes of hypothermia, including hypothyroidism and Addison's disease, when a patient fails to respond to rewarming measures with a rise in core temperature of at least 1 °C per hour.

ED Management

Classify the hypothermia as mild, moderate, or severe (see above). Passive rewarming is satisfactory for mild hypothermia. Remove all wet or cold clothing, place pre-warmed layers of blankets on the patient, give warm IV fluids (normal saline at maintenance), and administer warmed (47 °C; 116.6 °F) humidified oxygen.

A patient with moderate hypothermia requires active external rewarming with electric warming blankets, hot water bottles, heating pads, or warming beds. However, IV access must already be obtained and fluid therapy initiated before active rewarming is started. Otherwise, as vasodilation occurs during warming, the patient can become acutely hypotensive and develop a fatal cardiac arrhythmia.

Treat severe hypothermia with active core rewarming; use warmed nasogastric, peritoneal, or pleural lavage. For peritoneal dialysis infuse a commercial dialysate, normal saline, or lactated Ringer's solution heated to 40–45 °C (104–113 °F). Place two trocars (one for infusion and one for drainage) into the peritoneal cavity. Use a dose of 15 mL/kg, and leave the fluid in place for half-hour, then aspirate.

Because of the very low threshold for cardiac arrhythmias, handle a hypothermia victim as gently as possible. Rapidly assess the child's airway and breathing. Intubate if the patient requires a protected airway or has an oxygen saturation <85% while breathing warmed, humidified oxygen.

Continuously monitor the cardiac rhythm, and if the patient is hypotensive, give a 20 mL/kg fluid challenge of normal saline through a large-bore IV. If peripheral vasoconstriction interferes with obtaining venous access, insert a central femoral line or an IO, but avoid catheters that enter the heart since they may induce cardiac dysrhythmias. After obtaining access and before initiating IV fluids, obtain blood for CBC, electrolytes, BUN, creatinine, calcium, magnesium, amylase, osmolality, fibrinogen, CPK, and PT and PTT.

If the patient's fingerstick reveals hypoglycemia, give glucose (0.5–1.0 g/kg IV). Treat hypotension unresponsive to fluid boluses with a dopamine drip (start at 2–5 mcg/kg/min). Place a Foley catheter and send urine for dipstick and microscopic analysis.

Ventricular fibrillation and asystole (not bradycardia) are the only indications for chest compressions since external cardiac massage can induce fatal ventricular arrhythmias in profound hypothermia. Ventricular fibrillation may occur spontaneously when the core temperature is <28 °C (82.4 °F). If ventricular fibrillation is present, attempt defibrillation (2 J/kg first attempt, 4 J/kg the second attempt, then ≥4 J/kg [10 J/kg or the adult dose maximum (monophasic and biphasic)]). However, electrical defibrillation and standard advanced cardiac life support drug protocols are unlikely to be successful at core temperatures of 28–30 °C (82.4–86 °F). Medications that improve the chances of a return of spontaneous circulation include amiodarone IV/IO (5 mg/kg bolus), and epinephrine IV/IO (0.01 mg/kg of a 1:10,000 solution). Most atrial arrhythmias are benign and disappear with rewarming.

It can be especially difficult to distinguish between hypothermia and death. Therefore, continue all resuscitative measures until the patient's core temperature is >32 °C (89.6 °F).

Indications for Admission

- Hypothermia (mild, moderate, severe)

Bibliography

Brown DJ, Brugger H, Boyd J, Paal P. Accidental hypothermia. *N Engl J Med*. 2012;**367**(20):1930–1938.

Corneli HM. Accidental hypothermia. *Pediatr Emerg Care*. 2012;**28**(5):475–480.

Lantry J, Dezman Z, Hirshon JM. Pathophysiology, management and complications of hypothermia. *Br J Hosp Med (Lond)*. 2012;**73**(1):31–37.

Petrone P, Asensio JA, Marini CP. Management of accidental hypothermia and cold injury. *Curr Probl Surg*. 2014;**51**(10):417–431.

Rischall ML, Rowland-Fisher A. Evidence-based management of accidental hypothermia in the emergency department. *Emerg Med Pract*. 2016;**18**(1):1–18.

Inhalation Injury

Inhalation injuries account for up to 50% of fire-related deaths in the United States. There are four distinct clinical entities with inhalation injuries: thermal burns of the upper airway, smoke inhalation, carbon monoxide poisoning, and cyanide poisoning. The clinical presentations, treatments, and prognoses differ, and serious life-threatening complications can occur insidiously or rapidly.

Thermal Injury

Thermal burns from inhalation injuries almost never involve the lungs or lower airways because of the poor heat-carrying capacity of air and the excellent heat-dissipating capacity of the upper airway. However, lower parenchymal injury can occur with steam burns. Thermal injury above the glottis is very common and probably the most immediate life-threatening problem in a patient with inhalation injury. The extent of the injury may not be seen until 24 hours after the initial insult.

Smoke Inhalation

Many of the chemical components in smoke (aldehydes and organic acids), as well as soot and particulate matter, cause direct parenchymal injury when inhaled, resulting in acute pulmonary insufficiency, pulmonary edema, and bronchopneumonia.

Carbon Monoxide Poisoning

Carbon monoxide (CO) (pp. 228–229) poisoning is the most common cause of fire-related deaths. It is a colorless, odorless, tasteless gas produced by incomplete combustion of carbon-containing materials (wood, fuel, paper). CO binds to hemoglobin with an affinity approximately 250 times greater than oxygen, resulting in displacement of oxygen from hemoglobin and causing cellular anoxia affecting all organ systems.

Cyanide

Cyanide is released through incomplete combustion of acrylics, wool, and plastics and it is absorbed rapidly. Cyanide inhibits aerobic metabolism, reversibly binds with cytochrome oxidase, and inhibits the last step of mitochondrial oxidative phosphorylation, leading to a depletion of adenosine triphosphate.

Clinical Presentation and Diagnosis

Thermal Injury

Thermal injury of the upper airway causes laryngeal edema and laryngospasm which can occur at any time within the first 24 hours and cause total airway obstruction within minutes. Clinically, there is a history of exposure to smoke or fire in an enclosed space, in association with cough, tachypnea, hoarseness, stridor, or carbon-tinged sputum. Burns on the head, face, or neck and singed nasal hairs may also be present.

Smoke Inhalation

A patient with flame burns, the smell of smoke on the clothes, or a history of being in an enclosed smoke-filled room is at high risk for developing pulmonary injury from smoke inhalation. Hoarseness, wheezing, rales, or soot-tinged sputum may be early evidence of pulmonary insufficiency. However, the absence of these signs does not rule-out parenchymal damage, since a patient who appears symptom-free 1–2 hours post-inhalation may subsequently develop significant respiratory problems within a matter of hours. In general, pulmonary insufficiency with bronchospasm occurs in the first 12 hours post-inhalation, pulmonary edema occurs 6–72 hours post-inhalation, and bronchopneumonia occurs within five days post-inhalation. Since the ABGs and chest x-rays may not deteriorate until 12–24 hours post-inhalation, if there is a suspicious history, evaluate and treat the patient for smoke inhalation.

Carbon Monoxide Poisoning

The measured level of carboxyhemoglobin (COHb) correlates only moderately with the clinical picture and degree of CO poisoning. Mild symptoms include dizziness, headache, and GI symptoms. Moderate symptoms include syncope, chest pain, shortness of breath, and altered mental status. Severe symptoms include dysrhythmias, hypotension, non-cardiogenic pulmonary edema, seizures, coma, and ventilatory/cardiac arrest. The COHb level may not accurately reflect the degree of CO poisoning at the cellular level. Therefore, rely on the history and clinical presentation when assessing and managing an inhalation victim for CO poisoning.

Cyanide

Cyanide intoxication presents with altered mental status including seizures and coma. A lactate level ≥10 mmol/L associated with a change in mental status and/or cardiovascular instability suggests the diagnosis. Pulse oximetry is of little value because cyanide inhibits oxidative phosphorylation.

ED Management

Thermal Injury

Mental status changes, cough, tachypnea, hoarseness, stridor, carbon-tinged sputum, singed nasal hairs, or burns on the head, face, or neck are absolute indications for immediate direct visualization of the mouth and upper airway. This can be done in the ED with either a fiberoptic bronchoscope or a laryngoscope, but ensure that the personnel and equipment to perform an emergency intubation or tracheostomy are at the bedside. Upon visualization of the airway, the presence of erythema, edema, dried mucosa, or small blisters on the hard palate or mucosa of the upper airway are clear indications for elective early intubation. All the other signs and symptoms mentioned above are relative indications for elective intubation.

Expectant observation of a patient with a history of, or any signs or symptoms of smoke exposure, is appropriate only in a facility where emergency intubation and/or tracheostomy can be performed immediately. If intubation is required, sedate the patient, if necessary, but steroids are not useful. Elective tracheostomy significantly increases the morbidity and mortality of patients with smoke inhalation and is never indicated.

Smoke Inhalation

Provide humidified high-concentration oxygen by either a tight-fitting nonrebreather face mask or through an endotracheal tube. As with thermal injury of the upper airway, fiberoptic bronchoscopy is the standard diagnostic procedure for pulmonary injury. Treat wheezing with nebulized albuterol (0.03 mL/kg), and follow the progression of the pulmonary disease with serial ABGs and chest x-rays. Prophylactic antibiotics and steroids are contraindicated in treating inhalation injury. Good pulmonary hygiene, bronchodilators, and humidified oxygen are the mainstays of treatment.

Carbon Monoxide Poisoning

The management of CO poisoning is discussed in detail elsewhere (see Hyperbaric Oxygen Therapy, pp. 221–224). However, defer hyperbaric treatment if the patient has severe burns (>30% TBSA), needs PEEP for oxygenation, or requires pressors to maintain a blood pressure. In centers which do not have a hyperbaric chamber, contact the local poison control center for information as to the location of the nearest available hyperbaric center. If a hyperbaric chamber is not available, provide 100% oxygen for at least 24 hours to patients with severe CO poisoning, regardless of the COHb level. Obtain serial ABGs to follow and correct any acid–base derangements.

Cyanide

If cyanide poisoning is suspected, use the Lily Cyanide Antidote Kit that includes amyl nitrite, sodium nitrite, and sodium thiosulfate. However, if the patient has CO poisoning, only use the sodium thiosulfate, as nitrites will induce a methemoglobinemia which may exacerbate the hypoxia secondary to elevated carboxyhemoglobin. Alternatively, use hydro-xocobalamin (man-made vitamin B12a), which chelates with the cyanide molecule (1:1) to form cyanocobalamin or vitamin B12, which is excreted in the urine, causing a reddish color that can continue for up to 28 days. Cyanocobalamin does not affect oxygen-carrying capacity, although it can interfere with certain laboratory tests, including glucose, creatinine, and CPK. Contact the local Poison Control Center for appropriate pediatric dosing.

Indications for Admission
- Documented thermal injury of the upper airway
- Severe CO poisoning
- Smoke inhalation with upper or lower airway injury
- History of significant smoke or fire exposure in an enclosed area

Bibliography

Dries DJ, Endorf FW. Inhalation injury: epidemiology, pathology, treatment strategies. *Scand J Trauma Resusc Emerg Med*. 2013;**21**:31.

Enkhbaatar P, Pruitt BA Jr, Suman O, et al. Pathophysiology, research challenges, and clinical management of smoke inhalation injury. *Lancet*. 2016;**388**(10052):1437–1446.

Mintegi S, Clerigue N, Tipo V, et al. Pediatric cyanide poisoning by fire smoke inhalation: a European expert consensus. Toxicology Surveillance System of the Intoxications Working Group of the Spanish Society of Paediatric Emergencies. *Pediatr Emerg Care*. 2013;**29**(11):1234–1240.

Sheridan RL. Fire-related inhalation injury. *N Engl J Med*. 2016;**375**(5):464–469.

Walker PF, Buehner MF, Wood LA, et al. Diagnosis and management of inhalation injury: an updated review. *Crit Care*. 2015;**19**:351.

Lead Poisoning

Lead poisoning in children is usually the result of environmental lead exposure through chronic ingestion or inhalation. Young children are at risk of lead exposure through pica (ingestion of lead-based paint chips), lead-contaminated dust or dirt along heavily traveled roads, and water from lead-soldered plumbing. In addition, exposure to lead can occur through burning of automobile battery casings, improperly home-glazed ceramics, or certain folk medicines (e.g., Mexican folk remedies such as azarcon and greta or cosmetics such as kohl and surma). Despite widespread lead-screening programs, children who frequent inner-city EDs may have disproportionately elevated lead levels.

Clinical Presentation

The majority of patients are asymptomatic, but are brought to the ED because they have been observed eating paint chips or have an elevated microsample lead level noted during routine blood lead screening. Although acute lead poisoning is rare, consider it in the differential of vague, nonspecific signs and symptoms such as headaches, anorexia, abdominal pain, constipation, intermittent vomiting, listlessness, or irritability. With increasing levels, encephalopathy develops with persistent vomiting, drowsiness, clumsiness, ataxia, and seizures. Kidney damage results in a spectrum ranging from slight aminoaciduria to a full Fanconi syndrome. High lead levels are also associated with a microcytic anemia.

A mildly elevated blood lead level (<25 mcg/dL) is associated with decreased intelligence and impaired development. A lead level of 25–60 mcg/dL may cause headache, irritability, and anemia, while a lead level of 60–80 mcg/dL is associated with gastrointestinal symptoms and subclinical renal effects. With a level >80 mcg/dL there may be overt intoxication, with encephalopathy, increased intracranial pressure, and seizures.

Diagnosis

The risk for lead exposure is primarily determined by the patient's home environment. In most cases the nonspecific presentation may be mistaken for a viral syndrome. However, consider lead poisoning in a patient who lives in an older home (up to 1960), has a history of pica or iron-deficiency anemia, uses products from other countries (including spices, health remedies, or pottery), or has a family history of lead poisoning. Clinical features suggesting plumbism include persistent vomiting, listlessness, irritability, clumsiness, or loss of acquired developmental skills. Although rare, lead poisoning can also present as an acute encephalopathy, afebrile seizures, or signs of increased intracranial pressure. Also consider lead poisoning if there is evidence of child abuse or neglect.

Nonspecific laboratory findings include anemia (normocytic or microcytic), basophilic stippling, and the presence of radiopaque chips on abdominal x-ray.

ED Management

If lead poisoning is suspected (based on symptoms), obtain a venous blood lead level (BLL), as well as a CBC and iron studies to screen for a concomitant iron-deficiency anemia. Also order a plain abdominal radiograph (KUB) if the patient is symptomatic, or if there is a history of pica or the child was seen with paint chips in his or her mouth. If the KUB is positive (radiopaque particles in the intestinal tract), give a pediatric hypertonic phosphate enema, then repeat the x-ray.

Ask if the patient has pica and whether the child may have been exposed to environmental lead, such as previous residence in a country where lead exposure is common, use of products that contain lead, or an adult in the home works with, or has a hobby that involves exposure to, lead).

The management of acute encephalopathy (pp. 508–512), seizures (pp. 531–535), and increased intracranial pressure (pp. 527–529) are discussed elsewhere.

Management of Elevated Screening Microsamples

Treatment is indicated for a BLL ≥5 mcg/dL. Report an elevated BLL to the local Department of Health, including the patient's name, birthdate, address, and phone number.

BLL 5–14 mcg/dL

If the elevated BLL was from a capillary sample, send a confirmatory venous blood lead and arrange for re-testing within 1–3 months.

BLL 15–44 mcg/dL

Re-test the venous BLL within 1–4 weeks and consult with an expert regarding the treatment.

BLL ≥45 mcg/dL

Re-test venous BLL immediately, unless the child is encephalopathic. Once the elevated BLL is confirmed, arrange for chelation therapy in the hospital or at a lead-safe facility with expertise in treating lead poisoning.

Chelation Therapy

Asymptomatic and BLL 45–69 mcg/dL

Arrange for outpatient chelation, preferably with oral dimercaptosuccinic acid (succimer). Use 10 mg/kg PO q 8h on days 1–5, then 10 mg/kg PO q 12h on days 6–14.

Symptomatic Patient or Asymptomatic With BLL ≥70 mcg/dL

Admit the patient and treat with two drugs, oral succimer (as above) and, after 48 hours, $CaNa_2EDTA$ (edetate), 1000–1500 mg/m^2/day IV continuous infusion for five days. Obtain pretreatment electrolytes, calcium, creatinine, and a urinalysis.

Encephalopathy

Give IM British AntiLewisite (BAL) 3–5 mg/kg q 4h for 3–5 days, followed four hours later by $CaNa_2EDTA$ (as above) once urine output is established.

Follow-up
- Asymptomatic patient with a venous lead level <5 mcg/dL: repeat the BLL in 3–6 months
- Asymptomatic patient with a venous lead level 5–14 mcg/dL: repeat the BLL in 1–3 months
- Asymptomatic patient with a venous lead level 15–44 mcg/dL: repeat the BLL in 1–4 weeks
- Asymptomatic patient with a lead level >45 mcg/dL: repeat the BLL in 48 hours

Indications for Admission
- Any symptoms of lead poisoning
- BLL ≥70 mcg/dL
- Unable to assure a lead-safe environment at discharge

Bibliography

American Academy of Pediatrics. Recommendations on medical management of childhood lead exposure and poisoning. www.pehsu.net/_Library/facts/medical-mgmnt-childhood-lead-exposure-June-2013.pdf (accessed May 22, 2017).

Council on Environmental Health. Prevention of childhood lead toxicity. *Pediatrics.* 2016;**138**(1). pii: e20161493.

Dapul H, Laraque D. Lead poisoning in children. *Adv Pediatr.* 2014;**61**(1):313–333.

Etzel RA (ed.). *Handbook of Pediatric Environmental Health* (3rd ed). Elk Grove Village, IL: American Academy of Pediatrics, 2012; 439–454.

Nussbaumer-Streit B, Yeoh B, Griebler U, et al. Household interventions for preventing domestic lead exposure in children. *Cochrane Database Syst Rev.* 2016;**10**:CD006047.

Lightning Injuries

Lightning injuries are the third-most common cause of storm-related death in the United States (after flash floods and tornados). Lightning is a direct current estimated to produce up to 10,000–200,000 amperes and 20 million to 1 billion volts for a duration of several microseconds.

Lightning causes injury by direct strike, ground strike, side splash, and blunt trauma. About 3–5% of injuries are from a direct strike, which is the most serious, as the patient absorbs the entire charge. It most often occurs when the victim is in the open or in contact with metal objects. A ground strike occurs when the lightning strikes the ground near a person, so the closer the patient is to the ground strike, the more likely injury will ensue. A side splash injury (approximately 30% of injuries) occurs when lightning jumps from the primary site through the air to a person. Blunt injury is the result of the expansion and explosion of rapidly cooling air, and is estimated to occur in one-third of lightning strikes.

Electrical energy follows the path of least resistance, which are nerves and blood vessels, followed by muscle, skin and tendons. Bone and fat have the highest resistance. However, skin resistance, and therefore the extent of injury, depends on whether the skin is wet (decreased skin resistance, less penetration of deep tissues) or dry (increased skin resistance, more penetration of deep tissues).

Clinical Presentation

Lightning injuries frequently affect multiple organ systems. Cutaneous burns may range from minor first-degree to severe third-degree. Dermal ferning, or feathering burn, is a reddish erythema that appears within several hours of the injury and disappears in several days. It is characteristic of lightning injuries. Burns may also present in a linear or punctate fashion, but discrete entrance and exit burns are rare.

Signs of central nervous system involvement include mental status changes, amnesia, aphasia, paralysis, and seizures. Many types of brain injury have been documented, such as subdural and epidural hematoma and intraventricular hemorrhage.

Dysrhythmias, including ventricular fibrillation, ventricular tachycardia, asystole, and nonspecific ST–T-wave changes, may occur but usually resolve within 24 hours. Myocardial infarction is uncommon. Vascular instability may also occur, but resolves after several hours.

Possible pulmonary injuries include pulmonary contusions and hemopneumothorax. Muscle injury can result in rhabdomyolysis and myoglobinuria. Approximately one-half of lightning victims have an eye injury, including cataracts, retinal detachment or hemorrhage, or optic nerve injury. Cataracts are most frequently unilateral and may occur immediately after the lightning strike or as late as two years after. Otologic injuries include tympanic membrane rupture, which occurs in over 50% of victims, and middle ear hematoma. Hearing loss may be a late sequela.

Psychiatric effects are a special late consequence among children. These include anxiety, depression, sleep disturbances, separation anxiety, and secondary enuresis.

ED Management

The management of lightning strikes is basically the same as that for electrical injuries (pp. 214–217). This includes basic and advanced life support, a full trauma examination, and neurologic, renal, and dermatologic assessment. Pay special attention to the possibility of otologic and ophthalmologic injuries common to lightning strikes.

Follow-up

• Ophthalmologic and otologic follow-up in 2–3 days
• Psychiatric follow-up within one month

Indications for Admission

• Lightning strike victim with cardiovascular, neurologic, or renal injury (by history or direct observation in the ED)

Bibliography

Davis C, Engeln A, Johnson EL, et al. Wilderness Medical Society practice guidelines for the prevention and treatment of lightning injuries: 2014 update. *Wilderness Environ Med.* 2014;25(4 Suppl.):S86–S95.

Glatstein MM, Ayalon I, Miller E, Scolnik D. Pediatric electrical burn injuries: experience of a large tertiary care hospital and a review of electrical injury. *Pediatr Emerg Care.* 2013;29(6):737–740.

Sanford A, Gamelli RL. Lightning and thermal injuries. *Handb Clin Neurol.* 2014;120:981–986.

Thomson EM, Howard TM. Lightning injuries in sports and recreation. *Curr Sports Med Rep.* 2013;12 (2):120–124.

9 Gastrointestinal Emergencies

Sari Kay, Michelle Tobin, and Sandra J. Cunningham

Abdominal Pain

Abdominal pain is a common complaint in children. The extensive differential diagnosis (Table 9.1) necessitates a systematic approach to make an accurate diagnosis.

Clinical Presentation

Visceral pain receptors in the abdominal serosa responding to mechanical and chemical stimuli, such as stretching, tension, and ischemia, send signals to the spinal cord resulting in poorly localized, ill-defined pain. Upper gastrointestinal (GI) pathology manifests as epigastric discomfort; distal small bowel and proximal colonic diseases are perceived as periumbilical pain; and distal colonic pain is referred to the lower abdomen. Conversely, stimulation of the somatoparietal pain receptors in the parietal peritoneum causes localized pain on the same side and at the same dermatomal level as the source of the pain. Parietal pain is usually sharp, well-defined, and aggravated by movement or cough. Referred pain is similar to parietal pain, but occurs at a site distant to, but supplied by the same dermatome as, the involved organ. Non-GI causes, such as genitourinary infections and pneumonia, can also manifest as abdominal pain and must be considered on the differential for a patient with abdominal pain.

Diagnosis

Obtain a thorough history and assess for worrisome symptoms, such as weight loss, unexplained fevers, dysphagia, bilious emesis or hematemesis, chronic unexplained diarrhea, hematochezia or melena, poor growth or delayed puberty. Ask about the duration, quality, intensity, location, and radiation of the pain. Also note the response to defecation, urination, meals, and change in position. Determine if there is upper or lower GI bleeding, fever, vomiting, diarrhea, night or early morning awakening, weight loss, or growth failure. Inquire about respiratory, cardiovascular or urinary symptoms, stooling habits, menstrual cycle, testicular pain, sexual activity, and the possibility of pregnancy. Ask about past illnesses, medication, travel, trauma, family and social history, and exposure to animals or sick contacts.

Although a definitive diagnosis cannot always be made immediately, a primary goal is the early recognition of surgically correctable emergencies and potentially unstable conditions.

Start with assessing vital signs and then begin the examination with the non-threatening and painless components, leaving the abdominal and rectal examinations for the end.

Table 9.1 Differential diagnosis of abdominal pain

Diagnosis	Differentiating features
Gastrointestinal	
Appendicitis	Pain followed by vomiting
	Associated with low-grade fever and anorexia
	Pain starts periumbilical and migrates to RLQ
Bowel obstruction	Crampy pain which is usually periumbilical
	Associated with bilious vomiting and abdominal distention
Cholelithiasis	Colicky pain, typically RUQ
Cholecystitis	Pain RUQ, positive Murphy's sign
Constipation	Pain can be migratory and is relieved upon defecation
	Rectal vault filled with stool on digital rectal examination
Gastroenteritis	Vomiting prior to or simultaneously with abdominal pain
	Pain often relieved by vomiting or bowel movement
	Diarrhea may be prominent
	Fecal leukocytes or blood present if bacterial
Hepatitis	Tenderness on exam in RUQ
	May be jaundiced
Incarcerated hernia	Usually inguinal or umbilical
	Evidence of bowel obstruction
Inflammatory bowel disease	Recurrent episodes of pain
	Associated with bloody diarrhea
Intussusception	Pain and vomiting alternating with periods of lethargy
	Usually afebrile and may have guaiac positive stools
	80% of patients are <2 years old
Irritable bowel syndrome	Recurrent crampy lower abdominal pain
	Alternating episodes of nonbloody diarrhea and constipation
Lactose intolerance	Intermittent, crampy pain associated with dairy intake
Meckel's diverticulum	Painless LGI bleeding
	May perforate or lead to an intussusception, causing pain
Mesenteric adenitis	Diagnosis of exclusion
Necrotizing enterocolitis	Usually presents in the first few weeks of life
	Feeding intolerance, bloody stools and/or bilious vomiting
	Abdominal distention and/or erythema
	Pneumatosis intestinalis on x-ray
Pancreatitis	Pain is epigastric, may radiate to the back
Peptic ulcer/gastritis	Pain is usually epigastric, gnawing-like, worse with fasting
Volvulus	Distention, bilious vomiting

Table 9.1 (cont.)

Diagnosis	Differentiating features
Gynecological/genitourinary	
Endometriosis	Cyclical, usually pelvic pain, may have irregular menses
Ovarian cyst	Pain during or shortly after menses
Menstruation	Crampy pain that subsides on day 1–2 of menses
Mittelschmerz	Lower abdominal or pelvic pain
	Occurs around the time of ovulation
Pelvic inflammatory disease	Pain is usually lower in abdomen
	Vaginal discharge or bleeding
Pregnancy	Positive serum or urine pregnancy test
Torsion	Ovarian or testicular torsion may present at any age
	Abnormal cremasteric reflex in males
Hematology/oncology	
Henoch–Schönlein purpura	Pain may precede the rash, arthritis, and nephritis
Hemolytic-uremic syndrome	Pain accompanies microangiopathic hemolytic anemia
	Renal insufficiency or failure
Lymphoma	Solid tumor may cause bowel obstruction or intussusception
Porphyria	Vomiting and constipation
	Mental status changes, peripheral neuropathy
	Urinary complaints and hypertension
Sickle cell disease	Vaso-occlusive crisis or splenic sequestration
	Associated anemia
Metabolic/toxic	
Adrenal insufficiency	Chronic fatigue, weight loss
	Hypotension, hyperpigmentation
	Hyponatremia, hyperkalemia, hypercalcemia
Diabetic ketoacidosis	Polyuria, polydypsia, polyphagia
	Kussmaul respirations
Ingestion	Detailed history is key
Pulmonary/cardiovascular	
Heart failure	Typically associated with myocarditis
	Tachycardia, diffuse ST segment changes on EKG
Pneumonia (RLL)	Tachypnea and pulmonary rales are usually present

Table 9.1 (cont.)

Diagnosis	Differentiating features
Renal	
Hydronephrosis	If acute, pain more severe with associated nausea or vomiting
Nephrolithiasis	Colicky pain, typically flank and back
	Gross or microscopic hematuria
Urinary tract infection	Frequency, urgency, dysuria, flank pain, suprapubic tenderness
Miscellaneous	
Abdominal migraine	Acute intermittent non-colicky pain
	Resolves spontaneously over several hours
Functional pain	Recurrent attacks of abdominal pain in the school-aged child
	No vomiting, diarrhea, fever or weight loss
Musculoskeletal	Pain reproduced by palpating contracted abdominal wall muscles
Streptococcal pharyngitis	Pain associated with fever and exudative pharyngitis
	Cervical or submandibular lymphadenopathy
Splenomegaly	Typically associated with viral infection such as Epstein–Barr
Trauma	Duodenal hematoma, liver or spleen laceration, or renal contusion
	Consider abuse if proposed mechanism does not match injury

Quickly assess the patient's hydration status and cardiovascular/respiratory stability. Try to elicit and localize abdominal tenderness, as well as rebound tenderness or masses. A pelvic exam is necessary for all sexually active or postmenarchal females with lower abdominal pain. Perform a testicular examination for males.

In an infant, suspect an intra-abdominal surgical emergency such as malrotation with midgut volvulus or intussusception whenever there is a history of bilious or projectile vomiting and/or bleeding. The signs may be preceded or accompanied by irritability, poor feeding, and lethargy. Suspect a surgical condition if the physical examination reveals abdominal distension, a scaphoid abdomen, localized abdominal tenderness or guarding, a mass, high-pitched or absent bowel sounds, or if the patient is ill-appearing. A patient with peritoneal irritation will often remain motionless, whereas a patient with visceral pain is usually changing positions and writhing in discomfort.

ED Management

If the etiology of the abdominal pain is unclear and the patient has persistent, severe symptoms, obtain a CBC, electrolytes, liver function panel, amylase, lipase, inflammatory markers, urinalysis, and stool guaiac. Obtain a pregnancy test for any postmenarchal female. If the patient has been vomiting or is dehydrated, give a 20 mL/kg NS intravenous (IV) bolus, followed by maintenance fluids either IV or oral, if tolerated. Give one oral dose of ondansetron (8–15 kg: 2 mg; 6–30 kg: 4 mg; >30 kg: 8 mg). Obtain an abdominal ultrasound if there is suspicion for appendicitis, hepatobiliary disease, pancreatitis, renal disease, or pregnancy based on laboratory values.

See the specific sections for the work-up for other etiologies, such as appendicitis (pp. 241–244), cholelithiasis (pp. 260–263), hepatitis (pp. 268–272), intussusception (pp. 273–274), Meckel's diverticulum (pp. 282–283), ovarian cyst (pp. 323–325), and pancreatitis (pp. 238–241). If the work-up is inconclusive and the patient continues with severe or focal pain, admit for serial abdominal examinations. Further ED evaluation by pediatric surgery is warranted for focal pain or signs of peritonitis. Consult pediatric gastroenterology if surgical emergencies have been ruled out and the etiology is still unclear.

Follow-up

- No suspicion of a surgical condition, patient appears well, initial laboratory tests normal: primary care follow-up within one week

Indications for Admission

- Suspected surgical abdomen
- Dehydration or inability to take fluids
- Persistent, severe abdominal pain

Bibliography

Chang PT, Schooler GR, Lee EY. Diagnostic errors of right lower quadrant pain in children: beyond appendicitis. *Abdom Imaging*. 2015;**40**(7):2071–2090.

Huguet A, Olthuis J, McGrath PJ, et al. Systematic review of childhood and adolescent risk and prognostic factors for persistent abdominal pain. *Acta Paediatr*. 2016. DOI: 10.1111/apa.13736.

Kameda T, Taniguchi N. Overview of point-of-care abdominal ultrasound in emergency and critical care. *J Intensive Care*. 2016;**4**:53.

Kim JS. Acute abdominal pain in children. *Pediatr Gastroenterol Hepatol Nutr*. 2013;**16**(4):219–224.

Kulik DM, Uleryk EM, Maguire JL. Does this child have appendicitis? A systematic review of clinical prediction rules for children with acute abdominal pain. *J Clin Epidemiol*. 2013;**66**(1):95–104.

Leung A, Sigalet D. Acute abdominal pain in children. *Am Fam Physician*. 2003;**67**:2321–2326.

Smith J, Fox SM. Pediatric abdominal pain: an emergency medicine perspective. *Emerg Med Clin North Am*. 2016;**34**(2):341–361.

Acute Pancreatitis

Acute pancreatitis is a serious cause of abdominal pain in children. While pancreatitis is associated with many conditions, up to 30% of cases are idiopathic (Table 9.2). Premature activation of digestive enzymes, particularly trypsinogen, causes injury of the pancreatic acinar cells. This can precipitate a systemic inflammatory response, oxidative stress, edema, and, in severe cases, necrosis of the gland with associated multiorgan failure.

Clinical Presentation

The classic symptoms of acute pancreatitis are abdominal pain, nausea, vomiting, and anorexia. The pain is typically located in the epigastrium, right upper quadrant, or

Table 9.2 Etiologies of pancreatitis

Anatomic	Annular pancreas, pancreas divisum, sphincter of Oddi dysfunction
Biliary	Biliary sludge, choledochal cyst, cholelithiasis
Genetic	Hereditary pancreatitis, trypsinogen gene mutation,
Infections	Coxsackie B, echovirus, Epstein–Barr virus, hepatitis (A and B), HIV, influenza A, leptospirosis mumps, *Mycoplasma, Salmonella*
Mechanical	Blunt abdominal trauma (including child abuse), S/P ERCP
Medications	Alcohol, anticoagulants, azathioprine, borate, chlorthiazide, corticosteroids, cytarabine, ethanol, indomethacin, isoniazid, L-asparaginase, mercaptopurine, mesalamine, salicylic acid, tetracycline, valproic acid
Metabolic	Alpha-1 antitrypsin deficiency, diabetes, hypercalcemia, hypertriglyceridemia
Nutritional	Malnutrition, vitamin A and D deficiency
Systemic disease	Anorexia nervosa, cystic fibrosis, inflammatory bowel disease, juvenile idiopathic arthritis, polyarteritis nodosa, Reye syndrome, systemic lupus erythematosus
Other	Familial, idiopathic

periumbilical area, with radiation to the back or lower chest. Both the pain and vomiting are worsened by eating. Younger patients may present with subtle symptoms of vomiting, lethargy, and irritability. Other associated symptoms include fever, jaundice, diarrhea, or clay-colored stools.

On physical examination the patient is often tachycardic, and sometimes hypotensive early in the disease. There may be tenderness in the upper abdomen, and the patient may refuse to lie supine. Guarding, rebound tenderness, abdominal distension, and decreased bowel sounds can mimic an acute surgical abdomen. With severe hemorrhagic pancreatitis, serosanguinous fluid may track through fascial planes resulting in blue discoloration of the flanks (Grey-Turner sign) or the umbilicus (Cullen sign). Signs of ascites (shifting dullness, fluid wave) or pleural effusion (decreased bowel sounds, friction rub, dullness to percussion) may be present if the disease is advanced. Patients with severe acute pancreatitis will present in shock with signs and symptoms of multiorgan failure, including shortness of breath, oliguria, hemorrhage, or change in mental status.

Diagnosis

The diagnosis of acute pancreatitis is confirmed when the patient has two or three of the following findings:

- clinical symptoms consistent with acute pancreatitis including abdominal pain, nausea, vomiting, or back pain;
- serum amylase or lipase ≥3 times the upper limit of normal;
- radiographic (CT or ultrasound) evidence of acute pancreatitis.

Table 9.3 Causes of amylase elevation

Biliary

Bile duct obstruction

Cholecystitis

Intestinal

Appendicitis

Intestinal obstruction

Perforated peptic ulcer

Pancreatic

Acute or chronic pancreatitis

Pancreatic duct obstruction

Pancreatic tumor

Salivary

Parotitis

Salivary duct obstruction

Trauma

Miscellaneous

Burns

Diabetic ketoacidosis

Macroamylasemia

Pregnancy (ruptured ectopic)

Renal insufficiency

Lipase is more sensitive and specific than amylase in acute pancreatitis. A normal amylase does not rule-out acute pancreatitis, while an elevated amylase level can occur in a variety of other conditions (Table 9.3). In addition, the degree of elevation does not correlate with disease severity.

In suspected acute pancreatitis, obtain a CBC, electrolytes including glucose, calcium, magnesium, liver function tests (bilirubin direct and total, gamma-glutamyl transpeptidase [GGT], alanine aminotransferase [ALT], aspartate aminotransferase [AST], alkaline phosphatase), and a triglyceride level. Other laboratory abnormalities that occur with severe pancreatitis include hypocalcemia, hypomagnesemia, hyperglycemia, and hemoconcentration. If there is associated cholelithiasis, there may be elevations of direct bilirubin, GGT, and alkaline phosphatase.

Radiologic confirmation requires either abdominal ultrasound or a CT scan. Ultrasound can document the presence of a pancreatic pseudocyst, dilated ducts, cholelithiasis, abscesses, or ascites. Abdominal CT scan is helpful in suspected traumatic pancreatitis and can provide better visualization of masses, necrosis, and hemorrhage. Imaging can also detect associated injury to the liver, spleen, and duodenum. In patients with respiratory signs or symptoms, obtain a chest x-ray to assess the disease severity and to rule-out pleural effusions, ARDS, or pneumonia.

ED Management

The management of pancreatitis is supportive. Keep the patient NPO in an effort to "rest" the pancreas and prevent stimulation of pancreatic exocrine secretions. Start an IV and aggressively treat signs of hypovolemia with 20 mL/kg boluses of an isotonic solution (LR or NS). Closely monitor the patient's hydration status, as there may be ongoing leakage of fluid into the interstitial space. Provide sufficient fluid to maintain adequate circulation. Give an H_2 blocker IV to help prevent stress ulceration (ranitidine 8 mg/kg/day div q 8h, 50 mg/dose maximum; famotidine 0.6–0.8 mg/kg/day div q 12h, 40 mg/dose maximum). Reserve antibiotics for clinical signs of sepsis, necrotic pancreatitis, cholangitis, or multiorgan system failure.

Manage pain with morphine 0.05 mg/kg/dose IV or subcutaneously every 2–4 hours. Alternatives include fentanyl (0.5–1 mcg/kg/dose q 1–2h) or meperidine (0.5 mg/kg/dose q 2–4h), but with repeated doses there is the risk of the accumulation of neurotoxic metabolites, which may cause seizures. If the patient requires multiple doses of narcotic analgesia, use a fentanyl or morphine drip via a patient-controlled analgesia (PCA) pump.

Admission to an ICU is indicated for severe complications such as shock, impending renal failure, hypoxia, or significant metabolic derangements. In addition, supplemental calcium (see pp. 191–193), magnesium, and insulin may be needed.

Indications for Admission

- Acute pancreatitis

Bibliography

Pohl JF, Uc A. Paediatric pancreatitis. *Current Opinion Gastroenterol.* 2015;**31**:380–386.

Sathiyasekaran M, Biradar V, Ramaswamy G, et al. Pancreatitis in children. *Indian J Pediatr.* 2016;**83**(12):1459–1472.

Suzuki M, Sai JK, Shimizu T. Acute pancreatitis in children and adolescents. *World J Gastrointest Pathophysiol.* 2014;**5**(4):416–426.

Working Group IAP/APA Acute Pancreatitis Guidelines. IAP/APA evidence-based guidelines for the management of acute pancreatitis. *Pancreatology.* 2013;**13**(4 Suppl. 2):e1–15.

Appendicitis

Appendicitis is the most common childhood illness requiring emergency surgery, with a peak incidence in the second decade of life. It begins with obstruction of the appendiceal lumen, often secondary to an appendicolith or lymphoid hyperplasia, leading to distention. If not recognized in time, necrosis of the wall of the appendix occurs, followed by perforation and subsequent peritonitis. Early diagnosis is of paramount importance.

Clinical Presentation

In uncomplicated appendicitis (prior to rupture), there is a short history (usually <36 hours) of abdominal pain, anorexia, nausea, and vomiting. Early in the course colicky or persistent periumbilical pain is typical. The pain then shifts to the right lower quadrant where it is constant and severe. Low-grade fever (<38.3 °C;101 °F) is common, and a change in stool pattern occurs in about 15% of patients. Other symptoms may include dysuria or labial, testicular, or penile pain. Maintain a high index of suspicion, as many patients do not have a "classical" presentation.

On physical examination tenderness is greatest over McBurney's point (one-third of the distance along a line from the anterior superior iliac spine to the umbilicus). There may be positive psoas (pain on passive hip hyperextension consistent with retrocecal appendix) and/or obturator (pain on passive internal rotation of the thigh consistent with pelvic appendix) signs. In the case of a retrocecal appendix, the maximum tenderness and rigidity may remain in the periumbilical area or in the right flank. While palpating the left lower quadrant, discomfort may be elicited in the right lower quadrant (Rovsing's sign). Rigidity of the abdominal wall, diffuse tenderness, and involuntary guarding are suggestive of perforation.

Perforation occurs in 20–40% of patients and, although the incidence varies with age, it is seen most frequently in children under four years old. Other signs of rupture include pain for more than 36 hours, frequent vomiting, dyspnea secondary to elevation of the diaphragm, lethargy in the young child, and a temperature >38.5 °C (101.3 °F).

Diagnosis

A careful history and physical examination are the keys to diagnosing appendicitis. Defer the abdominal and rectal examinations for last. Gently palpate the abdomen beginning away from the right lower quadrant. If the patient's responses do not seem accurate, palpate the abdomen with the membrane of the stethoscope, as the child will believe that auscultation, and not palpation is being performed. Since appendicitis is a progressive disease, increasing abdominal pain, tenderness, and rigidity on serial physical examinations are highly suggestive of the diagnosis.

Try to elicit rebound tenderness which occurs with inflammation of the peritoneum. To do this in a younger child, shake or percuss the abdomen, tap firmly on the feet, or ask the patient to cough, jump down from the table, or hop. In an older patient, depress the abdomen for 5–10 seconds, then withdraw your hand suddenly. Rebound tenderness is confirmed by finding pain on release, rather than during direct pressure.

The differential diagnosis of appendicitis is extensive, as shown in Table 9.4. If the diagnosis remains unclear, perform a rectal examination. Right-sided tenderness is consistent with appendicitis, whereas hard stool in the vault is suggestive of constipation, which can mimic appendicitis, although some constipated patients will be fidgety or "dancing," and will not keep still. Also perform a pelvic exam and obtain urine for a pregnancy test in sexually active females and perform a genital exam, including the cremasteric reflex, to rule-out testicular torsion in a male.

ED Management

When the diagnosis is evident from the history and physical examination, make the patient NPO, start maintenance IV hydration with D_5 ½ NS, obtain a CBC, electrolytes, urinalysis, type and screen, and consult a surgeon. If there is evidence of intravascular depletion (orthostatic vital sign changes, delayed capillary refill, hypotension), give the patient a bolus of 20 mL/kg of NS or lactated Ringer's.

In general, abdominal x-rays are not necessary. However, a KUB may confirm constipation, or reveal an appendicolith (10% of cases), soft tissue mass, or focal ileus in the right lower quadrant consistent with the diagnosis of appendicitis.

Table 9.4 Differential diagnosis of appendicitis

Diagnosis	Differentiating features
Bacterial enteritis	Guaiac positive stools and fecal leukocytosis
Bowel obstruction	Crampy, periumbilical pain
	Abdominal distention
Cholecystitis	RUQ pain with positive Murphy's sign
Cholelithiasis	RUQ colicky pain
Constipation	Pain is nonmigratory and is relieved upon defecation
	Stool palpated in descending colon and ampulla
Diabetic ketoacidosis	Polyuria, polydypsia, polyphagia
	Kussmaul respirations
Intussusception	Pain and vomiting alternating with periods of lethargy
	Afebrile
	80% of patients are <2 years old
Ectopic pregnancy	Positive pregnancy test
	Vaginal bleeding
Functional abdominal pain	Recurrent attacks of abdominal pain
	No vomiting, diarrhea, fever, or weight loss
Henoch–Schönlein purpura	Pain may precede the rash
Hepatitis	RUQ tenderness and jaundice (variable)
Inflammatory bowel disease	Recurrent episodes of pain
	Bloody diarrhea and abdominal distention
Intrauterine pregnancy	Positive pregnancy test
Mesenteric adenitis	Diagnosis of exclusion
Pancreatitis	Epigastric pain that may radiate to the back
Pelvic inflammatory disease	Pain in lower abdomen
	Vaginal discharge or bleeding
Pneumonia	Tachypnea may be present
Testicular torsion	Tender, swollen, erythematous hemiscrotum
	Abnormal cremasteric reflex
Urinary tract infection	Frequency, urgency, dysuria, and flank pain
	Pyuria
Urolithiasis	Colicky pain with gross or microscopic hematuria
Viral gastroenteritis	Vomiting prior to, or simultaneously with, abdominal pain
	Abdominal pain relieved by vomiting or a bowel movement
	Diarrhea may be prominent

Perform an ultrasound to evaluate the appendix, although the findings may be limited in an obese patient. A diagnostic examination may show a fluid-filled, non-compressible, distended, tubular mass >6 mm. Perform a CT scan with IV contrast only if the diagnosis remains unclear or it is likely that the patient has an abscess. CT findings in acute appendicitis include: appendicular diameter of >6 mm; appendicolith; pericecal fat stranding; thickening of adjacent bowel walls; free peritoneal fluid; lymphadenopathy; and the presence of a phlegmon. However, MRI is preferred over CT scan if available, given its lack of radiation.

A mildly elevated WBC and CRP is supportive of a diagnosis of appendicitis and a WBC >15,000/mm^3 suggests rupture or another bacterial process (pneumonia, bacterial gastroenteritis). Do not delay surgical evaluation if these values are normal in a patient with a clinical picture that is suggestive of appendicitis. Obtain a chest x-ray if there is tachypnea, rales, other pulmonary signs, or an elevated WBC in a child with a negative abdominal CT scan.

Serum electrolytes may be helpful in patients with abdominal pain and dehydration. A low serum sodium (<130 mEq/L) may reflect third-spacing of fluids from the ileus associated with a ruptured appendicitis. A urinalysis is necessary to rule-out diabetic ketoacidosis (glycosuria and ketonuria) or a urinary tract infection (bacteriuria and pyuria). Although there can be WBCs in the urine with an appendicitis, bacteriuria is typically absent.

Once the diagnosis of appendicitis has been made, and agreed upon by the surgical team, start antibiotic therapy. If a non-perforated appendicitis is suspected, give cefoxitin (40 mg/kg; 2 g maximum) or cefotetan (30 mg/kg/day div q 12h; 6g/day maximum) IV, while awaiting appendectomy. If a perforated appendicitis is suspected, give broader antibiotic coverage to prevent or minimize intraperitoneal abscess formation. Use monotherapy with piperacillin-tazobactam (350 mg/kg/day divided q 6h; 3g/dose maximum; use 175 mg/kg/day for infants <6 months) IV.

The appropriate use of analgesia does not impair diagnostic accuracy. Give morphine subcutaneously or IV (0.1 mg/kg; 5 mg maximum for the initial dose; titrate subsequent doses based upon clinical effect). Do not use nonsteroidal medications such as ketorolac if there is a possibility of surgical intervention, as this class of drugs inhibits platelet function and can cause excessive bleeding.

When appendicitis cannot be excluded, admit the patient for IV hydration and observation and keep them NPO.

Follow-up

- If appendicitis seems highly unlikely, have the patient return in 6–8 hours, if still symptomatic, or sooner if the symptoms intensify. Prescribe a clear liquid diet and no analgesics.

Indications for Admission

- Suspected or confirmed appendicitis

Bibliography

Glass CC, Rangel SJ. Overview and diagnosis of acute appendicitis in children. *Semin Pediatr Surg.* 2016;25(4):198–203.

Hansen LW, Dolgin SE. Trends in the diagnosis and management of pediatric appendicitis. *Pediatr Rev.* 2016;37(2):52–57

Kulik DM, Uleryk EM, Maguire JL. Does this child have appendicitis? A systematic review of clinical prediction rules for children with acute abdominal pain. *J Clin Epidemiol.* 2013;66(1):95–104.

Moore MM, Kulaylat AN, Hollenbeak CS, et al. Magnetic resonance imaging in pediatric appendicitis: a systematic review. *Pediatr Radiol.* 2016;46(6):928–939.

Rentea RM, Peter SD, Snyder CL. Pediatric appendicitis: state of the art review. *Pediatr Surg Int.* 2017;33(3):269–283.

Seattle Children's Hospital. Appendicitis v.1.2. www.seattlechildrens.org/pdf/appendicitis-pathway .pdf (accessed June 20, 2017).

Assessment and Management of Dehydration

The most common causes of dehydration in children are vomiting (pp. 289–293) and diarrhea (pp. 255–260).

Clinical Presentation and Diagnosis

Dehydration is classified by the percentage of total body water lost: mild (<5%), moderate (5–10%), and severe (>10%). A variety of signs and symptoms and ancillary data help to distinguish the degree of dehydration (Table 9.5). The most objective measure is an acute change in weight from the premorbid state, which reflects fluid loss.

Table 9.5 Assessment of degree of dehydration

Signs/symptoms	Mild (<5%)	Moderate (5–10%)	Severe (>10%)
Abnormal skin turgor	–	+/–	+
Altered mental status	–	+/–	+
Capillary refill time >2 s	–	+/–	+
Decreased urine output	+/–	+	+
Depressed fontanelle	–	+	+
Dry mucous membranes	+	+	+
Hyperpnea	–	–	+
Hypotension	–	–	+
Orthostatic vital sign changes	–	+/–	+
Serum acidosis	–	+/–	+
Sunken eyeballs	–	+	+
Tachycardia	+/–	+	+
Urine specific gravity	Normal/high	Normal/high	High
Weak peripheral pulses	–	–	+

Goals are: ① stabilise VS ② replace Fluids
③ Correct lyte abnormalities.

ED Management

The management priorities are stabilization of the patient's vital signs, replenishment of the intravascular volume, and correction of electrolyte abnormalities.

No Dehydration

If the patient has diarrhea but is not dehydrated and appears well, give clear fluids to maintain hydration, as well as an age-appropriate diet as tolerated. Allow a breastfed infant to continue to nurse. If the patient also is vomiting, give small amounts of clear fluids (see Mild and Moderate Dehydration below). Confirm that all infants and children can tolerate oral fluids prior to discharge.

Mild and Moderate Dehydration *(oral hydration – if tolerated)*

A patient with mild or moderate dehydration can be orally rehydrated, if willing and able to tolerate fluids. *1st GUT rest for 30 – 60 mts,*

Vomiting *(Approx – 10–20 ml q 10 mts) for hr a reassess,*

If the patient has been vomiting, wait 30–60 minutes after the last episode to initiate oral fluids. Use an oral rehydration solution (ORS) containing 60–90 mEq/L of sodium and 20–25 g/L of glucose. Give an infant (<1 year of age) small (5–10 mL) aliquots and an older child a larger amount (10–20 mL) of fluid every 5–15 minutes, over the next hour, followed by reassessment of the hydration status. If a patient with gastroenteritis is unable to tolerate the fluid, give ~~one dose of ondansetron~~ (see p. 292). Once the patient looks well and has stopped vomiting, discharge him or her with written instructions on how to advance the diet by increasing the amount of ORS over 8–12 hours.

Diarrhea *50 ml (5% dehyn) / kg over 4 hrs.*

Start rehydration with an ORS. Give a total volume of 40–50 mL/kg in small aliquots (15–30 mL) over a 3–4 hour period, while doing hourly reassessments of hydration status. Failure of oral rehydration (inability to take adequate volume orally, excessive ongoing losses) is an indication for IV rehydration therapy. Once the initial rehydration is tolerated, resume giving milk (breast or formula) to an infant. If an infant has large, watery stools, supplement the milk with feedings of an ORS. For older infants and toddlers already taking solid foods, recommend an ORS, with a low-fat carbohydrate diet. ~~Anti-diarrheal compounds~~ and ~~anti-motility agents~~ have ~~no role~~ in the management of acute diarrhea.

Severe Dehydration

IV fluid restoration is necessary for ~~severe dehydration, shock, altered mental status~~ or if the patient is ~~unable to take fluids orally.~~

Initial Intravascular Restoration *20ml/kg over 20 mts, rept PRN.*

Initiate fluid resuscitation with a ~~20 mL/kg bolus~~ of normal saline or lactated Ringer's solution ~~over 20–30 minutes~~. Obtain blood for electrolytes, BUN, creatinine, lactate and glucose. Also obtain a urinalysis, and if the ~~urine~~ contains ~~large ketones~~ or if the child is ~~hypoglycemic, add 2 mL/kg of D25~~ (0.5 g/kg of glucose) to the bolus solution. After the first bolus, reevaluate the patient using parameters outlined in Table 9.5. If there is a poor

$$\frac{25}{100} \times 2\,ml = 0.5G.$$

[handwritten: Isonatremic 1st 8 hrs.]

[handwritten: Next 16 hrs m + ½ D   K 30 m Eg/L.]
[handwritten: <2 yrs D5 ⅓ NS > 2 yrs D5 ½ NS]

response to the initial bolus, repeat the infusion. Patients with renal or cardiac disease are at risk for developing congestive heart failure and patients with sickle cell disease are at risk for acute chest syndrome. Therefore, carefully and thoroughly assess their fluid status. If there is a poor response to three IV boluses, consider other associated organ disease, such as sepsis, myocarditis, and neurogenic shock, or the need for central venous monitoring before giving additional boluses. Following the restoration of adequate intravascular volume, assess the need for replacement of fluid and electrolyte deficits.

Calculate maintenance fluids using the Holiday–Segar method: *[handwritten symbol]*

- 100 mL/kg/day for the first 10 kg (1000 mL/day) or 4 mL/kg/h for the first 10 kg;
- 50 mL/kg/day for the next 10 kg (500 mL/day) or 2 mL/kg/h for the next 10 kg;
- 20 mL/kg/day for each additional kg or 1 mL/kg/h for each additional kilogram.

Replacement of Fluid and Electrolyte Deficits   *[handwritten: Isotonic Na (130 – 150)]*

Isotonic Dehydration -- In isotonic dehydration the serum sodium is between 130 mEq/L and 150 mEq/L. Estimate the percentage of dehydration either by physical signs and symptoms or, more accurately, if a recent premorbid weight is known. Multiply the percentage of dehydration by the weight of the child to calculate the fluid deficit (e.g., 10% dehydration × 20 kg child = a deficit of 2 L). Administer maintenance fluid requirements plus half of the deficit over the first 8 hours and the second half over the following 16 hours. Sodium requirements are 2–4 mEq/kg/day. In general, either D_5 ½ NS (≥2 years of age) or D_5 ⅓ NS (<2 years of age) is an adequate solution. Potassium requirements are 2–3 *[handwritten symbol]* mEq/kg/day. After the patient has voided, add potassium chloride (20–40 mEq/L) to the IV bag.

[handwritten: < 130 m Eg]

Hypotonic Dehydration -- Hypotonic dehydration occurs when salt losses exceed water losses or when water intake exceeds required salt intake. Hyponatremia is defined as serum sodium <130mEq/L. Use the following formula to calculate the sodium deficit to be added to the replacement fluids (see Hyponatremia, pp. 197–200):

$$\text{mEq sodium required for replacement} = (\text{desired sodium} - \text{measured sodium}) \times (\text{premorbid body weight in kg}) \times 0.6$$

Give the sodium replacement over four hours, but do not exceed a rate of correction of more than 0.5–1 mEq/h. An excessively rapid correction of the serum sodium may be associated with central pontine myelinolysis.

Symptomatic hyponatremia (seizures) requires a more rapid correction with hypertonic 3% saline. Three percent saline contains 513 mEq/L of Na, so that every 2 mL contains 1 mEq Na. One mL/kg of 3% NaCl will increase the plasma sodium by approximately 1 mEq/L. The initial goal is to raise the serum sodium by 5 mEq, which is usually sufficient to terminate the seizures; calculate the amount of 3% NaCl (mL) required as follows:

$$3\% \text{ NaCl (mEq/L)} = (125 - \text{measured Na}) \times \text{premorbid weight(kg)} \times 0.6$$

Multiply the results by 2 to determine the volume in milliliters.

Hypertonic Dehydration -- Hypernatremia is defined as a serum sodium >150 mEq/L. It occurs when solute-free water losses exceed salt losses or in the context of excessive salt intake. The degree of dehydration is more difficult to determine in these patients because the

[handwritten: > 150 mEg.]

extracellular fluid space is preserved. The skin may have normal turgor but feel doughy. Calculate the free water deficit as follows:

✳ Solute − free water deficit (mL) = (measured sodium − 145) × 4 mL/kg
× (premorbid weight in kg)

(Use 3 mL/kg for serum sodium >170 mEq/L.)

Because of the potential for neurologic complications, correct the serum sodium and free water deficit ~~slowly over 48 hours~~, with a daily sodium decrease of 10–15 mEq/L (approximately 0.5 mEq/h). In general, D_5 ½ NS is an appropriate solution. Add 40 mEq/L of potassium acetate after the patient voids (see Hypernatremia, pp. 188–191).

Calculation Examples

10 kg (Premorbid Weight) Child With 10% Isotonic Dehydration (Sodium = 140mEq/L)

Fluid deficit(L) = premorbid weight(kg) × %dehydration
Fluid deficit(L) = 10 kg × 0.10 = 1L
Maintenance fluid = 100 mL/kg/day = 1000 mL
Sodium deficit (mEq) = fluid deficit(L) × %Na from ECF × Na(mEq/L)in ECF
Sodium deficit = 1L × 0.6 × 140 mEq/L = 84 mEq
Maintenance sodium requirements = 3 mEq/kg/day = 30 mEq

Give half of deficit in the first 8 hours and the remaining half in the next 16 hours and divide the maintenance evenly over 24 hours.
First 8 hours:

Fluid deficit 500 mL + maintenance 333mL = 833 mL/8h = 104mL/h
Sodium deficit 42 mEq + maintenance 10mEq = 52mEq
Sodium concentration : 52 mEq/0.833L = 62 mEq/L

10 kg (Premorbid Weight) Child With 10% Hypotonic Dehydration (Sodium 115 mEq/L)

Fluid deficit and maintenance (as above)
Sodium deficit and maintenance (as above)
Additional sodium deficit = (desired Na mEq/L − measured Na mEq/L)
× %Na from ECF(L/kg) × weight(kg)
Additional sodium deficit = (135 − 115) × 0.6 × 10 = 120 mEq

Give half of deficit in the first 8 hours and the remaining half over the next 16 hours; divide the maintenance evenly over 24 hours.
First eight hours:

Fluid deficit and maintenance = 833 mL/8h = 104 mL/h(as above)
Sodium(deficit + maintenance) = 52 mEq(as above)
Additional sodium deficit = 60 mEq
Sodium concentration: (52 mEq + 60 mEq)/0.833L = 134 mEq/L

10 kg (Premorbid Weight) Child With 10% Hypertonic Dehydration (Sodium 160 mEq/L)

Fluid deficit and maintenance (as above)

Sodium maintenance (as above)

Solute-free water deficit = 4 mL/kg × weight(kg) × (measured Na − desired Na)

Solute-free water deficit = 4 mL/kg × 10kg × (160 − 145) = 600mL

Solute fluid deficit = total fluid deficit − free water deficit

Solute fluid deficit = 1000 mL − 600 mL = 400 mL(0.4L)

Solute sodium deficit = solute fluid deficit (L) × (%Na from ECF) × (desired Na mEq/L)

Solute sodium deficit = 0.4 L × 0.6 × 145 mEq/L = 35 mEq

Give half of the free water deficit + the total solute fluid deficit + solute sodium deficit + maintenance sodium and fluid divided over the first 24 hours.

Fluids:

$$300 \text{ mL} + 400 \text{ mL} + 1000 \text{ mL} = 1700 \text{ mL/day} = 71\text{mL/h}$$
$$\text{Sodium maintenance} + \text{solute sodium deficit} = 65 \text{ mEq}$$
$$\text{Sodium concentration}: 65 \text{ mEq}/1.7\text{L} = 38 \text{ mEq/L}$$

Follow-up

- Mild or moderate dehydration: primary care follow-up the next day or return to the ED if unable to tolerate oral fluids

Indications for Admission

- Significant ongoing fluid losses and/or inability to tolerate oral fluids
- Severe dehydration
- Hypotonic or hypertonic dehydration

Bibliography

Engorn B, Flerlage J. *Harriet Lane Handbook* (20th edn.). Philadelphia, PA: Elsevier, 2015; 246–267.

Florez ID, Al-Khalifah R, Sierra JM, et al. The effectiveness and safety of treatments used for acute diarrhea and acute gastroenteritis in children: protocol for a systematic review and network meta-analysis. *Syst Rev.* 2016;5:14.

Freedman SB, Pasichnyk D, Black KJ, et al. Gastroenteritis therapies in developed countries: systematic review and meta-analysis. *PLoS One.* 2015;**10**(6):e0128754.

Moritz ML, Avus JC. Misconceptions in the treatment of dehydration in children. *Pediatr Rev.* 2016;**37**:29–31.

Niescierenko M, Bachur R. Advances in pediatric dehydration therapy. *Curr Opin Pediatr.* 2013;**25** (3):304–309.

Parashette KR, Croffie J. Vomiting. *Pediatr Rev.* 2013;**34**(7):307–319.

Colic

Colic, also referred to as paroxysmal fussing of infancy, is a benign, self-limited process whose etiology and pathogenesis are poorly understood.

Clinical Presentation

Infants commonly present around 2–3 weeks of age with paroxysms of inconsolable crying. The behavior peaks between 6–8 weeks and typically resolves by three months of age, although in 30% of cases the symptoms extend into the fourth and fifth months of life.

In mild cases, the fussiness occurs only in the evening or has some other regular diurnal pattern. Babies with colic may exhibit rhythmic kicking, grimacing, and flatus. However, vomiting, diarrhea, constipation, and failure to thrive are not characteristic of colic. The key feature of colic is that between episodes the infant appears comfortable and alert. The crying may not respond to the parents' attempts at comforting or may cease only to resume when the infant is put down. Notably, the physical and neurologic examinations are normal. In the ED, the parents are concerned about the baby being ill, or they are exhausted and want relief.

Diagnosis

The key to making the diagnosis of colic is the parents' statement that the infant is perfectly fine between paroxysms. However, several conditions other than colic can present with only fussiness or excessive crying. See Table 9.6 for the differential diagnosis of colic.

Perform a complete physical examination. If the baby cries during the examination, offer a gloved finger or nipple or place the infant in the prone position or over your shoulder. When distracted, the colicky baby will appear alert and will suck vigorously on a nipple or pacifier. Upon gentle palpation, the abdomen is soft and nontender.

Table 9.6 Differentiating diagnosis of colic

Diagnosis	Differentiating features
Allergic colitis	Guaiac positive stools
Congenital glaucoma	Excessive tearing; abnormal red reflex
Congestive heart failure	Tachypnea and diaphoresis during feeding; failure to thrive
Constipation/diarrhea	Change in stooling pattern; anal fissure
Corneal abrasion	Conjunctival hyperemia, excessive tearing
Gastroesophageal reflux	Regurgitation; irritability related to feeds
Hair tourniquet syndrome	Swelling of a digit, penis, or clitoris
Incarcerated hernia	Mass in inguinal region
Infantile spasms	Attacks occur in clusters throughout the day
Infection/sepsis	Fever, vomiting, diarrhea, lethargy, or decreased feeding
SVT	Pallor, poor feeding
Testicular torsion	Swollen, erythematous hemiscrotum
Trauma/abuse	Swelling over affected site; decreased movement

ED Management

The goal of the ED examination is to rule-out other conditions that can present with colicky pain. Once the diagnosis is made, reassure the parents that the infant is not seriously ill and that colic is a self-limited phenomenon among otherwise well infants. There is no definite cure or universally accepted treatment for colic. Instead, the lack of a recognized etiology has led to the existence of a number of controversial remedies. Dispel any of the commonly held myths about colic, including that medications are beneficial, that infants are "spoiled" by excessive holding, and that colic is caused by parental inexperience and anxiety. Reassure the parents and offer them suggestions that may mitigate a crying attack, such as increased holding and rocking of the baby, more frequent feeding, use of a pacifier, and environmental changes (stroller ride, infant swing, car ride). Encourage the parents to burp the infant frequently during and after feeding if they are not already doing so. Finally, avoid anti-spasmodics and gripe water which have not been proven effective and may have side effects.

If there is suspicion of cow's milk allergy, refer the family to a primary care provider who may decide to change to an elemental formula. Advise nursing mothers to consume a dairy- and soy-free diet until follow-up with the primary care provider.

Follow-up

- Primary care follow-up within the week
- Arrange for psychosocial support if the family can no longer cope with the crying

Bibliography

Akhnikh S, Engelberts AC, van Sleuwen BE, L'Hoir MP, Benninga MA. The excessively crying infant: etiology and treatment. *Pediatr Ann.* 2014;**43**(4):e69–75.

Chua C, Setlik J, Niklas V. Emergency department triage of the "incessantly crying" baby. *Pediatr Ann.* 2016;**45**(11):e394–e398.

Johnson JD, Cocker K, Chang E. Infantile colic: recognition and treatment. *Am Fam Physician.* 2015;**92**(7):577–582.

Shamir R, St James-Roberts I, Di Lorenzo C, et al. Infant crying, colic, and gastrointestinal discomfort in early childhood: a review of the evidence and most plausible mechanisms. *J Pediatr Gastroenterol Nutr.* 2013;**57** (Suppl. 1):S1–S45.

Constipation

Constipation is a common problem in children and causes significant distress to the child and family. It is an acute or chronic condition in which bowel movements occur less often than usual and/or consist of hard, dry stools that are painful or difficult to pass. Only a small percentage of patients will have an organic etiology; the vast majority will have functional constipation. Constipation may be precipitated by various events such as traumatic toileting experience, illness, anal fissure, diet changes, or it may represent a behavioral problem (Table 9.7).

Clinical Presentation

The presentation of constipation varies somewhat with age. For an infant, constipation is often defined more by the stool consistency (hard, pellet-like stools) rather than frequency

Table 9.7 Etiologies of constipation

Functional/Idiopathic

Developmental	Cognitive impairment
	Attention-deficit disorder
Psychiatric	Depression
Reduced stool volume	Low-fiber diet; dehydration
	Underfeeding
Situational	Coercive toilet training
	Toilet phobia
	School bathroom avoidance
	Excessive parental interventions
	Sexual abuse

Organic

Abnormal musculature	Prune belly
	Gastroschisis
	Down syndrome
Anatomic malformations	Imperforate anus, anal stenosis
	Anteriorly displaced anus
	Pelvic mass
Drugs	Opiates, phenobarbital, sucralfate, antacids, antihypertensives, anticholinergics, antidepressants, sympathomimetics
Gastrointestinal	Milk protein allergy
	Hirchsprung's disease
	Gluten enteropathy
Metabolic	Hypothyroidism; hypercalcemia
	Cystic fibrosis
	Diabetes mellitus
Neuropathic	Spinal cord abnormalities (tethered cord, trauma)
	Static encephalopathy
Other	Heavy metal ingestion (lead)
	Vitamin D intoxication
	Botulism

as this can vary based on diet. Similarly, symptoms such as grunting or straining with the passage of soft stool does not represent constipation. In older children, constipation is characterized by hard, large, painful stools which may occur daily, but more commonly will pass once every several days. Patients may complain of abdominal pain (can be severe), nausea, vomiting, bloating, abdominal distention, blood in the stool, decreased appetite, and the family may report soiling of the underwear. Younger children may exhibit withholding behaviors as well. Some patients may also present with frequent urinary tract infections or enuresis.

Diagnosis

The differential diagnosis is broad (Table 9.7), although the vast majority of patients will have functional or idiopathic constipation, with no objective evidence of a pathologic condition. In most cases, a thorough history and physical examination is sufficient to both make the diagnosis and rule-out significant organic disorders.

It is important to ask the age of onset, duration of symptoms, and if there was passage of meconium within the first 24–48 hours of life. Delayed passage of meconium and constipation onset under one month of age raises suspicion for an organic cause, such as Hirschsprung's disease, and warrants further investigation. Additionally, ask about stool frequency and consistency, diet habits, withholding behaviors, soiling, toileting history, medication use, prior treatments for constipation, current social stressors, gait abnormalities, or weakness, as well as abdominal pain and distension, and whether there is blood in the stool.

On physical examination, determine if there is normal growth and development. The abdominal examination may be notable for palpable stool or distention. Perform a careful neurologic examination of the lower extremities and inspect the perianal region for skin tags, fissures, rash, soiling, anal wink, and the anal position. Examine the lumbosacral region for a sacral tuft or dimple suggestive of a spinal abnormality. A rectal examination is not required for the diagnosis of constipation but can be performed if the history is unclear or to evaluate for a fecal mass. Finally, imaging and laboratory testing is not required to diagnose constipation, although they may be used to rule-out other etiologies.

ED Management

The goals of the ED management are disimpaction (if necessary); counseling to improve behavior, toileting, and dietary habits; and the institution of maintenance medication(s) until diet and behaviors have been modified.

The choice of medication(s) depends upon the patient's age. For infants under one year old, dietary changes are usually all that are needed. Encourage increased fluid intake and the use of juices containing sorbitol (prune, pear) and mix the juice with water in a 1:1 ratio, titrating intake according to stool consistency. If this is unsuccessful, recommend lactulose. In children over one year of age, polyethylene glycol electrolyte (PEG) solution is usually helpful.

For impaction, prescribe a clean out with PEG solution (1–1.5 g/kg/day divided 2–3 times) per day for three days. If there is a fecal mass, administer an enema. Lactulose (1–2 g/kg 1–2 times per day) can also be used if PEG is not tolerated. Recommend maintenance medication with PEG 0.5–0.8 mg/kg/day following the clean out until follow-up with primary care provider.

See Table 9.8 for a summary of pharmacologic products indicated in the treatment of constipation. The most effective treatment is PEG, whereas the others are useful for enhancing the effectiveness of PEG therapy, rather than to be used as monotherapy.

Table 9.8 Treatment of constipation

Medication	Dose	Notes
Osmotic agents		
Lactulose	1–3 mL/kg/day in divided doses (70% solution)	Can cause flatulence and cramping
Magnesium citrate	<6 years 1–3 mL/kg/day div q day or bid ≥6–12 years: 100–150 mL/day div q day or bid ≥12 years: 150–300 mL/day div q day or bid	Can cause Mg poisoning in infants Not for maintenance use
PEG powder (Miralax)	Disimpact: 1–1.5 g/kg/day for 3 days Maintenance: 0.5–0.8 g/kg/day	Mix 17 g in 6–8 oz of liquid and divide bid or tid
Phosphate enema	6 mL/kg up to 135 mL (do not use if <2 years)	Risk of severe ↑phosphate with ↓calcium
Sorbitol	1–3 mL/kg/day in divided doses (70% solution)	Same as lactulose
Lubricant		
Mineral oil	Disimpact: 15–30 mL/year of age (240 mL max.) Maintenance (≥1 year): 1–3 mL/kg/day	Lipoid pneumonia if aspirated
Stimulants		
Bisacodyl (Dulcolax)	≥2 years 0.5–1 suppository	Abdominal pain; hypokalemia
Senna (8.8 mg/5 mL)	2–6 years 2.5–7.5 mL/day	Idiosyncratic hepatitis
	6–12 years 5–15 mL/day	Risk of melanosis coli
Stool softener		
Docosate sodium	<3 years 10–40 mg/day	Very bitter (give with tasty liquid)
	≥3–6 years 20–60 mg/day	Divide into 1–4 daily doses
	≥6–12 years 40–150 mg/day	
	≥12 years 50–400 mg/day	

Finally, encourage toilet-trained children to sit on the toilet with knees above the hips for 5–10 minutes, 2–3 times per day after meals. This schedule enhances the likelihood a patient is going to stool since food in the stomach triggers the gastrocolic reflex, which then causes an urge to stool.

Follow-up

- Constipation without impaction: primary care follow-up in 1–2 weeks
- Impaction: primary care physician in 3–5 days

Indications for Admission

- Severe constipation with emesis and dehydration
- Serious underlying disorder (Hirschsprung's disease)

Bibliography

Colombo JM, Wassom MC, Rosen JM. Constipation and encopresis in childhood. *Pediatr Rev.* 2015;**36**(9):392–401.

Montgomery DF, Navarro F. Management of constipation and encopresis in children. *J Pediatr Health Care.* 2008;**22**:199–204.

Orenstein SR, Wald A. Pediatric rectal exam: why, when, and how. *Curr Gastroenterol Rep.* 2016;**18**(1):4.

Paul SP, Broad SR, Spray C. Idiopathic constipation in children clinical practice guidelines. *Arch Dis Child Educ Pract Ed.* 2016;**101**(2):65–69.

Tabbers MM, DiLorenzo C, Berger MY, et al. Evaluation and treatment of functional constipation in infants and children: evidence-based recommendations from ESPGHAN and NASPGHAN. *J Pediatr Gastroenterol Nutr.* 2014;**58**(2):258–274.

Diarrhea

Diarrhea is the excessive loss of fluids and electrolytes in the stool resulting in decreased stool consistency and/or increased frequency (usually >3 stools/day). Acute diarrhea usually lasts <7 days, but not longer than 14 days, at which point it is defined as chronic diarrhea. Infection is the most common cause of acute diarrhea and is a major cause of morbidity and hospitalization worldwide. In developed countries, most gastroenteritis is caused by viral infection. Bacterial, parasitic, and protozoal illnesses are less frequent but not uncommon. In a viral infection, diarrhea is non-inflammatory and results from an enteropathy in which the death of mature villus-tip cells (responsible for disaccharide digestion and monosaccharide absorption) causes an osmotic diarrhea due to the malabsorption of sugars. The pathophysiology of bacterial diarrhea involves a combination of impaired water absorption due to an inflammatory process and often a secretory toxin produced by the bacteria. Invasive bacterial disease in the colon results in frequent, small, bloody, often mucoid stools known as dysentery. Occasionally, both toxic and inflammatory processes are active. Chronic diarrhea may be due to an infectious or noninfectious etiology.

Clinical Presentation

The symptoms and signs of gastroenteritis are vomiting, abdominal pain, and diarrhea. Some patients will have fever. A patient with chronic diarrhea may have these same symptoms, but there may be associated malnutrition and weight loss.

Diagnosis

Inquire about the onset and duration of the diarrhea, the frequency and volume, and if there is blood or mucus. Also ask if there has been fever or vomiting. Obtain a detailed dietary history and keep in mind that sorbitol in apple and grape juice may exacerbate diarrhea. Ask about the patient's urine output, general activity level, and if there has been recent travel or sick contacts.

For a patient with chronic diarrhea, ask about a family history of autoimmune disorders, including celiac disease and inflammatory bowel disease. Inflammatory bowel disease may present with or without bloody diarrhea and the patient may also have fever, weight loss, oral ulcers, arthralgia, rash (pyoderma gangrenosum or erythema nodosum), or uveitis. Celiac disease can present with abdominal pain, joint pain, poor growth, and rash (dermatitis herpetiformis), as well as the diarrhea. A neuroblastoma or ganglioneuroma may cause chronic watery diarrhea, while bulky, greasy, foul-smelling stools are associated with celiac disease, cystic fibrosis, and pancreatic insufficiency. See Table 9.9 for the more common causes of acute diarrhea and their differentiating features.

Table 9.9 Differential diagnosis of acute diarrhea

Diagnosis	Differentiating features
Antibiotic-related	C. difficile: fever, toxicity, pain
Appendicitis	Periumbilical then RLQ pain
	Vomiting predominates
Campylobacter	Watery or bloody stools
	Most <1 week duration, but can be prolonged IBD-like
	Sources: undercooked poultry, unpasteurized milk, pets
Enteric adenovirus	Peak age <4 years; year-round
Enterohemorrhagic E. coli	Peak age <5 years; summertime
	Watery, then bloody diarrhea; severe abdominal pain
	Can lead to HUS
	Sources: undercooked meat, unpasteurized milk/cider
Enterotoxigenic E. coli	Major cause of traveler's diarrhea
Giardia lamblia	Epidemics: daycare, contaminated water
Intussusception	Intermittent colicky abdominal pain
	Currant jelly stools
Milk protein allergy	Presents <3 months old with mucoid, bloody stools
Onset of chronic illness	IBD; celiac disease; cystic fibrosis
Norovirus (Norwalk virus)	Epidemic outbreaks; school-age to adults
	Watery, nonbloody diarrhea
	Can have headache, malaise, and myalgias

Table 9.9 (cont.)

Diagnosis	Differentiating features
Rotavirus	Peak age <2 years; wintertime
	Fever, vomiting, watery, nonbloody diarrhea
	Watery, nonbloody diarrhea
Salmonella (non-typhi)	Abdominal cramps; bloody diarrhea
	Bacteremia in 5–10% of infant cases
	Moderate abdominal pain; watery diarrhea
	Sources: contaminated meat/eggs/poultry; reptiles
Shigella	Risk factors: daycare or crowded conditions at risk
	Can have high fever; voluminous, bloody stools
	Seizures can occur early and precede the diarrhea
Toddler's diarrhea	Viral illness gastroenteritis weeks to months before
	Large stools with food particles; exacerbated by juice
Yersinia enterocolitica	More common in young children and in cooler climates
	Can mimic appendicitis in older children
	Afebrile; foul-smelling stools; flatulence; distention
	Sources: undercooked pork, unpasteurized milk, well water
Other infections	Associated with UTI, otitis media, sepsis, pneumonia
	Mucoid or bloody stools

ED Management

The goals of management include: (1) recognition, treatment, and prevention of dehydration; (2) prescription of dietary therapy that maximizes nutrient retention; (3) recognition of invasive or potentially invasive infections; and (4) management of the public health aspects of acute gastroenteritis.

Determination of hydration status is the first priority. Use the patient's premorbid weight, vital signs, and clinical characteristics (Table 9.5) to estimate the degree of dehydration. See pp. 246–249 for the management of dehydration.

Most patients will not benefit from laboratory or stool studies. However, if there is a history of persistent (more than two weeks) or bloody diarrhea, test the stool for fecal leukocytes and blood. Obtain a stool culture if the tests are positive or the illness suggests a bacterial etiology. With a viral diarrhea, malabsorbed sugars are present either as reducing substances or converted to acids, and fecal leukocytes are absent. If indicated (i.e., cohorting of patients during an epidemic, diagnosis unclear, unusually sick patient), send a stool sample for rapid enzyme immunoassay for rotavirus. If the stools are grossly bloody, obtain a culture for bacterial pathogens (*E. coli* O157:H7, *Salmonella, Shigella, Yersinia, Campylobacter, C. difficile* toxin). If available, send a gastrointestinal pathogen panel which detects multiple viral, parasitic and bacterial pathogens.

E. coli O157:H7 is responsible for 90% of cases of hemolytic-uremic syndrome (HUS) in the United States. HUS occurs 3–12 days after the onset of diarrhea and is characterized by a triad of microangiopathic hemolytic anemia, thrombocytopenia, and oliguria or anuria. Clinically the child is pale, irritable, and edematous. Obtain a CBC with platelet count, BUN, creatinine, and electrolytes if the patient has a prior *E. coli* O157:H7 infection or is suspected of having HUS.

Empiric antibiotic treatment of suspected bacterial gastroenteritis is rarely necessary. More importantly, antibiotic treatment has been epidemiologically linked to HUS and a worse outcome in *E. coli* O157:H7 infection and prolonged *Salmonella* excretion. The treatment of *E. coli* O157:H7 is supportive, but consult a nephrologist in the event that HUS develops.

Treat proven *Shigella* with trimethoprim-sulfamethoxazole (8 mg/kg/day of TMP div bid; 320 mg/day maximum) for five days. Treat moderate to severe *Campylobacter* with erythromycin (40 mg/kg/day div tid or qid; 2 g/day maximum) for 5–7 days. Guidelines for treating *Salmonella* in infants are presented in Table 9.10. Do not treat uncomplicated, noninvasive *Salmonella* infections unless the patient is less than three months of age, immunocompromised, has chronic gastrointestinal disease (inflammatory bowel disease, celiac disease), or has severe colitis.

Table 9.10 Management of infants less than one year with diarrhea not requiring hospitalization at the initial visit

	Age	Management
I. First evaluation		
A. Colitis (dysentery fecal WBCs)	0–12 months	Stool culture
		CBC and blood culture if <3 months or appears ill
B. No colitis or diarrhea <5 days	0–12 months	No stool culture
		Evaluate for nonbacterial causes if indicated
C. Exposure to *Salmonella*	0–3 months	Stool and blood cultures
		CBC
II. Follow-up evaluation		
A. Diarrhea ≥5 days	0–12 months	Stool culture
B. Stool culture positive[a] and blood culture positive	0–12 months	Admit[b] and treat with antibiotics[c]
C. Stool culture positive[a] and blood culture negative		
1. Toxic, ill, immunocompromised	0–12 months	Admit[b] and treat with antibiotics[c]
2. Febrile, well-appearing	≤3 months	Admit[b] and treat with antibiotics[c]

Table 9.10 (cont.)

	Age	Management
3. Febrile, improving	3–12 months	Blood culture
		TMP-SMX[d] (blood culture pending)
4. Afebrile, improving	≤3 months	Oral antibiotics[e]
D. Stool culture positive[a] but blood culture not obtained at first visit		See category IIC CBC and blood culture

[a] Stool culture positive for *Salmonella*.
[b] Includes evaluation for focal infection of meninges, bone, urinary tract, and other sites.
[c] Cefotaxime or ceftriaxone.
[d] 8 mg/kg/day of TMP div bid.
[e] Oral/TMP-SMX pending sensitivities. If under one month of age, consult an infectious disease specialist.
Adapted from *Pediatr Infect Dis J* 1988;7:620.

Treat *C. difficile*-associated pseudomembranous colitis for 10–14 days with PO or IV metronidazole (30 mg/kg/day div qid, maximum 2 g/day) or, alternatively, with oral vancomycin (40 mg/kg/day div qid, maximum 500 mg/day).

Have all family members practice meticulous handwashing during a diarrheal illness. Report enteric pathogen infection to the public health authorities. Exclude from daycare children with diarrhea that overflows the diaper, those with bloody stools until treated or resolved, and patients with *Shigella* or *E. coli* O517:H7 until stool cultures are negative.

In milk protein allergy, stool cultures are negative, and typically the bleeding stops after switching to an elemental formula (Nutramigen, Alimentum) or eliminating cow's milk from the mother's diet in a breastfed infant. In 20–40% of cases, there is cross-reaction with soy formula.

Continue to feed milk (formula or breast) to an infant, or an age-appropriate diet to a child, if the patient is not dehydrated or as soon as rehydration is complete. Guidelines do not exist for the use of a soy formula in acute infantile gastroenteritis with suspected temporary lactase deficiency. However, it is reasonable to prescribe a switch to a soy formula for an infant less than six months of age who develops dehydration, is malnourished (less than fifth percentile weight for height), has a significant underlying medical condition, or has diarrhea that does not improve on cow's milk formula after five days of illness.

As a general rule, do not recommend pharmacologic agents to treat acute diarrhea, although a probiotic containing *Lactobacillus rhamnosus* GG and *Saccharomyces boulardii* may be effective in reducing the duration of symptoms.

In a patient with chronic diarrhea and malnutrition, obtain a CBC, liver function panel, inflammatory markers, celiac screening (TTG IgA and total IgA) and stool studies for infection and malabsorption including culture, ova and parasites, leukocytes, reducing substances (carbohydrate malabsorption), fat, pancreatic elastase, and fecal alpha-1-antitrypsin (protein malabsorption).

Consult a pediatric gastroenterologist if there is concern for a noninfectious etiology or for diarrhea with malnutrition and/or weight loss. Endoscopic evaluation is often required for diagnosis of chronic noninfectious etiologies.

Follow-up

- Mild or no dehydration: contact primary care provider in 2–3 days
- Noninfectious chronic diarrhea: follow-up with pediatric gastroenterologist in 1–2 weeks

Indications for Admission

- >5% dehydration
- Failure of oral rehydration
- Electrolyte abnormalities or severe anemia
- Febrile infant less than three months of age with suspected or proven *Salmonella* enteritis
- *Salmonella* bacteremia
- Hemolytic-uremic syndrome complicating *E. coli* O157:H7 infection
- Severe infection with clinical toxicity caused by any enteric pathogen
- Suspected surgical abdomen

Bibliography

Bruzzese E, Lo Vecchio A, Guarino A. Hospital management of children with acute gastroenteritis. *Curr Opin Gastroenterol.* 2013;**29**(1):23–30

Guarino A, Ashkenazi S, Gendrel D, et al. European Society for Pediatric Gastroenterology, Hepatology, and Nutrition/European Society for Pediatric Infectious Diseases evidence-based guidelines for the management of acute gastroenteritis in children in Europe: update 2014. *J Pediatr Gastroenterol Nutr.* 2014;**59**(1):132–152.

Pfeiffer ML, DuPont HL, Ochoa TJ. The patient presenting with acute dysentery: a systematic review. *J Infect.* 2012;**64**(4):374–386.

Vandenplas Y. Probiotics and prebiotics in infectious gastroenteritis. *Best Pract Res Clin Gastroenterol.* 2016;**30**(1):49–53.

Zella GC, Israel EJ. Chronic diarrhea in children. *Pediatr Rev.* 2012;**33**(5):207–217.

Gallbladder and Gallstone Disease

Gallbladder disease in children and adolescents is increasing in prevalence. The patient may have calculous cholecystitis, which occurs when a gallstone obstructs the cystic duct or, less commonly, the common duct. Factors predisposing to gallstone formation are chronic hemolytic disorders (sickle cell, hereditary spherocytosis, etc.), prolonged parenteral nutrition, chronic liver disease, obesity, pregnancy, malabsorption (terminal ileal resection, Crohn's disease, cystic fibrosis, etc.) prolonged fasting or rapid weight reduction, antibiotics (ceftriaxone), chemotherapy, a history of abdominal surgery, and a family history of gallstone disease. Acute cholangitis can ensue if the obstruction leads to an acute bacterial infection.

An acutely distended, inflamed gallbladder can occur in the absence of an obstructing gallstone (acalculous cholecystitis). This presents as a postoperative complication or as a result of sepsis or systemic infection, trauma, Rocky Mountain spotted fever, typhoid fever, *Shigella*, viral gastrointestinal or respiratory infections. In 50% of cases, acalculous cholecystitis is idiopathic.

Acute hydrops of the gallbladder is an acute non-inflammatory swelling of the gallbladder without gallstones. It is primarily recognized as a complication of Kawasaki disease (5–20% of patients), but it also occurs in viral hepatitis, streptococcal pharyngitis, staphylococcal infection, Henoch–Schönlein purpura, nephrotic syndrome, mesenteric adenitis, and Sjögren's syndrome, and as a consequence of long-term parenteral nutrition.

Clinical Presentation

Biliary "colic" and acute cholecystitis both present with the sudden onset of crampy pain, which rapidly becomes severe. In biliary colic, the severe pain lasts for 1–3 hours and then moderates into a dull ache over 30–90 minutes. With cholecystitis, the severe pain persists for >6–12 hours. Most commonly, the pain is in the right upper quadrant or epigastrium, although it can be periumbilical or diffuse. In one-third of patients, the pain radiates to the back, scapula, shoulder, or arm. Associated symptoms include anorexia, nausea, vomiting, and low-grade fever. As the gallbladder inflammation progresses, there may be local peritoneal inflammation with associated peritoneal pain. Acalculous cholecystitis and acute hydrops of the gallbladder present in a similar manner.

On physical examination, an enlarged gallbladder can be noted in one-third of cases, and there is often guarding of the right upper quadrant. Murphy's sign (inspiratory arrest with deep palpation of the right upper quadrant) and Boas' sign (tenderness or hyperesthesia over the right scapula) may be appreciated. Only 15–20% of patients develop jaundice. Two-thirds of cases of acute cholecystitis resolve spontaneously over the course of 2–3 days, although there may be progression to gallbladder necrosis and perforation with either localized abscess formation or peritonitis.

Acute cholangitis presents with Charcot's triad, fever, jaundice, and RUQ abdominal pain.

Diagnosis

Obtain blood for a CBC, liver function tests, amylase, lipase, and electrolytes. Cholecystitis is associated with increased serum alkaline phosphatase and direct bilirubin, as well as leukocytosis.

An ultrasound is usually sufficient to make the diagnosis of gallbladder disease. Gallstones, thickening of the gallbladder wall, and a positive sonographic Murphy sign (tenderness over the gallbladder from pressure of the ultrasound probe) may be noted with cholecystitis. In acalculous disease there will be the same findings, but without gallstones. The ultrasound in hydrops will reveal a distended gallbladder in the absence of stones, and a normal wall thickness.

See Table 9.11 for the differential diagnosis of right upper quadrant pain, which is the most common symptom of gallbladder disease.

Table 9.11 Differential diagnosis of right upper quadrant abdominal pain

Diagnosis	Differentiating features
Biliary tract disease	
Cholecystitis	Low-grade fever, variable jaundice
	Positive Murphy's and/or Boas' signs
Choledochal cyst	Palpable mass, seen on ultrasound
Cholelithiasis	Pain may worsen with meals
Gallbladder disease	Pain radiates around to back/scapula
	Ultrasound is diagnostic
Hydrops	Fever is rare (except with Kawasaki)
	Palpable RUQ mass
Liver disease	
Hepatic abscess	Insidious pain, fever, leukocytosis, elevated CRP/ESR
Hepatitis	Hepatomegaly
	↑ ALT/AST (4–100 times normal)
Other diagnoses	
Appendicitis (retrocecal)	Fever, vomiting, rebound tenderness
Fitz–Hugh–Curtis	Positive gonorrheal and/or chlamydial cultures
	Signs of PID are variable
Pancreatitis	Pain radiates straight to back
	↑ Amylase and lipase
Peptic ulcer disease	Pain may be relieved with meals
Pyelonephritis	Fever, CVA tenderness, pyuria
Renal stones	Colicky pain, hematuria
RLL pneumonia	Tachypnea, fever, cough

ED Management

If gallbladder disease is suspected, make the patient NPO, secure an IV, obtain the blood tests mentioned above, and obtain an ultrasound. In questionable cases, consult with gastroenterology to arrange advanced imaging (MRCP and/or HIDA) scan.

If cholecystitis or hydrops is diagnosed, obtain surgical consultation, and provide analgesia with either ketorolac (0.5 mg/kg every 6 hours for 5 days, 120 mg/day maximum) or morphine (0.05–0.1 mg/kg/dose every 2–4 hours; maximum 2 mg/dose infant, 4–8 mg/dose child, 15 mg/dose adolescent). Urgent surgery is indicated for peritonitis, perforation, or progression of symptoms with worsening pain and fever while under observation.

Treat suspected infection with ampicillin/sulbactam (200 mg/kg/day divided every 6 hours, 8 g ampicillin/day maximum) or piperacillin/tazobactam (300 mg/kg/day divided every 8 hours, 16 g piperacillin/day maximum), but do not use ceftriaxone as it may cause sludging of the gallbladder contents.

Management of acute hydrops is usually supportive and concurrent with treatment of any associated illness.

Indications for Admission
- Suspected cholecystitis or hydrops of the gallbladder
- Cholangitis
- Severe biliary colic unresponsive to ED analgesia

Bibliography
Bennett GL. Evaluating patients with right upper quadrant pain. *Radiol Clin North Am.* 2015;**53**:1093–1130.

Poffenberger CM, Gausche-Hill M, Ngai S, et al. Cholelithiasis and its complications in children and adolescents. *Pediatr Emerg Care.* 2012;**28**(1): 68–76.

Rothstein DH, Harmon CM. Gallbladder disease in children. *Semin Pediatr Surg.* 2016;**25**(4):225–231.

Wylie R, Hyams J, Kay M. Diseases of the gallbladder. In *Pediatric Gastrointestinal and Liver Disease* (5th edn.). Philadelphia, PA: Elsevier; 2011; 977–989.

Gastrointestinal Bleeding
By definition, the source of an upper gastrointestinal (UGI) bleed is proximal to the ligament of Treitz and is almost always concerning and, occasionally, life-threatening. Alternatively, lower gastrointestinal (LGI) bleeding, defined as intestinal bleeding distal to the ligament of Treitz, is a common complaint during childhood. Most LGI bleeds are minor and not hemodynamically significant, although they are almost always alarming to parents.

Clinical Presentation
The clinical presentation for UGI and LGI bleeds differs, but there can be overlap and both demand a careful and coordinated approach. GI bleeding may present as:
- hematemesis, which is vomiting of bright-red blood or coffee-ground material;
- melena, which is a tarry black stool containing digested blood and is characteristically malodorous;
- hematochezia, which is bright-red blood per rectum usually indicative of colonic or rectal bleeding, but is also seen in severe and rapid UGI bleeding;
- occult blood loss which occurs without gross blood in the stool.

Clinically, the presentation of a GI bleed may range from asymptomatic anemia to dizziness, dyspnea, or hypovolemic shock. A patient with UGI bleeding characteristically has hematemesis, melena, or occult blood loss, while an LGI bleed more commonly presents with hematochezia, melena, or occult blood loss.

Diagnosis
Confirm that the red or black color in the emesis and/or stool is actually blood by obtaining a gastroccult (stomach contents) and/or hemoccult/guaiac (stool). Note that red-colored

foods (beets, artificially colored drinks) or medications may turn the stools red and that some foods (blueberries, spinach, licorice) and medications (iron supplements, Pepto-Bismol) can cause black-colored stools. False-positive gastroccult or guaiac can occur with recent ingestion of undercooked meat and peroxidase-continuing fruits and vegetables (cantaloupe, turnip, radish, horseradish).

Once the presence of bleeding is confirmed, the next step is to determine the source. For UGI bleeding, also consider non-GI sources, which are more common than true UGI bleeds. Ask about recent epistaxis, pharyngitis, dental work, orofacial trauma, and hemoptysis. If an infant is breastfeeding, ask about the condition of the mother's nipples (cracked or infected). In newborns, perform an Apt test to differentiate neonatal blood from possible swallowed maternal blood. Common etiologies of UGI and LGI bleeding based on age are found in Tables 9.12 and 9.13.

If there is a UGI source, determine if the patient has had fever, vomiting, or has taken any medications associated with UGI bleeding (nonsteroidal anti-inflammatories, anti-coagulants, corticosteroids). Establish if there is any family history of peptic ulcer disease, *Helicobacter pylori* infection, or inflammatory bowel disease. Peptic disease in young children may present atypically with generalized abdominal pain, nocturnal or early-morning pain, and pain related to meals (causing exacerbation or relief). Consider alcoholic gastritis in an adolescent. An antecedent history of splenomegaly or liver disease raises the possibility of esophageal varices. Ask about umbilical vein catheterization, omphalitis, or congenital anomalies as well.

For an LGI bleed, ask about recent fever, vomiting, diarrhea, or constipation. Inquire if there has been recent antibiotic use (suggesting pseudomembranous colitis), prior episodes of bleeding (polyp, Meckel's diverticulum, anal fissure), and weight loss or arthralgia (inflammatory bowel disease).

On physical examination, initially focus on the vital signs (including orthostatic changes) and signs of shock (skin color, temperature, capillary refill). Check the skin for petechiae (coagulopathy) or jaundice (liver disease). For a UGI bleed, examine the nose and oropharynx carefully for a source of bleeding and look for signs of liver disease (jaundice, hepatomegaly, caput medusa), which raises the concern for variceal bleeding. In a patient with an LGI bleed, look for abdominal masses (volvulus, intussusception), perioral pigmentation (Peutz–Jeghers syndrome), and purpura (Henoch–Schönlein purpura). Examine the perianal area looking for anal fissures (constipation) and anal tags (inflammatory bowel disease), and perform a rectal examination to check for polyps, masses, or fecal mass suggestive of constipation.

ED Management

Unstable Patient

The priority is the recognition and treatment of shock and stabilization of vital signs. Begin fluid resuscitation if there are any signs of volume depletion (orthostatic changes, skin color changes, tachycardia, prolonged capillary refill, and/or altered sensorium) or there is active bleeding. Elevate the patient's legs, start two large-bore IVs, and give an isotonic fluid bolus with 20 mL/kg of normal saline or Ringer's lactate. Obtain a stat CBC, chemistry, liver function panel, coagulation studies, and a type and cross. Correct any coagulation defects (pp. 353–357) with vitamin K, fresh frozen plasma, or platelets. Have packed RBCs available

Table 9.12 Differential diagnosis of UGI bleeding

Diagnosis	Differentiating features
Any age	
Coagulopathy	Petechiae and purpura
	Other bleeding sites
Esophagitis	Associated GERD, infection, immunosuppression
Gastritis/ulcer disease	*H. pylori*
	Stressed patient
	Medications (NSAIDs, steroids, anticoagulants)
Mallory–Weiss tear	Forceful or repeated vomiting or retching
UGI obstruction	Persistent vomiting, which can be bilious
	Abdominal distention, irritability
Neonate	
Breastfeeding	Mother with cracked nipples or mastitis
Hemorrhagic disease (HDN)	Presents on days 1–5 of life
	Breastfed baby born at home at risk
Milk protein allergy	Streaks of blood and mucous in stool; rash
Stress gastritis	Stressful delivery, serious infection, or anoxic event
Swallowed maternal blood	Apt test to differentiate fetal from maternal blood
Infant	
Arteriovenous malformation / hemangioma	May have associated cutaneous lesions
Congenital factor deficiency	Bleeding disproportionate to trauma
GI duplication	Presence of heterotopic mucosa can cause ulcer/bleeding
Reflux esophagitis	Regurgitation, vomiting, irritability, poor feeding
Child and adolescent	
Caustic ingestion	Drooling, oropharyngeal burns, refusal to swallow
Crohn's disease	Weight loss, low-grade fever
	Extraintestinal manifestations
Esophageal foreign body	Antecedent choking event, drooling, refusal to swallow
Esophageal varices	Voluminous/painless bleed
	Splenomegaly, caput medusae
Swallowed blood	Dental, nasal, pharyngeal, or pulmonary bleeding source
Trauma/duodenal hematoma	Blunt trauma may be trivial causing gradual obstruction

Table 9.13 Differential diagnosis of LGI bleeding

Diagnosis	Differentiating features
Allergic	Formula-fed infant
	Breastfed if mother is ingesting milk
Anal fissure	Blood-streaked stool or blood passed following defecation
	History of constipation
	May have sentinel skin tag
Coagulopathy	Petechiae, purpura, other bleeding sites
Colitis	Frequent bloody, mucoid stools
Duplication of the bowel	May contain ectopic gastric mucosa and mimic a Meckel's
Hemolytic-uremic syndrome	Follows acute diarrheal illness
	Commonly *E. coli* O157:H7
Hemorrhoids	Teens with constipation
	Infants with portal hypertension
Henoch–Schönlein purpura	Colicky abdominal pain; arthralgias; hematuria
	Symmetric purpuric rash on lower extremities, buttocks
Hirschsprung's disease	Fever, vomiting, abdominal pain; history of constipation
Infectious	Abdominal pain, tenesmus
Inflammatory	Fever, weight loss, poor growth
	Extraintestinal symptoms
Intussusception	Intermittent colicky abdominal pain; vomiting
	Sausage-shaped mass in RUQ while RLQ feels empty
	Currant jelly stools
Lymphonodular hyperplasia	Benign condition diagnosed during endoscopy
	Presents <10 years of age
Massive UGI bleeding	May occur with gastroesophageal varices, ulcers
Meckel's diverticulum	Painless voluminous bleeding
Pseudomembranous colitis	*Clostridium difficile* (+)
	Recent antibiotic treatment
Polyp	Painless bright-red blood
	May have mucocutaneous lesions
Vascular malformations	Painless bleeding
	May have cutaneous lesions
Volvulus, midgut	Bright-red or maroon bleeding in infant or toddler
	Possible bilious vomiting and abdominal mass

and give a transfusion if there is brisk bleeding associated with anemia and hemodynamic compromise (see pp. 353–357). Ensure that the patient stays NPO.

If a UGI bleed is suspected, give a dose of an IV proton pump inhibitor (PPI), such as omeprazole (2 mg/kg, maximum 40 mg) IV. It is no longer routine practice to perform nasogastric tube (NGT) lavage as a negative lavage does not definitively rule-out a UGI bleed and NGT insertion can be dangerous in the case of esophageal varices. In the rare instance in which persistent UGI bleeding is brisk enough to require ongoing transfusions, consult a pediatric surgeon and a gastroenterologist for recommendations for vasopressin or octreotide therapy (for esophageal varices), PPI drip (ulcerations), and to arrange for emergent measures to control the bleeding.

For an LGI bleed, obtain an abdominal x-ray if the bleeding is associated with vomiting or abdominal pain to look for signs of intestinal obstruction (intussusception, volvulus, duplication). Brisk painless bleeding is most often due to a Meckel's diverticulum. If the patient is having diarrhea, obtain a stool culture and stool lactoferrin. Test for *C. difficile* if there is a recent history of antibiotic use or recent contact with someone with the infection. Obtain a blood culture if the patient is less than three months of age and febrile. Nonemergent endoscopy is warranted for any patient with GI bleeding due to colitis, once infection has been ruled out.

Stable Patient

For UGI bleeding, if the patient is hemodynamically stable, obtain the same laboratory studies (see above), and start an H_2 antagonist (ranitidine 1 mg/kg IV q 8h, 50 mg maximum per dose) or a PPI (omeprazole 2 mg/kg, maximum 40 mg). Consult a pediatric gastroenterologist as a PPI drip may be required for moderate to severe bleeding. An upper endoscopy is indicated for ongoing bleeding, UGI bleeding accompanied by peptic symptoms, and a significant drop in hematocrit, regardless of the presence of active bleeding. If there are no signs of active bleeding, the patient is hemodynamically stable, and there are no significant laboratory abnormalities, prescribe an antacid or H_2 blocker (as above) and discharge the patient home with follow-up as outlined below.

Treat an anal fissure in a well-appearing infant less than one year of age with petrolatum to the anus at each diaper change, and use dietary measures to treat coexistent constipation. For an older child, treat coexistent constipation (pp. 253–255) and recommend follow-up with the primary physician.

For a breastfeeding patient with suspected cow's milk protein intolerance, recommend that the mother start a dairy- and soy-free diet. If the patient is formula-fed, switch to a protein hydrolysate formula (Alimentum, Nutramigen). Note that symptoms may persist for up to two weeks after dietary adjustment.

If a polyp is suspected (history of prior polyps, polyp seen or palpated, perioral pigmentation), refer to a pediatric gastroenterologist for further work-up.

The ED management of constipation, intussusception (pp. 273–274), volvulus (p. 237), Meckel's diverticulum (pp. 282–283), and gastroenteritis (pp. 255–260) are detailed elsewhere.

A patient with suspected colitis and stable vital signs and laboratory values can be discharged home with follow-up with the primary care physician and referral to a gastroenterologist if it is noninfectious.

Follow-up
- Hemodynamically stable patient without peptic symptoms or active bleeding: 2–3 days with primary physician
- Cow's milk protein intolerance: 2–3 days with primary physician
- Polyp (with stable vital signs): pediatric gastroenterologist in 1–2 weeks
- Colitis: primary care physician within one week, pediatric gastroenterology if noninfectious

Indications for Admission
- Signs of intravascular volume depletion, inability to stay hydrated
- Significant UGI or LGI bleeding
- Infants less than three months of age with fever and colitis
- Severe abdominal pain

Bibliography
Balachandran B, Singhi S. Emergency management of lower gastrointestinal bleed in children. *Indian J Pediatr.* 2013;**80**(3):219–225.

Freedman SB, Stewart C, Rumantir M, Thull-Freedman JD. Predictors of clinically significant upper gastrointestinal hemorrhage among children with hematemesis. *J Pediatr Gastroenterol Nutr.* 2012;**54** (6):737–743.

Owensby S, Taylor K, Wilkins T. Diagnosis and management of upper gastrointestinal bleeding in children. *J Am Board Fam Med.* 2015;**28**(1):134–145.

Pant C, Olyaee M, Sferra TJ, et al. Emergency department visits for gastrointestinal bleeding in children: results from the Nationwide Emergency Department Sample 2006–2011. *Curr Med Res Opin.* 2015;**31**(2):347–351.

Singhi S, Jain P, Jayashree M, Lal S. Approach to a child with upper gastrointestinal bleeding. *Indian J Pediatr.* 2013;**80**(4):326–333.

Hepatitis
Hepatitis is defined as an inflammatory response affecting the liver. This can manifest as a mild, self-limiting disease or it can progress to fulminant hepatic liver failure, cirrhosis, or hepatocellular carcinoma. As a result of vaccinations for both hepatitis A (HAV) and B (HBV), there has been a dramatic decrease in the number of patients with infectious hepatitis. Globally, however, hepatitis A is still the leading cause of acute liver failure.

Clinical Presentation
During the prodromal phase, viral hepatitis may resemble a flu-like illness or gastroenteritis, with fever, lethargy, anorexia, nausea, vomiting, and right upper quadrant abdominal pain. The spleen is usually not palpable. In addition, with HBV, urticaria, purpura, papular acrodermatitis (Gianotti-Crosti syndrome), arthralgias, or arthritis may also occur. Other etiologies can mimic this clinical presentation (Table 9.14). Infectious mononucleosis may manifest as isolated hepatitis or a syndrome that includes pharyngitis and splenomegaly. Lymphadenopathy occurs in Epstein–Barr virus, cytomegalovirus, and HIV infections.

Table 9.14 Etiologies of hepatitis

Autoimmune disease

Autoimmune hepatitis

Primary biliary cirrhosis

Systemic lupus erythematous

Bacterial infections

Leptospirosis

Syphilis

Typhoid fever

Hereditary/other

Alpha-1-antitrypsin deficiency

Cystic fibrosis

Inborn error of metabolism

Non-alcoholic fatty liver disease

Wilson's disease

Drug/toxin-induced

Acetaminophen toxicity

Anticonvulsants

Carbon tetrachloride

Ethanol

Isoniazid

Oral contraceptives

Rifampin

Sulfonamides

Viral infections

Cytomegalovirus

Epstein–Barr virus

Herpes simplex virus

Varicella zoster virus

Although most young children with acute hepatitis do not have jaundice, 30% of cases of HBV will present with jaundice. The icteric phase lasts 1–4 weeks, with complete recovery in the majority of patients. A prolonged cholestatic form is rare in children. In about 0.1–1% of all cases, a fulminant hepatitis results in hepatic coma and possibly death. Both HBV and hepatitis C (HCV) hepatitis can progress to chronic liver disease, cirrhosis and hepatocellular carcinoma. There is also a carrier state for HBV that can be asymptomatic or associated with chronic liver disease. Acute HCV progresses to chronic disease in up to 70% of patients and end-stage liver disease occurs in 10% of patients.

Diagnosis

If hepatitis is suspected, obtain a CBC, electrolytes, LFTs (including AST, ALT, total and direct bilirubin, albumin), coagulation profile, an acute hepatitis serology panel (hepatitis B surface antigen [HBsAg], surface antibody [anti-HBs], core antibody [anti-HBc]; IgM anti-HAV; anti-HCV/HCV PCR; and hepatitis E IgG/IgM, if the patient is from an endemic area). If HBV infection is suspected, obtain Hepatitis D Ag, anti-D IgM/IgG, and HIV testing.

If infectious hepatitis has been ruled out, consider other possible causes and obtain the following labwork: acetaminophen level, and heterophile antibody, ceruloplasmin, alpha-1-antitrypsin phenotype. If an autoimmune process is being considered, send antinuclear antibodies (ANA), anti-smooth muscle antibodies (ASMA), and anti-liver-kidney microsome antibodies.

Suspect HAV if the patient is in daycare, has traveled to an endemic area, or has a history of possible exposure to contaminated food or shellfish. The presence of anti-HAV IgM confirms HAV infection within the previous four weeks, while anti-HAV IgG implies infection that occurred more than four weeks prior to testing or successful immunization.

The primary test for diagnosing HBV is the surface antigen (HBsAg), which appears in the blood 4–6 weeks after exposure, but one week to two months before any elevation of the transaminases. HBsAg usually disappears 1–13 weeks after the onset of clinical disease. Persistence beyond six months defines chronic carriage or chronic hepatitis. Antibody to HBV surface antigen is protective, lasts indefinitely, and implies recovery from infection and absence of infectivity. It does not appear until there is resolution of the clinical hepatitis and is usually not measurable until several weeks after the disappearance of HBsAg. As a result, there can be a serologic "gap" when both HBsAg and anti-HBs are absent from the blood. This gap is filled by core antibody which is not protective. Anti-HBs can also indicate successful immunization when present without HBcAb. HBV serology is summarized in Table 9.15. Co-infection with HIV can alter disease progression, morbidity, and mortality related to HBV infection.

Table 9.15 Hepatitis B Serology

Stage of disease	HBsAg	anti-HBs	anti-HBc
Incubation	+	–	–
Acute illness	+	–	+
Early convalescence (serologic gap)	–	–	+
Resolved infection (<6 months ago)	–	+	+
Postrecovery (infection >6 months ago)	–	+	+
Chronic carrier	+	–	+
Post-vaccination	–	+	–

Abbreviations. HBsAg: hepatitis B surface antigen; anti-HBs: antibody to: hepatitis B surface antigen; anti-HBc: antibody to hepatitis B core antigen.

ED Management

The treatment is supportive, as there is no specific therapy for acute viral hepatitis. Intravenous hydration may be necessary for patients with severe vomiting. Treat a coagulopathy (INR >1.5 or PT >15) with vitamin K, 10 mg subcutaneously daily for three days. As prophylaxis against gastrointestinal bleeding give ranitidine (8 mg/kg/day div q 8h, 50 mg/dose maximum) or famotidine (0.6–0.8 mg/kg/day div q 12h, 40 mg/dose maximum). A fulminant course characterized by progressive jaundice and encephalopathy occurs in <1% of patients. See the section on liver failure (pp. 279–281) if the patient has coagulopathy, hypoglycemia, or encephalopathy, or returns to the ED with progressive jaundice.

Post-Exposure Prophylaxis

In the situation where the serologic status of the source of the exposure is unknown, promptly test the source for acute viral hepatitis serologies (HAV IgM, HBsAg, IgM anti-HbcAb, heterophile) and proceed with prophylaxis for hepatitis A or B, if indicated.

Hepatitis A Post-Exposure Prophylaxis

Give immune globulin (IG) within two weeks of exposure to all previously unimmunized household members or sexual contacts of a person who has serologically confirmed HAV infection. The dose is 0.02 mL/kg IM, 3 mL maximum, in each buttock for an infant or small child and 5 mL maximum in each buttock for an older child or adolescent. Also give IG to unimmunized daycare staff and attendees if one or more cases of HAV have been confirmed. Give the first dose of hepatitis A vaccine to all patients over one year of age. School contacts and health care personnel caring for the infected patient with HAV require good handwashing and stool precautions, not immune prophylaxis. When the index patient is known to be infected with HAV, serologic testing of contacts before IG administration is not necessary.

Hepatitis B Post-Exposure Prophylaxis

All previously unimmunized persons with direct (perinatal, sexual, or accidental percutaneous or mucosal exposure to blood or body fluids) exposure to an HBsAg-positive source require hepatitis B immune globulin (HBIG). The dose is 0.06 mL/kg IM (0.5 mL/dose for a neonate). Also give the first dose of hepatitis B vaccine, preferably within 24 hours of exposure or birth. Arrange to have the hepatitis B vaccine series completed using the age-appropriate dose and schedule. Only the hepatitis B vaccine series is indicated for household contacts of a known HBsAg-positive source or people who have had percutaneous or mucosal exposure to blood or body fluid with unknown HBsAg status.

Hepatitis C, D, E Post-Exposure Prophylaxis

There is no role for post-exposure prophylaxis in the case of hepatitis C, D, or E exposure.

Follow-up

- Suspected viral hepatitis: primary care follow-up in one week
- After HAV or HBV prophylaxis given: primary care follow-up in 2–4 weeks

Indications for Admission

- Fulminant hepatitis, with hypoglycemia, coagulopathy, encephalopathy, or vomiting precluding adequate oral intake

Bibliography

Chang M-H. Hepatitis B virus infection. In Suchy FJ, Sokol RJ, Balistreri WF (eds.) *Liver Disease in Children* (4th edn). Cambridge: Cambridge University Press, 2014:276–294.

Clemente MG, Schwarz K. Hepatitis. *Pediatr Rev.* 2011;32(8):333–340.

Komatsu H, Inui A. Hepatitis B virus infection in children. *Expert Rev Anti Infect Ther.* 2015;13 (4):427–450.

Matheny SC, Kingery JE. Hepatitis A. *Am Fam Physician.* 2012;86(11):1027–1034.

Rosenthal P. Hepatitis A and hepatitis B infection. In Suchy FJ, Sokol RJ, Balistreri WF (eds.) *Liver Disease in Children* (4th edn.). Cambridge: Cambridge University Press, 2014: 265–275.

Hepatomegaly

It is not unusual to palpate the liver below the costal margin in infants and young children, although a liver edge >3.5 cm below the costal margin in infants and >2 cm in children suggests hepatomegaly. Normal liver spans determined by percussion and palpation are 4.5–5 cm at one week of age, 7–8 cm for 12-year-old boys, and 6–6.5 cm for 12-year-old girls.

Clinical Presentation and Diagnosis

Apparent liver enlargement may be caused by downward displacement secondary to intrathoracic conditions (hyperinflation secondary to asthma or bronchiolitis, pneumothorax), subdiaphragmatic or retroperitoneal masses and thoracic deformities.

True liver enlargement results from inflammation, storage disorders, infiltrative processes, congestion, and obstruction. The most common cause of hepatomegaly is infectious mononucleosis or a mono-like syndrome (CMV, toxoplasmosis). Malaise, weakness, fever, pharyngitis, generalized lymphadenopathy, and splenomegaly are associated findings. Other common causes include viral hepatitis (vomiting, jaundice, dark urine, acholic stools), cirrhosis and chronic liver disease (jaundice, spider angiomata, splenomegaly, ascites, hemorrhoids), hemolytic anemias such as thalassemia (peculiar facies, jaundice), and congestive heart failure (tachypnea, rales, cardiomegaly, edema).

Serious but less common diseases include leukemia (pallor, bleeding, fever) and cystic fibrosis (failure to thrive, recurrent pulmonary illnesses). In the newborn consider congenital TORCH infection, neonatal hepatitis, and obstructive conditions (biliary atresia, choledochal cyst).

ED Management

If the patient does not appear seriously ill or jaundiced, a mono-like illness is most likely. Obtain a CBC with differential, heterophile antibody, liver function tests, and a hepatitis screen. If the diagnosis remains uncertain, refer the patient for further evaluation.

Jaundice, excessive vomiting, altered mentation, failure to thrive, and/or abnormal bleeding demand an immediate work-up. In addition to the laboratory tests mentioned above, obtain a PT, PTT, and glucose. Further evaluation is dictated by the clinical picture and may include a bone marrow aspiration, abdominal CT scan, liver–spleen scan, liver ultrasound, sweat chloride, alpha-1-antitrypsin assay and/or liver biopsy.

Follow-up
- Hepatomegaly without jaundice or ill appearance: primary care follow-up in one week

Indications for Admission
- Signs and symptoms of hepatic failure
- Severe vomiting that prevents adequate oral intake
- Suspicion of serious disease (leukemia, heart failure, cirrhosis, etc.) for evaluation and management

Bibliography

Clayton PT. Diagnosis of inherited disorders of liver metabolism. *J Inherit Metab Dis.* 2003;**26**:135–146.

Ebell MH, Call M, Shinholser J, Gardner J. Does this patient have infectious mononucleosis? The rational clinical examination systematic review. *JAMA.* 2016;**315**(14):1502–1509.

Mishra A, Pant N, Chadha R, Choudhury SR. Choledochal cysts in infancy and childhood. *Indian J Pediatr.* 2007;**74**:937–943.

Wolf AD, Lavine JE. Hepatomegaly in neonates and children. *Pediatr Rev* 2000;**21**:303–310.

Intussusception

Intussusception is the most frequent cause of intestinal obstruction in infants between three months and three years of age. Although it can occur at any age, 60% of patients are less than one year and 80% are less than two years of age. Anatomically, there is an invagination of one part of the bowel into the lumen of the distal adjoining part. The most common type is an ileocolic, but intussusception may occur at any level of the GI tract.

The majority of cases are idiopathic, although a lead point such as a polyp, lymphoma, Meckel's diverticulum, or bowel hematoma (as in Henoch–Schönlein purpura) is present in 5–10% of cases. A lead point is more likely in patients less than six months or more than six years of age. Mesenteric venous engorgement due to compression between the layers of the intussuscepted bowel causes mucous secretion and blood seepage, leading to the typical currant jelly stools. If the compression is not relieved, necrosis of the bowel with subsequent perforation and peritonitis can occur.

Clinical Presentation

Intussusception usually presents with the acute onset of intermittent abdominal pain and vomiting in a previously well infant. The classic triad of colicky abdominal pain, vomiting, and bloody stool is present in only about 25% of cases. The pain lasts 1–5 minutes, recurring every 5–20 minutes. During these paroxysms the baby may cry out, draw up his/her legs, and appear extremely uncomfortable. In between episodes the patient may initially appear well, but eventually becomes lethargic and apathetic. Vomiting follows the pain and, in the case of an ileoileal intussusception, may contain bile and suggests an intestinal obstruction.

Classic currant jelly stools are present early in only 10% of cases and are usually a late sign. In some cases, a currant jelly stool is found only with a rectal examination. Constipation, nonspecific diarrhea, and fever may also occur. With recurrent intussusception and spontaneous reduction, symptoms may be subacute or chronic over a period of a few days to weeks.

Initially the abdomen is soft between episodes of pain, but later it becomes distended and tender. In 85% of cases, a sausage-like mass can be palpated in the right abdomen. When the intussusception has progressed into the transverse colon, there may be absence of palpable viscera in the right lower quadrant (Dance's sign). An abdominal mass may be appreciated on rectal examination and stool for occult blood is positive in 75% of cases. Bowel sounds are initially hyperactive and then become hypoactive or absent.

Occasionally, intussusception can present with altered mental status as the most prominent sign.

Diagnosis

If the clinical suspicion of intussusception is high, prompt confirmation is necessary, as persistence of the intestinal obstruction may increase the child's risk for surgical intervention. The preferred imaging modality to confirm the diagnosis is abdominal ultrasound, looking for the target sign on transverse view and the pseudokidney sign on longitudinal view. In addition, color Doppler can assess the blood flow to the involved segment of bowel.

Prone and supine plain abdominal radiographs are a useful screening tool if ultrasound is not immediately available. Normally, the transverse colon and rectosigmoid are filled with air when a patient is supine; the ascending and descending colons are air-filled when prone. The inability to fill the ascending colon is highly suggestive of intussusception and the leading edge of the intussusceptum may be seen as a curvilinear density in the transverse colon.

Ultimately, a contrast enema, preferably with air, is both the diagnostic and therapeutic procedure of choice. In up to 90% of cases, the enema will reduce the intussusception.

ED Management

If intussusception is suspected, immediately notify a pediatric surgeon and radiologist. Insert an IV and give a bolus of 10–20 mL/kg of NS, followed by maintenance fluids. Obtain imaging to further support the diagnosis and then, if the patient is stable, obtain an air contrast enema as soon as possible. Surgery is indicated if the radiologist is unsuccessful at reducing the intussusception.

Small bowel – small bowel intussusception usually resolves spontaneously, without the need for a contrast enema.

Admit all patients with suspected or confirmed intussusception, as the immediate recurrence risk is about 10%. The majority of recurrent cases occur within the first 24 hours following reduction.

Indication for Admission

- Suspected or post-reduction intussusception
- Complications (perforation/peritonitis) secondary to intussusception

Bibliography

Gray MP, Li SH, Hoffmann RG, Gorelick MH. Recurrence rates after intussusception enema reduction: a meta-analysis. *Pediatrics.* 2014;**134**(1):110–119.

Jiang J, Jiang B, Parashar U, Nguyen T, Bines J, Patel MM. Childhood intussusception: a literature review. *PLoS One.* 2013;**8**(7):e68482.

Leeson K, Leeson B. Pediatric ultrasound: applications in the emergency department. *Emerg Med Clin North Am.* 2013;**31**(3):809–829.

Tareen, F, Mc Laughlin, D, Cianci, F, et al. Abdominal radiography is not necessary in children with intussusception *Pediatr Surg Int.* 2016;**32**:89.

Jaundice

The goals of the ED evaluation of the icteric child include rapid diagnosis of the acutely treatable causes of jaundice (sepsis, obstruction, metabolic disease), identification of patients in acute or impending liver failure (pp. 279–281), prophylaxis of susceptible contacts when icterus is caused by viral hepatitis, and reassurance when jaundice is physiologic or related to breastfeeding.

Jaundice is secondary to an increase in bilirubin, conjugated or unconjugated. This causes a yellow discoloration seen in the skin, eyes and mucous membranes. Jaundice can be due to an intrahepatic or extrahepatic disease process which leads to increased production or decreased excretion of bilirubin. These mechanisms may not be mutually exclusive.

Unconjugated hyperbilirubinemia is characterized by elevation of the indirect bilirubin fraction; the direct bilirubin is less than 20% of the total. Cholestasis is manifested by a direct bilirubin ≥1 mg/dL and/or a direct bilirubin that is ≥20% of the total bilirubin. By definition, cholestasis is pathologic and therefore requires further evaluation.

It is now standard practice for all newborns ≥35 weeks' gestation to have a jaundice risk assessment, which may include a serum or transcutaneous bilirubin measurement prior to discharge home from the nursery. As a result many neonates are being seen at 3–5 days of life for jaundice reassessment and/or bilirubin measurement.

Clinical Presentation

Neonates and Infants

In newborns, jaundice progresses in a cephalocaudal manner with increasing concentrations of total serum bilirubin.

Unconjugated Hyperbilirubinemia

Full-term, well-appearing neonates with unconjugated hyperbilirubinemia are likely to have physiologic jaundice, which peaks on the third day of life and then starts to decrease, typically resolving by ten days of life. The total bilirubin generally does not exceed 12 mg/dL at any time and the direct bilirubin is less than 2 mg/dL.

Breastfed infants may have prolonged unconjugated hyperbilirubinemia lasting several weeks. In general, under ten days of life, the jaundice is secondary to breastfeeding difficulty or dehydration. Afterwards it is caused by the breast milk itself. These infants have no evidence of blood group incompatibility, hemolytic disease, or infection.

Table 9.16 Most common hepatotoxins

Medications

Acetaminophen	Estrogens	Ketoconazole
Amiodarone	Haloperidol	Penicillins
Anticonvulsants	Halothane	Retinoids
Antineoplastics	Immunosuppressives	Sulfonamides
Aspirin	Isoniazid	Zidovudine
Erythromycin		

Environmental

Aflatoxins	Arsenic	Ma Huang/ephedra
Amanita mushroom	Carbon tetrachloride	

Conjugated Hyperbilirubinemia

Conjugated hyperbilirubinemia is never physiologic. Cholestasis is an indication of hepatocellular dysfunction, biliary obstruction, or a metabolic disorder. In infants, biliary atresia and neonatal hepatitis are the most common etiologies.

Children and Adolescents

Unconjugated Hyperbilirubinemia

The most common causes of unconjugated hyperbilirubinemia are hemolytic disorders. Gilbert's syndrome is characterized by mild, fluctuating unconjugated hyperbilirubinemia with levels of 2–5 mg/dL, normal liver function tests, and no evidence of hemolysis.

Conjugated Hyperbilirubinemia

Toxin-induced or viral hepatitis are the most common etiologies. Clinically apparent icteric hepatitis is most commonly caused by hepatitis A (HAV), hepatitis B (HBV), or hepatitis C (HCV) (see Acute Hepatitis, pp. 268–271). See Table 9.16 for a list of the most common hepatotoxins.

Diagnosis

Differentiate true icterus from carotenemia. Carotenemia is a nonpathologic accumulation of dietary carotene that causes yellow skin color in infants and toddlers without scleral icterus. In the jaundiced child, scleral icterus can be appreciated at a total serum bilirubin concentration of approximately 3.0 mg/dL, so that icterus is often noted before jaundice is appreciated.

In infants, unconjugated hyperbilirubinemia that does not fit the pattern of physiologic or breast milk jaundice and is not due to a hemolytic disorder (ABO incompatibility, glucose-6-phosphate dehydrogenase deficiency), excessive bruising, or a large cephalohematoma, may be caused by dehydration, polycythemia, hypothyroidism, infection (particularly UTI), or Crigler–Najjar syndrome.

See Table 9.17 for the differential diagnosis of jaundice. See pp. 268–271 for the diagnostic evaluation of suspected viral hepatitis.

Table 9.17 Differential diagnosis of jaundice

Diagnosis	Differentiating features
Unconjugated: neonates and Infants	
ABO/Rh incompatibility	Coombs positive
Breast milk jaundice	Presents after 4 days and may last for weeks
Crigler–Najjar syndrome	Presents 1–3 days of life
	Total bilirubin >15 mg/dL
Dehydration	Often due to poor breastfeeding (breastfeeding jaundice)
Hypothyroidism	Delayed stooling after birth
	Large fontanelles, macroglossia, umbilical hernia
Infection/sepsis	UTI can present with jaundice, which may be conjugated
Other hemolytic disorders	Coombs negative
Physiologic jaundice	Presents 1–3 days of life and resolves by 10 days
	Total bilirubin <15 mg/dL
Polycythemia	Plethora, lethargy/irritability, jitteriness
Sequestered blood	Bruising, cephalohematoma, CNS hemorrhage
Unconjugated: children and adolescents	
Gilbert syndrome	Intermittent jaundice
	Presents postpuberty when ill or stressed
Hemolytic disorders	Associated anemia
Conjugated: neonates and infants	
Biliary atresia	Presents in first 2 months of life, usually full-term
Choledochal cyst	Usually prenatal diagnosis
Congenital infection	CMV most common
	HIV, HSV, parvovirus B19, syphilis
Genetic/metabolic disease	Alpha-1 antitrypsin deficiency, cystic fibrosis, galactosemia
Neonatal hepatitis	Diagnosis usually requires liver biopsy
TPN cholestasis	Usually after two weeks of TPN
	Reverses when TPN stopped
Conjugated: children and adolescents	
Autoimmune hepatitis	(+) ANA and α-SMA, α-LKM-1, or α-SLA

Table 9.17 (cont.)

Diagnosis	Differentiating features
Cholelithiasis	Hemolytic disorder, obesity/weight loss, pregnancy
Dubin–Johnson syndrome	Presents postpuberty
	Worse with illness, stress, oral contraceptives
Hepatotoxins	See Table 9.16 for list of most common
Viral hepatitis	Prodrome of fever, vomiting
	RUQ pain then hepatomegaly
Wilson disease	Presents at 8–14 years
	Low serum ceruloplasmin

ED Management

Infants

If an infant is jaundiced, obtain total and direct bilirubin levels. Calculate the indirect or unconjugated bilirubin level by subtracting the direct bilirubin from the total bilirubin level. Well-appearing infants with unconjugated hyperbilirubinemia may be sent home if they have physiologic jaundice. Use an online resource such as www.bilitool.org to determine the management of hyperbilirubinemia in newborns.

If the infant has conjugated hyperbilirubinemia, obtain blood for culture, CBC, glucose, albumin, hepatic profile (including GGT), PT/INR, PTT, hepatitis serologies, thyroid function tests (if newborn screen is not readily available), and alpha-1-antitrypsin phenotype. Also obtain urine for culture, urinalysis, and reducing substances. Consult with a gastroenterologist, and admit the patient to facilitate the evaluation.

The diagnostic approach to the older child with suspected viral hepatitis is outlined elsewhere, although there is no specific therapy. See the section on liver failure (pp. 279–281) if the patient has coagulopathy, hypoglycemia, or encephalopathy, or returns to the ED with progressive jaundice.

Follow-up

- Breast milk or physiologic jaundice: primary care follow-up the next day

Indications for Admission

- Newborn requiring phototherapy
- Infant with conjugated hyperbilirubinemia
- Fulminant hepatitis, with hypoglycemia, coagulopathy, encephalopathy, or vomiting precluding adequate oral intake

Bibliography

Bilitool. www.bilitool.org (accessed June 7, 2017).

Brumbaugh D, Mack C. Conjugated hyperbilirubinemia in children. *Pediatr Rev.* 2012;**33**(7):291–302.

Fawaz R, Baumann U, Ekong U, et al. Guideline for the evaluation of cholestatic jaundice in infants: joint recommendations of the North American Society for Pediatric Gastroenterology, Hepatology, and Nutrition and the European Society for Pediatric Gastroenterology, Hepatology, and Nutrition. *J Pediatr Gastroenterol Nutr.* 2017;**64**(1):154–168.

Kaplan M, Bromiker R, Hammerman C. Hyperbilirubinemia, hemolysis, and increased bilirubin neurotoxicity. *Semin Perinatol.* 2014;**38**(7):429–437.

Khalaf R, Phen C, Karjoo S, Wilsey M. Cholestasis beyond the neonatal and infancy periods. *Pediatr Gastroenterol Hepatol Nutr.* 2016;**19**(1):1–11.

Maisels MJ. Managing the jaundiced newborn: a persistent challenge. *CMAJ.* 2015;**187**(5):335–343.

Liver Failure

Acute liver failure is a devastating disease. Rapid destruction of hepatocytes leads to progressive jaundice, coagulopathy, hypoglycemia, and encephalopathy. It is defined as uncorrectable coagulopathy despite treatment with vitamin K (INR >1.5 with encephalopathy, or INR >2 without encephalopathy, with no evidence of chronic liver disease in the past or at presentation). Although the list of etiologies of acute liver failure in childhood (Table 9.18) is long, in most cases no definite cause is found, especially in patients less than three years old.

Table 9.18 Causes of acute liver failure

Diagnosis	Differentiating features
Drugs/toxins	
Acetaminophen	↑AST/ALT to 400× normal
	Bilirubin normal
Amanita poisoning	Recent mushroom ingestion
	Severe GI symptoms
Anticonvulsants	Phenytoin, carbamazepine, phenobarbital
Idiosyncratic drug reaction	Herbals; green tea, weight loss agents, ephedra
Isoniazid	Affects <0.3% pts <20 years old
	Not dose-related
Genetic	
E. coli sepsis	(+) Urine reducing substances
Fatty acid oxidation defect	↑ Ammonia, nonketotic hypoglycemia
Galactosemia	Failure to thrive; cataracts,
Iron storage disease	Autosomal recessive; presents in adulthood
Mitochondrial disorders	Acidosis, ↑ammonia, ↑pyruvate/lactate, ↓glucose

Table 9.18 (cont.)

Diagnosis	Differentiating features
Tyrosinemia	Onset <6 months, cabbage-like odor
	Renal tubular acidosis
Wilson's disease	Hemolytic anemia
	Kayser–Fleischer rings, chorea, ataxia
	Immune dysregulation
Infectious	
Cytomegalovirus	Severe disease in immunocompromised host
Epstein–Barr virus	Severe disease in immunocompromised host
Hepatitis A–D	Infrequent, unless related to chronic infection
Herpes simplex virus	Usually no skin lesions, requires histology
Vascular	
Budd–Chiari syndrome	Abdominal pain, ascites, hepatomegaly
Ischemic hepatitis	CHF, shock, thrombosis, vasculitis
Other	
Autoimmune hepatitis	Evidence of chronic disease: ascites, spider angiomata
Malignancy	Metastatic disease
	Primary leukemia/lymphoma

Clinical Presentation

Patients initially present with jaundice, after a prodrome of nausea, vomiting, abdominal pain, anorexia, and malaise. In children, particularly infants, evidence of encephalopathy may be subtle and not apparent until the terminal stages of disease. Infants can present with poor feeding, increased irritability, and changes in sleep pattern. Older children can present with asterixis. Complications of acute liver failure include hypotension, cerebral edema, coagulopathy, acidosis, hypoglycemia, electrolyte disturbances, renal failure, and sepsis.

Hepatic encephalopathy is graded based upon changes in consciousness:

Stage 1: mild confusion, decreased attention, irritability, and reversal of sleep cycles.

Stage 2: drowsiness, personality changes, and intermittent disorientation.

Stage 3: gross disorientation, marked confusion, and slurred speech.

Stage 4: coma.

Diagnosis

Inquire about possible exposure to hepatitis through blood products, travel, and sexual activity. In infants also ask about exposure to herpes or cytomegalovirus. Take a detailed medication history, which includes the use of herbal remedies, weight loss products, glue sniffing, cocaine use, and exposure to industrial chemicals. Ask about previous infections and risks for HIV, as immunodeficient patients are at risk for severe hepatitis.

Pertinent physical examination findings including pruritus, ascites, palmar erythema, digital clubbing, cutaneous xanthoma, and prominent abdominal vessels are suggestive of chronic liver disease.

Perform a careful neurologic examination, looking for alteration in mental status and signs of increased intracranial pressure. Test for asterixis, a forward flapping of the hands when the patient's arms are extended and wrists are dorsiflexed. Smell the breath for fetor hepaticus (a musty, sweet, or fecal odor).

Obtain a CBC with differential, electrolytes, including magnesium and phosphorus levels, BUN, creatinine, and hepatic profile (AST, ALT, alkaline phosphatase, total bilirubin, direct bilirubin, total protein, and albumin), PT, PTT, INR, fibrinogen, type and hold, CPK, LDH, ammonia level, acetaminophen level, and a viral hepatitis panel, including CMV, HSV, and EBV. If clinically indicated, send a βhCG, HIV, serology for autoimmune hepatitis, ceruloplasmin, lactate, and pyruvate levels.

Patients can have electrolyte disturbances including hypoglycemia, hypokalemia, hyponatremia, hypophosphatemia, hyperammonemia, metabolic acidosis, and respiratory alkalosis.

ED Management

The priorities in the ED are the prompt recognition of acute liver failure and early management of potential complications, especially cerebral edema. Frequent assessment of the neurologic status is critical, as the patient may deteriorate rapidly. Elective intubation is indicated for a patient with grade 3 or 4 encephalopathy.

Insert an IV and infuse a glucose-based solution at a rate of 4–6 mg/kg/min. Correct any electrolyte abnormalities and closely monitor the patient's input and output. See pp. 453–455 for the treatment of acetaminophen ingestion.

Administer vitamin K (5–10 mg subcutaneously for three days, maximum rate of 1 mg/min) to patients with coagulopathy (INR >1.5 or PT >15). As prophylaxis against GI bleeding, also give either ranitidine (8 mg/kg/day div q 8h, 50 mg/dose maximum) or famotidine (0.6–0.8 mg/kg/day div q 12h, 40 mg/dose maximum). If there is active bleeding, the patient requires an invasive procedure (including central line placement), or if the patient's INR >7, give fresh frozen plasma to maintain an INR ≤1.5. In addition, give a platelet transfusion if the count is <50,000/mL or the patient has significant bleeding. Administer cryoprecipitate if the fibrinogen level is <100 mg/dL.

Admit the patient to an ICU where the multisystem complications of acute liver failure can be continually assessed and managed.

Indications for Admission

- Acute hepatic failure

Bibliography

Bhatia V, Bavdekar A, Yachha SK. Management of acute liver failure in infants and children: consensus statement of the pediatric gastroenterology chapter, Indian Academy of Pediatrics. *Indian Pediatr.* 2013;50:477–482.

Devictor D, Tissieres P, Durand P, Chevret L, Debray D. Acute liver failure in neonates, infants and children. *Expert Rev Gastroenterol Hepatol.* 2011;5(6):717–729.

Squires RH, Alonso EM. Acute liver failure in children. In Suchy FJ, Sokol RJ, Balistreri WF (eds.) *Liver Disease in Children* (4th edn.). New York: Cambridge University Press, 2014; 32–50.

Meckel's Diverticulum

Meckel's diverticulum is the most common intestinal malformation and the most frequent cause of massive lower gastrointestinal bleeding (LGI) in children. The rule of "2"s is commonly used to recall its features: it occurs in approximately 2% of the population; it is usually located within 2 feet of the ileocecal valve; it is 2 inches long; it presents before age 2 (50% of cases); and it is twice as common in males. About one-half of diverticula contain ectopic mucosa, usually gastric, but ectopic pancreatic, small bowel, or colonic mucosa can also be present.

Clinical Presentation

Clinical symptoms occur in 4–25% of cases of Meckel's diverticulum and are due to complications, including hemorrhage, obstruction, or diverticulitis. Bleeding occurs in 40–60% of symptomatic patients, secondary to ulceration of the ileal mucosa adjacent to the ectopic gastric tissue. Many children present with massive painless rectal bleeding; however, chronic blood loss or tarry stools can also occur.

Intestinal obstruction, presenting with abdominal pain and vomiting which can be bilious, occurs in 20% of symptomatic patients. This can be secondary to intussusception with the diverticulum acting as a lead point, volvulus around the fixed tip of the diverticulum, internal herniation, or incarceration in an inguinal hernia. One-half of cases of intussusception due to Meckel's diverticulum occur in infancy, with a presentation that is identical to idiopathic intussusception.

Diverticulitis and perforation occasionally occur, possibly secondary to peptic ulceration in older children. This presentation is clinically indistinguishable from acute appendicitis, although the area of most intense pain is closer to the midline.

Diagnosis and ED Management

The ED management, as well as the differential diagnosis, is dictated by the presenting symptom. (See Abdominal Pain, pp. 234–238; Lower Gastrointestinal Bleeding, pp. 263–268; Intussusception, pp. 273–274; and Acute Appendicitis, pp. 241–244).

A history of previous episodes of lower gastrointestinal bleeding is important, as many patients with a bleeding Meckel's diverticulum will have had a similar episode in the past. Perform a complete physical examination, although there are no specific findings in a patient with a Meckel's diverticulum.

ED Management

Once it has been established that the bleeding is coming from the lower gastrointestinal tract, insert a large-bore IV if there is active bleeding, orthostatic vital sign changes, tachycardia, or hypotension. Give fluid resuscitation with normal saline boluses (20 mL/kg) as needed. Obtain a CBC with differential, platelet count, type and cross-match, PT, and PTT.

If there is strong suspicion for a Meckel's, order a technetium-99m pertechnetate scintiscan (Meckel's scan) for a stable patient with painless LGI bleeding. It is a simple and noninvasive method for identifying a Meckel's diverticulum with ectopic gastric mucosa, with a sensitivity of 85–90% and a specificity of >95%. To increase the accuracy of the scan, give oral cimetidine (20 mg/kg/day), or for an emergency scan, subcutaneous pentagastrin (6 mcg/kg) prior to the procedure. Note there may be false-positives due to faulty technique, uptake at other sites of ectopic gastric mucosa (e.g., in a gastrogenic cyst), vascular anomalies, intestinal ulcerations, and some enteric duplications. There can also be false-negatives if the gastric mucosa mass in the diverticulum is insufficient or if scintigraphic activity is diluted due to brisk hemorrhage or bowel hypersecretion.

Notify a pediatric surgeon when there is strong suspicion for a Meckel's diverticulum as surgery may be required on an emergent basis, after correction of anemia or fluid and electrolyte imbalances.

Indications for Admission
- Positive Meckel's scan
- Significant LGI blood loss with evidence of hypovolemia
- Intestinal obstruction or suspected surgical abdomen

Bibliography

Al Janabi M, Samuel M, Kahlenberg A, Kumar S, Al-Janabi M. Symptomatic paediatric Meckel's diverticulum: stratified diagnostic indicators and accuracy of Meckel's scan. *Nucl Med Commun.* 2014;**35**(11):1162–1166.

Alemayehu H, Hall M, Desai AA, St Peter SD, Snyder CL. Demographic disparities of children presenting with symptomatic Meckel's diverticulum in children's hospitals. *Pediatr Surg Int.* 2014;**30** (6):649–653.

Huang CC, Lai MW, Hwang FM, et al. Diverse presentations in pediatric Meckel's diverticulum: a review of 100 cases. *Pediatr Neonatol.* 2014;**55**(5):369–375.

Sinha CK, Pallewatte A, Easty M, et al. Meckel's scan in children: a review of 183 cases referred to two paediatric surgery specialist centres over 18 years. *Pediatr Surg Int.* 2013;**29**(5):511–517.

Pyloric Stenosis

Pyloric stenosis is caused by hypertrophy of the pylorus muscle, causing progressive obstruction of the gastric outlet. It must always be considered in a young infant with nonbilious emesis, particularly in the absence of fever or diarrhea. It is five times more common in boys than girls, usually occurs in full-term infants, and in about 5–7% of cases there is a positive family history in a parent or sibling.

Clinical Presentation

Infants with pyloric stenosis usually present between 2–8 weeks of life with nonbilious, nonbloody emesis that is initially intermittent, and is often attributed to gastroesophageal reflux, overfeeding, or cow's milk intolerance. As the muscular hypertrophy progresses, the emesis becomes projectile or forceful, occurring after each feed. Parents often note that the infant appears hungry after vomiting and demands refeeding. As the vomiting continues, the infant can become dehydrated with poor weight gain and lethargy.

Diagnosis

The diagnosis can be confirmed by appreciating a small mobile mass ("olive") slightly above and to the right of the umbilicus. Palpate for the olive-size pylorus either during a feed or immediately after vomiting, when the abdominal musculature is relaxed. Peristaltic gastric waves, traveling from the left upper quadrant to the right lower quadrant may be seen after a feed and just before forceful emesis occurs.

Obtain an abdominal ultrasound to confirm the diagnosis and accurately measure the pylorus. A wall thickness >3 mm and a channel length >12 mm are diagnostic. If the ultrasound is negative or equivocal, but the clinical picture is suggestive of pyloric stenosis, repeat the study in 1–2 days to look for progression of the muscular hypertrophy. If ultrasound is unavailable, obtain an upper gastrointestinal radiographic contrast study. A dilated stomach with outlet obstruction and/or a narrowed, elongated pyloric channel that swings upward (string sign) confirms the diagnosis.

Because the obstruction is proximal to the ampulla of Vater, recurrent vomiting classically causes a hypokalemic, hypochloremic metabolic alkalosis. However, as a result of readily available ultrasound, the diagnosis is now being made in younger patients, so that these metabolic abnormalities are not always present at the time of diagnosis.

The most common alternative diagnoses are gastroesophageal reflux and improper feeding practices (large nipple hole, failure to burp the infant, etc.). The differential diagnosis is summarized in Table 9.19.

ED Management

If an olive is palpated, make the patient NPO, insert a nasogastric tube if there is persistent emesis, and obtain blood for a CBC, electrolytes, and type and hold. Start an IV and give a 20 mL/kg bolus of NS if the infant appears dehydrated. Otherwise, infuse a maintenance solution at a rate appropriate to the patient's weight and hydration status. Pyloromyotomy

Table 9.19 Differential diagnosis of pyloric stenosis

Diagnosis	Differentiating features
Adrenal insufficiency	Nonprojectile; ambiguous genitalia (female)
Antral web or atresia	Present in first week of life
Duodenal stenosis/atresia	Bilious vomiting; history of polyhydramnios
Gastroenteritis	Fever and/or diarrhea
Gastroesophageal reflux	Nonprojectile
Improper feeding practices	Nonprojectile; well-nourished
Increased ICP	Enlarging head circumference; split sutures
	VIth nerve palsy
Inborn error of metabolism	Lethargy; poor feeding; metabolic acidosis
Midgut volvulus	Bilious vomiting
	Guaiac positive stool
Sepsis	Fever, toxicity

is not urgent. Therefore, delay surgery until any fluid and electrolyte imbalances are corrected (chloride >100 mEq/L and bicarbonate <25 mEq/L).

If an olive is not appreciated, and the patient appears well-hydrated, observe the parent feeding an oral electrolyte maintenance solution. A patient who does not vomit can be discharged, with daily follow-up. If the patient vomits the feed or appears dehydrated, obtain radiographic studies and admit the infant to the hospital for further evaluation.

Follow-up
- Infant can tolerate oral fluids and does not appear dehydrated: the next day

Indications for Admission
- Suspected or confirmed pyloric stenosis
- Inability to tolerate oral feedings

Bibliography

Georgoula C, Gardiner M. Pyloric stenosis a 100 years after Ramstedt. *Arch Dis Child.* 2012;**97** (8):741–745.

Peters B, Oomen MW, Bakx R, Benninga MA. Advances in infantile hypertrophic pyloric stenosis. *Expert Rev Gastroenterol Hepatol.* 2014;**8**(5):533–541.

Ranells JD, Carver JD, Kirby RS. Infantile hypertrophic pyloric stenosis: epidemiology, genetics, and clinical update. *Adv Pediatr.* 2011;**58**:195–206.

Rectal Prolapse

Rectal prolapse is usually a benign, self-limited condition that occurs predominantly in the first four years of life, with the highest incidence in the first year. In younger patients it is most often secondary to anatomical variants, but patients four years of age or older are more likely to have an underlying condition that may require surgical repair.

Clinical Presentation and Diagnosis

Rectal prolapse appears as a sausage-shaped, dark red mass that protrudes from the anus. It occurs during defecation and often recedes spontaneously by the time the child reaches medical attention. An underlying or predisposing condition can usually be identified (see Table 9.20).

A protruding polyp or hemorrhoid can easily be differentiated from a prolapsed rectum by simple inspection, as they do not involve the entire anal circumference.

ED Management

Prolapsed tissue that is not reduced in a timely manner has an increased risk of edema, congestion, and development of ulcers. If the prolapsed rectum does not reduce spontaneously, lubricate the prolapsed tissue and gently reduce it manually. This may require steady pressure for several minutes. Afterwards, perform a digital rectal examination to confirm successful reduction. If the rectum re-prolapses, apply a piece of adhesive overlying the buttocks to keep the prolapse reduced

Table 9.20 Conditions associated with rectal prolapse

Anorectal anomalies	Inflammatory bowel disease
Celiac disease	Intractable cough (cystic fibrosis, pertussis)
Chronic constipation with straining	Milk protein allergy
Chronic diarrheal disease	Parasitic infection
Chronic malnutrition	Previous anorectal surgery
Cystic fibrosis	Rectal polyps
Ehlers–Danlos syndrome	Spinal cord lesions (myelomeningocele)
Hirschsprung's disease	Ulcerative colitis (pseudopolyps)
Increased abdominal pressure	

Adapted from, Cares K, El-Baba M. Rectal prolapse in children: significance and management. *Curr Gastroenterol Rep* 2016;18:22–28.

Perform careful physical and neurologic examinations, paying careful attention to the anus, spine, and lower extremities, as identification of a treatable underlying cause decreases risk of recurrence. Refer the patient to a primary care setting to arrange for serial stool collections for ova and parasites and, if there have been recurrent unexplained episodes of prolapse, order a sweat chloride test (to rule-out cystic fibrosis).

Follow-up
- Primary care follow-up within one week

Bibliography
Cares K, El-Baba M. Rectal prolapse in children: significance and management. *Curr Gastroenterol Rep.* 2016;**18**:22–28.

Hill SR, Ehrlich PF, Felt B, et al. Rectal prolapse in older children associated with behavioral and psychiatric disorders. *Pediatr Surg Int.* 2015;**31**(8):719–724.

Sun C, Hull T, Ozuner G. Risk factors and clinical characteristics of rectal prolapse in young patients. *J Visc Surg.* 2014;**151**(6):425–429.

Umbilical Lesions
Most umbilical lesions are benign. The umbilical cord begins to dry shortly after birth and typically separates completely and falls off by the end of the second week (mean 7–10 days). Delayed separation, defined as after three weeks of age, is most commonly caused by vigorous use of antiseptics to clean the cord and is rarely secondary to abnormal neutrophil function.

Clinical Presentation

Umbilical Hernia
An umbilical hernia presents as a bulging out of the umbilicus that is most prominent when the baby is crying or stooling. Umbilical hernias are common, they can be quite large, and

are more frequent among African-Americans. Most umbilical hernias will close by four years of age. The vast majority of umbilical hernias are painless, although occasionally a piece of mesentery can become incarcerated, causing local pain and tenderness.

Granuloma

The most common umbilical lesion is the persistence of granulation tissue at the site of cord separation. This presents as a soft, friable, reddish/pink mass protruding from the umbilicus. There may be a small amount of a blood-tinged discharge.

Omphalitis

Omphalitis is an infection of the umbilical cord stump or the surrounding tissue, caused by organisms that have colonized the area. In newborns, a small rim of erythema around the umbilicus can be normal. In contrast, omphalitis presents with a foul odor, drainage from the umbilicus, and erythematous streaking, particularly in the direction of the liver. The infant may have fever, irritability, decreased oral intake, and lethargy.

Persistent Omphalomesenteric Duct and Urachus

After the cord separates, a persistent omphalomesenteric duct may present with fecal drainage. A persistent urachus may manifest as drainage of urine from the umbilicus. Either remnant may also persist as a blind sinus with a purulent or egg-white discharge.

Diagnosis

Normally, once the umbilical cord separates, there is no erythema or tenderness of the surrounding skin, although there can be a small amount of blood-tinged, non-foul-smelling discharge.

Examine the umbilicus for any masses, erythema, and odor, and note the quality of the discharge, if any. Look for signs of local pain and tenderness, which could signify an incarcerated hernia or omphalitis. If the drainage smells like feces, consider a persistent omphalomesenteric duct, while a large amount of clear watery discharge suggests persistent urachus is possible. Purulent drainage or material resembling egg whites suggests a persistent sinus secondary to one of the two preceding conditions. A febrile and sick-appearing infant is more likely to have omphalitis.

ED Management

Umbilical Hernia

The treatment is education and reassurance since most umbilical hernias resolve without intervention. However, instruct the parents to seek medical attention if the hernia cannot be easily reduced. Surgical repair is not indicated until the child is at least four years old unless it is very large (>1.5 cm), as these are unlikely to close spontaneously. If the patient presents with an incarcerated hernia (very rare), manually reduce the incarcerated mesentery and arrange for surgical repair. Urgent surgical reduction is required if the hernia is not reducible or the bowel is strangulated (very rare).

Granuloma

Treat a small granuloma with cauterization using a silver nitrate stick. Moisten the stick with tap water and apply to the granuloma until the entire surface changes from a pinkish-red to a grayish color. Avoid contact with normal skin as silver nitrate can cause a chemical burn. Advise the family to not bathe the baby for several days and to keep the area dry. The silver nitrate application may be repeated every few days, as needed. If the mass is particularly large when first seen, tie a ligature (3-0 nylon) around the base, and see the patient again in one week. At that time, sever the granuloma at its base, and then cauterize the stump. Surgery may be required for a large granuloma which does not respond to these conservative measures.

Omphalitis

Omphalitis is potentially life-threatening. Perform a full sepsis work-up, including a culture of any discharge, admit the infant, and treat with IV nafcillin (100 mg/kg/day div q 6h). In communities with a high prevalence of methicillin-resistant *S. aureus*, use clindamycin (40 mg/kg/day div q 6h) or vancomycin (15–20 mg/kg/day div q 6–8h) instead. In cases of severe omphalitis (toxic-appearing, peritonitis), if the patient is not already receiving clindamycin, add anaerobic coverage with either clindamycin or metronidazole (30 mg/kg/day div q 8h). Note that severe omphalitis can progress to necrotizing fasciitis which can spread rapidly and require surgical debridement. Consult pediatric surgery if this is a concern.

Omphalomesenteric and Urachal Remnants

If a persistent omphalomesenteric duct or urachus is suspected, consult with a pediatric surgeon to confirm the diagnosis and arrange for management.

Delayed Cord Separation

If the presumed etiology is not excessive antiseptic use, obtain a CBC with differential. Regardless of the cause, instruct the parents to keep the cord dry and refer the infant to a primary care provider for follow-up within one week.

Follow-up

- Umbilical granuloma, delayed cord separation: primary care visit within one week
- Umbilical hernia: next routine primary care visit
- Omphalomesenteric and urachal remnants: follow-up with pediatric surgeon in one week

Indications for Admission

- Omphalitis
- Incarcerated or strangulated umbilical hernia

Bibliography

Hegazy AA. Anatomy and embryology of umbilicus in newborns: a review and clinical correlations. *Front Med.* 2016;**10**(3):271–277.

Hsu JW, Tom WL. Omphalomesenteric duct remnants: umbilical versus umbilical cord lesions. *Pediatr Dermatol.* 2011;**28**(4):404–407.

Sanyaolu LN, Javed M, Wilson-Jones N. A baby with a discharging umbilical lesion. *BMJ*. 2016;**355**: i5587.

Sarwar U, Javed M, Wright T, Dawson A, Wilson-Jones N. These umbilical lesions weren't granulomas after all. *J Fam Pract*. 2016;**65**(2):E1–E3.

Sherman JM, Rocker J, Rakovchik E. Her belly button is leaking: a case of patent urachus. *Pediatr Emerg Care*. 2015;**31**(3):202–204.

Vomiting

Vomiting is the expulsion of gastrointestinal contents through the mouth. It may have a protective function in eliminating ingested toxins and infectious agents. Vomiting can be classified as a primary, in which there is an underlying gastrointestinal cause, or secondary to another etiology, such as visceral pain or a systemic illness. Protracted vomiting may lead to complications such as dehydration, metabolic alkalosis, esophagitis, Mallory–Weiss tears, malnutrition, or dental problems.

Clinical Presentation

The presentation of vomiting varies greatly. Obtain a detailed history focusing on duration, onset, time of day, time frame in relation to food ingestion, associated symptoms (fever, nausea, diarrhea, abdominal pain, headache, vision changes, personality changes, irritability, or lethargy), medications, and travel history. Ask the family to describe the vomitus (bilious, food content digested/undigested, bloody, presence of fecal matter). Bilious emesis may indicate a surgical process and is an obstruction until proven otherwise.

The conditions associated with vomiting are listed in Table 9.21.

Diagnosis

The differential diagnosis of vomiting is summarized in Table 9.22.

ED Management

Vomiting

Assess the patient's hydration status and compare the current and premorbid weights, if available. Assess vital signs and hemodynamic status (orthostatic vital signs) and perform thorough physical and neurologic examinations.

The choice of laboratory testing, if any, depends on the history and physical examination. Perform a chemistry panel, assessing for electrolyte abnormalities and hydration status, a lipase level to rule-out pancreatitis, LFTs ± ammonia level for liver disease and a pregnancy test. Obtain a urinalysis testing for an infection, DKA, and hematuria for renal stones. If intestinal obstruction is suspected, obtain a flat and upright abdominal x-ray looking for air-fluid levels. If there is bilious emesis, make the patient NPO and decompress the stomach with a nasogastric tube; place the tube onto low, intermittent suction. Give appropriate IV fluid resuscitation and consult a pediatric surgeon.

Gastroenteritis usually responds to small sips of sugar-containing clear liquids (oral electrolyte solution, sweetened weak tea, decarbonated soda, fruit juice).

Table 9.21 Conditions associated with vomiting diagnoses

Vomiting characteristics

Abdominal pain not relieved	Cholecystitis, pancreatitis, appendicitis
Abdominal pain relieved	Peptic ulcer disease
Chronic small volume	Psychogenic, GER, rumination
Bilious	Obstruction distal to the ampulla of Vater
	Prolonged forceful vomiting
Bloody	(See Table 9.12: Differential diagnosis of UGI bleed)
During eating	Psychogenic, peptic ulcer disease
Early morning	↑ICP, pregnancy, psychogenic, uremia
Feculent	Distal GI obstruction, gastrocolic fistula
Forceless	Gastroesophageal reflux, overfeeding, rumination
Projectile	Pyloric stenosis, proximal GI obstruction, sepsis, ↑ICP

Associated sign/symptoms

Bulging fontanelle	Meningitis
Chronic without weight loss	Psychogenic
Diarrhea	Gastroenteritis, food intolerance, intussusception
	Inflammatory bowel disease
Epigastric pain	Pancreatitis, peptic ulcer disease
Failure to thrive	Congenital adrenal hyperplasia, celiac disease, severe GER, IBD, metabolic disorder
Fever	Gastroenteritis, appendicitis, cholecystitis, pancreatitis
	Inflammatory bowel disease
	Infection outside of GI tract (otitis, pharyngitis, UTI)
Headache	↑ICP, migraine, ↑ intraocular pressure
High-pitched bowel sounds	GI obstruction
Jaundice	Hepatobiliary disease, neonate with UTI
Mental status change	CNS disease, ingestion, uremia, intussusception, Reye's
RUQ abdominal pain	Cholecystitis, hepatitis, RLL pneumonia
Scars on knuckles, loss of dental enamel	Bulimia
Severe hypotension	Adrenal crisis, sepsis, severe dehydration
Surgical scars	GI obstruction due to adhesions
Unusual odor	Inborn error of metabolism, toxin induced, DKA, uremia
Visible bowel loops	GI obstruction

Abbreviations: DKA: diabetic ketoacidosis; GER: gastroesophageal reflux; GI: gastrointestinal; IBD: inflammatory bowel disease; ICP: intracranial pressure; RUQ: right upper quadrant; UGI: upper gastrointestinal; UTI: urinary tract infection

Table 9.22 Differential diagnosis of vomiting

Diagnosis	Differentiating features
CNS conditions	
Head trauma	Altered mental status, retrograde amnesia, headache
Increased ICP	Hypertension, bradycardia, VIth nerve palsy
	Focal neurologic exam
Migraine	Past history, aura, photophobia, motion sickness
Endocrine/metabolic diseases	
Adrenal crisis (CAH)	Hyperkalemia, hyponatremia, hypotensive shock
Diabetic ketoacidosis	Polyuria/dipsia/phagia, abdominal pain, ketotic breath
Hypercalcemia	Confusion, proximal muscle weakness, hyporeflexia
Inborn error of metabolism	Poor feeding, hepatomegaly, acidosis, hyperammonemia
Uremia	Renal failure, pruritus, ammonia breath, encephalopathy
Gastrointestinal diseases	
Cholecystitis	Low-grade fever, Murphy's sign, pain radiates to scapula
Food intolerance	Related to specific food intake
GER	Infant with forceless vomiting, fussiness, feeding aversion
Hepatitis	Hepatomegaly, +/- jaundice with dark urine/acholic stools
IBD	Poor growth, ↑ ESR, guaiac positive stools
Pancreatitis	Epigastric/RUQ pain radiates to back; high amylase/lipase
Peptic ulcer disease	Coffee-ground emesis, vomiting with meals relieves pain
Infectious diseases	
ENT infection	Pharyngitis, sinusitis, otitis media, URI, labyrinthitis
Food poisoning	Onset 1–6 h post-ingestion, brief illness
	Diarrhea in one-third of patients, afebrile
Gastroenteritis	Fever (high with bacterial), diarrhea, abdominal pain
Meningitis/encephalitis	Fever, mental status changes, signs of increased ICP
Respiratory infection	Post-tussive emesis
Sepsis	Toxic-appearing, lethargy, signs of shock
UTI/pyelonephritis	Urinary complaints may be absent in infants
Surgical conditions	
Appendicitis	Fever, anorexia, periumbilical then RLQ abdominal pain
Esophageal stricture	History of caustic ingestion, gradual swallowing difficulty
Foreign body/bezoar	Infant/toddler, developmentally delayed child
GI obstruction	Vomiting may be bilious

Table 9.22 (cont.)

Diagnosis	Differentiating features
Pyloric stenosis	2–8-week-old with projectile vomiting, ↑bicarbonate
Testicular/ovarian torsion	Scrotal or adnexal tenderness, severe pain
Miscellaneous	
Anaphylaxis	Multisystem (commonly skin, respiratory, cardiovascular)
Bulimia	Binging followed by purging, usually normal or overweight
Cyclic vomiting	Onset at 2–5 years, 2–3 day episodes; well in between
Munchausen by proxy	Frequent recurrent illnesses without a clear etiology
Nephrolithiasis	Colicky flank pain that radiates to the groin
Overfeeding	Forceless emesis in a thriving infant
Psychogenic vomiting	Associated with anxiety disorder or emotional distress
Pregnancy	Missed menses, vomiting may not be limited to morning
Rumination	Neurologically impaired child, weight loss
Toxic ingestions	Toddler or teen; abuse/suicide attempt

Abbreviations: CAH: congenital adrenal hyperplasia; ENT: ear, nose, and throat; ESR: erythrocyte sedimentation rate; GER: gastroesophageal reflux; GI: gastrointestinal; IBD: inflammatory bowel disease; ICP: intracranial pressure; RLQ: right lower quadrant; UGI: upper gastrointestinal; URI: upper respiratory infection

Antiemetics are not routinely indicated, but may be used in certain circumstances, such as postoperative vomiting, vomiting associated with chemotherapy, motion sickness, cyclic vomiting, or to prevent electrolyte abnormalities in severe persistent vomiting. Give one oral dose of ondansetron (8–15 kg: 2 mg; 16–30 kg, 4 mg; >30 kg, 8 mg) to children with acute gastroenteritis who do not tolerate oral rehydration in order to limit repeated vomiting and prevent hospitalization. Do not give an antiemetic prior to evaluation for a possible surgical abdomen.

Regurgitation

Regurgitation is the effortless passage of refluxate from the stomach into the esophagus. Most infants and children with regurgitation do not require acute treatment in the ED if there are no associated symptoms. The majority of infants with GER peak at 4–6 months and improve thereafter. Instruct the parents to give the infant small frequent feeds and to keep the baby upright after feeds. Thickening the formula with one teaspoon of oatmeal cereal per ounce may be helpful. For patients with associated eczema, failure to thrive, diarrhea, or constipation, consider milk protein allergy and obtain a stool guaiac. Infants and children with GER and associated failure to thrive, pulmonary disease, anemia, or esophagitis require further evaluation; consult a gastroenterologist.

If the patient is diagnosed with pyloric stenosis, make the patient NPO, place an IV and administer normal saline 20 cc/kg if the patient is dehydrated. Otherwise, infuse D5 ¼ NS to D5 ½ NS at maintenance. Once the patient is voiding well, add KCl to the fluid. The electrolytes need to be corrected before proceeding to surgery for a pyloromyotomy.

Follow-up

- Tolerating oral fluids and mild or moderate dehydration: primary care follow-up the next day or return to the ED if unable to tolerate clear fluids at home
- Tolerating oral fluids and not dehydrated: primary care follow-up within one week

Indications for Admission

- Significant ongoing fluid losses and/or inability to tolerate oral fluids
- Severe dehydration or altered mental status
- Suspected surgical abdomen, suspected or confirmed pyloric stenosis

Bibliography

Chandran L, Chitkara M. Vomiting in children. *Pediatr Rev.* 2008;**29**:183–192.

Jobson M, Hall NJ. Contemporary management of pyloric stenosis. *Semin Pediatr Surg.* 2016;219–224.

Wyllie R, Hyams JS, Kay M. *Pediatric Gastrointestinal and Liver Disease* (4th edn.). Philadelphia, PA: Elsevier, 2011; 88–105.

Chapter 10

Genitourinary Emergencies

Sandra J. Cunningham

Balanoposthitis

Balanitis is inflammation of the glans penis; posthitis is inflammation of the prepuce. Balanoposthitis, which is inflammation of both sites, occurs in up to 3% of uncircumcised boys. The etiology in most cases is poor hygiene and accumulation of smegma, which can lead to a secondary bacterial infection. In circumcised boys without residual foreskin or glans penis adhesions, balanitis may be secondary to contact dermatitis from urine, laundry soaps, powders, or ointments. In an adolescent with a retractable foreskin, risk factors are poor hygiene and sexually transmitted infections.

Clinical Presentation and Diagnosis

Balanoposthitis presents with erythema, edema, and pain of the distal phallus, particularly the glans penis. There may be secondary meatitis with resultant dysuria and reluctance to void. The foreskin will be more difficult to retract than it was prior to the onset of the inflammation and a discharge may be present. In severe cases, the cellulitis can extend down the shaft of the penis and onto the lower abdominal wall or the scrotum. Inguinal lymphadenopathy or adenitis is often present.

Recurrent episodes of posthitis can result in phimosis, whereas repeated episodes of balanitis may result in meatal stenosis, with a poor stream and dribbling of urine.

ED Management

Acute localized infections usually respond to frequent warm-water sitz baths followed by drying of the penis and the application of topical antibiotics (bacitracin tid or mupirocin bid) and topical antifungal cream (nystatin) bid for two weeks. Reinforce proper hygiene and the avoidance of forceful retraction of the foreskin. If there is voluntary retention, fever, or cellulitis extending onto the penile shaft, treat with oral antibiotics for seven days. Prescribe 40 mg/kg/day of either cephalexin (div bid) or cefadroxil (div bid), but in communities where MRSA is prevalent either use clindamycin (20 mg/kg/day div q 6h) or add trimethoprim-sulfamethoxazole (8 mg/kg/day of trimethoprim div bid) to one of the above regimens.

More severe infections with purulent discharge and widespread cellulitis require admission and treatment with parenteral antibiotics (nafcillin 150 mg/kg/day div q 6h) or clindamycin (30–40 mg/kg/day div q 6–8h).

Failure of balanoposthitis to respond to warm soaks and systemic antibiotics may be due to inadequate drainage secondary to phimosis. An urgent incision of the dorsal inner foreskin is indicated if there is a poor urinary stream or dribbling.

Follow-up

- Inability to void: immediate; otherwise primary care follow-up in one week

Indications for Admission

- Severe infection
- Urinary retention

Bibliography

Andreassi L, Bilenchi R. Non-infectious inflammatory genital lesions. *Clin Dermatol.* 2014;**32** (2):307–314.

Castagnetti M, Leonard, M, Guerra, L, Esposito C, Cimador, M. Benign penile skin anomalies in children: a primer for pediatricians. *World J Pediatr.* 2015;**11**(4):316–323.

Edwards SK, Bunker CB, Ziller F, van der Meijden W. 2013 European guidelines for the management of balanposthithis. *Int J STD AIDS.* 2014;**25**:615–626.

Randjelovic G, Otasevic S, Mladenovic-Antic S, et al. *Streptococcus pyogenes* as the cause of vulvovaginitis and balanitis in children. *Pediatr Int.* 2016;**59**(4):432–437.

Meatal Stenosis

Meatal stenosis is a narrowing of the urethral meatus, usually secondary to recurrent episodes of subclinical meatitis. Etiologies include ammoniacal diaper dermatitis (circumcised boys) and recurrent balanoposthitis (uncircumcised boys). Acquired meatal stenosis occurs very rarely in uncircumcised boys because the foreskin acts as a protective cover for the meatus. Congenital meatal stenosis is also very rare.

Clinical Presentation

Obstructive symptoms occasionally occur, including hesitancy, straining, urgency, frequency, and post-voiding dribbling. An abnormal urinary stream may be seen, with either spraying or upward deflection. There may be pain at the initiation of urination or burning at the meatus, although urinary retention is rare. If there is an associated meatitis, an erythematous, swollen meatus is noted, often with a purulent discharge.

Diagnosis

The diagnosis of meatal stenosis can be made upon direct observation of the urinary stream, although a narrowed meatus on visual inspection does not confirm the diagnosis.

ED Management

Treat purulent meatitis with warm-water sitz baths and oral antibiotics for seven days. Use 40 mg/kg/day of either cephalexin (div qid) or cefadroxil (div bid). Refer all patients to a urologist for confirmation of the diagnosis and further evaluation. Immediately consult a urologist for the rare case of acute urinary retention.

Follow-up

- Meatitis without retention: urology follow-up in 1–2 weeks

Indication for Admission

- Urinary retention

Bibliography

Godley SP, Sturm RM, Durbin-Johnson B, Kurzrock EA. Meatal stenosis: a retrospective analysis of over 4000 patients. *J Pediatr Urol.* 2015;**11**(38):e1–6.

Leslie JA, Cain MP. Pediatric urologic emergencies and urgencies. *Pediatr Clin North Am.* 2006;**53**:513–527.

Paraphimosis

Paraphimosis is entrapment of the foreskin behind the coronal sulcus of an uncircumcised or inadequately circumcised penis. It occurs when a tight foreskin is retracted proximal to the glans penis and then is not returned to its normal position. This produces a tourniquet effect with resultant venous congestion and edema of the glans.

Clinical Presentation and Diagnosis

On examination, there is edema and tenderness of the glans penis with a tight proximal collar of swollen tissue. The glans congestion will progress over time and skin color will change from the normal pink to blue to white (ischemia), with eventual gangrene. The penile shaft is unaffected. The constriction by the foreskin along with resultant edema may lead to urethral obstruction at the coronal level. The patient then complains of difficulty voiding and urinary retention. Direct erosion into the urethra rarely occurs.

ED Management

Place an ice bag on the foreskin and administer a topical (EMLA cream) or regional (penile block with lidocaine without epinephrine) anesthetic, and/or sedate the patient (see Sedation and Analgesia, pp. 712–722). Reduce the edema by applying manual circumferential compression for several minutes. Next, grasp the penile shaft with the index and third fingers of each hand, with the thumbs on the glans. Apply firm downward pressure on the glans against counter-pressure on the shaft, which will usually advance the foreskin back over the glans. Alternatively, following the application of EMLA cream with an occlusive dressing (30 min to 1 hour), inject 1 mL of hyaluronidase (150 U/mL) into one or more sites in the edematous prepuce. Resolution of the edema is almost immediate, and the foreskin can be gently retracted over the glans. It is critical to attempt to advance the most distal foreskin ring (the portion closest to the coronal margin). If this tight ring can be reduced, then the remainder of the foreskin will follow. Occasionally, there is tearing of the skin with bleeding, which can be controlled by compression. Instruct the patient to avoid retracting his foreskin for several days. Refer the patient to a urologist for follow-up and evaluation of the need for an elective circumcision.

If the paraphimosis cannot be reduced, consult a urologist immediately to perform a dorsal slit to release the constricting ring of tissue.

Follow-up

- Reducible paraphimosis: urology follow-up in 1–2 weeks

Bibliography

Chen J, Muhammad W. Reduction of paraphimosis. In Ganthi L (ed.) *Atlas of Emergency Medicine Procedures*. New York: Springer, 2016; 495–499.

Clifford ID, Craig SS, Nataraja RM, Panabokke G. Paediatric paraphimosis. *Emerg Med Australas*. 2016;**28**(1):96–99.

Ludvigson AE, Beaule LT. Urologic emergencies. *Surg Clin North Am*. 2016;**96**(3):407–424.

Vunda A, Lacroix LE, Schneider F, Manzano S, Gervaix A. Videos in clinical medicine: reduction of paraphimosis in boys. *N Engl J Med*. 2013;**368**(13):e16.

Phimosis

Phimosis is the inability to retract the tight foreskin over the glans penis. In 50% of uncircumcised boys the foreskin is retractable at one year of age, and 90% are retractable by four years. The remaining 10% may not become retractable until puberty. If associated infections (local or more proximally in the urinary tract) or voiding difficulties occur, correction may be indicated.

Clinical Presentation and Diagnosis

Acquired phimosis is a result of poor hygiene with inflammation of the glans. Accumulated smegma may form aggregates that appear as whitish, globular masses under the nonretractile foreskin. Associated inflammatory conditions may coexist, including balanoposthitis (pp. 294–296) and meatitis (pp. 295–296). With severe phimosis, the foreskin may balloon during voiding as the urine collects under it and then dribbles out from the tight opening. The adolescent may complain of pain on erection, secondary to tension on the foreskin from the glandular adhesions.

ED Management

Treat accumulated smegma without any associated infection with gentle retraction of the foreskin during bathing. Depending on the patient's age, if there is no infection, refer him to a urologist for consideration of elective circumcision. If there is ballooning of the foreskin with a dribbling urinary stream, or an associated UTI, consult a urologist. Gentle dilation may be necessary, after which an elective circumcision or preputial plasty (surgical widening of the phimotic ring) is indicated.

Follow-up

- Phimosis without associated difficulty voiding: urology follow-up in 1–2 weeks

Bibliography

Castagnetti M, Leonard M, Guerra L, Esposito C, Cimador M. Benign penile skin anomalies in children: a primer for pediatricians. *World J Pediatr*. 2015;**11**(4):316–323.

Hayashi Y, Kojima Y, Mizuno K, Kohri K. Prepuce: phimosis, paraphimosis, and circumcision. *Sci World J*. 2011 3(11):289–301.

Ludvigson AE, Beaule LT. Urologic emergencies. *Surg Clin North Am.* 2016;**96**(3):407–424.

Sneppen I, Thorup J. Foreskin morbidity in uncircumcised males. *Pediatrics.* 2016;**137**(5). pii: e20154340.

Priapism

Priapism is a sustained and painful penile erection that results from either increased arterial flow (high flow) or, more commonly, from decreased venous outflow (low flow). It most frequently occurs as a complication of sickle cell disease (pp. 370–375) with a reported incidence of 30% before the age of 20 years. It may also result from spinal cord injury, leukemic infiltration, medications, or trauma.

Clinical Presentation and Diagnosis

The patient presents with a sustained, painful erection. Urinary retention may result with a distended bladder palpable on examination. Persistence of the priapism can lead to corporal fibrosis, with resultant erectile dysfunction. In boys with sickle cell disease, other manifestations of the crisis may be present.

ED Management

Initial management includes analgesia or sedation, hydration, and oxygenation. If the patient has sickle cell disease, determine the percentage of HgbS. Consult with a pediatric hematologist to promptly arrange an exchange transfusion to reduce the HgbS to 30–35%. If the priapism persists in spite of adequate reduction of HgbS, consult a urologist to perform aspiration of blood from the corpora cavernosa, followed by irrigation with a dilute epinephrine solution. Most commonly, however, reduction of HgbS is sufficient to effect resolution of the priapism. On occasion, acute bladder drainage with a Foley catheter may be necessary.

Indication for Admission

- Priapism

Bibliography

Broderick GA. Priapism and sickle-cell anemia: diagnosis and nonsurgical therapy. *J Sex Med.* 2012;**9** (1):88–103.

Mockford K, Weston M, Subramaniam R. Management of high-flow priapism in paediatric patients: a case report and review of the literature. *J Pediatr Urol.* 2007;**3**:404–412.

Salonia A, Eardley I, Giuliano F, et al. European Association of Urology guidelines on priapism. *Eur Urol.* 2014;**65**(2):480–489.

Shigehara K, Namiki M. Clinical management of priapism: a review. *World J Mens Health.* 2016;**34**(1):1–8.

Subramaniam S, Chao JH. Managing acute complications of sickle cell disease in pediatric patients. *Pediatr Emerg Med Pract.* 2016;**13**(11):1–28.

Renal and Genitourinary Trauma

Renal Trauma

Blunt trauma, secondary to motor vehicle accidents, falls, and athletic injuries, is the major cause of renal injuries in children The pediatric kidney is particularly susceptible to injury due to the relative paucity of surrounding fat, its size in relation to surrounding organs, and an immature thoracic cage, which provides inadequate protection. An underlying congenital anomaly, including ureteropelvic junction obstruction, primary obstructive megaureter, or ectopic or solitary kidneys, is found incidentally in up to 20% of patients with traumatic hematuria. Associated intraperitoneal injuries occur in approximately 25% of cases of blunt and 80% of penetrating renal trauma.

Ureteral Trauma

Ureteral trauma is relatively uncommon, and when present is usually associated with multiple intra-abdominal injuries. Children are at higher risk for avulsion of the ureter at the junction of the renal pelvis (ureteropelvic junction), which is a relatively fixed point in the course of the ureter.

Bladder Trauma

The pediatric bladder is particularly susceptible to blunt trauma, especially from motor vehicle accidents. The majority of bladder injuries are associated with pelvic fractures.

Urethral Trauma

Urethral injury is usually the result of blunt trauma to the lower abdomen, a straddle injury to the perineum, or iatrogenic injury from urethral instrumentation.

Clinical Presentation

Renal Trauma

The patient will commonly present with flank pain, which may be localized or radiate to the ipsilateral groin. There may also be costovertebral tenderness, flank ecchymoses, extravasation of blood or urine into the perirenal tissues, or a palpable flank mass. Associated findings include ipsilateral rib fractures and fractured transverse processes of the vertebral bodies. Either gross or microscopic hematuria is nearly always present, although the degree of hematuria can be variable and does not correlate with the severity of the injury. In patients with vascular pedicle injuries, hematuria can be absent.

Ureteral Trauma

The early presentation of ureteral trauma is nonspecific and may be initially overlooked while attention is paid to other serious injuries. Hematuria is initially present in only 70% of cases. Later, there may be fever or flank or abdominal pain. A high level of clinical suspicion is required for early diagnosis.

Bladder Trauma

The majority of bladder injuries are associated with pelvic fractures. A child's bladder is more susceptible to injury because it sits higher in the abdomen. Also, a distended bladder is more vulnerable to blunt injury. A patient with a ruptured bladder presents with suprapubic and abdominal pain with tenderness on palpation, hematuria, and, with large tears, inability to void.

Urethral Injury

The male urethra is divided into anterior and posterior portions. Posterior urethral injuries are generally caused by severe blunt trauma and are usually associated with other significant injuries. Lower abdominal and pelvic swelling, tenderness, and ecchymosis are commonly seen, with hematuria and blood at the external meatus. With complete disruption of the urethra, the patient may be unable to void.

Anterior urethral injuries are usually isolated and are caused by direct blunt or penetrating trauma, instrumentation, or a straddle injury. The patient may have perineal ecchymosis, usually in a butterfly distribution, and scrotal hematomas. Bleeding from the meatus is the hallmark of urethral injury and may be associated with an inability to void.

Urethral injuries in females are uncommon due to the short length and mobility of the urethra.

Penile and Scrotal Injuries

Most penile injuries occur as a result of circumcision. The injuries vary from an inappropriate amount of skin removed to complete transection of the penis. Penile injuries due to blunt or penetrating trauma in childhood are rare, but may be associated with urethral injury. Penile and scrotal zipper injuries are common and usually present with skin avulsion, while tourniquet injuries to the penis can occur from hair or other objects forming a tight circumferential band.

Scrotal trauma secondary to straddle injuries (biking) or direct trauma (sporting event) can present with acute swelling, ecchymosis, hematocele, and testicular injury with disruption of the tunica albuginea. In severe cases, blood and/or urine extravasates into the upper abdominal wall and into the perineum along Colles' fascia.

Diagnosis and ED Management

Although hematuria is generally present, there is no consistent relationship between the number of red cells and the degree of urinary tract injury, particularly with renal injuries. In fact, the absence of blood does not exclude a major injury, such as a ureteral transection or an injury to the renal vasculature. Therefore, suspect a renal injury in any blunt trauma patient with gross or microscopic hematuria on urinalysis, or with signs or symptoms suggestive of renal injury (flank pain or hematoma, lower rib fracture, shock), particularly with rapid deceleration as the mechanism of injury. Renal imaging is indicated if the urinalysis has >50 RBCs per high-power field. Always consider the possibility of sexual abuse in a child presenting with trauma to the external genitalia.

Obtain immediate surgical and urologic consultation for a hemodynamically unstable patient. For the stable patient, arrange for a CT scan with contrast for proper staging of injuries and identification of any other associated intra-abdominal injuries.

Renal Trauma

If an isolated renal injury is likely, promptly obtain a CT scan of the abdomen and pelvis after administration of IV contrast.

Table 10.1 Staging of renal injuries

Grade	Findings	Treatment
1	Contusion with microscopic or gross hematuria	Bed rest
	No intraparenchymal laceration	Serial hematocrits
2	Subcapsular nonexpanding hematoma	Bed rest
	Confined to renal retroperitoneum	Serial hematocrits
	Laceration with a parenchymal tear <1 cm of cortex	
	No involvement of the collecting system	
	No extravasation of urine	
3	Laceration with parenchymal tear >1 cm	Bed rest
	No involvement of the collecting system	Serial hematocrits
	No extravasation of urine	
4	Laceration with extensive parenchymal injury	Ureteral stent
	Involvement of the collecting system	Possible renal exploration with reconstruction or nephrectomy
	Vascular damage to the hilar vessels	
5	Parenchymal destruction (shattered kidney)	Ureteral stent
	Hilar vascular injury with devascularization	Possible renal exploration with reconstruction or nephrectomy

The staging of renal injuries is shown in Table 10.1. Maintain the patient at bed rest with close hemodynamic monitoring and consult a urologist.

Ureteral Trauma

If a ureteral injury is suspected, obtain a CT scan (with contrast) of the abdomen and pelvis. Extravasation of the contrast is the hallmark of ureteral injury. Hydronephrosis, ureteral deviation, or lack of visualization of contrast in the distal ureter may also be noted. Consult a urologist to arrange emergent treatment, either intraoperative repair or urinary diversion with a nephrostomy tube. A preoperative retrograde pyelogram may be necessary to delineate the degree of injury.

Bladder Trauma

Inability to void, a distended bladder, and gross hematuria suggest a serious bladder injury. Consult a urologist immediately, as urethral integrity must be assured before catheterization is performed. Urethral disruption is suggested by a boggy mass palpated on rectal examination. A retrograde urethrogram is indicated in males. After evaluation of urethral integrity, obtain a gravity cystogram for all patients. Calculate the age-adjusted bladder capacity before administering the contrast material [in ounces; <2 years: 2 + (age in years × 2); ≥2 years: 6+ (age in years/2)]. Bladder injuries are classified by extravasation of contrast into either the extraperitoneal, intraperitoneal, or both spaces, particularly with penetrating trauma.

Treat a patient with extraperitoneal extravasation with either a suprapubic or urethral catheter. Intraperitoneal extravasation is an indication for intraoperative repair and suprapubic diversion of urine.

Urethral Injury

Blood at the urethral meatus indicates a urethral injury; consult a urologist to perform a retrograde urethrogram. Do not catheterize the patient before urethral integrity is fully evaluated, as catheterization can convert a partial disruption into a complete transection. After the level and degree of urethral injury are ascertained, suprapubic catheter placement is indicated for temporary urinary diversion pending more definitive repair on an emergent or expectant basis.

External Genital Trauma

Treat penile hair tourniquet with an ice bag to ease the pain and shrink the swelling. Application of soapy water to the hairs facilitates removal.

Wrap any size penile amputation in saline gauze, put it in a plastic bag, and place it on ice, with pressure and sterile dressings applied to the remaining shaft. Immediate reanastomosis surgery may be successful.

If gentle attempts to remove penile skin caught in a zipper are unsuccessful, inject 1% lidocaine (without epinephrine) into the foreskin. Then, the zipper can be closed, cut through at its base, and opened from the base, releasing the entrapped skin.

Apply sterile saline-soaked towels to an amputation or avulsion of scrotal skin and consult a urologist to determine the need for surgery. If there is a urethral foreign body, arrange for cystoscopy and transurethral extraction after percutaneous placement of a suprapubic catheter by a urologist.

Obtain a sonogram for suspected traumatic testicular torsion or testicular rupture.

Indications for Admission

- Abnormal CT scan (renal contusion, laceration, collecting system injury, major vessel injury)
- Penile or scrotal amputation
- Bladder or urethral contusion, laceration, or rupture
- Inability to void

Bibliography

Dangle PP, Fuller TW, Gaines B, et al. Evolving mechanisms of injury and management of pediatric blunt renal trauma: 20 years of experience. *Urology.* 2016;**90**:159–163.

LeeVan E, Zmora O, Cazzulino F, et al. Management of pediatric blunt renal trauma: a systematic review. *J Trauma Acute Care Surg.* 2016;**80**(3):519–528.

McClain Z, Bell DL. Adolescent male genitourinary emergencies. *Adolesc Med State Art Rev.* 2015;**26** (3):484–490.

McGeady JB, Breyer BN. Current epidemiology of genitourinary trauma. *Urol Clin North Am.* 2013;**40** (3):323–334.

Serafetinides E, Kitrey ND, Djakovic N, et al. Review of the current management of upper urinary tract injuries by the EAU Trauma Guidelines Panel. *Eur Urol.* 2015;**67**(5):930–936.

Viola TA. Closed kidney injury. *Clin Sports Med.* 2013;**32**(2):219–227.

Scrotal Swellings

A number of conditions can produce an acutely erythematous and tender hemiscrotum. Testicular torsion is the most serious and requires prompt diagnosis and surgical intervention.

Clinical Presentation

Testicular Torsion

Testicular torsion is caused by twisting of the spermatic cord leading to venous, lymphatic, and eventual arterial occlusion. Although testicular torsion can occur at any age, the peak is 14 years (range 12–18 years). There is another small peak among neonates. About 60% of patients experience the sudden onset of severe testicular or scrotal pain that may radiate to the groin or lower abdomen, often before awakening in the early-morning hours. Other symptoms include nausea, vomiting, and a wide-based gait. Younger patients may only complain of abdominal or inguinal pain.

On physical examination, there is hemiscrotal swelling and erythema. The involved testis may be elevated with a horizontal orientation. The hemiscrotal swelling does not transilluminate, elevation of the testicle does not diminish the pain (Prehn's sign), and the ipsilateral cremasteric reflex is absent in nearly all cases. There is no fever or dysuria, and in about half of the cases there is a history of subacute bouts of scrotal pain (previous intermittent torsion).

Torsion of the Testicular Appendage

The appendix testis is a mullerian duct remnant at the upper pole of the testicle. Torsion on its vascular pedicle can mimic testicular torsion, most often at 7–12 years of age. The patient will complain of pain and tenderness localized to the superior pole of the testis. In some cases, a characteristic bluish nodule, representing an infarcted appendage, can be seen through the thin scrotal skin (blue dot sign). More often, the blue dot is not evident until several days after the surrounding scrotal edema and erythema have resolved. The swelling does not transilluminate, although there may be an associated reactive hydrocele that does. The cremasteric reflex is not affected. Elevation of the testis does not relieve the pain, and there is no fever or urinary symptoms. Previous subacute episodes are uncommon.

Epididymo-Orchitis

Epididymo-orchitis is caused by the spread of an infection from the bladder or urethra to the epididymal and testicular ducts and tubules. It may be confused with a testicular torsion, although it is uncommon in boys <14 years of age. Etiologies in pre-adolescents include mumps, infectious mononucleosis, varicella, *Mycoplasma*, and Coxsackieviruses. When epididymitis occurs in non-sexually active boys, there may be a history of a urinary tract anomaly (ectopic ureter, vesicoureteral reflux), recent urethral instrumentation, or an associated urinary tract infection. In sexually active males, the most common etiologies are *Chlamydia* and *N. gonorrhea*, (pp. 330–341). Noninfectious epididymitis is uncommon.

Symptoms include the gradual onset of localized testicular, and possibly abdominal pain, nausea, vomiting, fever, and dysuria. On examination, there may be localized testicular or epididymal tenderness, non-transilluminating scrotal swelling, and a thickened epididymis. In pubertal boys, manual scrotal elevation often relieves the pain in epididymo-orchitis (Prehn's sign), but not in testicular and appendiceal torsions. The cremasteric reflex is unaffected.

Inguinal Hernia

Inguinal hernias are most common in the first year of life, especially among premature infants. The hernias are predominantly indirect, secondary to a patent processus vaginalis, and are more common on the right side. Males are affected ten times more often than females. Typically, recurrent episodes of painless, nonerythematous scrotal and inguinal swelling occur, often when the baby is crying or straining. Bowel sounds may be heard in the scrotum, and transillumination is variable. In females, an ovary may be palpated in the hernia sac. Incarceration within the inguinal ring can occur and presents with acute tenderness, erythema, and induration. Over the course of a few hours, strangulation (vascular compromise) occurs with eventual bowel obstruction and necrosis, causing vomiting, decreased bowel sounds, abdominal distention, and possible fluid and electrolyte imbalances.

Hydrocele

Hydroceles are most common during the first year of life, especially on the right side. The mass transilluminates, and the testicle is usually palpable posteriorly in the scrotum. The swelling generally involves only the scrotum and does not extend into the inguinal canal. Hydroceles are categorized according to whether the processus vaginalis is narrowly patent, permitting passage of peritoneal fluid (communicating) or obliterated (noncommunicating).

Communicating hydroceles typically present with recurrent episodes of painless, nonerythematous scrotal swellings that vary in size. It may be possible to completely reduce the hydrocele fluid by gentle pressure. Noncommunicating hydroceles are usually present at birth, are stable in size without waxing and waning, and are not reducible with gentle pressure.

Varicocele

A varicocele is a collection of dilated spermatic cord veins. They are virtually always found on the left side in adolescents. The patient may complain of a sensation of heaviness or dull ache in the scrotum but more often a varicocele is asymptomatic. Examination in the upright position reveals a nontender, nonerythematous scrotum with a "bag of worms" inside. Varicoceles enlarge with a Valsalva maneuver and decrease in the recumbent position.

Hematocele

A hematocele can occur after scrotal trauma or in association with a bleeding diathesis. A painful, bluish scrotal swelling is seen. When examination of the ipsilateral testis is difficult, scrotal ultrasound can assess the integrity of the involved testicle.

Testicular Tumor

Testicular tumors are unusual in young children, although they are the most common solid tumor in males 15–35 years of age. There is diffuse or localized unilateral testicular enlargement that is firm or rock hard, but painless. There can be an associated reactive hydrocele. If the tumor is secondary to leukemic infiltration, the mass can be bilateral.

Diagnosis

Although appendicular torsions and epididymo-orchitis may closely resemble a testicular torsion, the diagnosis in patients with acute hemiscrotal pain and swelling is testicular torsion until proved otherwise. If there is any suspicion of torsion, immediately obtain urologic consultation. Arrange for immediate surgery if the clinical signs and symptoms are consistent with testicular torsion. If the diagnosis is uncertain, imaging studies, if available within one hour of the patient's presentation, may help differentiate among the causes of an acute hemiscrotum. These include color Doppler ultrasound (decreased blood flow in testicular torsion, increased with appendicular torsion and epididymo-orchitis) and radio-isotope scrotal scanning (cold in testicular torsion, normal or hot in appendicular torsion, hot with epididymo-orchitis).

With appendicular torsion, pain and swelling may be localized to the superior testicular pole and a blue dot may be seen through the thin scrotal skin. Dysuria with pyuria and possible bacteriuria may occur in epididymo-orchitis, along with fever and an elevated WBC count.

Inguinal hernias, hydroceles, hematoceles, and varicoceles can usually be distinguished by the clinical findings. If a strangulated inguinal hernia cannot be ruled out, obtain an abdominal radiograph. Dilated intestinal loops with air-fluid levels may be seen along with a loop of bowel in the scrotum.

ED Management

Testicular Torsion

All suspected cases must be evaluated immediately by a urologist or general surgeon, as testicular survival depends on the duration and degree of ischemia. The testicular salvage rate approaches 100% if the patient is explored within six hours of the onset of symptoms, but it drops to 20% 12 hours after the onset of symptoms and 0% at 24 hours. Because it is not possible to accurately determine whether the torsion has been intermittent or complete, duration of symptoms for >24 hours is not a reason to defer surgery. The intermittent nature of the torsion increases the chance of survival despite a long duration. In preparation for surgery, make the child NPO and obtain a CBC, type and cross-match, and a urinalysis.

In extreme circumstances, when prompt surgical intervention is not possible, manual detorsion may be attempted after administering adequate sedation and analgesia. Two-thirds of cases of testicular torsion occur in the medial direction. Rotate the left testis 180–360° clockwise, or the right counterclockwise ("when in doubt, turn it out") until the torsion is relieved as documented by pain relief, lower position of the testis within the scrotum, or increased blood flow by Doppler. Surgery is still necessary, as retorsion often occurs acutely.

Torsion of Appendage Testis

Surgery is indicated when testicular torsion cannot be clinically excluded, or if unremitting swelling or pain continues for several days. Otherwise, treat symptomatically with analgesics and bed rest.

Epididymo-Orchitis

Treat the prepubertal male with antibiotics (trimethoprim-sulfamethoxazole, 8 mg/kg/day of TMP div bid or amoxicillin 40 mg/kg/day div tid) for ten days, analgesics, bed rest, and scrotal support. For epididymitis most likely caused by a sexually transmitted disease, treat with a single dose of ceftriaxone 250 mg IM plus doxycycline 100 mg PO bid for ten days.

Inguinal Hernia

An easily reducible hernia requires no acute treatment. Refer the patient to a surgeon so that elective repair can be arranged. The vast majority of incarcerated inguinal hernias can be manually reduced. Manual reduction and elective repair are less hazardous than operating on an incarcerated hernia. If the hernial sac contents cannot be easily pushed back into the abdomen, sedate the patient (pp. 712–722) and place him in the Trendelenburg position, with an ice bag on the hernia. After 30 minutes, attempt to push the hernia back into the abdomen by bimanual reduction. Apply pressure to the internal inguinal ring with one hand, while milking the entrapped gas and fluid of the incarcerated bowel into the intra-abdominal intestines with the other hand. This will usually facilitate reduction of the entire bowel. If reduction is successful, refer the patient for prompt elective repair. If reduction is not successful, admit the patient for correction of any fluid and electrolyte imbalances prior to emergency herniorrhaphy.

Hydrocele

Almost all noncommunicating hydroceles spontaneously resolve prior to 12 months of age. Thereafter, refer the patient to a urologist for possible correction. Refer patients with communicating hydroceles for elective surgical repair, and caution the parents about the possible presence of an associated inguinal hernia.

Varicocele

Refer the patient to a urologist for evaluation. There is a 20% risk of subsequent subfertility due to the effect of the varicocele on spermatogenesis. Prompt surgery is indicated in cases of loss of testicular volume.

Hematocele

Obtain an ultrasound to rule-out rupture of the tunica albuginea, which is an indication for surgical exploration. Otherwise, treat with rest and analgesia. If the patient has a bleeding diathesis, employ appropriate measures (pp. 353–357) and consult with a urologist.

Testicular Tumor

If there is any suspicion of a testicular tumor, obtain a scrotal ultrasound. If a mass is detected, obtain serum for βhCG, α-fetoprotein, and LDH, and immediately consult with a urologist.

Follow-up

- Appendiceal torsion: 2–3 days if the pain persists
- Epididymo-orchitis, incarcerated inguinal hernia, idiopathic scrotal edema: primary care follow-up in 7–10 days
- Hematocele: 3–5 days

Indications for Admission

- Suspected testicular torsion
- Incarcerated inguinal hernia

Bibliography

Bowlin PR, Gatti JM, Murphy JP. Pediatric testicular torsion. *Surg Clin North Am.* 2017;**97** (1):161–172.

Lambert SM. Pediatric urologic emergencies. *Pediatr Clin North Am.* 2012;**59**:965–976.

Mcconaghy JR., Panchal B. Epididymitis: an overview. *Am Fam Phys.* 2016;**94**(9):723–726.

Ta A, D'Arcy FT, Hoag N, D'Arcy JP, Lawrentschuk N. Testicular torsion and the acute scrotum: current emergency management. *Eur J Emerg Med.* 2016;**23**(3):160–165.

Workowski KA, Bolan GA. Sexually transmitted diseases treatment guidelines, 2015. *MMWR Recomm Rep.* 2015;**64**(RR-03):1–137.

Undescended Testis

Undescended testis (cryptorchidism) occur in 4% of term and up to 40% of boys born at ≤30 weeks' gestation. Spontaneous descent occurs in the majority over the first 6–12 months, after which time descent is unlikely. Histologic deterioration begins as young as one year of age and affects fertility, even in unilateral cases. Half are right-sided and approximately 30% are bilateral, predominantly in premature boys. An undescended testis is at higher risk for torsion, trauma, and, possibly, malignant degeneration. Referral to a urologist is warranted by one year of age.

Clinical Presentation and Diagnosis

Eighty percent of undescended testes are palpable in the groin (inguinal canal or in the superficial inguinal pouch) or in an ectopic location. There may be an associated inguinal hernia. Some of these testes are actually retractile, and will reenter the scrotum during a warm bath or can be milked into the scrotum without a tendency to spring back up to the groin when released.

Most impalpable testes are ultimately found within the abdomen or, on occasion, in the groin if atrophic or dysplastic. In the remaining cases there is unilateral or bilateral testicular absence, most commonly vanishing testis syndrome.

ED Management

Examine the child for other abnormalities, such as hypospadias or hernia. No acute treatment is necessary. Refer an infant under one year of age to a primary care provider, and instruct the parent to examine the scrotum while the child is in a warm bath. Refer patients at one year of age to a urologist. If an inguinal hernia is present, arrange for early surgical correction of the cryptorchidism and the hernia, regardless of the patient's age.

Bibliography

Braga LH, Lorenzo AJ. Cryptorchidism: a practical review for all community healthcare providers. *Can Urol Assoc J.* 2017;**11**(1–2 Suppl. 1):S26–S32.

Kurtz D, Tasian G. Current treatment options of undescended testes. *Curr Treat Options Peds.* 2016;2:43–51.

Radmayr C, Dogan HS, Hoebeke P, et al. Management of undescended testes: European Association of Urology/European Society for Paedatric Urology Guidelines. *J Pediatr Urol.* 2016;12:335–343.

Sepúlveda X, Egaña PL. Current management of non-palpable testes: a literature review and clinical results. *Transl Pediatr.* 2016;5(4):233–239.

Urethritis

Urethritis is an inflammation of the urethral mucosa caused by local irritation (chemical, infection, foreign body insertion). While infectious causes of urethritis are rare in prepubertal children, sexually transmitted infection is the most common etiology in sexually active adolescents.

Clinical Presentation and Diagnosis

Irritation

Perfumed soaps, bubble bath, or chlorine may cause a chemical irritation of the distal urethral and penile meatus. The patient presents with meatal pain, itching, and dysuria. The urine culture is negative.

Anatomic Abnormalities

A prolapsed urethra most commonly occurs in prepubertal African-American females. The prolapsed mucosa is visible as an edematous red or purple doughnut-shaped mass. The initial complaint may be painless bleeding or spotting.

Other abnormalities, such as urethral diverticulum, urethral polyp, and valve of Guérin, are uncommon. They usually present with difficulty voiding, gross hematuria, voiding pain at the dorsal glans penis, and blood spotting on the underpants.

Foreign Body

A urethral foreign body causes a bloody urethritis. There may be a clear history of insertion, the object may be palpable in the urethra, or it may be radiopaque.

Posterior Urethritis

This is a nonspecific urethral inflammation in boys 5–15 years old. It presents with urethral discharge, urethral bleeding, or terminal hematuria. The physical examination is normal, and routine cultures of the discharge and the urine are sterile.

Sexually Transmitted Urethritis

In males, gonorrhea, *Chlamydia* or *Ureaplasma* cause dysuria, urethral discharge, and occasionally epididymitis or prostatitis. In females, *Chlamydia* is associated with the acute urethral syndrome (dysuria, urgency, suprapubic tenderness, pyuria) or pelvic inflammatory disease (pp. 330–341).

Obtain a urinalysis and routine urine culture, and perform a Gram's stain and culture (*Gonococci, Chlamydia*) of the urethral discharge.

ED Management

Irritation
Discontinue the chemical irritant, if known, and if the symptoms are severe, give phenazo-pyridine hydrochloride (12 mg/kg/day div tid, 200 mg maximum dose) for one or two days, only.

Anatomic Abnormalities
Treat a prolapsed urethra with warm compresses or sitz baths, tid. Prescribe a topical estrogen cream bid for two weeks and arrange follow-up. Consult a urologist if marked edema causes voiding difficulty. Refer patients with gross hematuria in association with penile voiding pain to a urologist.

Foreign Body
Immediately consult a urologist.

Posterior Urethritis
Treat with ten days of antibiotics (<8 years: amoxicillin 40 mg/kg/day div tid; ≥8 years: trimethoprim-sulfamethoxazole, 8 mg/kg/day of TMP div bid). There is a high rate of recurrence, and bulbar urethral stricture can result. Therefore, refer the patient to a urologist.

Sexually Transmitted Urethritis
For children weighing <45 kg, treat with a single dose of ceftriaxone 125 mg IM followed by either PO azithromycin 20 mg/kg (1 g maximum) in a single dose, or a seven-day course of oral erythromycin (50 mg/kg/day div q 8h) or doxycycline 100 mg bid (>8 years of age). For children weighing ≥45 kg, treat with a single dose of ceftriaxone 250 mg IM plus azithro-mycin 1 g orally × 1 dose or doxycycline as above.

Follow-up
• Urethritis: primary care follow-up in 7–10 days

Indications for Admission
• Inability to void
• Urethral foreign body

Bibliography
Henderson L, Farrelly P, Dickson AP, Goya A. Management strategies for idiopathic urethritis. *J Pediatr Urol.* 2016;**12**(1):35.e1–5.

Jayakumar S, Pringle K, Ninan GK. Idiopathic urethritis in children: classification and treatment with steroids. *J Indian Assoc Pediatr Surg.* 2014;**19**(3):143–146.

Ludvigson AE, Beaule LT. Urologic emergencies. *Surg Clin North Am.* 2016; **96**:407–424.

Perkins MJ, Decker CF. Non-gonococcal urethritis. *Dis Mon.* 2016;**62**(8):274–279.

Urinary Retention

Urinary retention is defined as the inability to urinate for >12 hours. Acute urinary retention is rare in children. In the male infant, posterior urethral valves are the most common congenital cause of retention. Other etiologies include a urethral polyp, urethral stricture, urethral diverticulum, meatal stenosis, and fecal impaction. In the female infant, retention is most often secondary to a prolapsing ureterocele, urethral prolapse, labial inflammation and adhesions, or a foreign body.

Urinary retention can also be the presenting symptom of tumors (neuroblastoma, Ewing's sarcoma, sacrococcygeal teratoma). Infections (cystitis, urethritis, meatitis), iatrogenic or self-instrumentation, lower urinary tract stones, spinal cord lesions, medications (antihistamines, decongestants, bronchodilator, tricyclic anticholinergics, probantheline), and psychogenic retention are other causes of urinary retention. In addition, urinary retention and dysfunctional voiding may be the presenting symptoms of sexual abuse.

Clinical Presentation and Diagnosis

Urinary retention in a newborn male presents as dribbling or a poor stream. In the female a bulging introital mass may be seen, representing a ureterocele. In either sex, the bladder may be persistently palpable.

In older patients, urinary retention may present with urgency, hesitancy, frequency, dribbling, a poor stream, and a distended, palpable bladder. Dysuria (cystitis or urethritis), a urethral discharge (urethritis), or an inflamed, swollen urethral meatus (meatitis) may be present. Ensure that uncircumcised males do not have balanoposthitis or phimosis. Ask about a history of recurrent urinary tract infections.

Patients with spinal cord abnormalities usually have a visible deformity of the back (sacral dimple, tuft of hair, sinus). On neurologic examination, there may be altered lower extremity reflexes, decreased anal sphincter tone, a sensory level, or differential responses to sensory testing in the lower extremities compared with the upper extremities.

Psychosomatic retention usually occurs in females with no previous history of voiding abnormalities. The initiating stress factor is often unrecognized by the patient and parents, and no other congenital or acquired etiology can be found.

Consider the possibility of sexual abuse if the history and physical examination are not consistent with any other etiologies for urinary retention.

ED Management

Initially provide symptomatic treatment, such as a warm-water bath or viscous lidocaine for local inflammation. If unsuccessful, catheterize the patient. Obtain blood for BUN and creatinine and urine for urinalysis, and immediately refer all infants with dribbling, poor stream, or failure to void within 48 hours of birth to a urologist.

The management of cystitis (pp. 694–695), urethritis (p. 309), and meatitis (p. 295) is discussed elsewhere.

Treat retention secondary to urinary tract instrumentation with sitz baths tid and phenazopyridine hydrochloride (12 mg/kg/day div tid, 300 mg/dose maximum) for 1–2 days, but warn the family that the urine will turn orange. Discontinue any medication associated with retention.

If a spinal cord lesion is suspected, consult with a neurologist. Intermittent catheterization or an indwelling catheter may be required as a temporizing measure.

If psychosomatic retention is suspected, immediately refer the patient to a psychiatrist. Once again, temporary intermittent catheterization or an indwelling catheter may be required. The management of possible sexual abuse is discussed elsewhere (pp. 608–611).

In cases of urinary retention secondary to fecal impaction, rapid treatment of the impaction (see Constipation, pp. 253–254) leads to resolution of the urinary retention.

Indication for Admission

- Urinary retention that cannot be relieved in the ED

Bibliography

Ludvigson AE, Beaule LT. Urologic emergencies. *Surg Clin North Am.* 2016;**96**:407–424.

Marshall JR, Haber J, Josephson EB. An evidence-based approach to emergency department management of acute urinary retention. *Emerg Med Pract.* 2014;**16**(1):1–20.

Nevo A, Mano R, Livne PN, et al. Urinary retention in children. *Urol.* 2014;**84**:1475–1479.

Gynecologic Emergencies

Dominic Hollman, Elizabeth Alderman, and Anthony J. Ciorciari

Abnormal Uterine Bleeding

The average age of menarche in the United States is 12.8 years, which is approximately two years after breast budding and consistent with the Tanner IV stage of pubertal development. The normal interval between periods ranges from 21 to 35 days, with 3–7 days of bleeding. With normal menstrual flow, a girl uses 3–6 tampons or pads a day, and the average blood loss is 30–60 mL. Menstrual blood loss of >80 mL is abnormal and can lead to lower hemoglobin, hematocrit, and serum iron levels.

Abnormal uterine bleeding (AUB) is irregular, painless bleeding of endometrial origin. Most cases are secondary to anovulation, which is common during the first 2–3 years after menarche, although up to 20% may have anovulatory bleeding 4–5 years after menarche. The etiologies of abnormal vaginal bleeding are listed in Table 11.1.

Clinical Presentation

A typical pattern of AUB is prolonged or excessive flow alternating with periods of oligomenorrhea or amenorrhea. Pain, fever, chills, abdominal pain, and vaginal discharge are absent. Below are the definitions of the three clinical stages of AUB. Management is dependent on the severity of vaginal bleeding.

Mild AUB

With mild AUB the menses may be somewhat prolonged or the cycle shortened for 2–3 months. The hemoglobin and hematocrit are normal, >11 g/dL and >35%, respectively.

Moderate AUB

Moderate AUB is characterized by prolonged periods and an increased flow severe enough to cause a decrease in hemoglobin and hematocrit to 9–11 g/dL and 25–35%, respectively.

Severe AUB

Severe AUB results in significant decreases in the hemoglobin and hematocrit, to <9 g/dL and <25%, respectively. Clinical signs of acute blood loss (tachycardia, orthostatic vital sign changes, delayed capillary refill) with a hemoglobin <11 g/dL is also consistent with severe AUB.

Table 11.1 Etiologies of dysfunctional uterine bleeding

Bleeding disorders

Factor deficiencies

ITP

Platelet dysfunction

von Willebrand disease

Chronic illness

Chronic renal disease

Inflammatory bowel disease

Liver disease

Complications of pregnancy

Ectopic pregnancy

Implantation bleeding

Molar pregnancy

Spontaneous abortion

S/P termination of pregnancy

Endocrine disorders

Adrenal disorders

Pituitary adenoma

Polycystic ovarian syndrome

Thyroid disease

Medications and devices

Aspirin

Chemotherapy

Depo-medroxyprogesterone

Implantable contraception

IUD

Oral, ring, and patch contraceptives

Prednisone

Warfarin

Other gynecological

First intercourse

Sexual assault

Vaginal trauma

Sexually transmitted infections

Acute salpingitis

Cervicitis

Endometritis

Diagnosis

Abnormal uterine bleeding is a diagnosis of exclusion. Inquire about the age of menarche, date of last normal menstrual period, length of last menstrual period, frequency and regularity of menses, typical length of flow, the number of pads or tampons used, and when the period before the last menstrual period was and whether it was normal. Ask about other bleeding manifestations such as nosebleeds or easy bruisability, epistaxis, bleeding gums, hematuria, and, rarely, hematochezia. Ask about sexual activity (including genital trauma, history of pregnancy, history of sexually transmitted infections), foreign bodies (tampon use, self-insertion), contraceptive history (particularly oral contraceptives, depo-medroxyprogesterone acetate, intrauterine device [IUD], contraceptive patch, ring, or implant), medications used (aspirin, coumadin, antipsychotics, antidepressants, steroids), endocrine disorders (specifically symptoms related to thyroid disease, pituitary adenoma, or androgenizing symptoms such as acne or hirsutism, which may be associated with poly-cystic ovary syndrome), emotional stress, eating habits (including pica) and chronic illnesses.

Pregnancy (pp. 325–330) is suggested by a history of amenorrhea, but a positive serum βhCG confirms the diagnosis. Breast tenderness and an enlarged uterus may be noted. Salpingitis (p. 331) may present with a vaginal discharge, lower abdominal pain, fever, chills, cervical motion tenderness, and/or adnexal tenderness.

On physical examination, the priorities are the vital signs, manifestations of a bleeding diathesis, and the gynecologic examination. Check for orthostatic hypotension, bradycardia (hypothyroidism), tachycardia (hyperthyroidism, significant blood loss), delayed capillary refill (shock), petechiae or ecchymoses (bleeding diathesis), or evidence of a chronic illness such as cachexia or swollen joints.

Inspect the external genitalia to look for signs of trauma or bleeding sources. If the patient is sexually active, perform a speculum exam looking for evidence of trauma or infection (cervical discharge; cervical or intravaginal warts or herpes). Also perform a bimanual examination to check the cervix for tenderness on motion (salpingitis). Palpate the uterus to determine size and tenderness, and examine the adnexae for masses and tenderness. If the patient is not sexually active, but has abdominal pain, perform a recto-abdominal examination assessing for a pelvic mass. Obtain a pelvic ultrasound if the patient is pregnant, or there is abdominal or pelvic pain, suspicion of a tubo-ovarian abscess, or suspicion of an abdominal or pelvic mass or one is palpated.

ED Management

The management of AUB is almost exclusively based on the level of anemia caused by the vaginal bleeding. The goal of the work-up is to exclude other causes of bleeding that may require different ED management.

For all patients, obtain a CBC with platelet count, thyroid function tests (TSH and free T4), pregnancy test, and clotting studies (PT, PTT). If the patient is sexually active, also obtain a gonorrhea and chlamydia test, rapid plasma reagin (RPR), and a quanti-tative pregnancy test if the urine pregnancy test is positive. A type and cross-match is indicated for moderate, severe, or prolonged bleeding or orthostasis. Severe bleeding at menarche warrants testing for von Willebrand disease (von Willebrand factor [VWF] antigen, VWF activity and factor VIII activity), which may not manifest until that time. If the patient has signs of hyperandrogenism or is obese, or polycystic ovary syndrome is suspected, obtain a free and total testosterone, DHEAS, androstenedione, and sex hormone binding globulin, as once a girl begins hormonal treatment these parameters cannot be accurately assessed. If a pelvic mass is appreciated or ectopic pregnancy suspected, obtain an ultrasound.

Mild AUB

Observation and reassurance are all that are needed. Advise the patient to keep a menstrual calendar. Iron supplementation (325 mg/day of ferrous gluconate or multivitamin with iron) may be necessary, but the majority of these patients spontaneously convert to normal menstrual cycles within several months.

Moderate AUB

Treat with a monophasic combined oral contraceptive pill (COCP) with 30–35 mcg estrogen/varying progesterone (e.g., Sprintec, Ortho-Novum1/35, Lo-Ovral) if there is no contraindication to estrogen. These include migraine with aura, untreated hypertension, known clotting risk (e.g., antiphospholipid antibody), untreated hyperlipidemia, cardiovascular disease, history of a stroke or deep vein thrombosis, active liver disease, pregnancy, and breast cancer. If a first-degree relative has a clotting disorder, it is prudent to have the patient tested for hereditary hypercoagulable states such as Antithrombin III deficiency and Protein C and Protein S deficiency before prescribing an estrogen-containing OCP.

Always prescribe the 21-day pill pack, as taking the placebos of the 28-day pack will cause a withdrawal bleed. Give two pills per day until the follow-up visit with adolescent medicine or gynecology in one week. If the bleeding does not stop or slow significantly in two days, advise the patient to contact adolescent medicine or gynecology. Once the bleeding completely stops, the patient may be transitioned to one pill per day. Give the patient and parent/guardian detailed written instructions, as this regimen is complicated, and if not followed exactly may result in breakthrough bleeding. Also prescribe an oral antiemetic, such as prochlorperazine (10 mg q 6–8h 40 mg/day maximum) or ondansetron (15–30 kg: 4 mg bid; >30 kg: 8 mg bid).

If the patient has a contraindication to estrogen, prescribe medroxyprogesterone acetate (Provera) 10 mg PO daily, and give the first dose in the ED. Arrange follow-up with adolescent medicine or gynecology within one week. Eventually, these patients may be prescribed a progestin-only pill (depot-medroxyprogesterone acetate) or a long-acting reversible progestin-only contraceptive (IUD or implant).

When the patient is at the point of taking one OCP per day, add ferrous gluconate (325 mg tid) to treat the associated anemia. Starting the iron while the patient is taking more than one OCP per day may exacerbate the gastrointestinal side effects. At the follow-up visit, obtain a hemoglobin, and if it is >12 g/dL, allow a withdrawal bleed. A week after stopping the COCP, begin a new 28-day pill pack and cycle the patient for six months, or institute the progestin-only method outlined above for six months.

Severe AUB

The priority is restoration of adequate perfusion (see Shock, pp. 28–35) with 20 mL/kg boluses of isotonic crystalloid (normal saline or Ringer's lactate). A packed RBC transfusion (10 mL/kg) is indicated if the patient is symptomatic (tachycardia, dizziness), either at rest or standing, or remains orthostatic after the boluses. To stop the bleeding immediately, begin monophasic COCP (35 mcg estrogen) qid, if there are no estrogen contraindications. If the patient is bleeding profusely or is in shock, give a conjugated estrogen (Premarin), 25 mg IV over 20 minutes q 4–6h. This is usually effective after the first or second dose, but a maximum of four doses may be given. An antiemetic may be needed (as above). If the bleeding does not subside or increases after the third dose of Premarin, or the vital signs continue to deteriorate, consult a gynecologist to determine whether a dilation and curettage is indicated. Continue treatment with monophasic COCP as outlined for moderate AUB above. If the patient has a contraindication to estrogen, begin medroxyprogesterone acetate (Provera) 10 mg PO and tranexamic acid 1300 mg PO q 8h, and give the first dose immediately. Consult adolescent medicine and, if a bleeding diathesis exists, hematology/oncology.

Follow-up

- Mild AUB: routine primary care follow-up. Have the patient maintain a menstrual diary. Advise her to call her primary care provider if bleeding continues for another week.
- Moderate AUB: Refer the patient to an adolescent medicine specialist or gynecologist for follow-up within a week, but sooner (within 2–3 days) if the bleeding does not stop

Indication for Admission

- Severe AUB
- Moderate AUB with symptoms or signs of inadequate perfusion

Bibliography

American College of Obstetricians and Gynecologists. ACOG committee opinion no. 557: management of acute abnormal uterine bleeding in nonpregnant reproductive-aged women. *Obstet Gynecol.* 2013;**121**(4):891–896.

Bennett AR, Gray SH. What to do when she's bleeding through: the recognition, evaluation, and management of abnormal uterine bleeding in adolescents. *Curr Opin Pediatr.* 2014;**26**(4):413–419.

Deligeoroglou E, Karountzos V, Creatsas G. Abnormal uterine bleeding and dysfunctional uterine bleeding in pediatric and adolescent gynecology. *Gynecol Endocrinol.* 2013;**29**(1):74–78.

Gray SH. Menstrual disorders. *Pediatr Rev.* 2013;**34**(1):6–17.

Matteson KA, Rahn DD, Wheeler TL 2nd, et al. Nonsurgical management of heavy menstrual bleeding: a systematic review. *Obstet Gynecol.* 2013; **121**:632.

Breast Disorders

Common breast disorders include neonatal hypertrophy, premature thelarche (either alone or with precocious puberty), breast masses, breast abscesses, and gynecomastia.

Clinical Presentation

Neonatal Breast Hypertrophy

Neonatal breast hypertrophy occurs in up to two-thirds of normal newborns of both genders. It results from maternal hormonal stimulation, and presents as palpable breast tissue, present from birth, in an otherwise healthy infant. Occasionally, in female infants, there is also galactorrhea, clitoral hypertrophy, and a bloody vaginal discharge, also resulting from the effect of maternal hormones. Most cases resolve within a month, although breast hypertrophy may persist for several months.

Premature Thelarche

The mean onset of breast development in the United States is approximately ten years for white girls and nine years for African-American girls. Premature thelarche is defined as breast enlargement, in the absence of other signs of puberty, before seven years of age in white girls and six years of age in African-American girls. At times it is the result of neonatal breast hypertrophy failing to regress. Bilateral breast buds (2–4 cm) are present with no associated nipple or areolar change, nipple discharge, axillary or pubic hair, clitoral enlargement, acne, or growth spurt. The presence of any of these other findings suggests more significant pathology, including true precocious puberty, CNS disorders, ovarian tumors, and exogenous estrogens.

Breast Masses

Breast masses are a common source of fear and anxiety in the adolescent female, but most cases are benign, secondary to fibrocystic changes or physiologic breast tissue. While adolescents typically have dense breast tissue at baseline, fibrocystic changes can ensue, appearing as cord-like thickening that may present as "lumps." These "lumps" may become tender and enlarged prior to menses each month.

The most common discrete masses in adolescents are fibroadenomas. These are benign lesions that present as firm, rubbery, mobile masses with clearly defined borders. Other common benign findings include simple cysts, capillary hemangiomas, and fat necrosis.

Cystosarcoma phyllodes is a rare primary tumor that is usually, but not always, benign. The tumor is generally large (about 6 cm), and there may be overlying skin changes (tautness, retraction, necrosis). Invasive breast cancer (adenocarcinoma) is exceedingly rare in children and adolescents. A positive family history of breast cancer and prior radiation treatment are risk factors. The most common malignant breast masses in adolescents are metastases from other primary cancers, such as rhabdomyosarcoma, lymphoma, neuroblastoma, and melanoma.

Mastitis and Breast Abscesses

Mastitis (inflammation of the breast) and breast abscesses (a local accumulation of pus in the breast) are infections that can occur in newborns as well as adolescent females. *Staphylococcus aureus* is the most common pathogen in both age groups. In adolescents, abscesses are most frequent during lactation, while in non-lactating teenagers the etiology is unclear, but may be due to duct ectasia or metaplasia of the duct epithelium. Trauma or manipulation of the skin can also lead to infection. The abscess presents on the skin adjacent to the areola as a warm, erythematous, tender mass, which may be fluctuant. The patient may be febrile.

Gynecomastia

Nearly 50% of adolescent males undergo benign, usually bilateral, increase in the glandular and stromal tissue of the breast, generally at Tanner stages II–III. It results from an increase in estrogen that is usually part of normal adolescent development.

Gynecomastia resolves within 1–2 years. Persistence beyond adolescence may be pathologic, secondary to disorders that cause increased estrogen, decreased androgen, or abnormality at the receptors for estrogen or androgen. These include testicular, adrenal, or other hCG-producing tumors. Hypogonadotropic hypogonadism, androgen insensitivity, hyperthyroidism, hyperprolactinemia, liver disease, kidney disease, or obesity can also cause gynecomastia. Drug use, either medical (spironolactone, cimetidine, digoxin), or recreational (marijuana) are other etiologies.

Diagnosis

Neonatal Breast Hypertrophy

A history and physical examination, including a genital exam to assess for other signs of maternal estrogenization, are all that is required.

Premature Thelarche

A complete physical examination must be performed to rule-out true precocious puberty. Premature thelarche is the diagnosis if no other pubertal changes are present. Note the presence of secondary sexual characteristics, such as pubic hair, estrogenized vaginal mucosa, and clitoral enlargement. The presence of any of these findings is indicative of precocious puberty, not isolated premature thelarche.

Breast Masses

A breast examination is usually sufficient to diagnose fibrocystic changes and to distinguish an abscess from a true breast mass. If a cyst is suspected, schedule the patient to be reexamined after her next menstrual period, as the lesion will often disappear. If a discrete lesion persists, arrange for an ultrasound, which is the imaging modality of choice for evaluating breast masses in adolescents.

Mastitis and Breast Abscess

The diagnosis of mastitis is usually evident on inspection of the warm, tender, erythematous breast bud. An adolescent may have a history of a recent pregnancy and may or may not be lactating. A neonate may be febrile, although associated symptoms in infant mastitis are uncommon. If the area is fluctuant, presume the child has an associated abscess and arrange for aspiration. This can help confirm the diagnosis and provide a specimen for culture.

Gynecomastia

Gynecomastia can be differentiated from adipose tissue in that gynecomastia presents with a firm, rubbery, discrete mass that is usually <3 cm in diameter. The breast tissue is symmetrically located under the nipple/areolar complex. Although the subareolar nodule may extend beyond the margin of the areola, an asymmetric mass in relation to the areola is not consistent with benign gynecomastia.

In addition, examine the abdomen to evaluate for an adrenal tumor and the testicles to assess testicular volume (or presence of atrophy) and to palpate any masses.

ED Management

Neonatal Breast Hypertrophy

Reassurance, cool compresses, and avoidance of breast massaging are all that is necessary. Refer the infant to a primary care provider.

Premature Thelarche/Precocious Puberty

If there are no other signs of puberty, reassure the patient and family that the condition is not serious and refer the patient to a primary care physician for routine follow-up. If other signs of puberty are present, arrange for a pediatric endocrinology visit within one week.

Breast Masses

Reassurance is all that is needed for a patient with either physiologic or fibrocystic changes. If a cyst is palpated, arrange for follow-up with the patient's primary doctor after her period. If the lesion persists, or if there is a more concerning finding on examination, obtain an ultrasound and refer to either an adolescent medicine specialist or a surgeon.

Mastitis and Breast Abscesses

Infants <4 weeks old, or 4–8 weeks of age with either fever >100.6 °F (38.1 °C) or a "toxic" appearance, require a complete sepsis evaluation, hospitalization, and IV antibiotics (pp. 391–392). If a patient 4–8 weeks of age is afebrile and nontoxic, obtain a blood culture and admit for IV antibiotics.

Treat a patient >8 weeks of age with IV nafcillin (150 mg/kg/day div q 6h), oxacillin (100–200 mg/kg/day div q 6h; 12 g/day maximum), or cefazolin (100 mg/kg/day div q 6–8h; 6 g/day maximum). If MRSA is a concern or there is a life-threatening penicillin allergy, use IV vancomycin (8 weeks to 11 years of age: 10–15 mg/kg div q 6–8h; 1 g/dose maximum; ≥12 years of age: 10–15 mg/kg q 12h or 1 g IV q 12h) or IV clindamycin (40 mg/kg/day q 6h) for 7–10 days. Supportive care with warm packs and elevation of the breast are important adjuncts. If the patient has an abscess, prior to instituting antibiotic therapy arrange for a needle aspiration by an experienced pediatric or breast surgeon and send a specimen for culture to guide further therapy.

Treat afebrile, well-appearing, older children and adolescents with mastitis with cephalexin (40 mg/kg/day div q 6h or q 12h, respectively) for 7–10 days. If MRSA is a concern, either use clindamycin (20 mg/kg/day q 6h) or add trimethoprim-sulfamethoxazole (8 mg/kg/day of trimethoprim div bid). Warm compresses 4–6 times daily are an important adjunctive measure. Follow-up within 24 hours; if the mass enlarges or becomes fluctuant, or if the patient becomes febrile, admit her for intravenous antibiotics and possible incision and drainage (if an abscess has developed).

Gynecomastia

If the patient has findings consistent with pubertal gynecomastia (duration <2 years, Tanner stages II–III), no laboratory work-up is indicated. If there is concern that this is not benign gynecomastia, or if it has persisted for more than two years, obtain a urinalysis, electrolytes, BUN/creatinine, liver function tests, serum testosterone, estradiol, LH, and hCG, and refer the patient to their primary care provider.

Follow-up

- Breast abscess or mastitis in the older child: follow-up with primary care provider in 24 hours
- Breast mass: follow-up with adolescent medicine or surgery
- Premature thelarche, asymmetry or gynecomastia: follow-up with primary care provider
- Precocious puberty (premature thelarche associated with other secondary sexual characteristics): pediatric endocrinologist within one week

Indications for Admission

- Mastitis and breast abscess in the neonate and infant
- Breast abscess in the older child who has fever or is ill-appearing

Bibliography

Day CT, Kaplan SL, Mason EO, Hulten KG. Community-associated *Staphylococcus aureus* infections in otherwise healthy infants less than 60 days old. *Pediatr Infect Dis J.* 2014;**33**:98.

DiVasta AD, Weldon C, Labow BI. The breast: examination and lesions. In Emans SJ, Laufer MR, Goldstein DP (eds.) *Emans, Laufer and Goldstein's Pediatric & Adolescent Gynecology* (6th edn.). Philadelphia, PA: Lippincott Williams & Wilkins, 2012; 405.

Frazier AL, Rosenberg SM. Preadolescent and adolescent risk factors for benign breast disease. *J Adolesc Health.* 2013;**52**(5 Suppl.):S36–S40.

Kaneda HJ, Mack J, Kasales CJ, Schetter S. Pediatric and adolescent breast masses: a review of pathophysiology, imaging, diagnosis, and treatment. *AJR Am J Roentgenol.* 2013;**200**(2):W204–W212.

Valeur NS, Rahbar H, Chapman T. Ultrasound of pediatric breast masses: what to do with lumps and bumps. *Pediatr Radiol.* 2015;**45**(11):1584–1599.

Dysmenorrhea

Dysmenorrhea (painful menstruation) is very common in teenagers and may be a response to elevated levels of prostaglandin. The majority of cases are classified as primary dysmenorrhea, which generally do not present at menarche and are not associated with significant pelvic pathology. In secondary dysmenorrhea there is pelvic pathology, most often salpingitis, endometriosis, or genital tract obstruction secondary to a congenital malformation of the uterus or vagina.

Clinical Presentation

Primary Dysmenorrhea

Primary dysmenorrhea usually presents within 6–12 months of menarche. Typically, colicky suprapubic pain begins several hours before or after the start of a period. The pain may radiate to the back or down the thighs. In 50% of patients there may be nausea, vomiting, diarrhea, and migraine headaches. The symptoms can last from a few hours to several days and there is often a family history of dysmenorrhea.

Secondary Dysmenorrhea

Secondary dysmenorrhea generally presents years after menarche, although dysmenorrhea with the first menses may be a sign of a congenital anomaly with a gynecologic outflow tract obstruction. As in primary dysmenorrhea, the pain occurs during menstruation. There may be a history of pelvic inflammatory disease, vaginal discharge, abdominal or pelvic surgery, menorrhagia, or endometriosis, or an IUD might be in place.

Diagnosis

The most important aspect in managing a girl with lower abdominal pain who is peri-menstrual is to determine if she has primary or secondary dysmenorrhea. Additionally, non-gynecologic causes of lower abdominal pain must be ruled out (see Abdominal Pain, pp. 234–238).

Obtain a menstrual history, including age of menarche, last menstrual period, regularity of menses, frequency and severity of the pain, and its relation to the periods. Ask about a history of vaginal discharge, sexual activity, IUD use, previous pelvic inflammatory disease, or abdominal/pelvic surgery. Ask about family or personal history of dysmenorrhea.

Perform a complete physical examination to exclude any gastrointestinal or urinary causes of lower abdominal pain, such as appendicitis, gastroenteritis, constipation, inflammatory bowel disease, renal colic, or urinary tract infection. Perform an external vaginal examination to assess hymenal patency. If secondary dysmenorrhea is suspected in a girl who is not sexually active, perform a recto-abdominal examination to assess for a pelvic mass, which usually reflects uterine enlargement. If the patient is sexually active, perform a pelvic examination, looking for causes of secondary dysmenorrhea, including cervical motion tenderness, an IUD, and adnexal or uterine enlargement or tenderness. A pelvic sonogram may be helpful when a bimanual examination cannot be performed, or is

Table 11.2 Differential diagnosis of dysmenorrhea

Diagnosis	Differentiating features
Congenital anomalies	Cyclical lower abdominal pain at menarche or in an amenorrheic patient
Ectopic pregnancy	Positive βhCG
	Unilateral adnexal mass
Endometriosis	Pain starts before bleeding and persists beyond
	Uterus/ovaries tender or enlarged
Imperforate hymen	Bulging vaginal mass with no patent hymen
	Patient is ≥Tanner III without history of menses
Intrauterine pregnancy	Positive βhCG
	Enlarged uterus (greater than pear or orange sized)
Ovarian cyst/tumor	Mass palpated on bimanual or recto-abdominal exam
Salpingitis	Fever, cervical motion tenderness, vaginal discharge
	Adnexal enlargement/tenderness (can be unilateral)

inconclusive or unreliable. Obtain a pregnancy test for all patients who have had previous menses, or if a girl is Tanner III, or more mature, with no previous menses. See Table 11.2 for the differential diagnosis of dysmenorrhea.

ED Management

Primary Dysmenorrhea

Oral prostaglandin synthetase inhibitors (nonsteroidal anti-inflammatories) are effective in 70–100% of patients. Use ibuprofen (Motrin, Advil) 400–600 mg q 6h, naproxen (Anaprox 550 mg first dose, then 275 mg q 12h; Aleve 440 mg first dose, then 220 mg q 12h), or mefenamic acid (Ponstel), 500 mg first dose, then 250 mg q 6h.

Since a patient with primary dysmenorrhea ovulates monthly and therefore has regular cycles, have the patient keep track of her menses with a menstrual calendar or the calendar on her cell phone. Advise the patient to start the medication one day before the onset of each period, beginning with a loading dose taken with food. If one nonsteroidal anti-inflammatory agent is ineffective, try an alternative. Side effects include nausea, dizziness, dyspepsia, and gastric irritation. These medications are contraindicated in patients with ulcers and aspirin allergy; use with caution in patients taking anticoagulants or with liver or kidney disease.

Other treatments that may be helpful include heating pads, exercise, a low-salt diet, a well-balanced diet, and reduction of stress. Suppression of ovulation by oral contraceptives is effective, but reserve this therapy for the primary care setting, where appropriate follow-up can be arranged.

Secondary Dysmenorrhea

Refer the patient to a gynecologist to treat the underlying cause. If a patient has a congenital anomaly causing obstruction with hematocolpos, consult with a gynecologist to determine if immediate surgical intervention is indicated. The management of salpingitis is discussed on pp. 337–340. If endometriosis is suspected, refer the patient to a gynecologist to arrange for laparoscopic confirmation of the diagnosis, followed by hormone therapy.

Follow-up

- Primary dysmenorrhea: primary care follow-up before the next period
- Secondary dysmenorrhea: gynecological follow-up before the next period

Bibliography

Allen LM, Lam AC. Premenstrual syndrome and dysmenorrhea in adolescents. *Adolesc Med State Art Rev.* 2012;**23**(1):139–163.

De Sanctis V, Soliman A, Bernasconi S, et al. Primary dysmenorrhea in adolescents: prevalence, impact and recent knowledge. *Pediatr Endocrinol Rev.* 2015;**13**(2):512–520.

Emans S. Dysfunctional uterine bleeding. In Emans SJ, Laufer MR, Goldstein DP (eds.) *Emans, Laufer, Goldstein's Pediatric & Adolescent Gynecology* (6th edn.). Philadelphia, PA: Lippincott Williams & Wilkins, 2012; 270–286.

Peacock A, Alvi NS, Mushtaq T. Period problems: disorders of menstruation in adolescents. *Arch Dis Child.* 2012;**97**(6):554–560.

Ovarian Emergencies

Ovarian masses are common causes of lower abdominal and pelvic pain, particularly in adolescents. The vast majority of these masses are benign, with the majority being functional cysts, such as follicular, corpus luteum, and theca-lutein types. However, many cysts are asymptomatic, and the incidence of ovarian cysts may be underestimated. They may be noted incidentally on an ultrasound performed for other indications.

Ovarian neoplasms are uncommon in children and adolescents. They represent 1% of the malignant neoplasms discovered in girls ≤17 years of age.

Ovarian torsion can occur with normal ovaries, or in the context of an ovarian mass or cyst. Ovarian masses are a major risk factor for torsion, implicated in 50–95% of cases. The risk for torsion increases with increased size of the mass, (>5 cm). In younger children, the presence of a long ligament increases the risk of torsion, and they are less likely to have an ovarian cyst or mass than postpubertal females. Ovarian torsion is a surgical emergency.

Clinical Presentation

Ovarian Cysts

In young children, ovarian cysts typically present as a mass noted by a parent or clinician. Pain is typically present, ranging from dull and achy to severe pain that can mimic appendicitis or peritonitis. The pain may also be intermittent, suggestive of a partial torsion. In adolescents, pain is usually the presenting complaint, along with menstrual irregularities. If the cyst is hormonally active, there may be premature breast development or vaginal bleeding. There may also be precocious puberty, as in McCune–Albright syndrome.

In all age groups, nausea and vomiting, as well as a "full" bloated feeling may be present. If the cyst is large, there may be mass effect on the bladder or bowel, causing voiding or stooling changes. In such cases, malignancy is a concern.

When a cyst ruptures, the fluid or blood within the peritoneum can cause pain and irritation. Depending on the volume of blood, patients may experience lightheadedness or other signs of hemodynamic instability.

Ovarian Torsion

Ovarian torsion presents with the sudden onset of moderate to severe pelvic pain, which is typically unilateral. It occurs in both young girls and adolescents, commonly in the setting of an ovarian mass, though this may not be known at the time of presentation. The patient may have nausea and vomiting, and possibly fever, as well as signs of peritonitis. The patient may have a recent history of similar, intermittent symptoms (representing partial torsion) which had spontaneously resolved prior to the current symptoms.

Diagnosis

Ovarian Cysts

Obtain a detailed medical history, including current symptoms, occurrence of similar symptoms in the past, and any pertinent past medical/surgical or social history. In younger girls, ask about any early signs of puberty, such as vaginal bleeding or the presence of breast development or pubic hair. In adolescents, a menstrual history is important, including date of last menstrual period, age at menarche, length and duration of cycle, and presence of irregular or excessive bleeding. Obtain a sexual history, as sexually transmitted infection is an important cause of pelvic pain. Review any current medications (including hormonal birth control methods). Upon review of systems, new onset of constipation or urinary retention might be a sign of an ovarian cyst or mass.

Check vital signs for hemodynamic instability, which may be associated with a ruptured cyst, and perform a detailed abdominal examination. In sexually active females a pelvic exam is indicated, particularly a bimanual examination, to assess ovarian size, presence of a mass, and signs of infection (such as pelvic inflammatory disease). In younger girls and virginal adolescents, perform a recto-abdominal examination instead.

Laboratory work-up includes a urine or serum pregnancy test if the patient has attained menarche or is pubertal (pregnancy can occur prior to menarche). Obtain relevant STI testing in sexually active patients, including gonorrhea and chlamydia, as well as an RPR and HIV testing. In patients with signs of hemodynamic instability or peritoneal signs, obtain a CBC, as well as a type and screen, as these patients may need surgical intervention.

The definitive diagnostic imaging study for ovarian masses is pelvic ultrasound, which can detail both the size and the character of the mass. Ultrasound can identify follicular cysts, corpus luteal cysts, and more complex masses and tumors, including teratomas and masses suspicious for malignancy. If a cyst has ruptured, fluid may be seen in the pelvis. A large amount of fluid may indicate hemorrhage from the ruptured cyst.

Further laboratory testing may be indicated depending on ultrasound findings. A gynecology consult is indicated for cysts ≥6 cm, if a malignancy is suspected, or the ultrasound results are equivocal.

Ovarian Torsion

In addition to the history and physical examination for a cyst, ask about any previous or current history of ovarian mass. Perform the same laboratory evaluation as above.

Pelvic ultrasound with Doppler is the imaging modality to diagnose torsion. Aside from noting any ovarian or adnexal masses, Doppler is important to evaluate blood flow. Absent or impaired flow within the ovary is diagnostic of torsion and vascular compromise, although the absence of an ovarian mass on ultrasound does not exclude the diagnosis of torsion. Ultrasound may also diagnose other conditions that may present similarly to torsion, such as ectopic pregnancy, a cyst or mass without torsion, and tubo-ovarian abscess.

ED Management

Ovarian Cysts

Management depends on the size and character of the cyst, as well as the symptomatology. Manage small, follicular cysts (<6 cm) conservatively, with observation and pain control, as most of these simple cysts resolve spontaneously. A combined oral contraceptive pill is an option, which also has the benefit of preventing new cysts from forming. If a symptomatic patient has a cyst ≥6 cm, consult a gynecologist to arrange cystectomy. If a patient with a large simple cyst (6–10 cm) is asymptomatic, observation is an option, but consult gynecology for evaluation and follow-up. In all cases, the patient and parent must be instructed to return to the ED if significant abdominal pain recurs.

Corpus luteal cysts can grow to 5–12 cm, but most regress spontaneously, and can be managed with observation and pain control, along with oral contraceptives. They typically do not require surgical intervention unless the patient has pain or peritoneal signs, although large cysts are at increased risk for torsion. Sonographic findings of more complex cysts or masses require gynecology consult.

Manage ruptured ovarian cysts conservatively with observation, pain control, and rest if symptoms are mild, the cyst is small, and the patient is hemodynamically stable. For large cysts (>6 cm), severe pain, or evidence of hemorrhage (clinical or radiographic), urgent gynecology consultation is necessary for possible surgical intervention.

Ovarian Torsion

Ovarian torsion is a surgical emergency. Consult gynecology urgently, as early surgical intervention can restore blood flow to the ovary, and preserve the ovary and ovarian function. Depending on the findings at surgery, cystectomy, salpingo-oophorectomy, or oophoropexy may be performed.

Follow-up

- Simple or corpus luteal cyst; ruptured cyst without peritoneal signs or hemodynamic instability: primary care provider or adolescent medicine specialist within one week

Indications for Admission

- Ovarian cyst: ovarian surgery is indicated (large or symptomatic mass, ruptured cyst with associated hemodynamically instability, malignancy)
- Ovarian torsion

Bibliography

Berlan ED, Emans SJ, O'Brien RF. Vulvovaginal complaints in the adolescent. In Emans SJ, Laufer MR, Goldstein DP (eds.) *Emans, Laufer, Goldstein's Pediatric and Adolescent Gynecology* (6th edn). Philadelphia, PA: Lippincott Williams and Wilkins, 2012; 42–95.

Reddy J, Laufer MR. Advantage of conservative surgical management of large ovarian neoplasms in adolescents. *Fertil Steril.* 2009; **91**:1941.

Rousseau V, Massicot R, Darwish AA, et al. Emergency management and conservative surgery of ovarian torsion in children: a report of 40 cases. *J Pediatr Adolesc Gynecol.* 2008; **21**:201.

Trager JDK. Vulvar dermatology. In Emans SJ, Laufer MR, Goldstein DP (eds.) *Emans, Laufer, Goldstein's Pediatric and Adolescent Gynecology* (6th edn.). Philadelphia, PA: Lippincott Williams and Wilkins, 2012; 381–404.

Pregnancy and Complications

Approximately 57 of 1000 women 15–19 years of age in the United States become pregnant each year. Spontaneous abortions complicate 8–31% of pregnancies, and approximately 2% are ectopic.

Clinical Presentation

Knowing whether a patient is pregnant is essential in evaluating her complaints and determining management. The first step is to interview the teenager privately and assure her that the discussion is confidential. Often the pregnant patient presents with vague complaints of "abdominal pain" or "not feeling right" because she does not want her family to suspect the possible pregnancy. The patient may not realize or may deny that she is pregnant. Also, she may not volunteer the information that she has missed a period or had unprotected intercourse.

During early pregnancy, a teenager may report "missing" her period or that it was "different" (longer or shorter than usual). Fatigue, dizziness, syncope, nausea with or without vomiting (especially in the morning), urinary frequency, and weight gain may be noted by two weeks. Nipple discharge (colostrum) can occur as early as six weeks.

On examination, the breasts have darkened areolae and enlarged nipples. Often, there is protrusion of Montgomery's glands. Findings on pelvic examination depend on the time elapsed since the first day of the last normal period. At five weeks the examination may be normal; at 6–7 weeks there may be softening of the uterus at the junction of the cervix (Hegar's sign); at 6–8 weeks the cervix and vaginal mucosa may have a bluish tinge due to venous congestion (Chadwick's sign) and the uterus may be soft and slightly enlarged; and by 8–12 weeks the fetal heart may be heard with Doppler. At 12 weeks, the globular uterus can be palpated at the level of the pubic symphysis; at 16 weeks at the midpoint between the symphysis and umbilicus; and at 20 weeks at the level of the umbilicus. However, the best way to estimate gestational age is to use a "pregnancy wheel." This tool will give an approximate gestational age based upon the first day of the patient's last period and the usual interval between her periods.

Threatened Abortion

With a threatened abortion, the history is compatible with early pregnancy. There is vaginal bleeding with or without pain. On examination, the os is closed and there is no tissue found in the vault. While there may be uterine and/or adnexal tenderness, cervical motion tenderness is notably absent.

Imminent Abortion

With an imminent abortion the cervix is dilated or open. The bleeding and pain are typically more severe than would be expected from a threatened abortion.

Inevitable Abortion

An inevitable abortion resembles an imminent abortion, except that there are products of conception protruding from the dilated or open cervix.

Incomplete Abortion

In an incomplete abortion, some placental tissue still remains in the uterus. The vaginal bleeding is usually heavy and the patient may complain of severe abdominal pain.

Complete Abortion

There is full passage of the products of conception. The patient may be asymptomatic on presentation but will likely have a history of abdominal pain, vaginal bleeding, and passage of tissue.

Missed Abortion

A missed abortion is a fetal death in utero before the 20th week, but with the pregnancy retained. If the patient knew she was pregnant, she may report that she does not feel fetal movement. Abdominal pain and/or vaginal bleeding are possible, but unlikely.

Ectopic Pregnancy

An ectopic pregnancy occurs when the blastocyst implants in a location other than the uterus; the vast majority are in the fallopian tubes. Major predisposing factors include pelvic inflammatory disease, prior pelvic or abdominal surgery, or prior ectopic pregnancy. However, about half of patients who have an ectopic pregnancy do not have an identifiable risk factor.

The classic presentation is a history of a delayed menstrual cycle, with symptoms of early pregnancy, followed by abdominal pain and mild to moderate vaginal bleeding. A late or missed period occurs in 75% of patients, followed by vaginal spotting or bleeding. Brisk or heavy bleeding is uncommon. The vast majority of patients will complain of abdominal pain which can be of any severity and in any location in the abdomen or pelvis. Up to 5–10% of patients may complain of fever.

Physical examination findings include abdominal and pelvic tenderness and cervical motion tenderness. An adnexal mass is found in up to 50%. If the ectopic pregnancy has ruptured, the patient may present with signs of hypovolemic shock.

Diagnosis

Pregnancy tests detect the presence of human chorionic gonadotropin (hCG) in the blood or urine. The standard urine pregnancy test is 99% sensitive and specific, detecting 25 mIU/mL of hCG. In normal pregnancies it may be positive as early as 3–4 days after implantation and virtually always by the expected date of the missed period. However, if the urine is not sufficiently concentrated there may be a false-negative finding.

The serum hCG by radioimmunoassay can be positive within seven days of conception (before a period has been missed). In most intrauterine pregnancies, the quantitative serum hCG will double every 1.5–2.3 days (about 36–55 hours). The doubling will slow somewhat when the level is >10,000–20,000 mIU/mL; however, by this time ultrasonography is diagnostic.

With an ectopic pregnancy, the hCG does not rise as fast. However, a single hCG measurement is of limited value, since the exact gestational age is often not known and there is some overlap in the range of hCG levels found in the two conditions. Therefore, obtain serial hCG determinations two days apart. Doubling of the hCG within 48 hours suggests an intrauterine pregnancy. A slower doubling time, or a rise of less than 66% over two days suggests, but does not confirm, an ectopic pregnancy. Up to 10–15% of normal pregnancies will have an abnormal serum hCG doubling time, and as many as one-third of

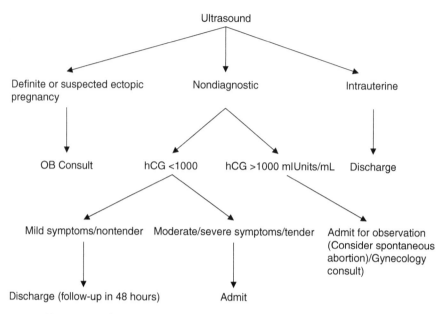

Figure 11.1 Management of suspected ectopic pregnancy.

ectopic pregnancies will have what is considered to be a normal serum hCG doubling time (>66% over two days).

The serum progesterone is useful for diagnosing an ectopic pregnancy. In a normal pregnancy, the level is >25 ng/mL, while a level <5 ng/mL is highly associated with an ectopic pregnancy. Values between 5–25 ng/mL are indeterminate. In this situation, obtain a diagnostic ultrasound.

It is not always safe to wait two days to confirm the diagnosis. Using transabdominal ultrasound, a normal intrauterine pregnancy can be detected with an hCG >6500 mIU/mL. However, transvaginal ultrasound is far more sensitive (90–95%) and can confirm the presence of a gestational sac at an hCG of 1000–1500 mIU/mL. However, discriminatory values will differ across medical centers. The diagnostic and therapeutic approach of ectopic pregnancy is summarized in Figure 11.1.

The differential diagnosis of ectopic pregnancy includes a normal pregnancy with another cause for the abdominal or pelvic pain. These include gynecologic conditions which may complicate pregnancy and can be evaluated by ultrasound, such as an ovarian cyst, ovarian or tubal torsion, or ruptured corpus luteum. Alternatively, the pathology may be non-gynecologic, such as an appendicitis, cholecystitis, or a renal stone.

ED Management

The priority is expedient diagnosis and management of an ectopic pregnancy. Suspect an ectopic pregnancy in any pubertal female with vaginal bleeding and/or lower abdominal pain, especially if her period is late. Perform a pelvic examination; any abnormality suggests the possibility of an ectopic pregnancy. Immediately arrange for gynecologic consultation, obtain blood for hCG, CBC, type and cross-match, insert a large-bore IV, and monitor the patient carefully, with frequent vital signs and serial hematocrits.

If a ruptured ectopic is likely (peritoneal signs, orthostatic vital sign changes, positive FAST [focused assessment with sonography for trauma], or falling hematocrit associated with a positive hCG), immediately consult with a gynecologist.

If a ruptured ectopic is not likely and the patient is not in shock, obtain an ultrasound and hCG and follow the management plan outlined in Figure 11.1. If the ultrasound is nondiagnostic and the hCG is <1000 mIU/mL, admit the patient if the symptoms (abdominal pain, cervical tenderness) are moderate or severe. If the patient has no abdominal tenderness, she may be discharged if reliable follow-up is guaranteed for outpatient serial hCG measurements every 48 hours. A normal increase suggests an intrauterine pregnancy, which must be confirmed by transvaginal ultrasound. Obtain obstetrical consultation for any patient with an abnormal hCG rise or no uterine pregnancy on ultrasound.

If the hCG is >1000 mIU/mL and the ultrasound is nondiagnostic, admit the patient for observation (possible spontaneous abortion) and obstetrical consultation. If the ultrasound is not immediately available, admit the patient for close observation, serial hCG measurements, and possible laparoscopy. Culdocentesis is indicated only if transvaginal ultrasound is not available. It is very specific: nonclotting blood in the cul-de-sac mandates surgical exploration. However, sensitivity is poor as "dry taps" can occur and straw-colored fluid excludes only a ruptured ectopic.

Consult an obstetrician to attempt medical management of a confirmed ectopic pregnancy if the fetus is <4 cm on ultrasound and the patient is hemodynamically stable. Single-dose methotrexate therapy will terminate >95% of ectopic pregnancies when the hCG is <5000 mIU/mL; it is more than 80% effective when the hCG is 5000–15000 mIU/mL.

Manage threatened abortions expectantly, with instructions to return for reevaluation if the bleeding continues for 48 hours or there are worsening symptoms. In such cases, hospitalize the patient and obtain a type and cross-match in case a transfusion becomes necessary (hemoglobin <7.0 g/dL; symptoms of hypovolemia not relieved by crystalloid fluid resuscitation).

Admit a patient with an imminent, inevitable, or incomplete abortion and consult with a gynecologist for dilation and curettage. In the ED insert a large-bore IV and obtain a CBC and a type and hold. Order a type and cross-match and begin fluid resuscitation with isotonic crystalloid (pp. 32–35) if the patient is symptomatic of acute blood loss. If the blood loss is severe (with an estimated need of four units of blood), also give platelets and fresh frozen plasma.

Discharge a patient with a complete abortion, unless there are signs of serious blood loss. In that case, insert a large-bore IV and obtain a CBC and type and cross-match.

Check the Rh status for any patient with a threatened, imminent, inevitable, complete, incomplete, or missed abortion or an ectopic pregnancy. If she is Rh negative, IM RhoGAM is required. Give a mini-dose (50 mcg) during the first trimester; use 300 mcg beyond the first trimester.

If a normal intrauterine pregnancy is diagnosed, make an appointment for the teenager (and her partner) to be seen within the next few days in an adolescent gynecology or family planning clinic for appropriate counseling and management. Social work referral may also be indicated.

Follow-up

- Possible ectopic pregnancy, without abdominal tenderness: at once for dizziness or abdominal pain; otherwise in 48 hours

Indications for Admission

- Ectopic pregnancy (confirmed or probable)
- Ectopic pregnancy unlikely (nondiagnostic ultrasound, hCG < 1000 mIU/mL), but follow-up not guaranteed
- Ultrasound nondiagnostic and hCG <1000 mIU/mL, but patient has moderate or severe abdominal pain or cervical motion tenderness
- Ultrasound nondiagnostic and hCG >1000 mIU/mL
- Imminent, inevitable, or incomplete abortion
- Severe acute blood loss

Bibliography

Barash JH, Buchanan EM, Hillson C. Diagnosis and management of ectopic pregnancy. *Am Fam Physician*. 2014;**90**(1):34–40.

Committee on Adolescence. Addendum: adolescent pregnancy – current trends and issues. *Pediatrics*. 2014;**133**(5):954–957.

Connolly A, Ryan DH, Stuebe AM, Wolfe HM. Reevaluation of discriminatory and threshold levels for serum β-hCG in early pregnancy. *Obstet Gynecol*. 2013;**121**(1):65–70.

Institute of Obstetricians and Gynaecologists, Royal College of Physicians of Ireland and Directorate of Clinical Strategy and Programmes, Health Service Executive. Clinical practice guideline: the diagnosis and management of ectopic pregnancy. www.hse.ie/eng/about/Who/clinical/natclinprog/o bsandgynaeprogramme/ectopicpregnancy.pdf (accessed June 20, 2017).

Yen S, Goyal MK, Hillard P. Adolescent gynecologic emergencies. *Adolesc Med State Art Rev*. 2015;**26** (3):473–483.

Sexually Transmitted Infections

In the United States, one in four teenagers will have a sexually transmitted infection (STI) before graduating from high school. Pelvic inflammatory disease (PID) is a common infection of young women which can have serious sequelae and significant morbidity.

PID is usually a polymicrobial infection caused by bacteria ascending from the vagina and cervix. *Neisseria gonorrhoeae* and *Chlamydia trachomatis* are responsible for many cases, and are present in as many as 50% of patients. These organisms can also cause cervicitis, urethritis, epididymitis, or proctitis.

Treponema pallidum, the agent responsible for syphilis, can cause severe systemic disease with long-term sequelae. Herpes simplex virus (HSV) is the agent responsible for the majority of genital ulcers in the United States, and while treatable, is incurable. Several strains of human papillomavirus (HPV) have been associated with cervical cancer. More commonly in adolescents, certain other strains of HPV cause genital warts. The HPV vaccine helps prevent infection by up to nine of the most common strains, seven of which cause cervical cancer. There is no cure for human immunodeficiency virus (HIV), but treatments continue to evolve. *Trichomonas* is a protozoan that causes vaginal discharge and inflammation.

Clinical Presentation

Cervicitis

Cervicitis can occur with *N. gonorrhoeae* and/or *C. trachomatis* infection. Other pathogens include *Ureaplasma, Mycoplasma, Bacteroides*, and *E. coli*. It is often associated with purulent discharge (especially gonorrhea), though it can be asymptomatic. On examination, the cervix is erythematous and friable, but there is no cervical motion tenderness.

Urethritis

Urethritis is the most common manifestation of STI in males, but it also occurs in females. Commonly, males with urethral infection are asymptomatic, although dysuria and a urethral discharge may occur. Classically, purulent discharge is associated with infection by *N. gonorrhea*. Non-gonococcal urethritis is most often caused by *C. trachomatis*, but many other organisms can be responsible, especially *Ureaplasma* and *Mycoplasma*. In females, chlamydia can cause an acute urethral syndrome with dysuria, urgency, suprapubic tenderness, and pyuria without hematuria or bacteriuria.

Epididymitis

Males may present with testicular pain and swelling, associated with epididymitis. This may mimic a testicular torsion. *N. gonorrhea* and *C. trachomatis* are the most common responsible organisms, but it may also occur after a viral infection.

Pelvic Inflammatory Disease

PID is an ascending infection of the upper genital tract. The term PID encompasses the diagnoses of endometritis, salpingitis, oophoritis, tubo-ovarian abscess, and peritonitis. It is often polymicrobial, with *C. trachomatis* and *N. gonorrhea* as the most common causes, although *Mycoplasma, Ureaplasma, Peptostreptococcus, Gardnerella, E. coli*, and others are also implicated. Often no causative organism is identified.

Patients can present with a spectrum of symptoms, from nonspecific lower abdominal pain to frank peritonitis. Other symptoms often include vaginal discharge, dyspareunia, irregular vaginal bleeding, and nausea and vomiting. Severe cases may present with high fever, shaking chills, and signs and symptoms of possible peritonitis (abdominal pain on cough or ambulating, tenderness to abdominal percussion, abdominal rigidity).

On pelvic examination, at least one of the following are present: cervical motion tenderness, adnexal tenderness, or uterine tenderness. A purulent cervical discharge may be noted, and there may be evidence of acute cervicitis. The WBC, ESR, and CRP may all be elevated.

In contrast, a common presentation is less dramatic, with lower abdominal pain and history of vaginal discharge as the only complaints. The patient may be afebrile, without significant vaginal discharge, and with a relatively normal WBC, ESR, and/or CRP. See Table 11.3 for a summary of diagnostic criteria for pelvic inflammatory disease.

Proctitis

Proctitis occurs most commonly in males who engage in receptive anal intercourse. Patients may present with a history of constipation, anal itching, rectal fullness, pain with defecation,

Table 11.3 Pelvic inflammatory disease diagnostic criteria

Minimum criteria (one or more must be present)

Cervical motion tenderness

Uterine tenderness

Adnexal tenderness (unilateral or bilateral)

Additional criteria (increases specificity of diagnosis)

Temperature (oral) >101 °F (38.3 °C)

Abnormal cervical or vaginal mucopurulent discharge

Abundant WBCs on saline microscopy of vaginal secretions

Elevated ESR

Elevated CRP

Laboratory documentation of cervical infection with *N. gonorrhea* or *C. trachomatis*

Note: Consider the patient's risk profile for acquiring STDs when deciding to initiate empiric treatment for PID. Adapted from Centers for Disease Control. Sexually transmitted diseases treatment guidelines, 2015 (updated July 27, 2016). *MMWR Recomm Rep.* 2015;64(RR-03):1–137.

change in bowel habits, or blood in stool. Mild local disease is common and may be accompanied only by an abnormal stool smear (leukocytes present).

Genital Herpes

Genital herpes is the most common cause of genital ulcers in the United States. Both HSV-2 and HSV-1 infections are implicated in genital outbreaks, but HSV-2 is more likely to cause recurrent outbreaks. The incubation period for primary infections can range from 2–12 days. Initially, vesicles appear, which then rupture within several days to become small, painful ulcers. The patient may complain of dysuria (due to contact of urine with the lesion) in addition to local burning. Inguinal nodes may enlarge and be tender, and about two-thirds of patients complain of a headache, fever, myalgias, and malaise. Some initial infections present only with the vesicles/ulcers, without the other symptoms. Symptoms may last up to three weeks. Recurrent herpes eruptions are less severe and shorter in duration (3–5 days).

Genital or Anogenital Warts

Condylomata acuminata, or anogenital warts, are caused by the human papillomavirus (HPV), commonly types 6 and 11. They can be located in most sites in the anogenital area, typically around the vaginal introitus or the penis, but can occur elsewhere, including the cervix, vagina, urethra, perineum, perianal skin, anus, and scrotum. Rarely, they may be caused by autoinoculation (i.e., if an adolescent has a wart on the hand). Anogenital warts are classically described as cauliflower-like growths, but they may be flat, papular, or pedunculated. Most are asymptomatic, but they may cause itching, burning, pain, or bleeding.

The HPV vaccine protects against wart-causing types 6 and 11, as well as several cancer-causing types, including 16 and 18, which cause the majority of changes on Pap smears and cervical cancer.

Trichomoniasis

Trichomoniasis, caused by *Trichomonas vaginalis*, is a sexually transmitted infection that most commonly causes vaginitis (pp. 343–346).

Syphilis

The hallmark of primary syphilis is the chancre, which develops 2–12 weeks after exposure. It appears as a painless ulcer with a smooth, clean base, raised indurated borders, and scanty yellow discharge. In males the chancre (usually 3 mm to 3 cm in size) is most frequently seen on the penis, scrotum, anus, lips, or in the mouth. In females, it occurs on the vulva, vagina, cervix, or urethra, lips, or in the mouth. Fifty percent of patients have more than one chancre, and enlarged, firm, painless regional lymph nodes are seen in 60–80% of patients. Untreated, the chancre resolves in 3–7 weeks, and the signs of secondary syphilis may appear 4–10 weeks after the primary lesion appears.

Several skin (and mucous membrane) eruptions are typical of secondary syphilis. Commonly, there are nonpruritic, well-demarcated, brownish red macules, papules, or pustules symmetrically distributed on the trunk and extremities. These are often found on the palms and soles, which distinguishes them from most other rashes.

Condylomata lata are highly contagious, flat, moist, pink papules that occur in warm, moist intertriginous areas. When the maculopapules involve the mucous membranes in the mouth, they appear as shallow gray ulcers called mucous patches. Other signs of secondary syphilis include "moth-eaten" alopecia and nontender, firm or rubbery lymphadenopathy. Constitutional symptoms, including low-grade fever, headache, fatigue, sore throat, weight loss, arthralgias, and myalgias, occasionally accompany the above findings.

Latent syphilis is an asymptomatic period of varying lengths, which may occur after the symptoms of secondary syphilis resolve. Tertiary syphilis is marked by neurodegenerative changes, blindness, and cardiac, auditory, or gummatous lesions.

Chancroid (*Haemophilus Ducreyi*)

Chancroid causes painful genital ulcers. It typically presents as single or multiple lesions, often with ragged edges and tender inguinal nodes. It is relatively uncommon in the United States, usually occurring in outbreaks, but it may be underdiagnosed.

Lymphogranuloma Venereum

Lymphogranuloma venereum (LGV) presents with tender inguinal or femoral lymphadenopathy ("buboes"). It is caused by three serotypes of *C. trachomatis* (L1, L2, L3). While it is also associated with ulcers, these are usually transient, and the patient typically seeks medical attention for late sequelae, such as large inguinal nodes or rectal strictures. LGV is rare in the United States and more often seen in males. In Europe, LGV proctitis is seen in men who have receptive anal sex.

Pubic Lice

Pediculosis pubis (p. 129) usually presents with itching in the pubic region, or a patient may notice lice or nits (eggs) in their pubic hair.

Diagnosis

When a patient presents with lower abdominal pain, obtain a thorough adolescent history, without the parent present. Important questions to ask include those regarding sexual activity, including most recent sexual intercourse, number of new partners in the previous three months, number of lifetime partners, types of sexual activity (vaginal, oral, anal), history of previous sexually transmitted infections (STI), and condom use.

Cervicitis

A cervicitis may be diagnosed clinically via visualization of cervical inflammation or mucopurulent discharge from the cervical os, or if there is friability of the cervix on swab collection. In order to distinguish between cervicitis and PID (see below) in a symptomatic patient, perform a pelvic examination, which allows for direct visualization of the cervix, as well as a bimanual examination to assess for cervical motion or adnexal tenderness, which are consistent with the diagnosis of PID. Also send a cervical swab to evaluate for gonorrhea and chlamydia. Most often, cervicitis secondary to *N. gonorrhea* or *C. trachomatis* is diagnosed by laboratory testing of either a cervical swab obtained in the context of a pelvic exam, or via screening with a urine nucleic acid amplification test (NAAT).

Urethritis

Send a urine NAAT for the diagnosis of gonorrhea and chlamydia in males. Alternatively, insert a urethral swab to obtain specimens for NAAT. In refractory cases, send culture of urethral secretions and first-void urinalysis to test for *T. vaginalis.*

Epididymitis

Send a urine NAAT for *N. gonorrhea* and *C. trachomatis.* Alternatively, obtain a urethral swab for NAAT. Send a urinalysis to assess for pyuria or bacteriuria.

Pelvic Inflammatory Disease

The priorities are to identify PID, which is a clinical diagnosis, and to rule-out an ectopic pregnancy. A history of new or multiple sexual partners, previous sexually transmitted infections, or a report of inconsistent or absent condom use increases the likelihood of PID as the diagnosis. Ask the patient about her menstrual history, including the time of her last menstrual period. Also ask about the presence of irregular bleeding, which can suggest infection. Given the morbidity associated with untreated PID (sterility, increased risk of ectopic pregnancy, chronic pelvic pain), it is important to have a low index of suspicion in diagnosing PID.

Perform a careful abdominal examination. Look for evidence of pregnancy and surgical scars on the abdomen. A crucial part of the physical assessment of a patient suspected of having PID is the pelvic examination. An external exam is important to evaluate for evidence of other STIs (herpes, warts). The speculum exam allows the provider to examine the cervix for signs of cervicitis, assess discharge amount and character, and obtain samples for laboratory evaluation. Bimanual examination is a key component. Begin treatment for PID if the patient has cervical motion tenderness, uterine tenderness, and/or adnexal tenderness, if other diagnoses can be ruled out.

Although PID can be definitively diagnosed via laparoscopy, this is invasive and rarely indicated. Pelvic ultrasound may be useful to diagnose a tubo-ovarian abscess but may miss endometritis or salpingitis.

In the differential diagnosis of PID, also consider gastroenteritis (diarrhea), inflammatory bowel disease (weight loss, bloody stools, change in bowel pattern), acute appendicitis (right lower quadrant pain and tenderness), urinary tract infection (suprapubic or flank pain, dysuria, bacteriuria in association with pyuria), right lower lobe pneumonia (cough, tachypnea, rales, right upper quadrant pain) and, rarely, cholecystitis (right upper quadrant pain). The pelvic exam may be abnormal in any condition that can cause peritonitis. Always consider an ectopic pregnancy and send a pregnancy test when there has been amenorrhea or abnormal menses preceding the episode.

Fitz-Hugh–Curtis syndrome (perihepatitis) occurs in up to 20% of patients with PID and presents with right upper quadrant pain, occasionally accompanied by right-sided pleuritic chest and shoulder pain and normal liver function tests. Less commonly, a patient may have Fitz-Hugh–Curtis syndrome without symptoms of PID. The causative organisms are the same as those for PID, although *N. gonorrhea* or *C. trachomatis* may or may not be identified on cervical or urine diagnostic testing.

Proctitis

Perform a thorough anal inspection to assess for external lesions (HSV, HPV, hemorrhoids), as well as a rectal examination to assess for tenderness. Send a urine NAAT (or cervical swab in females), and a rectal swab for gonorrhea and chlamydia cultures. NAAT swabs for gonorrhea and chlamydia may be more sensitive than culture, but are not currently FDA-approved for rectal samples.

Herpes

Maintain a reasonably high index of suspicion, as herpes lesions may be misdiagnosed as folliculitis, dermatitis, latex allergy, or medical illnesses that present with genital ulcers, such as EBV, Behçet's disease, or Crohn's disease. Viral culture or PCR assay of an active lesion are now the gold standards for diagnosis, although PCR is more sensitive than culture. Swab the vesicular fluid or ulcerated lesions, or send vesicular scrapings. Serum testing for HSV-1 and HSV-2 antibodies is not as useful, as a positive serology only indicates that an infection has occurred at some time in the past. Typing HSV does have some relevance for patient counseling in that HSV-2 is more likely to recur.

Genital Warts

Genital warts are diagnosed by inspection; HPV testing is not recommended. Arrange for a biopsy if the patient is immunocompromised, the diagnosis is in doubt, or there is no response to treatment.

Syphilis

Suspect all genital lesions of being syphilis. Chancres can be confused with chancroid (multiple soft, tender ulcers; very tender contiguous adenopathy), granuloma inguinale (red, beefy, granulating painless lesion without adenopathy), lymphogranuloma venereum (transient vesicular, papular, or pustular ulceration with markedly enlarged tender nodes), or lichen planus (annular flat-topped papules). Also, rule-out herpes (multiple, superficial, painful lesions), pyogenic granuloma (single, painful, erythematous lesion that often looks like ground beef), molluscum contagiosum (grouped, umbilicated, flesh-colored papules, similar lesions elsewhere on the body), and condyloma accuminatum (dry, single or clustered, warty lesions). The maculopapular eruption of pityriasis rosea is not present on the palms and soles, although it can otherwise resemble the rash of secondary syphilis. The scaly plaques of psoriasis can be on the penis and elsewhere on the body.

If syphilis is suspected, send a non-treponemal serologic test for syphilis (RPR or VDRL). Approximately 25% of patients with primary syphilis have a negative RPR or VDRL, especially within the first 3–5 weeks after the initial infection. Therefore, if syphilis is likely and the RPR or VDRL is negative, send a treponemal serologic test (FTA-ABS), which has greater sensitivity than the VDRL or RPR. If the VDRL or RPR is positive, follow this with a confirmatory treponemal test (FTA-ABS or TP-PA), as false-positive non-treponemal tests occur in several medical conditions unrelated to syphilis (measles, chicken pox, mumps, HSV, viral pneumonia, pregnancy, malaria, SLE, hemolytic anemia, HIV).

The non-treponemal antibody titer correlates with disease activity: A four-fold rise in titer (e.g., 1:8 to 1:32) is diagnostic of active infection, while a four-fold drop confirms treatment response. Treponemal tests remain positive throughout life for 75–85% of patients, so they cannot be used to assess treatment response. Samples of tissue or exudates from lesions may also be sent for darkfield microscopy or direct fluorescent antibody (DFA) for the definitive diagnosis of syphilis.

Chancroid and LGV

A high index of suspicion is necessary for making these diagnoses. The diagnosis of chancroid is made clinically by excluding syphilis and herpes, as it is extremely difficult to culture *Haemophilus ducreyi*. LGV is diagnosed by clinical suspicion or *C. trachomatis* culture.

Pubic Lice

The diagnosis of lice is made by inspection. Live lice appear as small (1–4 mm), moving particles resembling dandruff flakes, and nits are firmly attached to the side of hair shafts. Nits fluoresce (white or gray) under a Wood's lamp.

ED Management

The antibiotic treatment of STIs is summarized in Table 11.4. Obtain a pregnancy test for all females before initiating any antibiotic treatment.

Cervicitis

Treat afebrile patients on an outpatient basis with oral antibiotics. Schedule a follow-up office visit within one week of completing therapy, and emphasize both the avoidance of intercourse until the patient's partner is cultured and treated, and the use of condoms to prevent both future infections and pregnancy. Check local state laws to see if expedited partner treatment for chlamydia is permitted.

Urethritis

Treat a male with presumptive or definite urethritis and schedule primary care follow-up visit in one week. The partner(s) must also be tested and treated. Treat a female with acute urethral symptoms for chlamydial urethritis, and schedule a follow-up office visit.

Table 11.4 Treatment of sexually transmitted infections

Chlamydia trachomatis: Urethritis, cervicitis, and proctitis (for epididymitis and pelvic inflammatory disease, see below)

Preferred regimens

Azithromycin 1 g PO as one dose *or* doxycycline[1] 100 mg PO bid × 7 days

Alternative Regimens (all for 7-day course)

Erythromycin 500 mg PO qid *or* ofloxacin[2] 300 mg PO bid *or* levofloxacin[2] 500 mg PO daily

Neisseria gonorrhea: Urethritis, cervicitis, pharyngitis, and proctitis (for epididymitis and pelvic inflammatory disease, see below)

Preferred regimens

Ceftriaxone 250 mg IM *or* cefixime 400 mg PO *plus* azithromycin 1 g PO × 1

Alternative regimens

Gemfloxacin 320 mg PO × 1 *or* gentamicin 240 mg IM × 1 *plus* azithromycin 2 g PO × 1[3]

Epididymitis

Preferred regimen

Ceftriaxone 250 mg IM once *plus* doxycycline[1] 100 mg PO bid × 10 days

Alternative regimen

Ofloxacin[2] 300 mg orally twice a day for 10 days[4] *or* levofloxacin[2] 500 mg orally once daily for 10 days[4]

Pelvic inflammatory disease: inpatient

Preferred regimens

Cefoxitin 2 g IV q 6h *or* cefotetan 2 g IV q 6h *plus* doxycycline[1] 100 mg PO *or* IV q 12h, until improved

Clindamycin 900 mg IV q 8h *plus* gentamicin 2 mg/kg IV once, *followed by* gentamicin 1.5 mg/kg IV q 8h, until improved

Alternative regimen

Ampicillin/sulbactam 3 g IV q 6h plus doxycycline[1] 100 mg PO or IV q 12h, until improved

Once the patient is improved on any of these regimens: give doxycycline[1] 100 mg PO bid to complete a 14-day course.

If the patient does not improve in first 48–72 hours: add metronidazole 500 mg PO bid to the above regimens

Pelvic inflammatory disease: outpatient

Preferred regimen

Ceftriaxone 250 mg IM once, *plus* doxycycline[1] 100 mg PO bid × 14 days *with or without* metronidazole 500 mg PO bid × 14 days

Alternative regimens

Cefoxitin 2 g IM once *plus* probenecid 1 g PO once, *plus* doxycycline[1] 100 mg PO bid × 14 days *with or without metronidazole* 500 mg PO bid × 14 days

Table 11.4 (cont.)

An alternative third-generation cephalosporin (ceftizoxime, cefotaxime) *plus* doxycycline[1] 100 mg PO bid × 14 days *with or without* metronidazole 500 mg PO bid × 14 days

Ofloxacin[2] 400 mg PO bid × 14 days *with or without* metronidazole 500 mg PO bid × 14 days

Levofloxacin[2] 500 mg PO daily × 14 days *with or without* metronidazole 500 mg PO bid × 14 days

Herpes simplex

First episode

Acyclovir 400 mg PO tid × 7–10 days *or* 200 mg PO 5 times/day × 7–10 days *or* valacyclovir 1 g PO bid × 7–10 days

or famciclovir 250 mg PO tid × 7–10 days

Recurrent

Acyclovir 400 mg PO tid × 5 days *or* 800 mg PO bid × 5 days *or* 800 mg PO tid × 2 days *or* valacyclovir 500 mg PO bid × 3 days

or 1 g PO daily × 5 days *or* famciclovir 125 mg PO bid × 5 days *or* 1 g PO bid × 1 day

Daily suppressive therapy

Acyclovir 400 mg PO bid *or* valacyclovir 500 mg to 1 g PO daily *or* famciclovir 250 mg PO bid

Genital warts (HPV)

External anogenital warts: patient-applied

Podofilox 0.5% solution or gel: apply to visible warts bid for 3 days, followed by 4 days of no therapy

May repeat for up to four cycles

Imiquimod 5% cream: apply to warts once daily at bedtime, 3 times a week for 8–16 weeks

Instruct patient to wash with soap and water 6–10 hours later

Sinecatechins 15% ointment: apply tid (0.5 cm strand to each wart) for no longer than 16 weeks; do not wash off after use

External anogenital warts: provider-administered

Podophyllin resin[5] 10–25% in compound tincture of benzoin; apply to wart(s) once weekly and allow to air-dry

Trichloroacetic acid (TCA) or bichloroacetic acid (BCA) 80–90%. Apply to wart(s) once weekly and allow to air-dry

Cryotherapy with liquid nitrogen or cryoprobe; repeat every 1–2 weeks

Surgical removal or intralesional interferon or laser surgery

Intra-anal warts

Cryotherapy with liquid nitrogen or TCA or BCA 80–90% (as above) or surgical removal

Vaginal warts

Cryotherapy with liquid nitrogen (avoid cryoprobe for risk of vaginal perforation/fistula formation) or TCA or BCA 80–90% (as above) or surgical removal

Table 11.4 (cont.)

Cervical warts

Cryotherapy with liquid nitrogen or TCA or BCA 80–90% (as above) or surgical removal in consultation with a specialist

Refer to a gynecologist for cervical exophytic warts, as precancerous changes must be ruled out via biopsy before treatment

Urethral meatus warts

Cryotherapy with liquid nitrogen or surgical removal

Trichomoniasis

Preferred regimen
Metronidazole 2 g PO in one dose

Alternative regimens

Tinidazole 2 g PO in one dose *or* metronidazole 500 mg PO bid × 7 days

Syphilis

Primary, secondary, and early latent (<1 year)

Preferred regimen

Benzathine penicillin G 2.4 million units IM as a single dose

Alternative regimens

Doxycycline[1] 100 mg PO bid × 14 days *or* tetracycline 500 mg PO 4 times daily × 14 days

Late–latent (duration >1 year) and tertiary

Preferred regimen

Benzathine penicillin G 2.4 million units IM weekly × 3 weeks

Alternative regimen

Doxycycline[1] 100 mg PO bid × 4 weeks *or* tetracycline 500 mg PO qid × 4 weeks

Chancroid

Azithromycin 1 g PO once *or* ceftriaxone 250 mg IM once *or* ciprofloxacin[2] 500 mg PO bid × 3 days *or* erythromycin 500 mg PO tid × 7 days

Lymphogranuloma venereum (LGV)

Preferred regimen

Doxycycline[1] 100 mg PO bid × 21 days

Alternative regimen

Erythromycin 500 mg PO 4 times daily × 21 days

Pediculosis

Preferred regimen

Permethrin 1% cream (or pyrethrins with piperonyl butoxide): apply to pubic area and leave for 10 minutes, then wash out

Wash affected clothing and bedding.

Alternative regimens

Table 11.4 (cont.)

Malathion 0.5% lotion applied for 8–12 hours and washed off *or* ivermectin 250 mcg/kg, repeat in 2 weeks

Note: if the infestation persists despite above treatment, use lindane[6] shampoo (apply for 4 min)

[1] Use only if >8 years old and not pregnant.
[2] Quinolones are no longer recommended as first-line treatment for uncomplicated gonococcal infections. They may be used in PID treatment if cephalosporins are unavailable and the community prevalence and individual risk of gonorrhea is low.
[3] Azithromycin 2 g PO × 1 as monotherapy for uncomplicated gonococcal infection may be effective, but is not recommended by the CDC due to increasing resistance.
[4] For acute epididymitis most likely caused by enteric organisms or with negative gonococcal culture or NAAT.
[5] Limit application to <0.5 mL podophyllin or to an affected area <10 cm^2 per session.
[6] Use only if other treatments fail. Risk of toxicity (seizure, aplastic anemia) is low with the recommended four-minute exposure.
Adapted from Centers for Disease Control and Prevention. Sexually transmitted diseases treatment guidelines, 2015 (updated July 27, 2016). *MMWR Recomm Rep.* 2015;64(RR-03):1–137. www.cdc.gov/std/tg2015/

Epididymitis

Treat with an oral outpatient regimen and schedule primary care follow-up visit in 72 hours.

Pelvic Inflammatory Disease

Since PID is a clinical diagnosis, initiate antibiotic therapy immediately once the laboratory assessment is completed. Obtain a GC/chlamydia sample via either cervical swab or urine test. Also send a wet preparation to evaluate for trichomoniasis, bacterial vaginosis, and yeast. Obtain an RPR screen for syphilis and a urine hCG, and offer HIV testing. Obtain a CBC, along with either an ESR or CRP, as elevation(s) are indicative, though not specific, for PID. If the patient has right upper quadrant pain consistent with Fitz-Hugh–Curtis syndrome, obtain LFTs. Since Fitz-Hugh–Curtis syndrome is a perihepatitis, the LFTs will be normal, while elevations suggest another diagnosis (hepatitis, gall bladder disease). A pelvic sonogram is indicated if tubo-ovarian abscess is suspected, or if the patient does not improve despite treatment.

Admit the patient for IV therapy if she is ill-appearing, pregnant, vomiting and unable to tolerate food or drink, at high risk of noncompliance, has previously failed outpatient therapy, has a tubo-ovarian abscess, or if surgical emergency (e.g., appendicitis) cannot be ruled out. If the diagnosis is in doubt, obtain an adolescent medicine or gynecology consult.

If the patient is to be treated with an outpatient antibiotic regimen, it is important to arrange a follow-up visit within 48–72 hours for reevaluation via bimanual examination. Also, remind the patient that the sexual partner(s) must be evaluated and treated. If the patient is not currently using hormonal contraception, this is an opportunity to offer it.

Proctitis

Treat proctitis on an outpatient basis and schedule primary care follow-up in one week.

Herpes

Treatment of primary herpes will shorten the duration of symptoms, decrease the amount of viral shedding, and prevent the formation of new lesions. It is not curative, nor does it prevent later recurrences. Refer the patient for primary care follow-up in one week, at which time suppressive therapy can be discussed.

Genital Warts

Treat with patient-applied regimens and arrange for follow-up in one week with an adolescent medicine provider, gynecologist, or dermatologist. Alternatively, refer to one of the above physicians for provider-applied treatments, such as podophyllin, trichloro-acetic acid, or cryotherapy.

Syphilis

Treat as an outpatient and schedule a primary care follow-up visit in one week. Arrange for the evaluation and treatment of all sexual partners, and remind the patient to avoid sexual activity until that time. Of note, the Jarisch–Herxheimer reaction may occur within the first 24 hours of treatment for syphilis. It is characterized by fever, headache, myalgia, tachycardia, and mild hypotension, and can occur in the treatment of primary, secondary, and early latent syphilis. In pregnant women, the reaction may cause early labor or fetal distress, but this risk is not a contraindication to treatment.

Chancroid

Clinical response to the treatment of chancroid can be seen within seven days. Evaluate and treat any individuals with whom the patient had sexual contact within ten days preceding the onset of symptoms.

Lymphogranuloma Venereum

Treat on an outpatient basis and schedule primary care follow-up in one week.

Pubic Lice

Treat on an outpatient basis and schedule primary care follow-up in one week.

Follow-up
- Pelvic inflammatory disease: adolescent medicine, gynecology, or ED follow-up in 48–72 hours for repeat bimanual examination
- Epididymitis: follow-up in 72 hours for reevaluation
- Cervicitis, proctitis, urethritis, chancroid, primary or recurrent herpes, LGV, pubic lice: primary care follow-up in one week
- Genital warts: adolescent medicine, gynecology or dermatology follow-up in 1–2 weeks
- Syphilis: one week for follow-up

Indications for Admission
- Pelvic inflammatory disease: ill appearance, unable to tolerate oral intake, concurrent pregnancy, tubo-ovarian abscess, uncertain diagnosis (i.e., cannot rule-out appendicitis), prior treatment failure, high likelihood of noncompliance

Bibliography

Centers for Disease Control and Prevention. Recommendations for the laboratory-based detection of *Chlamydia trachomatis* and *Neisseria gonorrhoeae* – 2014. *MMWR Recomm Rep.* 2014; **63**(RR-02):1–19.

Sauerbrei A. Optimal management of genital herpes: current perspectives. *Infect Drug Resist.* 2016;**9**:129–141.

Woods JL, Scurlock AM, Hensel DJ. Pelvic inflammatory disease in the adolescent: understanding diagnosis and treatment as a health care provider. *Pediatr Emerg Care.* 2013;**29**(6):720–725.

Workowski KA, Bolan GA, Centers for Disease Control and Prevention. Sexually transmitted diseases treatment guidelines, 2015. *MMWR Recomm Rep.* 2015;**64**(RR-03):1–137.

Vaginal Discharge and Vulvovaginitis

Vulvovaginitis is a common problem in prepubertal and pubertal girls. Prepubertal girls are particularly susceptible to vulvovaginitis secondary to irritation by soaps, chemicals, and clothing because of their thin vulvar epithelium and the lack of estrogenic stimulation. In addition, they are prone to poor hygiene and contamination with bowel flora, due to the proximity of the anus to the vaginal opening. In pubertal girls, sexual activity is the major etiologic factor of vulvovaginitis, and vaginal discharge is a common presenting complaint. In both prepubertal and pubertal girls, the wearing of nonabsorbent nylon underwear or tights, nylon bathing suits, ballet leotards, or tight-fitting jeans also provide an environment conducive for bacterial infection, particularly in hot weather.

Clinical Presentation

Prepubertal Girls

Nonspecific Vaginitis

Up to 75% of prepubertal vaginitis is nonspecific. This includes chemical vulvovaginitis, most commonly from harsh soaps or bubble bath. These girls present with vulvar and/or vaginal inflammation that is generally low-grade but persistent. There may be associated dysuria, pruritus, and discharge. If there is no obvious etiology for the complaint and a culture is obtained, it will be negative or grow normal flora (lactobacilli, *Staphylococcus epidermidis*).

Bacterial Infections

Specific bacterial infections occur most often with respiratory, enteric, or sexually trans-mitted infections. Group A *Streptococcus* vulvovaginitis can result from self-inoculation from a nasopharyngeal or a skin infection, and causes a distinctive bright red appearance to the vulva and/or peri-anal areas. *Staphylococcus aureus* can cause a vaginal infection in association with impetigo of the vulva or buttocks. *Haemophilus influenzae* and *Streptococcus pneumoniae* are other common infections of the respiratory tract that can cause vulvovaginitis.

Enteric organisms, such as *Shigella*, can cause a bloody discharge, usually in a girl who has recently had gastroenteritis. *Escherichia coli* may be found in the flora of asymptomatic prepubertal girls, but it is more common in those with complaints of vulvovaginitis.

Sexually Transmitted Infections

Infections with *Neisseria gonorrhea* and *Chlamydia trachomatis* present with copious green or yellow purulent discharge, which may be associated with labial swelling, dysuria, and genital pruritus. The vagina may be inflamed and excoriated. Suspect child abuse and alert Child Protective Services whenever a sexually transmitted disease is diagnosed in a prepubertal child. Although there is often no report of sexual contact in these cases, nonsexual acquisition of these organisms is exceedingly rare. Herpes infection of the vulva may be due to autoinoculation from an oral lesion and might not be sexually transmitted. *Trichomonas* infection is rare in prepubertal girls, but its presence is suspicious for sexual abuse.

Candidal Infection

Candida vulvovaginitis is rare in prepubertal girls, unless the child has recently finished a course of antibiotics, has diabetes, is immunosuppressed, or wears diapers.

Foreign Body

A vaginal foreign body produces a foul-smelling discharge which can be bloody. Toilet paper remnants are the most common objects found.

Pinworm

Pinworm (*Enterobius vermicularis*) presents with pruritus of the anus and/or vulva. It can also occur in adolescents but is much more common in younger children.

Pubertal Girls

In addition to vulvar or vaginal irritation, a discharge is extremely common. It may be associated with pruritus, foul odor, or dysuria, often in association with pyuria. Symptoms of vulvovaginitis may occur with STIs (gonorrhea, *Chlamydia*, *Trichomonas*), infections not usually associated with sexual contact (*Candida*, bacterial vaginosis), or a foreign body, or it may be physiologic leukorrhea.

Gonorrhea and Chlamydia

Adolescents may complain of a vaginal discharge, although the infection most often presents as a cervicitis. Abdominal pain along with discharge may indicate pelvic inflammatory disease (see pp. 331–335).

Trichomonas Vaginalis

Trichomoniasis is a relatively common sexually acquired infection caused by the motile, flagellated parasite *Trichomonas vaginalis*. A green-gray, thin, malodorous discharge occurs, often associated with pruritus or dyspareunia. There may also be abdominal pain, post-coital bleeding, and/or dysuria.

Candida Albicans

Candida is a common cause of vaginitis in the general adolescent population. Diabetes mellitus, immunosuppression, a recent course of antibiotics, pregnancy, obesity, and tight-fitting undergarments are risk factors. Sexual activity rarely plays a role in transmission and partners do not routinely need treatment.

Candida presents with a thick, white, cheesy discharge in association with pruritus, inflammation, and edema of the vulva, which can be associated with dysuria and/or dyspareunia. Alternatively, the discharge may be thin and watery.

Bacterial Vaginosis

Bacterial vaginosis (BV) is a common cause of vaginal discharge and inflammation, caused by a complex alteration of the microbial flora in the vagina. It results from an increase in the concentration of (among others) *Gardnerella vaginalis*, anaerobic organisms such as *Bacteroides* and *Mobiluncus* species, and *Mycoplasma hominis*, in association with a decrease in normal hydrogen peroxide-producing flora such as *Lactobacillus*. BV classically presents with a grayish-white, thin, malodorous discharge. The characteristic "fishy" odor is caused by the overgrowth of the above organisms, resulting in increased vaginal pH and the subsequent production of amines. Evaluate the patient for possible PID if there is associated lower abdominal pain.

Foreign body

In adolescents, a retained tampon is the most common object causing vaginitis. A foul-smelling, purulent discharge that may be bloody is typically present.

Contact Reaction

A contact vaginitis may be caused by soap, bubble bath, douche, perfume, or contraceptive foam or jelly.

Physiologic Leukorrhea

Adolescents may sometimes complain of a clear-white or mucoid discharge, either prior to menses or at mid-cycle. The discharge is nonpathologic, composed of epithelial cells and endocervical mucus. There is no evidence of inflammation.

Psychosocial Etiologies

With psychosocial issues, such as sexual molestation and school phobia, the patient's complaints are not consistent with the objective findings.

Diagnosis

Priorities on the physical examination are the breasts (Tanner stage), abdomen (tenderness, pregnancy, mass), and inguinal area (lymphadenopathy). Next, inspect the introitus for Tanner stage, inflammation, swelling, presence of discharge, and signs of trauma.

The vaginal examination of the prepubertal child may be challenging, but most often can be accomplished without sedation or anesthesia. Reassure the child that the examination will not hurt and ask the mother to remain in the room. Have the child lie supine, with her feet together and her knees apart ("frog-leg" position). Alternatively, in an older child, use the lithotomy position. In some children, the examination is more easily performed with the patient lying prone, in a knee–chest position, with the buttocks in the air and the knees 6–8 inches apart. Instruct her to relax and let her belly sag downward (a pillow may be placed below the abdomen), then gently spread the labia to view the vagina.

In an adolescent, an external genital exam is necessary. If she has complaints of abdominal pain, or has a high-risk history for having acquired a sexually transmitted disease, a speculum exam is indicated, but defer it if she is virginal. If the discharge is bloody, purulent, or particularly foul-smelling, carefully inspect the vagina for a foreign body. If a foreign body is suspected in a virginal female, palpate the vagina during a rectal exam.

Perform a wet prep on a sample of every vaginal discharge. After the specimen is obtained with a cotton swab, place it in a test tube containing a small amount of room-temperature saline. Place several drops of this solution on a slide, and observe under high power. Budding yeast are seen with candidal infection, with pseudohyphae noted; these may be more easily visualized after adding 10% potassium hydroxide (KOH). Trichomonads appear as live, flagellated, motile organisms. Examine the wet prep within 15 minutes of preparation to decrease the chance of *Trichomonas* losing their motility, swelling, or bursting. The wet prep is positive in up to 83% of *Candida* infections and 70% of *Trichomonas* infections. If *Trichomonas* infection is suspected, a pelvic examination is indicated, with further testing as below. BV is likely if three out of the following four criteria are met:

- presence of a homogeneous white non-inflammatory discharge adherent to the vaginal walls;
- discharge pH ≥ 4.5;
- the odor of the discharge sample becomes fishy or amine-like with the addition of KOH (positive "whiff test");
- the wet prep has clue cells (epithelial cells stippled with dark granules) noted in at least 20% of cells.

See Table 11.5 for a summary of the differences between candidal infection, BV, and trichomoniasis.

If a pelvic examination is indicated, obtain a cervical swab to test for gonorrhea and *Chlamydia*, as well as *Trichomonas* via NAAT, if available. If no (internal) pelvic exam was performed, send a vaginal swab or a urine sample for gonorrhea, *Chlamydia* and

Table 11.5 Differential diagnosis of vaginal discharge in pubertal girls

	Discharge	Vaginal pH	Whiff test*	WBCs	Wet prep
Bacterial vaginosis	White, gray, green Malodorous	>4.5	Present	Rare	>20% clue cells
Candida	"Cottage cheese"	≤4.5	Absent	Rare to ↑	Pseudohyphae or budding yeast
Trichomoniasis	Odorless, white, gray, green	Often >4.5	Possible	Can be ↑	Motile, flagellated trichomonads

* Whiff test: amine odor after the addition of 10% KOH
Adapted from Sexually transmitted infections. In Strasburger VC, Brown RT, Braverman PK, et al. (eds.) *Adolescent Medicine: A Handbook for Primary Care*. Philadelphia, PA: Lippincott Williams and Wilkins. 2006.

Trichomonas. In men, a urine NAAT for *Trichomonas* may be available (in addition to gonorrhea and *Chlamydia*), depending on laboratory validation.

ED Management

Prepubertal Girls

Nonspecific Vaginitis

Treat with warm-water sitz baths once or twice per day. Discuss proper hygiene techniques, such as front-to-back wiping, use of cotton underwear, not wearing tight-fitting pants, and avoiding wearing wet clothing (such as bathing suits). Recommend applying a small amount of an emollient (petrolatum, A&D) to protect the vulvar skin. If symptoms persist after 2–3 weeks reevaluate the patient for the possibility of a foreign body or infection. Prescribe amoxicillin (40 mg/kg/day div tid) or amoxicillin-clavulanate (45 mg/kg/day of amoxicillin div bid) for ten days if there is a purulent discharge despite negative cultures.

Gonorrhea and *Chlamydia*

In the prepubertal age group, a positive test for gonorrhea or *Chlamydia* is indicative of sexual abuse. For gonorrhea, treat with a single dose of IM ceftriaxone (<45 kg: 25–50 mg/kg 125 mg maximum; ≥45 kg: 250 mg). If the patient has an allergy to beta-lactams, consult with a pediatric infectious disease specialist to determine the appropriate treatment. Treat *Chlamydia* with erythromycin (<45 kg: 50 mg/kg/day div qid × 14 days; ≥45 kg: azithromycin 1 g orally in a single dose). Doxycycline is an alternative for a patient >8 years of age (100 mg bid for seven days). Report the case to the Child Protection Services.

Other Bacterial Etiologies

If the culture is positive, treat with a culture-specific antibiotic for 7–10 days.

Foreign Bodies

Usually, removal can be accomplished with forceps. On occasion, sedation or general anesthesia is required.

Pinworms

If pinworms are suspected by a history of rectal itching or characteristic adult thread-like worms are seen on the stool, treat with mebendazole (p. 389).

Pubertal Girls

Candida Albicans

Treat with topical azole (clotrimazole, miconazole, or terconazole) vaginal creams or suppositories for one week. In complicated patients (immunosuppressed, diabetic, pregnant), prescribe a 10–14-day course. Topical azoles may weaken condoms or diaphragms. As an alternative, give a single PO dose of fluconazole (150 mg); a longer course may be necessary for complicated patients (above). Advise the patient to avoid pantyhose and tight clothes. Continue treatment during menses, but it is generally not necessary to treat sexual partner(s).

Trichomonas

Treat with one oral dose of metronidazole (2 g) or tinidazole (2 g). Alternatively, prescribe metronidazole 500 mg PO bid for seven days. Advise the patient to avoid alcohol during treatment and for 72 hours afterwards, since alcohol consumption while taking metronidazole can lead to nausea, vomiting, flushing, and tachycardia. As trichomoniasis is a sexually transmitted disease, treat all sexual partners.

Bacterial Vaginosis

Treat with oral metronidazole 500 mg bid for seven days and advise against alcohol consumption (as above). Alternative regimens are metronidazole 0.75% gel, one applicator intravaginally daily for five days, or clindamycin 2% cream, one full applicator intravaginally nightly for seven days. It is not necessary to treat sexual partner(s). Oral metronidazole is indicated for symptomatic pregnant women and asymptomatic pregnant women at risk for pre-term delivery.

Foreign Bodies

These can usually be removed with forceps or via warm saline irrigation.

Contact Reaction

Avoidance of the offending agent is usually all that is required. Treat severe pruritus with diphenhydramine (5 mg/kg/day div q 6h) or hydroxyzine (2 mg/kg/day div tid). A low- to mid-potency topical corticosteroid cream (i.e., hydrocortisone 1% or triamcinolone 0.025–0.1%) for 2–3 days and sodium bicarbonate baths (2–4 tablespoons of baking soda in the tub) may also help.

Physiologic Leukorrhea

No treatment is necessary, aside from reassurance, although panty liners may be helpful.

Psychosocial Etiologies

Have an experienced interviewer speak with the patient to attempt to ascertain if sexual molestation has occurred. Refer all patients without a definite etiology to a primary care provider.

Follow-up

- Prepubertal girl with nonspecific vaginitis, or culture-proven bacterial vaginitis: primary care follow-up in 7–10 days
- Pubertal girl with vaginitis: primary care follow-up

Indications for Admission

- Suspected sexual abuse, if the patient's family is unable to provide the necessary support
- Severe vulvovaginitis with urinary retention or systemic signs (fever, toxicity)

Bibliography

Berlan ED, Emans SJ, O'Brien RF. Vulvovaginal complaints in the adolescent. In Emans SJ, Laufer MR, Goldstein DP (eds.) *Emans, Laufer, Goldstein's Pediatric and Adolescent Gynecology* (6th edn). Philadelphia, PA: Lippincott Williams and Wilkins, 2012; 42–95.

Trager JDK. Vulvar dermatology. In Emans SJ, Laufer MR, Goldstein DP (eds.) *Emans, Laufer, Goldstein's Pediatric and Adolescent Gynecology* (6th edn.). Philadelphia, PA: Lippincott Williams and Wilkins, 2012; 381–404.

Van Der Pol B, Williams JA, Taylor SN, et al. Detection of *Trichomonas vaginalis* DNA by use of self-obtained vaginal swabs with the BD ProbeTec Qx assay on the BD Viper system. *J Clin Microbiol.* 2014;**52**(3):885–889.

Workowski KA, Bolan GA, Centers for Disease Control and Prevention. Sexually transmitted diseases treatment guidelines, 2015. *MMWR Recomm Rep.* 2015;**64**(RR-03):1–137.

Chapter 12

Hematologic Emergencies

Mark Weinblatt

Anemia

Red cell production is driven by oxygen availability to tissues and oxygen requirements, thus varying greatly with age, activity, and environmental circumstances, such as altitude. The lower limits of normal hemoglobin levels range from 9.5 g/dL at three months of age to 11 g/dL in the teenager

Clinical Presentation

The signs and symptoms of anemia result from the decreased oxygen-carrying capacity of the blood and depend on the degree of anemia and acuteness of onset. Exercise intolerance, pallor, headache, fatigue, tachycardia, and systolic murmurs may occur with moderate anemia. Severe or rapidly developing anemia can cause nonexertional dyspnea, dizziness, orthostatic vital sign changes, cardiac gallop, syncope, hypotension, and heart failure.

Diagnosis

After determining that a patient is anemic for age with a CBC with red-cell indices, a reticulocyte count, and examination of the peripheral smear, the most expeditious way of narrowing the differential diagnosis is using an algorithm based on the red cell size (see Table 12.1). Microcytic anemias are due to delayed or abnormal hemoglobin formation, with disorders of the iron, globin chain, or porphyrin ring components. These disorders typically have decreased MCV, with a peripheral blood smear revealing hypochromic red cells. To further establish a diagnosis, consider additional testing such as iron and ferritin levels, hemoglobin electrophoresis, and a lead level. The Menser index (MCV in fL divided by the red blood cells [RBC] in millions: MCV/RBC) can help differentiate among the microcytic anemias. If the ratio is less than 11:1, thalassemia minor is likely, while a ratio greater than 14:1 suggests iron deficiency, lead intoxication, or anemia of chronic disease.

The uncommon macrocytic anemias with MCV >100 fL beyond the newborn period result from delayed nuclear maturation or elevated fetal hemoglobin content.

The normocytic anemias comprise the largest differential. The reticulocyte count and some additional features of the red cells can help establish the diagnosis.

Red Cell Shape

Variations in red cell shape include sickle cells (both crescent and "box car" shapes); target cells, often seen in hemoglobinopathies (especially Hgb C disease and the microcytic

Table 12.1 Differential diagnosis of anemia

Microcytic

Anemia of chronic disease

Chronic lead poisoning

Copper deficiency

Iron deficiency

Sideroblastic anemia

Thalassemia

Macrocytic

Diamond–Blackfan syndrome

Dyserythropoietic anemia

Fanconi's anemia

Folic acid deficiency

Hypothyroidism

Liver disease

Myelodysplasia

Vitamin B12 deficiency

Normocytic: ↓reticulocytes

Acquired aplastic anemia

Chronic renal disease

Drug suppression

Leukemia

Neuroblastoma

Transient erythroblastopenia

Viral marrow suppression

Normocytic: ↑reticulocytes

Acute blood loss

G-6-PD deficiency

Hemoglobin C disease

Immune hemolytic anemia

Infectious agents (e.g., malaria)

Mechanical or thermal damage

Pyruvate kinase deficiency

Sickle cell disease

Spherocytosis, elliptocytosis

Splenic sequestration

thalassemia syndromes) and liver disease; burr cells (renal disease, hemolysis); spherocytes (spherocytosis, ABO immune hemolysis); and schistocytes (hemolysis).

Color

Polychromasia occurs with increased RBC production in association with decreased life span or marrow recovery. This is usually indicative of an elevated reticulocyte count.

Inclusions

There may be Howell–Jolly bodies (decreased splenic function); basophilic stippling (thalassemia, lead poisoning, some enzyme deficiencies); or parasites (malaria, babesiosis).

History

A thorough history, including ethnicity, family background, and diet, is important in refining the etiology of anemia. Iron-deficiency anemia can be caused by excessive intake of cow's milk in infants or by restricted diets containing no reliable source of iron in older children. A complete lack of fresh vegetables might lead to folate deficiency. Unusual cravings, such as pagophagia and pica, are occasionally seen in patients with iron deficiency, and may further complicate the picture (e.g., causing ingestion of lead-containing paint chips).

A history of recent infections may suggest EBV or *Mycoplasma*-induced hemolysis, or parvovirus suppression of the bone marrow (particularly in patients with chronic hemolytic disorders). Inquire about blood loss, such as epistaxis, irregular menstrual bleeding, hematuria, or gastrointestinal bleeding. A history of unexplained or prolonged bleeding may suggest a hemostatic disorder, such as mild von Willebrand disease, that is contributing to anemia. Ask about chronic medical problems and inflammatory disorders, such as juvenile rheumatoid arthritis, inflammatory bowel disease (IBD), or gastrointestinal (GI) complaints (abdominal pain or bloating, chronic diarrhea) that might suggest celiac disease. Recurrent episodes of jaundice suggest hemolytic disorders such as G-6-PD deficiency, hemoglobinopathies, and spherocytosis. A patient with a hemolytic disorder may have a positive family history for anemia, intermittent jaundice, cholecystectomy in a young person, or non-traumatic splenectomy (hereditary spherocytosis, sickle cell disease, and some enzyme deficiencies). Ask about medication use, since many medications can suppress erythropoiesis (e.g., sulfa drugs and anticonvulsants) or trigger hemolysis in patients with G-6-PD deficiency.

Physical Examination

On examination, a healthy, vigorous child is more likely to have mild iron-deficiency anemia, thalassemia trait, or a mild chronic hemolytic anemia. A patient with a malignancy, severe malnutrition, severe chronic disease, or bone marrow infiltration usually appears ill. Jaundice, often accompanied by abdominal pain, splenomegaly and dark urine, is frequently seen in hemolytic processes. Untreated or undiagnosed thalassemia major or intermedia is often associated with frontal bossing, malar prominence, hepatosplenomegaly, and dental malocclusion. Generalized lymphadenopathy and hepatosplenomegaly are frequent features of myeloproliferative disorders and malignancies, especially leukemia and lymphoma. Petechiae, purpura, and multiple ecchymoses can be expected in hemostatic disorders. Orthopedic anomalies may suggest Fanconi's anemia (abnormal radii or thumbs) or Diamond–Blackfan syndrome (triphalangeal or bifid thumbs).

Iron Deficiency

Iron deficiency is the most likely diagnosis in an otherwise well child with mild-to-moderate microcytic, hypochromic anemia. While inadequate dietary intake of iron is the most common cause of iron deficiency in a young child, blood loss is more likely in an older child or adolescent.

ED Management

Iron Deficiency

Treat with oral ferrous sulfate, 6 mg/kg/day of elemental iron divided tid between meals. Give with juice (vitamin C enhances iron absorption), but not with milk, which impairs iron absorption. If there is difficulty with administration, give the iron as a single daily dose. Or, for young children, recommend iron gummies (15 mg ferrous fumarate = 5 mg elemental iron). A rise in hemoglobin and reticulocyte count after one week confirms both the diagnosis and adherence to the regimen. Lack of response suggests an incorrect diagnosis, ongoing blood loss, incorrect dose, malabsorption, or noncompliance with medication. Advise the patient or parents that GI complaints, particularly constipation and darkening of stools, may result from iron therapy. For occasional epigastric discomfort, divide the iron doses into smaller volumes at more frequent intervals or administer with food (not milk). Admit a patient with severe anemia and consult with a hematologist to consider a single dose of intravenous iron sucrose (0.5 mg/kg), which is a safe and well-tolerated preparation that facilitates a more rapid correction of anemia.

Blood Loss

Blood loss, particularly when acute, may require treatment with packed RBCs, especially if the patient is symptomatic (pronounced tachycardia, orthostatic hypotension, syncope). Do not rely solely on the level of the hematocrit to decide if a transfusion is necessary, since children often tolerate extremely low red cell counts without exhibiting any symptoms, if the anemia developed slowly. Consider associated clinical findings, such as resting heart rate and respiratory rate, as well as the likelihood of a further imminent decrease in the hematocrit in bleeding conditions. Other diseases that might warrant a transfusion include disorders associated with decreased erythrocyte production as seen in either bone marrow failure (aplastic anemia, transient erythroblastopenia of childhood, nutritional anemias, and drug-induced marrow suppression) or marrow replacement (leukemia, neuroblastoma, histiocytosis, storage disorders). Consult a pediatric hematologist before giving blood to these patients (see Transfusion Therapy, pp. 377–378).

Autoimmune Hemolytic Anemia

Initially treat with prednisone (2.5 mg/kg/day) after consultation with a pediatric hematologist. Packed red cell transfusions might be required, but this disorder can be associated with a high risk of transfusion reactions.

The treatment of most primary hematologic etiologies of anemia, other than iron deficiency, lead intoxication, and bleeding, usually requires consultation with a pediatric hematologist.

Follow-up

- Iron-deficiency anemia: one week, for a hemoglobin and reticulocyte count; sooner if the initial hemoglobin is extremely low and there is significant tachycardia

Indications for Admission

- Significant cardiovascular or cerebral symptomatology (syncope, tachycardia, heart failure)
- Acute blood loss requiring transfusion
- Pancytopenia or suspicion of a malignancy
- Acute Coombs positive or extrinsic hemolytic anemia with hemoglobin <8 g/dL
- Chronic hemolytic disease with acute reticulocytopenia and significant fall in hematocrit (aplastic crisis seen in sickle cell disease and spherocytosis)
- Severe glucose-6-phosphate dehydrogenase (G-6-PD) deficiency with exposure to oxidant stress (e.g., infections, mothballs, sulfonamides, antimalarials)
- Hemoglobin <5 g/dL

Bibliography

Brugnara C, Oski FA, Nathan DG. Diagnostic approach to the anemic patient. In Orkin SH, Nathan DG, Ginsburg D, et al. (eds.) *Nathan and Oski's Hematology of Infancy and Childhood* (8th edn.). Philadelphia, PA: Saunders Elsevier, 2014; 293–307.

Gallagher PG. Diagnosis and management of rare congenital nonimmune hemolytic disease. *Hematology Am Soc Hematol Educ Program*. 2015;**2015**:392–399.

Hartung HD, Olson TS, Bessler M. Acquired aplastic anemia in children. *Pediatr Clin North Am*. 2013;**60**(6):1311–1336.

Kett JC. Anemia in infancy. *Pediatr Rev*. 2012;**33**(4):186–187.

Lopez A, Cacoub P, Macdougall IC, Peyrin-Biroulet L. Iron deficiency anaemia. *Lancet*. 2016;**387** (10021):907–916.

Nathan DG, Ginsburg D, Look AT, Fisher DE, Lux SE (eds.) *Nathan and Oski's Hematology of Infancy and Childhood* (8th edn.). Philadelphia, PA: Saunders Elsevier, 2014; 293–307.

Hemostatic Disorders

Thrombocytopenia involves a decrease in the number of circulating platelets secondary to underproduction, as in marrow failure (aplasia, infections, or drugs) or marrow replacement (leukemia, storage disorders, histiocytosis); increased peripheral destruction (immune thrombocytopenic purpura [ITP], hypersplenism, infections, hemangiomas); ineffective production (myelodysplasia); or microangiopathic processes (hemolytic-uremic syndrome, disseminated intravascular coagulation ([DIC]).

Platelet dysfunction can also cause bleeding manifestations. These disorders of platelet function can be acquired (uremia; ingestion of aspirin or nonsteroidal anti-inflammatory medications) or inherited (von Willebrand disease, storage pool disorder).

Coagulation factors are necessary for the formation of fibrin strands at bleeding sites. Hemorrhage can occur when any of these proteins are either decreased in amount or dysfunctional. Factor activity is decreased in inherited deficiencies (hemophilia [factor VIII or IX] and von Willebrand disease), vitamin K deficiency (normal newborns, sodium warfarin [Coumadin] therapy, prolonged oral antibiotic therapy), liver failure, and disseminated intravascular coagulation (DIC).

The endothelium is responsible for the production of factor VIII and prostacyclin (a platelet inhibitor) and the insulation of coagulation factors and platelets from exposure to underlying collagen. Dysfunction of the endothelial system is observed in vasculitis (lupus, Henoch–Schönlein purpura) and infections (meningococcemia, *Rickettsia*, dengue fever).

Clinical Presentation

The presenting complaint of hemostatic disorders may vary greatly, depending on the location, acuity, and severity of bleeding. Platelet abnormalities are commonly associated with petechial or mucosal bleeding that occurs immediately after the trauma and will often respond to local pressure. With ITP, skin and mucosal bleeding often follow a benign viral illness or measles vaccination. Patients with coagulation factor abnormalities, particularly the hemophilias, may have delayed, posttraumatic deep tissue hemorrhages into muscles and joints. In the first few weeks of life, a coagulopathy may present with delayed, persistent bleeding from the circumcision site or the umbilical stump. Abrasions and tooth extractions respond poorly to local pressure and can continue to ooze and bleed for days. Bleeding secondary to vasculitis (such as Henoch–Schönlein purpura) usually presents as palpable purpura.

Diagnosis

Suspect a bleeding disorder in a child who presents with a history of bruising or bleeding that is out of proportion to the level of trauma, bleeding in unusual locations, spontaneous hemorrhage, and prolonged or recurrent bleeding. Ask about a family history of inherited hemorrhagic disorders, such as hemophilia A and B (X-linked), factor XI deficiency (autosomal recessive), and von Willebrand disease (usually autosomal dominant), or unexplained significant bleeding, particularly if a blood transfusion was necessary. A seriously ill child may have leukemia (pallor, fever, fatigue, hepatomegaly, lymphadenopathy), hemolytic-uremic syndrome (lethargy, diarrhea, oliguria), liver disease (vomiting, jaundice, hepatomegaly, dark urine, acholic stools), or DIC.

The diagnosis can be facilitated by a few simple screening tests. Platelet count; prothrombin time (PT) or international normalized ratio (INR), which assess the extrinsic clotting system (factor VII, plus the factors in the common pathway [I, II, V, X]); and partial thromboplastin time (PTT) for the intrinsic system (factors VIII, IX, XI, XII, plus the factors in the common pathway [I, II, V, X]) (see Tables 12.2 and 12.3).

ED Management

Give a patient with vitamin K deficiency who is actively bleeding 5–10 mg of vitamin K by slow IV infusion. Correction of coagulation factor levels begins within hours, with marked improvement by 24 hours. Treat severe bleeding with an infusion of fresh frozen plasma to rapidly correct the deficiencies. If there is a history of warfarin ingestion, a repeat administration of vitamin K might be necessary.

Treat thrombocytopenic conditions with local pressure to superficial bleeding sites. If this is unsuccessful, or the platelet count is <50,000/mm^3, obtain a type and crossmatch and consult a pediatric hematologist. Treat a patient with documented ITP and

Table 12.2 Differential diagnosis of bleeding disorders

Platelet count*	Prothrombin time*	Partial thromboplastin time*	Diagnoses
Normal	Prolonged	Normal	Circulating antibodies
			Coumadin ingestion
			Factor VII deficiency
			Mild liver disease
			Mild vitamin K deficiency
Normal	Normal	Prolonged	Circulating antibodies
			Factor VIII, IX, XI, or XII deficiency
			Heparin effect
			von Willebrand disease
Decreased	Prolonged	Prolonged	Congenital heart disease
			DIC
			Severe liver disease
Decreased	Normal	Normal	Thrombocytopenia
Normal	Prolonged	Prolonged	Dysfibrinogenemia
			Factor II, V, or X deficiency
			High-dose heparin or warfarin therapy
			Moderate liver disease
			Vitamin K deficiency
Normal	Normal	Normal	Child abuse and trauma
			Connective tissue disease
			Factor XIII deficiency
			Henoch–Schönlein purpura and other vasculitides
			Platelet dysfunction (inherited and acquired)
			Renal failure
			Vitamin C deficiency
			von Willebrand disease

* Normal values: platelet count: 150,000–300,000/mm^3; PT: <13 seconds or within 2 seconds of control or INR <1.2; PTT: <35–39 seconds or within 5 seconds of control.

Table 12.3 Differential diagnosis of thrombocytopenia

Diagnosis	Differentiating features
Drug induced	Taking antibiotics for 1–2 weeks
Epstein–Barr virus	Fever, fatigue, pharyngitis, splenomegaly
Fanconi's anemia	Short stature, abnormal thumbs, café-au-lait spots, macrocytosis
Gaucher's disease	Family history; bone pain, pathologic fractures, splenomegaly
Histiocytosis	Eczema, chronic otitis, bone lesions, hepatosplenomegaly
HIV	Adenopathy, recurrent infections, bruising, pallor, lymphopenia
HUS	Bloody diarrhea, lethargy, oliguria, pallor, jaundice
ITP	Extensive bruising and petechiae in a well-appearing child
	↑ MPV
	RBCs and WBCs are normal
Kasabach–Merritt syndrome	Enlarged portions of extremities, bleeding
Leukemia	Fever, bruising, pallor, adenopathy, abnormal white cells
Malaria	High fever, jaundice, splenomegaly, foreign travel
May–Hegglin anomaly	Family history of bruising and petechiae
	↑↑ MPV
	WBC inclusions
Meningococcemia	Fever and toxicity; palpable purpura, hypotension
Neuroblastoma	Fever, lower extremity weakness, abdominal mass
Osteopetrosis	Infant with severely impaired vision; bruising, splenomegaly,
Thrombocytopenia-absent radii	Bleeding from birth, abnormal forearms
Wiskott–Aldrich syndrome	Infant boy with eczema, frequent infections, ↓ MPV

serious, life-threatening bleeding with high-dose intravenous gamma globulin (0.5–1.0 g/kg over 4–5 hours) or high-dose corticosteroids (methylprednisolone 20–40 mg/kg over 1 hour), while awaiting consultation with a hematologist. A platelet transfusion will not raise the platelet count but can slow life-threatening bleeding. A patient who is Rh positive can also be treated with WinRho, 50 mcg/kg. For a patient with thrombocytopenia caused by decreased production (leukemia, other marrow failure syndromes), transfuse single-donor apheresis platelets (see Transfusion Therapy, pp. 377–378).

Replace deficient clotting factors as soon as possible. As a general rule, 1 unit/kg of factor VIII will raise a patient's factor level by 2%. Always consult with a hematologist before treating a coagulopathy patient with factor replacement, as the selection and dose of the factor product varies greatly and several synthetic, long-acting products are now available. Factor VII concentrate will often treat a variety of coagulopathies. Avoid giving aspirin and other medications that can inhibit proper platelet function to any child with a bleeding diathesis.

Obtain a CT scan of the head for a patient with a hemostatic disorder who has a moderate or severe headache or any neurologic symptoms (irritability, lethargy, vomiting, ataxia, loss of consciousness) after head trauma.

Follow-up
- Patient with ITP: repeat platelet count in 1–3 days, depending on the initial platelet count
- Patient treated with factor VIII: next day, or in 2–3 days if a long-acting factor concentrate was used

Indications for Admission
- Massive bleeding that causes hypovolemia or requires transfusion of packed RBCs
- Suspected or proven intracranial, intrathoracic, or abdominal hemorrhage
- Hemophiliacs or patients with other severe hemostatic disorders who sustain significant head trauma (e.g., lethargic, skull fracture, abnormal neurologic finding, or loss of consciousness)
- Significant hematemesis, hematochezia, or hematuria
- Severe inherited coagulopathy with gross hematuria, large laceration, or severe abdominal pain
- Clinical features suspicious for marrow replacement, DIC, hemolytic-uremic syndrome, or hepatic failure
- Generalized petechial or purpuric eruption in an acutely ill febrile child

Bibliography
Branchford B, Di Paola J. Approach to the child with a suspected bleeding disorder. In Orkin SH, Nathan DG, Ginsburg D, (eds.). *Nathan and Oski's Hematology of Infancy and Childhood* (8th edn.). Philadelphia, PA: Elsevier Saunders, 2014; 999–1009.

Branchford BR, Monahan PE, Di Paola J. New developments in the treatment of pediatric hemophilia and bleeding disorders. *Curr Opin Pediatr.* 2013;**25**(1):23–30.

D'Orazio JA, Neely J, Farhoudi N. ITP in children: pathophysiology and current treatment approaches. *J Pediatr Hematol Oncol.* 2013;**35**(1):1–13.

Labarque V, Van Geet C. Clinical practice: immune thrombocytopenia in paediatrics. *Eur J Pediatr.* 2014;**173**(2):163–172.

van Herrewegen F, Meijers JC, Peters M, van Ommen CH. Clinical practice: the bleeding child. Part II: disorders of secondary hemostasis and fibrinolysis. *Eur J Pediatr.* 2012;**171**(2):207–214.

van Ommen CH, Peters M. The bleeding child. Part I: primary hemostatic disorders. *Eur J Pediatr.* 2012;**171**:1–10.

Infection and the Immunocompromised Host
The hallmark of an immunocompromised patient is an increased susceptibility to infection, including increased frequency, duration, and severity, as well as infection caused by unusual pathogens.

Clinical Presentation

Although symptoms will vary with the organism and site of infection, immunocompromised patients often have recurrent respiratory infections and repeated severe bacterial illnesses (sepsis, pneumonia, meningitis). Persistent lymphadenopathy and hepatosplenomegaly are common findings in these disorders. Many patients have chronic diarrhea with some form of malabsorption and failure to thrive (IgA deficiency, exocrine pancreatic insufficiency). A variety of skin lesions can be seen, including eczema (Wiskott–Aldrich syndrome), pyoderma (cyclic neutropenia, Kostmann's syndrome, Job syndrome), and diffuse dermatitis (chronic granulomatous disease).

HIV infection presents in a variety of ways: lymphadenopathy, hepatosplenomegaly, and failure to thrive in an infant with maternal risk factors; a multiply-transfused child with interstitial pneumonitis; or a child with poorly responsive immune thrombocytopenic purpura.

Although most children with sickle cell disease are identified early in life by newborn hemoglobinopathy screening, a Caucasian child of Mediterranean background with unsuspected sickle cell disease may present with frequent bouts of unexplained bone pain, leukocytosis, and a chronic hemolytic anemia.

Lymphoma in an adolescent can cause adenopathy, fever, weight loss, splenomegaly, and herpes zoster or prolonged varicella infection.

Diagnosis

Prior to proceeding with an extensive immunologic evaluation, try to differentiate the immunodeficient child from one with frequent colds and normal immunologic function. Children can have 8–10 respiratory infections in any given year, but these are usually mild, self-limited, occasionally accompanied by fever, but with complete recovery between bouts. Allergy is more likely in children with repeated or persistent infections limited to the upper respiratory tract. An incompletely treated sinusitis or enlarged tonsils/adenoids are frequent underlying causes of recurrent upper respiratory infections. Likewise, infections limited to a particular organ suggest specific disease entities: cystic fibrosis, foreign body, collagen vascular diseases, or bronchiectasis with recurrent pneumonia; cow's milk sensitivity, celiac disease, and IBD with chronic diarrhea and failure to thrive. Many chronic diseases predispose patients to frequent infections (rheumatic disorders, chronic renal disease, sickle cell disease, diabetes, nutritional deficiencies, malignancies). Finally, a history of blood product administration to the patient or parent, intravenous drug abuse, or high-risk sexual activity raises the possibility of HIV infection.

ED Management

If the child has had either two or more serious infections (pneumonia, meningitis, sepsis, osteomyelitis) in a short period of time or an infection with an unusual pathogen, obtain a CBC with differential and platelet count, ESR, and quantitative immunoglobulins. In addition, evaluate cell-mediated immunity by measuring T-cell subsets and consider skin testing (*Candida*, streptokinase-streptodornase, mumps, and purified protein derivative [PPD]). Assume that any patient with a history of treatment with chemotherapeutic drugs for malignancy or autoimmune disorders, or with immunosuppressive medications (corticosteroids for asthma or IBD; infliximab or adalimumab for IBD) is at high risk for infections. Consult a pediatric hematologist or immunologist for further evaluation with specific definitive tests.

When a patient with a known immunodeficiency or neutrophil disorder presents with a fever (>38.6 °C, 101.5 °F), a conservative approach is necessary. Obtain a CBC and cultures of the blood, urine, and any wounds prior to initiating treatment. If there are central nervous system symptoms, perform a lumbar puncture with additional fluid to evaluate for unusual organisms (mycobacteria, India ink stain for *Cryptococcus*, viral encephalitis panel [including herpes]) in addition to the standard culture, cell count, glucose, and Gram stain.

Treat an ill-appearing neutropenic patient with a combination of an aminoglycoside such as tobramycin or gentamicin (6 mg/kg/day IV div q 8–12h) *and* either a semisynthetic penicillin (piperacillin/tazobactam 250 mg/kg/day IV div q 6h) *or* ceftazidime (100 mg/kg/day IV div q 8h) *or* meropenem (60 mg/kg/day IV div q 8h) for adequate *Pseudomonas* coverage. Cefepime (100 mg/kg/day IV div q 12h) can be used for monotherapy in a patient who does not appear seriously ill or unstable.

Treat a child with defective cell-mediated immunity who has fever and respiratory symptoms with trimethoprim-sulfamethoxazole (20 mg/kg/day of TMP div q 6h) along with broad-spectrum antibiotics, as listed above. Treat patients with splenic dysfunction with ceftriaxone or cefuroxime (100 mg/kg/day). If the patient has a very high fever or a toxic appearance, add vancomycin (60 mg/kg/day div q 6h) to cover resistant *Pneumococcus* and *Staphylococcus*. Consult a hematologist for patients with neutrophil disorders who have serious infections, as granulocyte transfusions or granulocyte colony stimulating factor (G-CSF), 5 mg/kg/day, may be indicated. With the advent of more resistant organisms such as vancomycin-resistant enterococcus and methicillin-resistant *S. aureus*, other antibiotic combinations often need to be explored with an infectious disease expert or hematologist.

Often a well-appearing child can be managed as an outpatient after receiving broad-spectrum antibiotics and a period of observation in the ED. Cefepime, with or without a 24-hour dose of aminoglycoside, is one option for the neutropenic patient, with follow-up the following day.

Follow-up

- Immunocompromised patient with low-grade fever not treated with antibiotics: next day, if still febrile

Indications for Admission

- Fever (>38.5 °C, 101.5 °F) in a patient with a granulocyte count <500/mm³, a documented phagocytic defect, or other immunodeficiency, after *consultation with a hematologist*
- Immunocompromised patient with pneumonia, an abscess, or localized infection (e.g., otitis, cellulitis) not responding to initial antibiotic therapy
- Patient with sickle cell disease under two years old with fever >39 °C (102.2 °F); older patient with high fever (>39.5 °C, 103.1 °F)
- Suspected malignancy
- Immunocompromised patient with a toxic appearance, regardless of the temperature
- Varicella or herpes zoster infection in a child with defective cell-mediated immunity

Bibliography

Alvarez E, Chamberlain LJ, Aftandilian C, Saynina O, Wise P. Pediatric oncology discharges with febrile neutropenia: variation in location of care. *J Pediatr Hematol Oncol.* 2017;**39**(1):e1–e7.

Henry M, Sung L. Supportive care in pediatric oncology: oncologic emergencies and management of fever and neutropenia. *Pediatr Clin North Am.* 2015;**62**(1):27–46.

Lehrnbecher T, Phillips R, Alexander S, et al. Guideline for the management of fever and neutropenia in children with cancer and/or undergoing hematopoietic stem-cell transplantation. *J Clin Oncol.* 2012;**30**(35):4427–4438

Manji A, Lehrnbecher T, Dupuis LL, Beyene J, Sung L. A systematic review and meta-analysis of anti-pseudomonal penicillins and carbapenems in pediatric febrile neutropenia. *Support Care Cancer.* 2012;**20**(10):2295–2304.

Phillips RS, Bhuller K, Sung L, et al. Risk stratification in febrile neutropenic episodes in adolescent/ young adult patients with cancer. *Eur J Cancer.* 2016;**64**:101–106.

Steele RW. Managing infection in cancer patients and other immunocompromised children. *Ochsner J.* 2012;**12**(3):202–210.

Leukemia and Lymphoma

The most common pediatric malignancy is acute lymphoblastic leukemia (ALL); among solid tumors, lymphomas are second only to brain tumors in frequency.

Clinical Presentation

Leukemia

The presenting symptoms of ALL usually result from the absence of normal hemato-poietic elements, along with the proliferation and accumulation of abnormal cells. Clinical findings are related to the degree of anemia (pallor, fatigue, lightheadedness, palpitations), thrombocytopenia (petechiae, purpura, epistaxis), and neutropenia (infections). Other signs and symptoms include joint or bone pain, hepatosplenomeg-aly, lymphadenopathy, skin nodules, and gingival hypertrophy. CNS involvement can be asymptomatic. Alternatively, there can be symptoms related to elevated intracranial pressure (headache, vomiting, irritability, visual disturbances) or unusual constella-tions of findings such as an isolated cranial nerve paresis or the "hypothalamic syndrome" (marked hyperphagia with weight gain, personality changes). Leukemic infiltration in organs such as the testes, kidneys, and ovaries can lead to firm, painless enlargement.

Hodgkin's Lymphoma

Hodgkin's lymphoma in children and adolescents most commonly presents with either firm, nontender, asymptomatic lymphadenopathy (particularly the cervical, supraclavicu-lar, mediastinal or para-aortic nodes) or, less commonly, with constitutional symptoms (fever, night sweats, cough, weight loss). Pruritus rarely occurs in children, and complica-tions such as jaundice and superior vena cava obstruction are uncommon. There may be a history of prolonged varicella or herpes zoster.

Non-Hodgkin's Lymphoma

The non-Hodgkin's lymphomas may also present with isolated, nontender, firm lympha-denopathy, but children more frequently have widespread disease. A primary mediastinal mass may cause dyspnea, cough, pleural effusion, and superior vena cava obstruction (respiratory distress; distended veins in neck and arms). Children can have primary tumors in Waldeyer's ring, presenting with tonsillar involvement misdiagnosed as a peritonsillar abscess. Primary gastrointestinal lymphomas (Peyer's patches of the distal ileum) can cause asymptomatic abdominal distention, vomiting and diarrhea, intussusception, or intestinal obstruction. Burkitt's lymphoma can present with retroperitoneal or mesenteric tumors and occasionally with involvement of the maxillary sinus, but jaw masses are uncommon in the United States.

Diagnosis

In addition to cytopenia, the hallmark of leukemia is the presence of large numbers of primitive leukocytes (blasts) in the blood and bone marrow. While metastatic neuroblas-toma may also replace the bone marrow with malignant cells, these cells do not appear in the peripheral blood.

Most often confused with leukemia and lymphomas are infectious mononucleosis and mono-like syndromes (cytomegalovirus, toxoplasmosis), which can present with fever, lymph-adenopathy, hepatosplenomegaly, cytopenias, and immature leukocytes on blood smear. However, these cells can usually be distinguished from leukemic blast cells. Pertussis can induce a profound leukocytosis ($>100,000/mm^3$) and neutropenia, but the cells are mature and anemia is not usually present. Children with ITP do not appear chronically ill, the platelets are usually large, and cytopenia of other cell lines is absent. Storage disorders (Gaucher's disease) may also present with hepatosplenomegaly and pancytopenia. A lymphoma-like picture can be seen with sinus histiocytosis, diphenylhydantoin therapy, and, rarely, in Kawasaki syndrome. A node biopsy is indicated if there is weight loss or supraclavicular lymphadenopathy, or the node is nontender, firm, and progressively enlarging.

ED Management

If leukemia or lymphoma is suspected, obtain a CBC with differential, platelet count, reticulocyte count, heterophile antibody or monospot test, electrolytes, liver function tests, lactic dehydrogenase, a blood culture, and chest film. Consult with a pediatric hema-tologist-oncologist.

Follow-up

• Asymptomatic patient with lymphadenopathy: 7–10 days
• Mild pancytopenia: repeat CBC in 3–4 days

Indications for Admission

• Blasts on peripheral smear with pancytopenia
• WBC $>100,000/mm^3$
• Mass pressure on a vital structure

Bibliography

Alexander S, Ferrnando AA. Pediatric lymphoma. In Orkin SH, Nathan DG, Ginsburg D, et al. (eds.) *Nathan and Oski's Hematology of Infancy and Childhood* (8th edn.). Philadelphia, PA: Elsevier Saunders, 2014; 1626–1674.

Allen CE, Kelly KM, Bollard CM. Pediatric lymphomas and histiocytic disorders of childhood. *Pediatr Clin North Am.* 2015;**62**(1):139–165.

Brugières L, Brice P. Lymphoma in adolescents and young adults. *Prog Tumor Res.* 2016;**43**:101–114.

Cooper SL, Brown PA. Treatment of pediatric acute lymphoblastic leukemia. *Pediatr Clin North Am.* 2015;**62**(1):61–73.

Madhusoodhan PP, Carroll WL, Bhatla T. Progress and prospects in pediatric leukemia. *Curr Probl Pediatr Adolesc Health Care.* 2016;**46**(7):229–241.

Lymphadenopathy

Palpable lymph nodes are a common finding and may be normal or a sign of minor or life-threatening disease. Lymph nodes are not usually palpable until a few months of age. Afterward there is a steady increase in the body's normal lymphoid tissue, so that by puberty nearly 100% of children will have at least some palpable nodes, most commonly in the cervical and inguinal areas. A variety of factors must be considered when deciding whether to pursue a work-up for enlarged nodes.

Clinical Presentation

Generalized Lymphadenopathy

Generalized lymphadenopathy is defined as enlargement in at least three noncontiguous lymph node regions. It is always abnormal, and usually nonlymphoid features of the primary disease process are evident (fever, rash, pharyngitis, arthritis, arthralgia, bruising, pallor, hepatosplenomegaly, etc.). The most common etiology is infection, particularly viral disease like infectious mononucleosis or mono-like illnesses (cytomegalovirus, toxoplasmosis). Other infectious etiologies include the exanthematous viral infections of childhood (measles, rubella, varicella), enteroviruses (echo, Coxsackie), tuberculosis, hepatitis B, syphilis, malaria, and HIV. Noninfectious causes include rheumatoid diseases (idiopathic juvenile arthritis, systemic lupus erythematosus), serum sickness, drug reactions (diphenylhydantoin), sarcoidosis, storage diseases, and eczema. Malignancies and related disorders to consider include leukemia, lymphoma, and histiocytosis.

Localized Lymphadenopathy

Reactive Adenopathy

Localized lymphadenopathy is most often a response to a regional infection. The location often suggests the underlying infection. Reactive cervical enlargement is most common, frequently secondary to a viral upper respiratory infection, pharyngitis, or otitis media. Occipital lymphadenopathy occurs in response to scalp conditions such as seborrhea, tinea capitis, and pediculosis; preauricular enlargement can be secondary to conjunctivitis and acne; and submandibular and submental nodes may enlarge with infection of the gingiva, teeth, buccal mucosa, pharynx, and tongue. Axillary lymphadenopathy can be caused by cat scratch fever, rat bite fever, or a recent immunization, while inguinal involvement occurs with venereal diseases (syphilis, gonorrhea, lymphogranuloma venereum, chancroid) and lower extremity infections. Since the supraclavicular nodes drain from the lungs and mediastinum, enlargement here is always a concern. Etiologies include infections (tuberculosis, histoplasmosis, coccidioidomycosis), neoplasms (lymphomas), and sarcoidosis. For any node site, a proximal cellulitis, dermatitis, or local pyogenic infection will cause reactive enlargement.

Adenitis

A second category of local lymphadenopathy is primary infection of the node, or adenitis. Most often this is bacterial in origin. The most common organisms are *Staphylococcus aureus* and group A *Streptococcus*, although anaerobes, tuberculosis, atypical mycobacteria, and HIV are other etiologies to consider.

Diagnosis

A complete history and physical examination are necessary to locate a primary infection, document a local adenitis, or diagnose a disease causing generalized lymphadenopathy. Note that any fever, weight loss, rash, jaundice, arthritis, arthralgias, bruising, pallor, pharyngitis or upper respiratory symptoms, hepatosplenomegaly, contact with contagious diseases, history of a cat scratch or rat bite, and sexual activity. When examining the involved node(s) there are six features to consider:

Location

Significant generalized lymphadenopathy always warrants further investigation, as does supraclavicular or axillary adenopathy. Isolated cervical, inguinal, and occipital nodes are less commonly pathologic.

Size

Generally, nodes larger than 1 cm in diameter are abnormal. However, cervical nodes may be 2–3 cm in diameter without an associated serious underlying disease.

Rate of Enlargement

Rapid enlargement is most commonly caused by an infection, either an adenitis or a reactive hyperplasia. Slow growth suggests a malignancy or a systemic disease.

Mobility

A node fixed to adjacent structures or matted to other nodes suggests an infiltrative disease that demands further evaluation. A freely mobile node is generally benign.

Consistency

Soft, shotty nodes are usually normal or represent reactive enlargement. Adenitis causes fluctuance, while malignancy is associated with hard, rubbery nodes.

Overlying Skin

Bacterial adenitis causes erythema and warmth of the overlying skin. Adherence of the skin to the node occurs in cat scratch fever and atypical *Mycobacterium* infection. A reactive node does not affect the overlying skin.

Table 12.4 Differential diagnosis of lymphadenopathy

Diagnosis	Differentiating features
Cat scratch	Fever, history of contact with kitten Localized lymphadenopathy proximal to scratch wound
Epstein–Barr virus	Pharyngitis, fatigue, splenomegaly, atypical lymphocytes Generalized lymphadenopathy
Enterovirus	Summertime; fever, petechia, hand–foot–mouth rash, aseptic meningitis
HIV	Opportunistic infections, bruising, lymphopenia
Histoplasmosis	Fever, flu-like illness, cough, chest pain
Hodgkin's disease	Rubbery nodes, fever, night sweats, weight loss, cough
Juvenile idiopathic arthritis	Fever, joint pains, fleeting rash Elevated ESR/CRP, anemia
Kawasaki disease	Strawberry tongue, conjunctivitis Thrombocytosis
Langerhans histiocytosis	Fever, chronic otitis, hepatosplenomegaly, eczema
Leukemia	Fever, bone pain, pallor, bruising, hepatosplenomegaly, Anemia, abnormal white cells
Lyme disease	Fever, "bullseye" rash, joint pains, headaches
Neuroblastoma	Abdominal mass, fever, bone pain
Rocky Mountain spotted fever	Tick bite, fever, rash on distal extremities, splenomegaly
Rubella	Maculopapular rash, joint pains
Systemic lupus erythematosus	Adolescent girl with facial rash, joint pains
Streptococcus	Fever, headache, cervical adenopathy
Tuberculosis	Fever, cough, weight loss, pulmonary lesions
Tularemia	Animal contact; fever, chills, skin ulceration, tender nodes

While abnormality of any one of these characteristics might not be worrisome, multiple abnormalities (e.g., a firm, fixed, supraclavicular node) are suspicious for an underlying serious disorder, particularly a malignant disease, and requires further investigation. See Table 12.4 for the differential diagnosis of lymphadenopathy.

ED Management

Generalized Lymphadenopathy

If infectious mononucleosis is suggested by the clinical findings (fever, fatigue, pharyngitis, hepatosplenomegaly), obtain a CBC with differential (to look for atypical lymphocytosis or monocytosis) and a monospot or heterophile antibody test to confirm the diagnosis. However, in a child under six years old with active mononucleosis, the heterophile is likely to be negative, so obtain EBV serology, including IgM. Treatment is supportive (bed rest, acetaminophen as needed). Instruct the patient to avoid contact sports if there is significant splenomegaly because of the risk of splenic rupture. Admission and steroid therapy (prednisone 2 mg/kg/day div bid) are indicated for neurologic symptoms (encephalitis, Guillain-Barré syndrome, transverse myelitis), respiratory distress, massively enlarged tonsils, or cytopenias.

For other situations, the clinical picture guides the evaluation, although in general a CBC with differential, ESR, liver function tests, VDRL, hepatitis B antigen, heterophile antibody, PPD, and chest film are often indicated. If any risk factors are present, obtain HIV serology.

Localized Lymphadenopathy

Reactive Adenopathy
In most cases a contiguous infection will be found and reactive adenopathy diagnosed. Treat the primary infection appropriately. The reactive node(s) will shrink as the infection resolves.

Adenitis
Treat an adenitis with 40 mg/kg/day of cefadroxil (div bid) or cephalexin (div qid). Alternatives include cefprozil (20 mg/kg/day div bid) or azithromycin (12 mg/kg/day). Warm compresses applied for 15–30 minutes every 3–4 hours are an important adjunct. Reevaluate the patient in 48–72 hours. If there has been a response, continue the antibiotic for a full ten-day course. If there has been no change in the node in an otherwise asymptomatic child, change the antibiotic to clindamycin (20 mg/kg/day div qid) or amoxicillin-clavulanate (875/125 formulation, 45 mg/kg/day of amoxicillin div bid) and follow-up in two days. However, if there is no improvement and the patient appears ill, or if the node continues to enlarge, obtain a CBC and blood culture and admit for further evaluation (including surgical consultation) and parenteral antibiotics (nafcillin 150 mg/kg/day div q 6h, ceftriaxone 100 mg/kg/day div q 12h, clindamycin 40 mg/kg/day div q 6h, or cefazolin 75 mg/kg/day div q 8h). If malignancy is suspected at any time because of a change in the nature of the node, lack of response to treatment, or associated physical or laboratory findings, request an immediate oncology consultation for node biopsy and/or other definitive diagnostic procedures.

Follow-up
- Adenitis treated with oral antibiotics: two days

Indications for Admission
- Systemic toxicity
- Suspicion of a malignancy or AIDS, to facilitate the work-up and management
- Adenitis unresponsive to oral antibiotics

Bibliography

Clarke RT, Van den Bruel A, Bankhead C, et al. Clinical presentation of childhood leukaemia: a systematic review and meta-analysis. *Arch Dis Child.* 2016;**101**(10):894–901.

Ebell MH, Call M, Shinholser J, Gardner J. Does this patient have infectious mononucleosis? The rational clinical examination systematic review. *JAMA.* 2016;**315**(14):1502–1509.

King D, Ramachandra J, Yeomanson D. Lymphadenopathy in children: refer or reassure? *Arch Dis Child Educ Pract Ed.* 2014;99(3):101–110.

Penn EB Jr, Goudy SL. Pediatric inflammatory adenopathy. *Otolaryngol Clin North Am.* 2015;48 (1):137–151.

Rosenberg TL, Nolder AR. Pediatric cervical lymphadenopathy. *Otolaryngol Clin North Am.* 2014;47 (5):721–731.

Sahai S. Lymphadenopathy. *Pediatr Rev.* 2013;34(5):216–227.

Oncologic Emergencies

Aggressive chemotherapy has dramatically increased the response and cure rates for malignancies, but is associated with significant adverse effects. While these complex treatment regimens are usually administered by pediatric oncologists, patients often present to the ED with complications. It is crucial for the ED staff to recognize potential and existing problems related to the cancer therapy.

Chemotherapeutic agents share many common side effects, including myelosuppression, nausea, and alopecia, but each drug has the potential for specific toxicities (Table 12.5). Consult a pediatric oncologist during the evaluation of a patient receiving treatment for a malignancy who presents to the ED with possible side effects.

The most common serious problems are fever, acute neurologic symptomatology, superior vena cava obstruction, respiratory distress, metabolic derangements, and intestinal perforation.

Clinical Presentation

Since malignant diseases and their treatments are associated with immunodeficiency and neutropenia, patients are particularly susceptible to infectious complications, typically manifested by fever >38.6 °C (101.5 °F). The immunodeficient patient with pneumonia might be suffering from an opportunistic infection (*Pneumocystis, Aspergillus, Candida, Legionella*). An absolute neutrophil count <500/mm^3 places the patient at risk for Gram-negative and fungal infections. Indwelling central venous catheters increase the risk of staphylococcal and streptococcal infections. Cultures are most important since the range of infection is very broad.

Acute neurologic symptomatology may result from spinal cord or nerve root compression or from intracranial involvement. Spinal cord or nerve root compression can cause back pain, lower extremity weakness and sensory loss, and bladder and bowel dysfunction. Headache, vomiting, and isolated cranial nerve paresis can result from intracranial involvement.

A patient with lymphoma or leukemia who presents with a mediastinal mass is at risk for superior vena cava obstruction with dyspnea, edema of the head and neck, and prominence of the superficial veins on the upper body. Mediastinal masses may also compress the tracheobronchial tree and cause respiratory distress.

A patient who develops mucositis, particularly in combination with prolonged neutropenia, is at risk for typhlitis and intestinal perforation. The possibility increases with superimposed diarrhea and steroid use. Because of the decreased inflammatory response and neutropenia, a perforation may present without the classic physical findings of peritoneal irritation, although there may be abdominal pain, fever, and distention.

Table 12.5 Side effects of chemotherapy

Drug	Potential adverse effects
Asparaginase	Allergic reactions, anaphylaxis, pancreatitis, fever, coagulopathy, hepatotoxicity
Avastin	Abdominal pain, headache, GI bleeding, nausea, diarrhea, neuropathy, epistaxis
Bleomycin	Fever, chills, allergic reactions, vomiting, pulmonary fibrosis, mucositis
Brentuximab	Peripheral neuropathy, myelosuppression, fatigue, URI symptoms, fever, cough
Busulfan	Myelosuppression, pulmonary fibrosis, glossitis, skin darkening
Carboplatin	Myelosuppression, nausea and vomiting, ototoxicity, fatigue, nephrotoxicity
Carmustine (BCNU)	Myelosuppression, vomiting, nephrotoxicity, mucositis, phlebitis, fever, pulmonary fibrosis
Chlorambucil	Myelosuppression, nausea and vomiting, diarrhea, pulmonary fibrosis, skin rash
Cisplatin	Nausea and vomiting, nephrotoxicity, neurotoxicity, hypomagnesemia, ototoxicity, hepatotoxicity
Clofarabine	Myelosuppression, fever/chills, diarrhea, nausea and vomiting, hepatotoxicity
Cyclophosphamide	Myelosuppression, vomiting, SIADH, hemorrhagic cystitis, immunosuppression, cardiotoxicity, skin darkening
Cytosine arabinoside	Myelosuppression, vomiting, hepatotoxicity, mucositis, conjunctivitis, fever, neurotoxicity
Dacarbazine	Myelosuppression, vomiting, hepatotoxicity, blistering
Dactinomycin	Myelosuppression, vomiting, hepatotoxicity, mucositis, blistering
Dasatinib	Fluid retention, thrombocytopenia, headache, musculoskeletal pain, thrombosis, arrhythmia
Daunorubicin	Myelosuppression, cardiotoxicity, blistering, mucositis, diarrhea
Dexamethasone	Weight gain, hypertension, diabetes, moodiness
Doxorubicin	Myelosuppression, vomiting, cardiotoxicity, blistering, mucositis, diarrhea
Etoposide	Myelosuppression, vomiting, hypotension, hepatotoxicity
Fludarabine	Myelosuppression, vomiting, diarrhea, blurred vision, mucositis, fatigue
5-Fluorouracil	Myelosuppression, vomiting, diarrhea, mucositis, headache, dermatitis
Gemcitabine	Myelosuppression, nausea and vomiting, hepatotoxicity, flu-like illness

Table 12.5 (cont.)

Drug	Potential adverse effects
Hydroxyurea	Myelosuppression, nausea and vomiting, mucositis, diarrhea
Idarubicin	Myelosuppression, vomiting, cardiotoxicity, blistering, diarrhea
Ifosfamide	Myelosuppression, vomiting, nephrotoxicity, neurotoxicity, hemorrhagic cystitis
Imatinib	Fluid retention, nausea, fatigue, musculoskeletal pain, thrombocytopenia
Irinotecan	Myelosuppression, vomiting, severe diarrhea, abdominal pain, headache
Lomustine (CCNU)	Myelosuppression, vomiting, hepatotoxicity, nephrotoxicity, anorexia
Mechlorethamine	Myelosuppression, vomiting, blistering, phlebitis, diarrhea, mucositis
Melphalan	Vomiting, mucositis, pulmonary fibrosis
6-Mercaptopurine	Myelosuppression, vomiting, hepatotoxicity
Methotrexate	Myelosuppression, vomiting, mucositis, hepatotoxicity, neurotoxicity, nephrotoxicity
Mitoxantrone	Myelosuppression, cough, GI bleeding, mucositis, diarrhea, headache
Prednisone	Weight gain, hypertension, diabetes, moodiness
Procarbazine	Myelosuppression, vomiting, diarrhea, neurotoxicity, fever, mucositis, myalgias
Rituximab:	Fever, chills, headache, hypotension, nausea, angioedema, anaphylaxis, myalgia
Sirolimus	Headache, peripheral edema, dermatitis, immunosuppression, myelosuppression
6-Thioguanine	Myelosuppression, vomiting, hepatotoxicity, mucositis
Thiotepa	Myelosuppression, mucositis, neurotoxicity
Topotecan	Myelosuppression, vomiting, abdominal pain
Tretinoin	Abdominal pain, muscle pain, constipation, anorexia
Vinblastine	Myelosuppression, vomiting, blistering
Vincristine	Peripheral neuropathy, SIADH, constipation, seizures
Vinorelbine	Myelosuppression, neuropathy, anorexia, constipation

A patient with a large tumor burden and rapidly proliferating disease is at risk for significant metabolic derangements, including hyperuricemia (oliguria), hyperkalemia (muscle weakness, and peaked T-waves, PR prolongation, and QRS widening on the ECG), and hypocalcemia (tetany, laryngospasm, carpopedal spasm, seizures).

Diagnosis and ED Management

For all febrile (>38.6 °C, 101.5°F) oncology patients, obtain a CBC with differential, urinalysis, chest x-ray (if there are respiratory symptoms or chest pain), and cultures of the throat, blood, urine, and wound (if any). If there is granulocytopenia (<1000/mm^3), consult the oncologist and consider admitting the patient for IV antibiotics pending culture results. The ultimate choice of antibiotic is best determined after checking the sensitivities of the local hospital flora. See p. 359 for initial antibiotic guidelines.

The treatment of varicella exposure in a patient with a negative history (and negative varicella titers) is zoster-immune globulin (VZIG; VariZIG®), 1 vial/10 kg (five vial maximum) given within four days of exposure. There is no benefit of VZIG if the patient is seen four or more days after the exposure. Regardless of VZIG treatment, if clinical varicella develops, admit the patient and treat with IV acyclovir (500 mg/m^2 IV q 8h) or valacyclovir.

If spinal cord compression is suspected, plain films of the spine may be helpful, but definitive diagnosis usually requires an MRI scan or, rarely, a myelogram. A patient with signs of intracranial involvement requires an emergent CT or MRI. If a mass lesion is found, immediately consult with a neurologist, neurosurgeon, and an oncologist. Urgent treatment is required with some combination of radiation therapy, dexamethasone, and surgical intervention.

The diagnosis of superior vena cava obstruction is confirmed by finding an anterior mediastinal mass on chest film or chest CT. Obtain a CBC with differential, platelet count, and serum creatinine while awaiting consultation with an oncologist. Secure IV access in a lower extremity to avoid aggravating the condition with intravenous fluids directed toward the superior vena cava. The treatment is chemotherapy, steroids, and, less commonly, radiation.

Treat elevation of uric acid (>5 mg/dL) with hydration (twice maintenance) and allopurinol (250 mg/m^2/day); add alkalinization of the urine with sodium bicarbonate (1–2 mEq/kg) if there is greater concern about tumor lysis. If the uric acid is >8 mg/dL, treat with rasburicase (0.15 mg/kg/day). Treat hyperkalemia > 6 mEq/L (pp. 186–187) with kayexalate enemas (1 g/kg). If the hyperkalemia is associated with ECG changes (peaked T-waves), give insulin (0.1 units/kg IV) and glucose (0.5 g/kg IV). If there is an associated QRS widening or PR lengthening, also give calcium chloride (20 mg/kg IV over 3–5 min). Dialysis is indicated for a serum potassium >7.5 mEq/L. Treat hypocalcemia (p. 193) <7.5 mEq/L with 75 mg/kg/day of elemental oral calcium, div q 6h, and amphojel 500 mg PO to lower the phosphorus.

If intestinal perforation is suspected, obtain an upright or right and left lateral decubitus films of the abdomen looking for free air. A CT scan often confirms the diagnosis. Immediately treat with broad-spectrum antibiotics (as for febrile patient, see above), including additional anaerobic coverage (metronidazole 30 mg/kg/day, div q 6h or piperacillin/tazobactam 250 mg/kg/day div q 6h). Carefully monitor the blood pressure, since these patients can rapidly develop both hypovolemia and septic shock. Treat hypotension (pp. 20–28) expeditiously with isotonic fluid and packed red cell transfusions, along with vasopressors. Consult a surgeon to arrange for possible emergency laparotomy.

Indications for Admission

- Fever (>38.6 °C, 101.5 °F) and granulocytopenia (<750/mm^3), unless the oncologist recommends outpatient management
- Pneumonia, or evidence of any serious infection (e.g., hypotension, toxic appearance)
- Clinical varicella
- Spinal cord compression, CNS disease, superior vena cava obstruction, airway obstruction
- Significant complication of therapy or serious metabolic derangement (uric acid >10 mg/dL; potassium >6 mEq/L; calcium <7.5 mEq/L)
- Suspected intestinal perforation

Bibliography

Henry M, Sung L. Supportive care in pediatric oncology: oncologic emergencies and management of fever and neutropenia. *Pediatr Clin North Am.* 2015;**62**(1):27–46.

Mullin EA, Gratias E. Oncologic emergencies. In Orkin SH, Nathan DG, Ginsburg D, et al. (eds.) *Nathan and Oski's Hematology of Infancy and Childhood* (8th edn.). Philadelphia, PA: Elsevier Saunders, 2014; 2267–2291.

Prusakowski MK, Cannone D. Pediatric oncologic emergencies. *Emerg Med Clin North Am.* 2014;**32** (3):527–548.

Sickle Cell Disease

The sickle cell syndromes are inherited disorders characterized by a chronic hemolytic anemia of variable severity, as well as recurrent obstruction of the microvasculature.

Clinical Presentation

Children with sickle cell disease (SCD) may present with a constellation of signs and symptoms, termed crises.

Vaso-occlusive Crisis

The most frequent complication of sickle cell disease is the vaso-occlusive crisis, which is secondary to obstruction of blood flow caused by sickled red blood cells in capillaries and small veins. Virtually all organ systems can be affected by sickling. Patients typically present with severe pain, fever, and symptoms that can mimic many infectious and inflammatory disorders. A common finding is bone pain in multiple sites, particularly the extremities and back. Other presentations may include priapism, respiratory distress, limp, hematuria, acute hemiplegia (stroke), acute visual impairment caused by retinal vein occlusion or proliferative retinopathy, and leg ulcers. Right upper quadrant pain and jaundice occur in older children secondary to cholelithiasis from chronic hemolysis. In children under two years of age, vaso-occlusive crises often take the form of dactylitis, or the "hand–foot" syndrome, with pain and swelling in the hands, feet, fingers, and toes.

Aplastic Crisis

Aplastic crises are manifested by worsening anemia and reticulocytopenia. These crises, lasting 7–10 days, usually follow viral infections (particularly parvovirus B19) that transiently suppress the bone marrow. Patients present with fatigue, lightheadedness, tachycardia, and palpitations. With parvovirus B19 infection, the patient may have a prodrome of fever, malaise, and myalgias, but the characteristic rash is usually absent.

Sequestration Crisis

Splenic sequestration crises, with pooling of RBCs in a rapidly enlarging spleen, can complicate homozygous sickle cell, but more often occurs in young patients doubly heterozygous for HbS and another abnormal hemoglobin, such as β-thalassemia (S-Thal) or hemoglobin C (S-C disease). The patient may present with cold clammy skin, a protuberant tense abdomen, marked tachycardia, extreme pallor, and profound hypotension, as well as a large left-sided abdominal mass (spleen). If unrecognized, deterioration can be rapid with a fatal outcome.

Hyperhemolytic Crisis

A hyperhemolytic crisis, with a falling hematocrit, increasing jaundice, and markedly elevated reticulocyte counts (>20%), is rare and may in reality be the resolving phase of an aplastic crisis. Increased hemolysis with a rise in bilirubin can also be seen in patients with concurrent G-6-PD deficiency.

Megaloblastic Crisis

A megaloblastic crisis, due to folate depletion, is rare and may be diagnosed by finding hypersegmented neutrophils and pancytopenia.

Infection

Infections account for many of the serious problems in patients with SCD. Hyposplenism (initially functional, then anatomic) in conjunction with decreased antibody production, decreased serum-opsonizing activity, vaso-occlusion, and defective neutrophil function places these children at risk for fulminant overwhelming sepsis, particularly with encapsulated organisms such as *Streptococcus pneumoniae*. They are also at increased risk for meningitis, pneumonia, pyelonephritis, and osteomyelitis (particularly *Salmonella*). While the polyvalent pneumococcal vaccine does not reliably prevent serious pneumococcal infections in children under two years of age, Prevnar conjugate vaccine, in conjunction with prophylactic penicillin, is very effective in young infants, and decreases the incidence of life-threatening pneumococcal disease.

Diagnosis

Most children with sickle cell disease are diagnosed in the neonatal period with mandatory newborn hemoglobinopathy screening tests. However, test an undiagnosed child who presents with any of the classic sickle cell symptomatology noted above for SCD. Confirm the screening test with hemoglobin electrophoresis to determine the particular form of the disease (S-S, S-C, S-Thal). Suspect the diagnosis in an asymptomatic patient whose peripheral blood picture reveals anemia, sickle cells, and reticulocytosis (>5%). In addition, the smear will often contain target cells, "helmet" cells, polychromasia, and Howell–Jolly bodies.

A major diagnostic problem in children with SCD is in determining the cause of certain symptomatology, in particular differentiating between infection and infarction. A vaso-occlusive crisis is always a diagnosis of exclusion. Leukocytosis (>18,000–25,000/mm^3) is typical in SCD, and fever may not be helpful in distinguishing the different entities. Particular difficulties are seen with the symptoms described below.

Bone Pain

Differentiating between bone infarcts and osteomyelitis can be very difficult, particularly when only one site is involved. Plain films and bone scans are often unreliable, necessitating needle aspiration to obtain a specimen for culture. Elevated serum inflammatory markers (CRP, ESR) and an increased number of bands (>10% of the total WBC) on peripheral smear may indicate an infection, but are not 100% sensitive. Aseptic necrosis of the head of the femur or humerus presents with bone pain and, in most cases, abnormal radiographs of the affected limb. An MRI scan is often necessary to detect early osteonecrosis.

Right Upper Quadrant Abdominal Pain

Consider hepatitis (especially for patients on chronic transfusion therapy), hepatic infarction, and cholelithiasis in patients with severe right upper quadrant pain, fever, and elevated bilirubin. With hepatic infarcts, abnormal liver chemistries, as a rule, return to baseline in a much shorter amount of time (days) than with hepatitis, while an abdominal sonogram usually detects biliary stones. While right lower lobe pneumonia, rib infarcts, intestinal wall infarcts, and renal disorders (pyelonephritis and papillary necrosis) can all cause pain in the same location, other physical and laboratory findings, including urinalysis and radiographs, help to differentiate among these conditions.

Chest Pain and Respiratory Distress

Patients with acute chest syndrome can deteriorate rapidly and occasionally require assisted ventilation. The major differential is between vaso-occlusion (pulmonary infarct) and infection (pneumonia). Fever, leukocytosis, and similar radiographic and auscultatory findings occur with both diseases. In addition, the two conditions can coexist and one can lead to the other, so it is prudent to treat for both entities. A ventilation–perfusion scan may differentiate between the two, although generally therapy will not be any different regardless of the results, so this test is not usually necessary. Finally, chest pain can be secondary to rib infarcts and abdominal disorders.

ED Management

Vaso-occlusive Crisis

Hydroxyurea is now widely used to increase the fetal hemoglobin level and thus prevent sickling. However, since there is no safe, effective antisickling agent to abort acute crises, therapy consists of treatment of the triggering event and potentiating factors, and supportive care including the following.

Vigorous Hydration

The patient often presents with decreased plasma volume secondary to fever, vomiting, and chronic hyposthenuria. In addition to ad lib oral intake, administer several hours of intravenous hydration at a twice-maintenance rate, except for a patient with a pulmonary infarct (use no more than maintenance fluids since these patients can rapidly develop pleural effusions and worsening respiratory status). The type of fluid is controversial, but D_5 ½ NS or D_5 ¼ NS is satisfactory.

Sodium Bicarbonate

Add sodium bicarbonate (1 mEq/kg) to the solution *only* if a marked metabolic acidosis is present (pH <7.20).

Analgesics

For mild vaso-occlusive crises, give aspirin (15 mg/kg), ibuprofen (10 mg/kg), or for a teenager 5 mg oxycodone plus 325 mg acetaminophen (Percocet) q 3–4h is an alternative. Ketorolac (0.5 mg/kg q 6h), a potent non-narcotic analgesic that is less likely to cause respiratory depression, is another excellent alternative. Occasionally, for more severe pain, a single injection of dilaudid or morphine (0.1 mg/kg), in conjunction with ketorolac and a few hours of vigorous hydration can prevent hospital admission. Vigorous analgesic therapy upon presentation to the ED may decrease the need for hospitalization.

Antipyretics

Fever leads to further dehydration and sickling, so treat with aspirin (15 mg/kg q 4h), ibuprofen (10 mg/kg q 6h), or acetaminophen (15 mg/kg q 4h).

Radiograph

If the patient is limping, obtain radiographs of the hip to rule-out aseptic necrosis of the femoral head. If positive, restrict weight bearing and consult with an orthopedist and hematologist.

Oxygen

Oxygen therapy has not been shown to be of benefit for the management of most painful crises, and in fact may be detrimental since there can be a "rebound" crisis with an outpouring of sickle cells from the bone marrow after oxygen administration is discontinued. Indications for supplementary oxygen include severe anemia, pneumonia or pulmonary infarction (particularly if there is documented hypoxia), and shock from infection or splenic sequestration.

Aplastic Crisis

If the patient has not yet begun to recover, as manifested by a brisk reticulocytosis, follow the hemoglobin closely; these patients often have little reserve. A transfusion is usually necessary if the hematocrit is <15% with a reticulocyte count <1%.

Sequestration Crisis

Do not give rapid IV boluses of dextrose or saline, which can cause pulmonary edema. The critical treatment is transfusion of packed RBCs. If the patient is hypotensive, immediately infuse plasmanate (10–20 L/kg) if packed RBCs are not available, followed by a rapid transfusion(s) of packed red cells in 5 mL/kg aliquots, if the hematocrit is <15%; do not transfuse to a hematocrit >25%. This is one instance where rapid red cell transfusion can be life-saving.

Megaloblastic Crisis

If the hematocrit is >20%, the absolute granulocyte count >1000/mm^3, and the platelet count >50,000/mm^3, administer folic acid 1 mg/day. Repeat the blood count in 4–7 days. For more pronounced cytopenia, the dose can be increased up to 5 mg/day.

Fever

For a patient more than two years of age in no distress, with a temperature <38.9 °C (102 °F) and no obvious source for the fever, obtain a blood culture, CBC, ESR, and a urinalysis. Obtain a urine culture if the patient has symptoms of dysuria, frequency or urgency, or if the urinalysis is suspicious for a UTI. If there is no marked left shift and the absolute band count is <3000/mm³, send a non-ill-appearing patient home to take oral antibiotics (<15 years: amoxicillin-clavulanate [875/125 formulation], 45 mg/kg/day of amoxicillin div bid *or* cefdinir 14 mg/kg/day div q day or bid; >15 years penicillin VK 250 mg qid). Give one dose of ceftriaxone (50 mg/kg IM) and observe for several hours before discharge from the ED. Arrange for follow-up in 24 hours, or sooner if the temperature goes higher.

Admit the patient with a temperature >39.4 °C (10 3 °F). Also admit any toxic-appearing patient and a child younger than two years with a temperature >38.9 °C (102 °F). Treat with IV ceftriaxone (100 mg/kg/day div q 12h). For a patient taking hydroxyurea (which can cause neutropenia), broad-spectrum antibiotic coverage is indicated (p. 359) if the absolute neutrophil count is <500/mm³. Add vancomycin for a toxic-appearing child.

In addition to the basic fever work-up, if there are any respiratory symptoms or chest pain, obtain a chest film, regardless of the auscultatory findings. Admit and treat any sickle cell patient with a pulmonary density as having a possible pneumonia. Administer ceftriaxone (100 mg/kg/day div q 12h), oxygen if hypoxic, and a red cell transfusion, and if the patient is older than five years of age, add azithromycin (10 mg/kg, once on day 1, followed by 5 mg/kg/q day on days 2–5) for possible *Mycoplasma* infection. If there is any suspicion of an osteomyelitis (fever, swelling, point tenderness of a single bone), consult an orthopedist and arrange for a needle aspiration for Gram's stain, cell count, and culture. Indications for a lumbar puncture include a febrile irritable infant under two years of age and a lethargic older patient with a temperature >39.4 °C (103 °F) and no fever source.

Acute Chest Syndrome

Monitor the oxygen saturation and give supplemental oxygen and a packed RBC transfusion to a hypoxic patient. For milder episodes, pain medication and incentive spirometry are useful to prevent deterioration.

Follow-up

- Vaso-occlusive crisis: next day
- Megaloblastic crisis: 4–7 days
- Patient older than two years with temperature <38.9 °C (102 °F): 24 hours, or sooner if the temperature goes higher

Indications for Admission

- Serious symptoms, including acute hemiplegia, gross hematuria, acute visual disturbance, severe right upper quadrant pain, or respiratory distress
- Splenic sequestration or aplastic crisis with hematocrit <15%
- Patient younger than two years with temperature >38.9 °C (102 °F), older child with sudden temperature >39.4 °C (103 °F) with or without an identifiable source
- Severe or prolonged vaso-occlusive crisis with pain unresponsive to usual therapeutic measures
- Irritable infant with hand–foot syndrome, particularly if not taking oral fluids well

- Clinical pneumonia or any newly discovered pulmonary density on chest film
- Severe megaloblastic crisis (hematocrit <20%, platelet count <50,000/mm^3, or granulocyte count <1000/mm^3)

Bibliography

Heeney ME, Ware RE. Sickle cell disease. In Orkin SH, Nathan DG, Ginsburg D, et al. (eds.) *Nathan and Oski's Hematology of Infancy and Childhood* (8th edn.). Philadelphia, PA: Elsevier Saunders, 2014; 675–714.

Kanter J, Kruse-Jarres R. Management of sickle cell disease from childhood through adulthood. *Blood Rev.* 2013;27(6):279–287.

Meier ER, Miller JL: Sickle cell disease in children. Drugs. 2012; 72(7):895–906.

Miller AC, Gladwin MT. Pulmonary complications of sickle cell disease. *Am J Respir Crit Care Med.* 2012;185(11):1154–1165.

Yawn BP, Buchanan GR, Afenyi-Annan AN, et al. Management of sickle cell disease: summary of the 2014 evidence-based report by expert panel members. *JAMA.* 2014;312(10):1033–1048.

The Abnormal CBC

Table 12.6 The abnormal CBC

Finding	Diagnoses
RBC abnormalities	
Microcytic	Iron deficiency, the thalassemias, sideroblastic anemias (including lead poisoning), porphyrias, the anemia of chronic inflammation
Normocytic	Marrow failure or replacement, immune and extrinsic hemolysis, acute blood loss, hemoglobinopathies, membrane disorders, enzyme deficiencies
Macrocytic	Vitamin B12 and folic acid deficiencies, liver disease, hypothyroidism, inherited aplastic anemia or pure red cell hypoplasia
Platelet abnormalities	
Increased size	Immune thrombocytopenic purpura, Bernard–Soulier syndrome, May–Hegglin anomaly
Decreased size	Wiskott–Aldrich syndrome, leukemias
Absence of color	Storage pool disorders
White cell abnormalities	
↑ Mature granulocytes	Infections, inflammation, stress reactions
↑ Immature cells	Leukemia
Leukopenia	Viral infections, overwhelming bacterial infections, drug suppression, marrow failure or marrow replacement.
Atypical lymphocytes	Viral infections (EBV, CMV)
Increased eosinophils	Parasitic infection, allergic disorders
Basophilia	Chronic myelogenous leukemia
Inclusions (Döhle bodies)	Serious infections, May–Hegglin anomaly

Bibliography

Farruggia P. Immune neutropenias of infancy and childhood. *World J Pediatr*. 2016;**12**(2):142–148.

Teachey DT, Lambert MP. Diagnosis and management of autoimmune cytopenias in childhood. *Pediatr Clin North Am*. 2013;**60**(6):1489–1511.

Walkovich K, Boxer LA. How to approach neutropenia in childhood. *Pediatr Rev*. 2013;**34** (4):173–184.

Thrombophilia

There are a number of inherited and acquired disorders that may present in childhood and predispose patients to thrombosis and abnormal clot formation. Three proteins – Protein C, Protein S, and Antithrombin III – are important in preventing abnormal clot formation. DNA mutations, including the Factor V Leiden and Prothrombin mutations, are important causes of thrombosis, and antiphospholipid syndrome is a possibility in any patient presenting with thrombosis. Elevated plasminogen activator inhibitor 1 and factor VIII are other predisposing factors.

Thrombocytosis can occur with a variety of conditions, as the platelet count often behaves as an acute phase reactant. Thrombocytosis may be seen in children with recent infections, major physical stress, or as a "rebound" phenomenon after a period of bone marrow suppression. Underlying disorders associated with thrombocytosis include malignancies (chronic myelogenous leukemia, neuroblastoma), Kawasaki syndrome, sarcoid, chronic inflammatory disorders (IBD), chronic hemolytic disorders, and iron deficiency. Primary idiopathic thrombocytosis is a rare condition that can sometimes be a precursor to leukemia. A platelet count >1,000,000/mm^3 may require treatment because of the risk of thrombosis.

Clinical Presentation

The patient will often present with swelling and pain in an extremity, most commonly the legs. Sometimes a distinct firm "cord" can be palpated, but more commonly there will be painful swelling, sometimes with overlying erythema. The swelling can be significant, with a marked asymmetry when comparing both extremities. A pulmonary embolus presents with sudden onset of respiratory distress and tachypnea, typically with chest pain and areas of decreased breath sounds on auscultation.

A possible sinus thrombosis is suggested by persistent severe headaches with a history of inflammation or infection in the head and neck area. A patient with acute onset of neurologic symptoms and a scan that demonstrates an infarct requires an evaluation for thrombophilia. A patient with swelling, numbness, and a cold upper extremity is highly suspect for thoracic outlet syndrome.

Diagnosis

If there is a suspicion of thrombophlebitis of an extremity, a Doppler study can assess patency of the vasculature. On occasion, MRI of the vessels can add more detail to the evaluation, particularly for thrombosis of deep veins. For a patient with respiratory symptoms, particularly if there is also suspicion of a thrombus in an extremity, a spiral CT scan of the chest will usually demonstrate the affected areas. D-dimers are typically elevated in a patient with thrombosis, and they can be markedly elevated with pulmonary embolism.

Ask about any history of indwelling catheters, particularly in the neonatal period or in patients with PICC lines or indwelling central venous catheters. Dehydration, birth control pills, and prolonged periods of immobilization can lead to localized stasis and thrombosis.

To evaluate the patient for a possible underlying predisposition, after consultation with a hematologist, obtain a CBC, PT, PTT, anticardiolipin antibodies; factor VIII activity; lupus anticoagulant; Protein C, Protein S, and Antithrombin III levels; Factor V Leiden; and prothrombin mutations.

ED Management

The presence of a thrombus warrants rapid intervention to prevent propagation and worsening symptoms. For patients with elevated platelet counts, give antiplatelet medications to reduce the risk of thrombus formation, including aspirin (often just one baby aspirin every other day) and dipyridamole (50–75 mg, 2–3 times per day). If a thrombus of the lower extremity is detected, institute anticoagulation promptly, preferably with low molecular weight heparin (1 mg/kg every 12 hours). Thrombolysis is another option, particularly for life-threatening pulmonary emboli and large deep vein thromboses, but this should be undertaken by vascular surgeons and interventional radiologists experienced in dealing with these situations.

Consult with a hematologist to initiate the work-up for a possible underlying predisposition for thrombophilia. Obtain a CBC, PT, PTT, anticardiolipin antibodies; factor VIII activity; lupus anticoagulant; Protein C, Protein S, and Antithrombin III panels, and Factor V Leiden, in addition to other tests that the consult suggests.

Indications for Admission

- Suspicion or confirmation of venous thrombosis
- Suspicion or confirmation of pulmonary embolus

Bibliography

Holzhauer S, Goldenberg NA, Junker R, et al. Inherited thrombophilia in children with venous thromboembolism and the familial risk of thromboembolism: an observational study. *Blood*. 2012;**120** (7): 1510–1515.

Klaassen IL, van Ommen CH, Middeldorp S. Manifestations and clinical impact of pediatric inherited thrombophilia. *Blood*. 2015;**125**(7):1073–1077.

Tolbert J, Carpenter SL. Common acquired causes of thrombosis in children. *Curr Probl Pediatr Adolesc Health Care*. 2013;**43**(7):169–177.

Tormene D, Gavasso S, Rossetto V, Simioni P. Thrombosis and thrombophilia in children: a systematic review. *Semin Thromb Hemost*. 2006;**32**:724–728.

Yang JY, Chan AK: Pediatric thrombophilia. *Pediatr Clin North Am*. 2013;**60**(6):1443–1462.

Transfusion Therapy

Criteria for transfusions vary, depending on the underlying condition, the desired effect, and the risks of transfusion versus the anticipated benefits. Each 1 mL/kg of packed cells raises the hematocrit approximately 0.7%. If the patient has a slowly evolving moderately severe anemia requiring red cell transfusion, appropriate compensatory mechanisms, and a normal blood pressure, transfuse a maximum volume of 10–15 mL/kg of packed red cells slowly, over 2–3 hours. For very severe, chronic, or well-compensated anemias, administer the blood in smaller 5 mL/kg aliquots, with several hours between transfusions to allow for the vascular compartment to remove excess fluid. A diuretic, such as furosemide (0.5 mg/kg IV), may be required between transfusions to prevent volume overload and heart failure. When treating acute or ongoing blood loss, particularly if there is hypovolemia or hypotension, administer the blood rapidly. This situation includes splenic sequestration crises in patients with chronic hemolytic anemias, such as sickle cell disease and spherocytosis.

For multiply-transfused patients or patients who have experienced prior febrile, non-hemolytic transfusion reactions, use leukocyte-depleted RBCs to decrease the likelihood of transfusion reactions. Request irradiated red cells for any immunodeficient patient, including neonates, patients with malignancies or immunodeficiency diseases, bone marrow transplant candidates, and patients on immunosuppressive therapy. Irradiation destroys lymphocytes that might cause serious graft-versus-host disease in the recipient.

Premedicate the patient with acetaminophen (15 mg/kg) to decrease the risk of febrile non-hemolytic transfusion reactions. For a patient with a history of frequent reactions, particularly if urticarial, give diphenhydramine (1 mg/kg PO or 0.5 mg/kg IV) and/or corticosteroids (hydrocortisone 1 mg/kg PO or IV). A patient with an autoimmune hemolytic anemia who requires transfusions poses additional difficulties. It may be impossible to find a completely compatible donor unit, so the least reactive unit is often the only alternative. If a cold antibody is present, infuse the RBCs through an intravenous fluid warmer to decrease the amount of hemolysis. Because of the high risk of reactions, administer high-dose steroids (hydrocortisone 1–1.5 mg/kg IV) prior to and every 3–4 hours during the transfusion.

Platelet transfusions can help stop bleeding in a thrombocytopenic patient who is not producing platelets (leukemia, aplastic anemia), but are of little value in patients with ITP, unless there is ongoing, severe internal bleeding. Generally, use single-donor apheresis platelets to expose the patient to fewer donors with a lessened risk of antibody sensitization and possible infection. Always premedicate the patient since reactions to platelet transfusions are more common than those associated with transfused RBCs.

Bibliography

Lacroix J, Tucci M, Du Pont-Thibodeau G. Red blood cell transfusion decision making in critically ill children. *Curr Opin Pediatr*. 2015;**27**(3):286–291.

Parker R. Transfusion in critically ill children: indications, risks, and challenges. *Crit Care Med*. 2014;**42**(3):675–690.

Sloan SR. Transfusion medicine. In Orkin SH, Nathan DG, Ginsburg D, et al. (eds.) *Nathan and Oski's Hematology of Infancy and Childhood* (8th ed). Philadelphia, PA: Elsevier Saunders, 2014; 1127–1166.

Chapter 13

Infectious Disease Emergencies

Keri A. Cohn, Michael E. Russo, Carmelle Tsai, and
Alexandra M. Vinograd

Botulism

Botulism is a neuroparalytic disease caused by a neurotoxin elaborated by *Clostridium botulinum*, a Gram-positive, spore-forming, obligate anaerobe whose natural habitat is the soil. Botulinum toxin is tasteless, odorless, and extremely toxic. It acts by irreversibly blocking the release of acetylcholine in peripheral somatic and autonomic synapses as well as at the motor end plates.

Infants lack the *Clostridium* inhibiting bile acids and protective bacterial flora found in the normal adult intestinal tract, so botulism spores can germinate in the intestinal tract. There are approximately 100 cases of infant botulism annually in the United States, with a peak incidence between 2–4 months of age. Honey consumption and parental employment at construction sites are significant risk factors.

In contrast, in older children, botulism usually occurs after the ingestion of preformed toxin in spoiled food. Raw, home canned, or inadequately prepared foods may be contaminated with the toxin, which is heat labile. Heating food to the boiling point destroys the toxin, but the bacterial spores are resistant to heat and may survive the home-canning process. Canned fish, vegetables, and potatoes have been implicated in outbreaks of botulism.

In wound botulism, *C. botulinum* grows in the injured tissue and produces toxin. Most cases of wound botulism in the United States occur either in intravenous drug users or children with compound extremity fractures.

Clinical Presentation

Infantile botulism begins gradually, 2–4 weeks after ingestion of the spores. Breastfed infants are infected later than formula-fed infants, and breastfeeding may moderate the severity of the illness. Constipation is often the first symptom, followed by weak cry, weak suck, drooling, difficulty feeding, dysphagia, loss of head control, signs of descending cranial nerve palsies, and hypotonia. Progressive paralysis can lead to respiratory failure.

After infancy, botulism manifests as a symmetric, descending, flaccid paralysis, without fever. Symptoms of food-borne botulism begin within 12–36 hours of ingestion of contaminated food. The patient develops blurred vision, diplopia, ptosis, ophthalmoplegia, dysarthria, and dysphagia. Autonomic signs include constipation, dry mouth, postural hypotension, urinary retention, and pupillary dilation with a sluggish or absent light reflex. Nausea and vomiting may also occur in one-third of patients. A descending weakness follows, which, in severe cases, may involve the respiratory muscles. Weakness is usually bilateral, but may be asymmetric. The sensory nerves and mentation are notably spared.

After a 4–14-day incubation period, the presentation of wound botulism is similar to food-borne botulism. There may be fever, but not nausea and vomiting. The wound may exhibit no signs of infection.

Diagnosis

The initial diagnosis is clinical, and CSF studies may be normal. The diagnosis can be confirmed by analyzing suspected food, serum, gastrointestinal contents/stool, or wound exudates for evidence of toxin or organisms. However, do not delay treatment while waiting for laboratory confirmation.

Other causes of paralysis include Guillain-Barré syndrome (ascending paralysis with an elevated CSF protein), poliomyelitis (asymmetric involvement, fever, CSF pleocytosis), myasthenia gravis (muscle fatigability, reversal of ptosis with edrophonium), spinal muscular atrophy (severe weakness, absent DTRs, tongue fasciculations), and tick paralysis (rapidly progressive generalized paralysis, absent DTRs, normal CSF protein, possible dysesthesias). In a febrile infant who is lethargic and feeding poorly, consider bacterial sepsis or meningitis. Metabolic causes of acute weakness include hypokalemia, hypo- and hypercalcemia, and hypo- and hyperthyroidism

ED Management

Admit the patient to an ICU for monitoring, as respiratory arrest from ascending paralysis can occur at any time. If clinically indicated (focal neurologic examination; signs of increased intracranial pressure), obtain a CT or MRI of the head.

The mainstay of therapy is supportive. Give human-derived antitoxin (BIG-IV; BabyBIG), which is produced and distributed by the California Department of Public Health (24-hour telephone number: 510-231-7600; www.infantbotulism.org). Equine-derived heptavalent botulinum antitoxin is available from the CDC for older children and adults.

Although antibiotics are not necessary to eradicate the bowel colonization of infants, treat wound botulism with antitoxin and antibiotics (penicillin or clindamycin). If sepsis cannot be excluded, obtain a CBC, blood culture, and lumbar puncture, and start age-appropriate empiric antibiotics (see pp. 391–394). Do not use aminoglycosides because they may potentiate the effects of the toxin. Notify the state health department of any suspected cases of botulism.

Indications for Admission

- Suspected botulism

Bibliography

American Academy of Pediatrics. Botulism and infant botulism. In Kimberlin DW, Brady MT, Jackson MA, Long SA (eds.) *Red Book: 2015 Report of the Committee on Infectious Diseases* (30th edn.). Elk Grove Village, IL: American Academy of Pediatrics, 2015; 294–297.

Centers for Disease Control and Prevention. Botulism. www.cdc.gov/botulism (accessed June 6, 2017).

Pifko E, Price A, Sterner S. Infant botulism and indications for administration of botulism immune globulin. *Pediatr Emerg Care.* 2014;30(2):120–124.

Proverbio MR, Lamba M, Rossi A, Siani P. Early diagnosis and treatment in a child with foodborne botulism. *Anaerobe.* 2016;39:189–192.

Rosow LK, Strober JB. Infant botulism: review and clinical update. *Pediatr Neurol*. 2015;**52** (5):487–492.

Chikungunya

Chikungunya is transmitted to humans by the *Aedes* mosquito. In Swahili, the name means "to become contorted," describing the characteristic joint pain that is part of the disease. Travelers returning from Africa, Asia, parts of Central/South America, islands in the Indian Ocean, the Western and South Pacific, and the Caribbean are at risk. Local transmission can occur if infected travelers return to an area where *Aedes* mosquitoes exist.

Clinical Presentation

The incubation period is generally 2–4 days (range 1–12 days). The disease presents with the sudden onset of high fever, arthralgias, myalgias, headaches, photophobia, and variable rash. The arthralgias are usually symmetrical, polyarticular, and frequently involve the fingers, wrists, ankles, elbows, toes, and knees. Joint swelling is common, especially of the ankles and wrists. While the other symptoms resolve in 1–2 weeks, the arthralgias commonly persist or recur for months or years. Atypical, severe disease is associated with neurologic complications, including encephalitis and febrile seizures, and/or multiorgan failure and death.

Diagnosis

Consider Chikungunya, as well as dengue fever, in a patient with fever and arthralgias or arthritis who has traveled to an endemic area within 15 days of symptom onset. Laboratory diagnosis includes viral isolation in culture, detection of viral RNA via RT-PCR, the presence of IgM antibodies, or a four-fold increase in IgG in paired samples.

ED Management

Treatment is supportive, including NSAIDS for management of arthralgias.

Follow-up

- Primary care in one week

Indications for Admission

- Neurologic complications
- End-organ complications

Bibliography

American Academy of Pediatrics. Arboviruses. In *Red Book: 2015 Report of the Committee on Infectious Diseases*. Elk Grove Village, IL: American Academy of Pediatrics, 2015; 240–246.

Burt FJ, Rolph MS, Rulli NE, Mahalingam S, Heise MT. Chikungunya: a re-emerging virus. *Lancet*. 2012;**379**(9816):662–671.

Centers for Disease Control and Prevention. Chikungunya. wwwnc.cdc.gov/travel/diseases/chikungunya (accessed June 2, 2017).

Madariaga M, Ticona E, Resurrecion C. Chikungunya: bending over the Americas and the rest of the world. *Braz J Infect Dis*. 2016;**20**(1):91–98.

Patterson J, Sammon M, Garg M. Dengue, Zika and chikungunya: emerging arboviruses in the new world. *West J Emerg Med*. 2016;**17**(6):671–679.

Pineda C, Muñoz-Louis R, Caballero-Uribe CV, Viasus D. Chikungunya in the region of the Americas: a challenge for rheumatologists and health care systems. *Clin Rheumatol*. 2016;**35**(10):2381–2385.

Dengue Viruses

Dengue viruses are transmitted to humans by certain species of *Aedes* mosquitoes, so that most infections are contracted during travel to tropical and subtropical areas. The incidence of travel-associated dengue has increased during the past decade due to epidemics in tropical regions, including Puerto Rico, the Caribbean, and Latin America. There are four serotypes and infection with one serotype does not provide immunity to the other serotypes.

Clinical Presentation

The typical incubation period is 4–7 days. The course ranges from asymptomatic infection to mild febrile illness to a severe and fatal hemorrhagic disease. Initial symptoms include fever for 3–7 days, abdominal pain, nausea and vomiting, cough, headache, retro-orbital pain, constipation, body aches, and joint pain ("breakbone fever"). On physical examination the patient may have a relative bradycardia, hepatomegaly, conjunctival injection, pharyngeal erythema, lymphadenopathy, and mild hemorrhagic manifestations such as petechiae. Approximately half of patients describe a variable rash, often macular, that starts on the trunk and spreads to the face and extremities. A second rash that results in desquamation may present after recovery from severe dengue.

The most severe infections cause dengue hemorrhagic fever (DHF) or dengue shock syndrome (DSS), with vascular leak. DSS presents at the time of initial defervescence, often when it seems that the patient is improving. Warning signs include abdominal pain, vomiting, clinical fluid accumulation (pleural effusions, ascites), mucosal bleeding, altered mental status, hepatomegaly, and/or a rising hematocrit (reflecting hemoconcentration) with a falling platelet count. DSS is heralded by a narrow pulse pressure (<20 mmHg). It can progress rapidly, resulting in irreversible shock and death. Rare complications include myocarditis, hepatitis, and neurologic symptoms. Laboratory abnormalities may include severe liver dysfunction, hypoproteinemia, elevated PTT, and decreased fibrinogen. The critical phase lasts 48–72 hours and is followed by the recovery phase. The patient can develop a second variable rash that resolves with desquamation over 1–2 weeks.

Diagnosis

Include dengue in the differential diagnosis of any febrile patient who lives in or who has traveled to a dengue-endemic area within two weeks and has at least two of the following criteria:

- nausea/vomiting
- rash
- aches and pains
- positive tourniquet test (>10 petechiae/inch^2 distal to a BP cuff inflated midway between systolic and diastolic)

- any warning signs: abdominal pain/tenderness, persistent vomiting, clinical fluid accumulation, mucosal bleeding, lethargy or restlessness, liver enlargement >2 cm, and an increase in hematocrit with concurrent rapid decrease in platelet count

Criteria for severe dengue include severe plasma leakage resulting in shock or fluid accumulation with respiratory distress, severe bleeding, and severe organ impairment (liver, CNS, cardiac, other organs)

In acute disease, the diagnosis can be confirmed with a dengue RT-PCR. If molecular detection is not available, obtain paired acute and convalescent phase testing for anti-dengue antibodies.

ED Management

The management of dengue is supportive. A patient with suspected dengue who can tolerate oral fluids can be managed at home, with daily follow-up and strict instructions to return if bleeding or the warning signs develop. Hospitalize any patient with warning signs, for close monitoring for vascular leak syndrome. Treat dengue shock with careful administration of isotonic crystalloid solutions to maintain cardiovascular stability while avoiding volume overload. Avoid aspirin, nonsteroidal anti-inflammatories (NSAIDS), and other anticoagulants due to the risk of hemorrhagic complications.

Indications for Admission

- Suspected dengue fever with any warning signs

Bibliography

Centers for Disease Control and Prevention (CDC). Dengue. www.cdc.gov/dengue (accessed June 2, 2017).

Gubler DJ, Ooi EE, Vasudevan S, Farrar J. *Dengue and Dengue Hemorrhagic Fever*. Boston, MA: CAB International, 2014.

Muller DA, Depelsenaire AC, Young PR. Clinical and laboratory diagnosis of dengue virus infection. *J Infect Dis.* 2017;**215**(Suppl. 2):S89–S95.

Nedjadi T, El-Kafrawy S, Sohrab SS, et al. Tackling dengue fever: current status and challenges. *Virol J.* 2015;**12**:212.

Simmons CP, Farrar JJ, Chau NV, Wills B. Dengue. *N Engl J Med.* 2012;**366**(15):1423–1432.

Encephalitis

Approximately 20,000 cases of encephalitis occur in the United States each year, most of which are mild. Enteroviruses (enterovirus, echovirus, Coxsackieviruses) are the cause of epidemics in the summer and fall. Sporadic cases of encephalitis are secondary to the herpes simplex viruses (HSV-1 and -2), arthropod-borne viruses (St. Louis encephalitis, California encephalitis, eastern, western, Venezuelan equine encephalitis, and West Nile [WNV] virus), and other herpes viruses (Epstein–Barr, cytomegalovirus, varicella zoster).

Bacterial causes include *Haemophilus influenzae, Neisseria meningitides, Streptococcus pneumoniae,* and *Mycobacterium tuberculosis,* although these organisms more often cause meningitis (pp. 422–425). Spirochetal infections include *Treponema pallidum, Leptospira* species, and *Borrelia burgdorferi* (Lyme disease). Other non-viral causes of encephalitis include *C. pneumoniae, Mycoplasma pneumoniae, M. hominis,* and *Coccidiodes immitus.* Additionally, *Toxoplasma gondii, Cryptococcus neoformans,* and *Listeria monocytogenes* can cause encephalitis in an immunocompromised patient.

Post-infectious encephalitis is thought to be an autoimmune phenomenon initiated by viral (influenza, varicella, measles) or bacterial (*Mycoplasma*) pathogens in children with symptoms of CNS inflammation in the absence of an acute bacterial or fungal infection. Characteristically, there is a latent phase between the acute illness and the onset of neurologic symptoms.

Clinical Presentation

Encephalitis most commonly begins as an acute systemic illness with fever and headache. Most patients have diffuse disease with behavioral or personality changes, altered level of consciousness, or generalized seizures. Some patients may have localized findings, such as ataxia, cranial nerve defects, hemiparesis, or focal seizures. Alternatively, there may be high fever, convulsions with bizarre movements, and hallucinations alternating with periods of clarity. Nuchal rigidity, if present, is less pronounced than with meningitis.

Herpes Viruses

Approximately 50% of newborns with HSV infection have CNS involvement. Morbidity and mortality depend on whether the infant has isolated CNS involvement or disseminated disease. Encephalitis in an older child or adolescent is usually secondary to HSV-1, which presents with fever, focal or generalized seizures, focal neurologic signs, and altered level of consciousness. Epstein–Barr virus encephalitis causes a focal encephalopathic disease in conjunction with fever, pharyngitis, lymphadenopathy, atypical lymphocytosis, and a positive heterophile test. Varicella encephalitis follows the distinctive exanthem and may lead to nystagmus, dysarthria, and cerebellar ataxia.

Arthropod and Mosquito Borne

These infections are transmitted by mosquitoes and ticks, and outbreaks occur primarily during the summer and fall seasons. Human WNV has been reported throughout the continental United States. The vector is mosquitoes that prey on birds and humans are the principal vectors. After an incubation period of 3–6 days, there is an abrupt onset of a febrile, flu-like illness. In addition, there may be conjunctivitis, retrobulbar pain, and a maculopapular rash that spreads from the trunk to the extremities and head. In contrast to adults, CNS involvement is rare in children. Other severe complications of WNV include hepatitis, pancreatitis, myocarditis, and hepatosplenomegaly.

Enteroviruses

Enteroviral infection usually occurs in the summer. Following a prodrome of fever and upper respiratory tract symptoms, the patient develops acute neurologic findings such as confusion, altered level of consciousness, or irritability. Neurologic manifestations are usually global rather than focal, although flaccid paralysis may occur. Other possible manifestations include photophobia and a macular or petechial rash.

Post-infectious

A patient with measles parainfectious encephalitis presents during recovery from the acute illness with the abrupt onset of fever, neurologic symptoms, and altered mental status. Approximately 50% of patients have seizures.

Diagnosis

Obtain a detailed history, including whether there has been any antecedent viral infection, systemic symptoms, ill contacts, or exposure to mosquitoes, ticks, or animals. Inquire about the immunologic status of the patient, recent travel or immunizations, and the possibility of accidental exposure to heavy metals or pesticides. Perform a thorough physical examination looking for rashes, lymphadenopathy, focal neurologic abnormalities, cerebellar signs, and evidence of increased intracranial pressure (including fundoscopy). Have a high index of suspicion for neonatal HSV infection in an acutely ill infant <21 days of age.

ED Management

Perform a lumbar puncture to exclude bacterial meningitis unless there are focal neurologic signs or evidence of increased intracranial pressure. In such a case, give the first doses of empiric antibiotics for suspected bacterial meningitis (see Table 13.8), and arrange for a CT scan of the head prior to performing the lumbar puncture. HSV is associated with hemorrhagic inflammation of the temporal lobe and sylvian fissure.

Send the CSF for Gram stain, cell count, protein, glucose, culture, rapid antigen identification test, viral culture, and if tuberculosis is a possibility, acid fast stain, culture and/or PCR for *Mycobacterium*. The CSF in viral encephalitis is usually clear, and the leukocyte count can range from none to several thousand with a polymorphonuclear predominance early in the course. The protein is normal to moderately elevated, and the glucose is initially normal (see Table 13.7).

Obtain a CBC, platelet count, electrolytes, BUN, creatinine, glucose, blood culture, and a urinalysis. If specific viral etiologies are being considered, send urine, stool, CSF, and throat swabs for viral diagnostic tests and sera for viral titers. In particular, if HSV or enterovirus is a possibility, send CSF for PCR, which is 98% sensitive and 94% specific. In several states, the Department of Health offers additional CSF testing for a PCR panel (along with serological testing) of most likely pathogens for cases of encephalitis with additional testing (arbovirus or West Nile serology), as the history warrants.

Admit patients with encephalitis for close observation of vital signs and fluid status. Treat for bacterial meningitis pending culture results. Better outcomes after neonatal HSV infection are strongly associated with a shorter interval between diagnosis and initiation of treatment. If herpes is suspected, treat with acyclovir (≤14 days: 20 mg/kg q 12h; >14 days to <3 months: 20 mg/kg q 8h; ≥3 months to 12 years: 10–15 mg/kg q 8h; ≥12 years: 10 mg/kg q 8h)

During enteroviral epidemics in the summer and fall, a patient older than six years of age who develops meningitis without encephalitis with a stable presentation (mild to moderate headache that responds to acetaminophen or ibuprofen, nontoxic appearance, CSF with a monocytic pleocytosis and normal chemistries) can be discharged for supportive care. Admit any patient with nuchal rigidity, unresponsive moderate to severe headache, lethargy, or inability to maintain hydration.

Follow-up

- Nontoxic patient with probable enteroviral infection: daily with primary care physician

Indications for Admission

- Non-enteroviral encephalitis or meningoencephalitis

Bibliography

Barzon L, Pacenti M, Sinigaglia A, et al. West Nile virus infection in children. *Expert Rev Anti Infect Ther.* 2015;**13**(11):1373–1386.

Jain S, Patel B, Bhatt GC. Enteroviral encephalitis in children: clinical features, pathophysiology, and treatment advances. *Pathog Glob Health.* 2014;**108**(5):216–222.

James SH, Kimberlin DW. Neonatal herpes simplex virus infection: epidemiology and treatment. *Clin Perinatol.* 2015;**42**(1):47–59.

Sanders JE, Garcia SE. Pediatric herpes simplex virus infections: an evidence-based approach to treatment. *Pediatr Emerg Med Pract.* 2014;**11**(1):1–19.

Song JL, Wang VJ. Altered level of consciousness: evidence-based management in the emergency department. *Pediatr Emerg Med Pract.* 2017;**14**(1):1–28.

Enteric Parasitic Infections

Roundworms, hookworms, whipworms, and treadworms (*Strongyloides*) are found throughout the world in communities where the soil is contaminated by eggs or larvae. While uncommon in the United States, these infections can occur when there is breakdown of hygiene or sanitation or, more commonly, in immigrants and travelers returning from endemic regions.

Clinical Presentation

Pinworms

Pinworm (*Enterobius vermicularis*) is the most common helminth infection in the United States. Pinworms are acquired from ingestion of eggs, which hatch in the duodenum and migrate to the cecum where they mature over 4–6 weeks. Gravid adult females migrate to the perineum where they lay eggs. Person to person and fomite (toys, bedding, etc.) to person transmission are common, as the eggs remain viable for 2–3 weeks in the environment. Autoinfection may occur, either from reingesting eggs or when hatched pinworms crawl back into the anus. Anal pruritus is the most common complaint, although pinworms can be asymptomatic. Vulvitis can rarely occur if a worm migrates into the vagina. There is no tissue migration of the larvae and no eosinophilia.

Roundworms

Roundworm (*Ascaris lumbricoides*) is one of the most common nematode infections worldwide, but it is relatively uncommon in the United States. The worms enter the body through ingestion of eggs, which hatch in the small intestine. Larvae then migrate by lymphatics or venules into the portal and then systemic circulation, ultimately arriving at the lungs, penetrating the pulmonary capillaries, and entering the airway. The larvae mature in the lungs for 10–14 days and then travel up the bronchial tree to the throat, where they are swallowed and mature into adults in the small intestine. Patients may develop Loeffler's syndrome, presenting with fever, cough, dyspnea, hemoptysis, and pulmonary eosinophilia, during the larval migration through the lungs. Adult worms (15–35 cm) in the intestine are usually asymptomatic, but they can cause intermittent abdominal pain and may sometimes be vomited up or passed in stool. Other less common complications are intestinal obstruction, blockage of the bile or pancreatic ducts, appendicitis, intussusception, and volvulus. *Ascaris* can affect the nutritional status of infected children by causing malabsorption of fats, proteins, and carbohydrates.

Hookworms

Hookworm (*Necator americanus* and *Ancyclostoma duodenale*) was previously widespread in the southeastern United States, but is now less common. The infection is typically acquired through penetration of the soles of the feet by the larvae. This causes a papulovesicular dermatitis sometimes referred to as "ground itch" that lasts for 1–2 weeks. The larvae enter the circulatory system where they penetrate the pulmonary alveoli, ascend the bronchial tree to the throat, and are then swallowed. Migrating worms may cause Loeffler's syndrome, an eosinophilic pneumonitis. Approximately 4–12 weeks after exposure, the larvae attach to the mucosa of the small intestine causing mild abdominal pain, nausea, and anorexia. Blood loss occurs secondary to parasite mediated destruction of capillaries in the intestinal mucosa and may cause a hypochromic, microcytic anemia and hypoalbuminemia. Eosinophilia is common.

Strongyloidiasis

Strongyloides stercoralis is found in tropical regions and the southeastern United States. Filariform (parasitic) larvae in contaminated soil invade the skin. They migrate via the circulatory system to the lungs and then up the tracheobronchial tree and into the intestinal tract.

There is a spectrum of illness due to *Strongyloides stercoralis*. Acute strongyloidiasis can present with a local reaction at the site of larval entry. This dermatitis can occur almost immediately and may last up to several weeks. Pulmonary symptoms (Loeffler's syndrome) may develop as larvae migrate through the lungs. Gastrointestinal symptoms (diarrhea, anorexia, abdominal pain) may occur about two weeks after infection. Larvae are detectable in the stool 3–4 weeks after infection. Chronic infection is most often asymptomatic, but has been associated with intermittent vomiting, diarrhea, constipation, and recurrent asthma.

Hyperinfection is a rare syndrome of accelerated autoinfection generally secondary to immunocompromise, most commonly associated with HTLV-1 infection or corticosteroid use. Patients may have diarrhea, abdominal pain, ileus, or small bowel obstruction. Massive larvae penetration through the lungs results in pulmonary hemorrhage and infiltrates on chest x-ray. Hyperinfection is often complicated by bacteremia and/or meningitis with enteric bacteria.

Whipworm

Trichuris trichuria is found throughout tropical regions and in the southeastern United States. It has a simple lifecycle in which ingested eggs develop in the intestine. There is no tissue invasion stage, so eosinophilia is rare. Infections are usually asymptomatic, although heavy infections can cause nausea, vomiting, diarrhea, abdominal distention and tenderness, rectal prolapse, and occasionally intestinal bleeding.

Entamoeba Histolytica

Entamoeba histolytica is found worldwide, but is most common in areas with poor sanitation. It is transmitted via fecal–oral ingestion of mature amebic cysts. Infection is usually asymptomatic, although there can be a spectrum of disease from asymptomatic intraluminal infection/colonization to colitis to extraintestinal infection. Patients with amebic colitis typically present with a several-week history of gradual onset of abdominal pain and tenderness, diarrhea, and bloody stools. Fever is usually absent or low grade. The presentation can occasionally mimic inflammatory bowel disease. Patients with liver abscesses complain of right upper quadrant pain and fever, generally without colitis. Though rare, spread to the lungs, pleura, and skin can occur by direct extension. Treatment is indicated for asymptomatic patients to prevent transmission to others and progression to symptomatic disease.

Diagnosis

The diagnosis of most parasitic infections can only be made if the possibility is considered. Recent travel to or emigration from endemic areas makes infestation more likely. A history of chronic or bloody diarrhea, dysentery, weight loss, or cutaneous eruptions suggests the possibility of a parasitic infection. Eosinophilia suggests roundworms, hookworms, or strongyloidiasis. Occasionally the patient or parent will report seeing a worm in the stool, vomitus, sputum, or perianal region. Often the physical examination is not helpful in determining the diagnosis.

A history of anal pruritus, particularly if multiple close contacts have similar symptoms, is suggestive of pinworm infestation. If confirmation is necessary, the cellotape (unfrosted Scotch tape) test can demonstrate parasite eggs under a microscope. Specialized collection kits are also available. The sensitivity of the test increases when performed in the morning prior to the first bowel movement or washing and if multiple samples are collected on different days. Stool samples are not helpful.

Roundworm, hookworm, and whipworm are diagnosed by finding eggs in a fresh stool specimen ("stool for ova and parasites"), with increased yield if three successive morning specimens are submitted. Refrigerate stool that cannot be examined within one hour. Additionally, adult *Ascaris* may sometimes be brought in by a child's family and can be identified based upon its size and gross physical characteristics.

Strongyloides larvae are excreted in low volumes in stool and is therefore difficult to diagnose by stool examination (ova and parasites). Specialized processing of stool can aid in diagnosis, while an enzyme immunoassay for *Strongyloides* IgG is very sensitive but it cannot differentiate between current or past infection and can also cross-react with other parasitic infections. Consultation with the microbiology laboratory or an infectious disease specialist will assist in making the diagnosis.

Entamoeba histioloytica is morphologically indistinct from *Enantomoeba dispar*, a non-pathogenic amoeba that can also be found in stool. Antigen tests or PCR on stool specimens can distinguish between the two. In extraluminal disease such as liver abscess, the organism may not be found in the stool, but an enzyme-linked immunosorbent assay (EIA) antibody test is very sensitive. Conversely, the EIA antibody test does not perform well in luminal disease and cannot distinguish between current and past infection. The diagnosis and management of enteric parasitic infections is summarized in Table 13.1.

Table 13.1 Diagnosis and treatment of enteric parasitic infections

Diagnosis	Treatment
Pinworms	
Presumptive or Scotch tape-test	Pyrantel pamoate (≥2 years of age 11 mg/kg) × 1, repeat in 2 weeks Albendazole and mebendazole are effective but much more expensive. Treat household members if repeated infection Bathe, change underwear, and wash bedding daily
Ascarasis[a]	
Ova and parasites	Albendazole (≥1 year of age): 400 mg once Mebendazole (≥ 2 years of age): 100 mg BID for 3 days or 500 mg × 1 Ivermectin (≥15 kg): 150–200 mcg/kg once
Hookworms[a]	
Ova and parasites	Albendazole (≥1 year of age): 400 mg once Mebendazole (≥ 2 years of age): 100 mg BID for 3 days or 500 mg × 1 Pyrantel pamoate (≥2 years of age): 11 mg/kg daily × 3 days
Whipworms[a]	
Ova and parasites	Albendazole (≥1 year of age): 400 mg daily × 3 days Mebendazole (≥ 2 years of age): 100 mg BID × 3 days Ivermectin (≥15 kg): 200 mcg/kg/day × 3 days)
Strongyloides	
Ova and parasites EIA[b]	Ivermectin (>15 kg): 200 mcg/kg/day × 2 days Albendazolec (≥1 year of age): 400 mg bid × 7 days
Enantomoeba histiolytica	
Ova and parasites antigen PCR[d] EIA if extraluminal	Asymptomatic: iodoquinol 40 mg/kg/day div tid × 20 days or paromomycin: 25–35 mg/kg/day div tid × 7 days Symptomatic: metronidazole (35–50 mg/kg/day div tid × 7–10 days) or tinidazole (≥3 years of age): 50 mg/kg daily × 3–5 days) followed by either iodoquinol or paromomycin (as above)

[a] Repeat ova and parasites testing two weeks after therapy for test of cure.
[b] Enzyme-linked immunosorbent assay.
[c] Albendazole is less effective than ivermectin for *Strongyloides*.
[d] Polymerase chain reaction.

ED Management

Although a pinworm infection may be treated on the presumptive evidence of rectal itching in the absence of local pathology, treat other parasitic infections only if positive identification is available. Otherwise, arrange for the collection of specimens and refer the patient for primary care follow-up. Note that albendazole was briefly discontinued and then reintroduced to the United States as a patented 100 mg chewable tablet that is much more expensive than previous formulations.

Refugee populations who have not had presumptive treatment prior to arrival in the United States may require empiric treatment. See the CDC guidelines for further

$38°C = 100·4°F.$

recommendations (www.cdc.gov/immigrantrefugeehealth/guidelines/domestic/intestinal-parasites-domestic.html#figure1).

Some laboratories may report the presence of non-pathogenic protozoa in the stool. These are harmless, are not associated with disease, and do not require any therapy. The Centers for Disease Control and Prevention has a list of these protozoa as well as a handout to discuss with patients' families to allay their concerns (www.cdc.gov/parasites/nonpath protozoa/).

Follow-up
- Primary care follow-up at the completion of therapy

Indications for Admission
- Dehydration or severe weight loss
- Extraintestinal amoebiasis
- Strongyloidiasis in immunocompromised patients

Bibliography
American Academy of Pediatrics. Drugs for parasitic infections. In Kimberlin DW, Brady MT, Jackson MA, Long SS (eds.) *Red Book: 2015 Report of the Committee on Infectious Diseases.* Lake Grove, IL, American Academy of Pediatrics, 2015; 927–956.

Choudhuri G, Rangan M. Amebic infection in humans. *Indian J Gastroenterol.* 2012;**31**(4):153–162.

Giovannini-Chami L, Blanc S, Hadchouel A, et al. Eosinophilic pneumonias in children: a review of the epidemiology, diagnosis, and treatment. *Pediatr Pulmonol.* 2016;**51**(2):203–216.

Hansen C, Paintsil E. Infectious diseases of poverty in children: a tale of two worlds. *Pediatr Clin North Am.* 2016;**63**(1):37–66.

Knopp S, Steinmann P, Keiser J, Utzinger J. Nematode infections: soil-transmitted helminths and *Trichinella. Infect Dis Clin North Am.* 2012;**26**(2):341–358.

Starr MC, Montgomery SP. Soil-transmitted helminthiasis in the United States: a systematic review – 1940–2010. *Am J Trop Med Hyg.* 2011;**85**(4):680–684.

Weatherhead JE, Hotez PJ. Worm infections in children. *Pediatr Rev.* 2015;**36**(8):341–352.

① < 2mths - 100·4°F, > 2mths 101·4°F. Imm· defy

Evaluation of the Febrile Child   101·4 × 1 or 100·4 × 3 /24hrs

Fever is one of the most common causes for a visit to the ED. For the purpose of ED evaluation, one set of fever definitions based on an increased risk of severe disease include:

- ≤56 of age: 38.0 °C (100.4 °F);
- >56 days of age: 38.5 °C (101.3 °F);
- immunocompromised patient: 38.5 °C (101.3 °F) once or 38.0 °C (100.4 °F) three times within 24-hour period (one hour apart).

Fever may be the presenting sign for a viral illness, a minor bacterial infection, or a life-threatening bacterial process. Rarely, fever may be the presenting sign of collagen vascular disease, drug intoxication, or malignancy. In many cases, the etiology of the fever remains unclear even after a thorough history and physical examination.

The priority is the identification of the child with a serious bacterial illness (SBI). Despite efforts to develop reliable methods for diagnosis, these patients may be clinically

MC, SBI in febrile infant is UTI

indistinguishable from children with self-limited viral diseases, and they may have no localizing signs whatsoever. The widespread use of the *Haemophilus influenza* type b vaccination and conjugate pneumococcal vaccine has led to a dramatic decline in the incidence of occult bacteremia in children and invalidated previously published management guidelines for the evaluation of nontoxic-appearing febrile children aged three months to three years. The most common SBI in the febrile young infant is now a urinary tract infection. ✻

Clinical Presentation

⑥ · Clinical Impression
Alertness, playfulness, interaction
Color, Hydration, Consolability

Clinical impression is a component of every strategy for evaluating febrile infants and young children. The best-known tool is the Yale Observation Scale (YOS), an objective scoring system based on the child's alertness, playfulness, interaction with the environment, color, state of hydration, quality of cry, and ability to be consoled (www.thecalculator.co/health/Yale-Observation-Scale-for-Infant-Fever-Calculator-922.html). In the young infant (<8 weeks), however, the clinical presentation has been shown to be neither sensitive nor specific for identifying which patient is at risk for SBI. Furthermore, focal infections in young infants typically do not present with localized findings. Meningeal signs may be absent despite the presence of meningitis. The older the patient, the more reliable the clinical impression becomes as a predictor of serious underlying illness and the more likely that the patient has specific localizing signs of illness.

Diagnosis

<8 wks - clinical exam is unreliable.
eg Meningitis w/o meningial signs.

Clinical impression and physical examination are the mainstays of diagnosis in older children. Laboratory tests help predict the risk of serious infection when the results of the clinical evaluation is equivocal or known to be unreliable, as in the case of the young infant (<8 weeks). However, because of the low prevalence of bacteremia, the positive predictive value of any single test remains very low.

High risk: Imm. defg, V-P shunt, Central lines
Unusual organism suspected.

ED Management

The management of the well-appearing febrile infants and children is summarized below by age. Modify these guidelines and use a more conservative approach in high-risk patients, including but not limited to the immunocompromised host, children with cerebrospinal fluid shunts or other indwelling lines, or if unusual pathogens are suspected. An ill-appearing child in any age group warrants a full sepsis evaluation and empiric antibiotics.

Under 28 Days of Age

Toxic - Complete Sepsis w/u & Empiric ATB,
Ell

Since clinical impression is unreliable in young infants, perform a full evaluation for sepsis including a complete blood count (CBC) with differential count, blood and urine cultures, urinalysis, and lumbar puncture (LP) for cell count, glucose, protein, Gram's stain, and culture. Obtain urine by catheter insertion or suprapubic aspiration. A chest radiograph is indicated if there are respiratory signs or symptoms. *Ampicillin & Cefotaxime*

Regardless of the initial test results, give empiric antibiotics (ampicillin and cefotaxime) and admit pending culture results. Ampicillin doses (IV/IM) are: <1 week of age: 75–150 mg/kg/day div q 8h (use 200–300 mg/kg/day div q 8h if group B streptococcal meningitis is suspected); >1 week of age: 100–200 mg/kg/day div q 6h (use 300 mg/kg/day

Respy Signs or Symptoms -, Consider, chest X ray.

also, consider HSV & Acyclovir Rx.

div q 4–6 hours if group B streptococcal meningitis is suspected). Cefotaxime doses (IV/IM) are: <1 week: 100–150 mg/kg/day div q 8–12h; 1–4 weeks: 150–200 mg/kg/day div q 6–8h. If meningitis is suspected, use 200 mg/kg/day div q 6h, but give higher doses (225–300 mg/kg/day div q 6–8h) in combination with vancomycin for meningitis due to penicillin-resistant S. pneumoniae.

Most patients in this age group with HSV infection are afebrile or hypothermic. Add empiric acyclovir (<35 weeks postconceptional age: 20 mg/kg every 12 hours; ≥35 weeks postconceptional age: 20 mg/kg every 8 hours) if HSV is suspected in patients who are ill-appearing, or present with abnormal neurological status, a vesicular rash, hepatitis, and/or a maternal history of primary HSV infection

28–56 Days of Age

The evaluation of the well-appearing 28- to 56-day-old varies by institution. Regardless of whether there is an identifiable source of infection, obtain a urinalysis, urine culture, CBC, and a blood culture, as well as a chest x-ray if the patient has signs or symptoms of respiratory illness. If the patient has diarrhea, send stool to evaluate for white blood cells, as well as a culture. Infants with clinical bronchiolitis, or documented RSV or influenza, have a much lower rate of SBI than infants without bronchiolitis, although there is still a risk of a urinary tract infection.

Low risk

Classify infants as *low-risk* if they are well-appearing, with normal vital signs after defervescence, and they meet all of the following criteria:

- full-term birth (>37 weeks' gestation);
- no chronic medical conditions;
- no prolonged NICU stay;
- no antibiotics within 72 hours;
- WBC >5000/mm^3 and <15,000/mm^3;
- urinalysis with ≤10 WBC per high-power field and no bacteria;
- band:neutrophil ratio <0.2;
- if sent, ESR <30 mm/h or a CRP < 1;
- if diarrhea is present, stool is heme negative and has ≤5 WBC per high-power field;
- normal chest radiograph (if obtained).

Recently developed protocols now suggest a stepwise approach to guide the need for an LP in these patients, as the risk of meningitis is very low in this population. Infants who meet all the above criteria for low risk for SBI may be managed as outpatients, with close follow-up and without expectant antibiotic therapy. A more conservative approach, including an LP, is appropriate when there is any uncertainty regarding the use of the stepwise approach. If the LP is negative, these infants may also be managed as outpatients without antibiotics.

Perform a full sepsis evaluation, including an LP, if the patient is ill-appearing or does not meet low-risk criteria. Admit these infants to the hospital and start empiric antibiotics with cefotaxime (IV/IM) 100–200 mg/kg/day div q 6–8h. Use higher doses (150–225 mg/kg/day div q 6–8h) for infections outside the CSF due to resistant S. pneumoniae. Treat for HSV in infants with abnormal neurological status, a vesicular rash, hepatitis or a maternal history of primary HSV infection (acyclovir 60 mg/kg/day IV div q 8h). Obtain CSF samples *prior* to the initiation of antibiotics unless the infant is too ill-appearing to delay treatment.

*Bronchiolitis
RSV
Influenza.*

*SBI - less likely
but UTI is possible.*

maternal Ig Infn, Neonate—Vesicles, Neurologic disease, Hepatitis

An exception is an infant who does not meet the low-risk criteria, but has clinical bronchiolitis and/or documented RSV or influenza, in whom the LP may be deferred if the plan is to admit without empiric antibiotics.

56–90 Days of Age

Clinical impression is slightly more reliable in this age group. If the patient is well-appearing, with otherwise normal vital signs, and no fever source found on careful examination, evaluate for a urinary tract infection. Obtain a chest radiograph if there are any concerning respiratory signs or symptoms, including tachypnea. Admit infants with suspected focal infections, such as otitis media, UTI, or pneumonia, and start treatment with IV/IM ceftriaxone. If the patient is ill-appearing, perform a full sepsis evaluation, begin empiric treatment with ceftriaxone 100 mg/kg/day div q 12h (IV/IM), and admit to the hospital.

If the patient is being discharged, the priorities are careful and frequent follow-up and parental vigilance for clinical deterioration. Give the parents specific guidelines for controlling the fever (15 mg/kg of acetaminophen q 4h), and for assessing the child at home (increased irritability or lethargy, decreased PO intake) and provide for a follow-up visit within 24–48 hours, or sooner if the patient seems worse to the parents.

90 Days to 36 Months of Age   *3 mths – 3 yrs.*

Clinical impression continues to be more reliable in this age group and the patient may present with localizing symptoms. Additionally, the widespread use of the *Haemophilus influenza* B (HIB) and conjugate pneumococcal vaccine (PCV-7) has reduced occult bacteremia rates to <1%. It is important to verify the child's immunization status to stratify their risk, as the following recommendations apply to patients who are fully immunized.

The well-appearing child with otherwise normal vital signs may be discharged home with close follow-up and parental vigilance for clinical deterioration. Screen for a urinary tract infection in males under one year of age or females with fever without a source for >2 days. *r/o UTI— males <1 yr, Females w/o Source a fever > 2 days*

If a febrile child is irritable, but has no signs of poor perfusion, administer an antipyretic (acetaminophen: <6 months of age: 15 mg/kg per dose q 6h; ≥6 months of age: 15 mg/kg per dose q 4h; *or* ibuprofen: >6 months of age: 10 mg/kg dose q 6h) and reevaluate in one half-hour. If the child is well-appearing and vital signs have normalized after defervescence, discharge home is appropriate. If the child is well-appearing but the vital signs do not normalize (i.e., persistent tachycardia) further evaluation may be warranted to exclude a SBI or myocarditis. Admit ill-appearing infants younger than six months of age with any focal bacterial infection, other than otitis media.

Any child who appears toxic requires immediate further evaluation based on the presenting symptoms and severity of disease, which may include CBC, blood culture, urinalysis, urine culture, chest x-ray, and possibly an LP.

≥36 Months of Age   *> 3 yrs*

Older children may be able to vocalize their symptoms and the clinical examination is generally reliable. The well-appearing patient with otherwise normal vital signs may be discharged home with follow-up if symptoms persist. Children who are not toilet trained are at higher risk of urinary tract infections. Obtain a screening urinalysis if a female has fever >39 °C (102 °F) without a source for >2–3 days.

Consider UTI – males <1 yr, Females i fever > 2 days x w/o a focus.

Follow-up

- 4–8 weeks: daily, until cultures are negative (ideally with the primary care provider)
- 8 weeks to 6 months: every 1–2 days, until afebrile (ideally with the primary care provider)
- ≥6–36 months: 24–48 hours
- >36 months: 2–3 days, if still febrile

Indications for Admission

- All infants <4 weeks of age with a temperature >38.0 °C (100.4 °F)
- Infants <56 days of age who do not meet low-risk criteria
- Most infants <6 months of age with focal bacterial infection other than otitis media
- Toxic-appearing child regardless of age or degree of fever

Bibliography

Arora R, Mahajan P. Evaluation of child with fever without source: review of literature and update. *Pediatr Clin North Am.* 2013;**60**(5):1049–1062.

Greenhow TL, Hung YY, Herz AM, et al. The changing epidemiology of serious bacterial infections in young infants. *Pediatr Infect Dis J.* 2014;**33**(6):595–599.

Hamilton JL, John SP. Evaluation of fever in infants and young children. *Am Fam Physician.* 2013;**87**:254–260.

Mathias B, Mira JC, Larson SD. Pediatric sepsis. *Curr Opin Pediatr.* 2016;**28**(3):380–387.

http://pediatrics.aappublications.org/content/pediatrics/suppl/2012/07/11/peds.2012-0127.DCSuppl emental/peds.2012-0127SupplementaryData.pdf

Fever of Unknown Origin

Fever of unknown origin (FUO) is defined as temperature higher than 38 °C (100.4 °F), for eight or more days, without a definitive diagnosis. Do not confuse FUO with "fever without a source," which is of shorter duration. In addition "pseudo-FUO" can occur when back-to-back episodes of self-limited infections are perceived by parents as one prolonged fever episode.

Clinical Presentation

The evaluation begins with a thorough, if not exhaustive, history and physical examination (Table 13.2), the results of which will guide the laboratory work-up. Determine the fever duration, height, pattern (sustained, relapsing, recurrent), and method of temperature-taking. Ask about any constitutional symptoms (weight loss, sweating) or associated symptoms, as well as travel (dengue, malaria) or unusual exposures (HIV), ethnic or genetic background (familial fever disorders), and exposure to medications (drug fever).

Diagnosis

Obtain an initial battery of tests, including a CBC with differential and peripheral smear, inflammatory markers (CRP and/or ESR), comprehensive metabolic panel, urinalysis, and

Table 13.2 History and physical examination findings in FUO

Finding	Common possible diagnoses
Abdominal pain, vomiting, diarrhea	Bacterial enteritis Inflammatory bowel disease Intra-abdominal abscess
Arthritis/arthralgia	Rheumatologic disorders
Diaphoresis	Dysautonomia Hyperthyroidism
Lymphadenopathy: general	Mono-like illness Oncologic process
Lymphadenopathy: localized	*Bartonella* *Mycobacterium*
Limb/bone pain	Leukemia/oncologic process Osteoarticular infection
Nasal discharge	Sinusitis
Rash	Idiopathic rheumatoid arthritis Kawasaki disease Preventable childhood diseases Typhoid fever
Red eyes	Autoimmune diseases Kawasaki disease

chest radiograph, as well as urine and aerobic and anaerobic blood cultures. Perform tuberculin skin testing, if indicated. Use the results of the history, physical examination, and basic laboratories to obtain additional tests. These may include:

- serology: EBV, CMV, parvovirus, and *Bartonella*, HIV;
- chemistry: uric acid, LDH, ferritin – concern for oncologic process or hemophagocytic lymphohistiocytosis (HLH);
- ANA, rheumatoid factor, C3/C4/CH50 – concern for an autoimmune process;
- immunoglobulins, antibody titers to known vaccines – concern for an immunodeficiency;
- echocardiogram – concern for Kawasaki disease or infectious endocarditis;
- MRI – concern for osteomyelitis;
- abdominal ultrasound, CT, or MRI – concern for abscesses, tumors, and lymphadenopathy (e.g., psoas abscess, liver abscess).

At the same time, consult with the appropriate subspecialist (infectious diseases, rheumatology, oncology, cardiology, gastroenterology, etc.).

ED Management (While the Diagnosis is Pending)

Do not give empiric antibiotics or other treatments (e.g., steroids) if the patient is clinically stable. These may mask or delay the diagnosis. If the patient is not stable or appears toxic, however, admit and initiate broad-spectrum antibiotic therapy (see pp. 391–393). In addition, stop all non-essential medications.

Follow-up

- Primary care in 24–48 hours. However, direct communication with the primary care provider (or subspecialist, if needed) prior to ED discharge is essential

Indications for Admission

- Unstable vital signs, toxic or ill appearance
- Dehydration requiring intravenous fluids
- Abnormal findings on diagnostic testing that require urgent further evaluation
- Inadequate outpatient follow-up or further work-up cannot be addressed as an outpatient

Bibliography

Antoon JW, Potisek NM, Lohr JA. Pediatric fever of unknown origin. *Pediatr Rev.* 2015;**36**(9):380–391.

Arora R, Mahajan P. Evaluation of child with fever without source: review of literature and update. *Pediatr Clin North Am.* 2013;**60**(5):1049–1062.

Rigante D, Esposito S. A roadmap for fever of unknown origin in children. *Int J Immunopathol Pharmacol.* 2013;**26**(2):315–326.

Seashore CJ, Lohr JA. Fever of unknown origin in children. *Pediatr Ann.* 2011;**40**(1):26–30.

Sherman JM, Sood SK. Current challenges in the diagnosis and management of fever. *Curr Opin Pediatr.* 2012;**24**(3):400–406.

HIV-Related Emergencies

Human immunodeficiency virus (HIV) can be transmitted via sexual contact, mucous membrane contact with contaminated bodily fluids, percutaneous exposure from contaminated sharp instruments or needles, and contaminated blood products (essentially eliminated in the United States), as well as from mother-to-child (either in utero, during delivery, or during breastfeeding). Optimal management during pregnancy, delivery, and the postpartum period has reduced the risk of transmission to the infant to less than 1% in many areas, but there are still about 100 perinatally infected infants born in the United States each year. Victims of rape or sexual abuse and teenagers engaging in unprotected sex may also present to the ED for HIV counseling, testing, and post-exposure chemoprophylaxis.

Clinical Presentation and Diagnosis

Previously Unknown Infection

Previously unrecognized perinatal transmission may present in infancy or childhood as failure to thrive, recurrent invasive bacterial infections, recurrent or recalcitrant oropharyngeal candidiasis, unexplained lymphadenopathy or hepatosplenomegaly, and/or chronic diarrhea. Adolescents with non-perinatally acquired acute HIV may present with a mononucleosis-like illness, including fever, malaise, headache, pharyngitis, rash, and generalized lymphadenopathy lasting 5–7 days. Therefore, routinely assess the sexual history and transmission risk factors (blood transfusion, needle sharing, needle sick, unprotected intercourse [especially receptive anal]) in adolescents presenting with this clinical picture, as many may not be forthcoming with this information.

In patients over 24 months of age, the diagnostic test of choice, including for possible acute infection, is a fourth-generation combined HIV-1 p24 antigen and HIV-1/2 antibody test. HIV RNA can be detected several days before antigenemia. Therefore, it can be used if clinical suspicion of acute retroviral syndrome remains, despite a negative fourth-generation test. The RNA NAAT can also be falsely positive, so confirmation then requires evidence of seroconversion. In perinatally exposed infants, maternal antibodies may be detectable in the infant until 24 months of age. Thus, in this age group, when the mother is known to be HIV-positive, order a qualitative HIV DNA or RNA NAAT.

Known HIV Infection

In the combined antiretroviral therapy (cART) era, most children with known HIV are well-controlled, and opportunistic infections are uncommon. Poor adherence to therapy, particularly during adolescence, increases the risk of opportunistic infections. HIV infection is staged (in addition to stage-defining infections) by age-specific CD4 count ranges (Table 13.3). If a child's recent CD4 count is unknown, one can generally predict severe immunodeficiency if they are being prescribed prophylactic antimicrobials such as trimethoprim-sulfamethoxazole (TMP-SMX) (for *Pneumocystis jiroveci* pneumonia [PJP] when given beyond one year of age) or azithromycin or clarithromycin (for *Mycobacterium avium* complex).

For patients who have moderate (Stage 2) to severe (Stage 3) immunodeficiency, consult a pediatric HIV specialist for a differential diagnosis of potential opportunistic infections during acute illness. Two specific opportunistic infections bear mentioning.

Pneumocystis Jiroveci Pneumonia

As a consequence of cART and the widespread provision of prophylaxis, PJP has become increasingly rare. The peak incidence is 3–6 months of age, although all infants under one year of age with HIV are prescribed PJP prophylaxis regardless of CD4 count. It is rare outside of infancy unless the child has a very low CD4 count (Stage 3). It may present rapidly or insidiously with varying symptoms of fever, cough, dyspnea, and poor feeding. Tachypnea is almost universally present and may be out of proportion to the degree of adventitious breath sounds. Quiet tachypnea or widespread crackles are typical, as is hypoxia. The typical radiologic findings begin as mild bilateral perihilar infiltrates, which progresses to a diffuse interstitial pattern. However, chest radiographs may be normal or just show hyperinflation early in illness. Serum lactate dehydrogenase (LDH) levels are often

Table 13.3 Age-specific CD4 counts

Stage	<1 year of age		≥1–5 years of age		≥6 years of age	
	CD4 count (cells/microliter	CD4%	CD4 count (cells/microliter)	CD4%	CD4 count (cells/microliter	CD4%
1	≥1500/mm^3	≥34%	≥1000/mm^3	≥30%	≥500/mm^3	≥26%
2	750–1499/mm^3	26–33%	500–999/mm^3	22–29%	200–499/mm^3	14–25%
3 (AIDS)	<750/mm^3	<26%	<500/mm^3	<22%	<200/mm^3	<14%

elevated, and can be used as a screening laboratory test in the ED, but the LDH is not sensitive nor specific for PJP. Direct fluorescence antibody (DFA) testing of lower respiratory specimens is more sensitive and specific than conventional stains such as GMS (silver) stain.

Oropharyngeal and Esophageal Candidiasis

Oropharyngeal candidiasis is still relatively common in HIV-infected children. In patients with good immune function, it will generally present and respond to therapies in the same way as in uninfected children. Esophageal candidiasis usually occurs with severe immunosuppression (CD4 <100 cells/microliter) with symptoms of fever, odynophagia/dysphagia, poor feeding, or emesis. Oropharyngeal candidiasis is usually concomitantly present with esophageal candidiasis, but may occasionally be absent in children on cART.

ED Management

Acute Febrile Illness

Well-appearing children with HIV who have adequate immune function (as evidenced by a high or Stage 1 CD4 count and no recent history of recurrent invasive bacterial infections) have a slightly higher risk of acute otitis media, community-acquired pneumonia, and possibly bacteremia than their HIV-negative peers. Therefore, ED management is similar to uninfected children for the age group and vaccination status. In patients with Stage 2 or 3 illness (or unknown CD4 counts), consult with a pediatric infectious disease or HIV specialist for recommendations on work-up.

Chronic Fever Without Focus

The goal of the ED evaluation is to evaluate for possible bacterial infection. Obtain a CBC, liver function tests, ESR and CRP, urinalysis, chest x-ray, and blood, urine, and stool cultures. Admit the patient for further diagnostic evaluation. In patients with Stage 2 or 3 illness (or unknown CD4 counts), consult with a pediatric infectious disease or HIV specialist.

Oropharyngeal and Esophageal Candidiasis

Treat mild oropharyngeal candidiasis with topical therapy such as clotrimazole troche 10 mg 4–5 times daily or nystatin suspension 4–6 mL four times daily for 7–14 days. Treat moderate or severe oropharyngeal candidiasis with fluconazole 6–12 mg/kg/day (400 mg maximum) PO for 7–14 days. If the child has symptoms concerning for concomitant esophageal candidiasis, obtain a fungal culture of scrapings from the oropharynx (to confirm *Candida* species and susceptibility), start fluconazole 6–12 mg/kg/day (600 mg maximum); it can be given PO if the child can tolerate it. In either case, consult an infectious disease specialist for fluconazole refractory disease or known fluconazole-resistant species of *Candida*.

PJP

If PJP is suspected, consult a pediatric HIV specialist. Start TMP-SMZ (20 mg/kg/day of TMP div q 6h) and also give prednisone (2 mg/kg/day div q 12h, 80 mg/day maximum) if recommended by the HIV specialist. If the child is able to produce sputum or is intubated, send a lower respiratory tract for PJP stains (the specific stain will vary by institution) and DFA. Consult a pediatric HIV specialist to determine the use of steroids in mild PJP.

Follow-up
- Well-appearing patients with a clearly identified focus (i.e., otitis media, urinary tract infection): pediatric HIV specialist in 24–48 hours

Indications for Admission
- Suspected PJP
- Suspected *Candida* esophagitis associated with poor oral intake
- Febrile illness in a patient with Stage 2 or 3 HIV

Guidelines for Managing Blood and Body Fluid Exposures
The efficacy of HIV post-exposure prophylaxis following nonoccupational exposures (nPEP) is unclear and guidelines rely heavily upon indirect inferences from data such as occupational exposures as well as expert opinion. Consult with a pediatric infectious diseases or HIV specialist if your institution does not have an nPEP policy. Factors that may increase the risk of HIV transmission include sexually transmitted diseases, acute and late-stage HIV infection, and high viral load. Factors that may decrease the risk include condom use, male circumcision, antiretroviral treatment, and pre-exposure prophylaxis. Accidental needlestick injuries following exposure to discarded needles, such as in parks or alleyways, are associated with a negligible risk for HIV exposure and to date there are no reported cases of HIV transmitted through this mechanism. The CDC guidelines can be found at: www.cdc.gov/hiv/risk/estimates/riskbehaviors.html.

ED Management
General considerations and specific elements necessary for a rational and consistent approach to HIV PEP after potential HIV exposure in children and adolescents are outlined in Figure 13.1 and Tables 13.4 and 13.5. In cases involving no- or low-risk exposures, reassure the caregiver that the child will not contract HIV infection and that post-exposure chemoprophylaxis is not necessary. For an individual presenting to the ED more than 72 hours following an exposure, chemoprophylaxis is not indicated, although exceptions may be made for high-risk exposures. In this case, or if selection of alternative prophylactic drug regimens is indicated, consult a local HIV expert. If local expertise is not available, advice may be obtained 9 a.m. to 12 a.m. (EST) from the National Clinicians' Consultation Center PEP line at 1-888-HIV-4911. Federal, state, and local HIV PEP guidelines are subject to modification based upon the epidemiology of HIV in the community, resource availability, and the continued advancement of knowledge in this complex area. Refer to https://aidsinfo.nih.gov for the most up-to-date national guidelines. Obtain a fourth-generation antigen/antibody blood (not oral) test at baseline prior to starting nPEP.

There are few data on nPEP following sticks from discarded needles or human bites. However, HIV is a relatively fragile virus and there have been no reported cases of transmission from sticks with discarded needles in the community. The exposure may be higher risk with a penetrating injury (particularly into a vessel), a large hollow-bore needle,

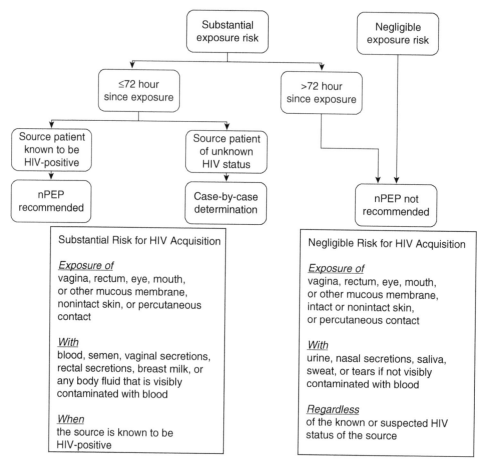

Figure 13.1 Risk assessment for nPEP.
Centers for Disease Control. Updated guidelines for antiretroviral post-exposure prophylaxis after sexual, injection drug use, or other nonoccupational exposure to HIV: United States, 2016, p 23. www.cdc.gov/hiv/pdf/programre sources/cdc-hiv-npep-guidelines.pdf.

or visible blood on the needle, and if there is a high HIV seroprevalence in the community where the stick occurred. Saliva has a low load of HIV and bites generally represent a negligible exposure risk. The exception is saliva contaminated with blood.

Bibliography

American Academy of Pediatrics. Human immunodeficiency virus infection. In Kimberlin DW, Brady MT, Jackson MA, Long SS (eds.) *Red Book: Report of the Committee on Infectious Diseases* (30th edn.). Elk Grove, IL: American Academy of Pediatrics, 2015; 453–476.

Centers for Disease Control and Prevention. HIV risk behaviors. www.cdc.gov/hiv/risk/estimates/ri skbehaviors.html (accessed June 5, 2017).

Centers for Disease Control and Prevention. Updated guidelines for antiretroviral postexposure after sexual, injection drug use, or other nonoccupational exposure to HIV – United States, 2016. www.cdc.gov/hiv/pdf/programresources/cdc-hiv-npep-guidelines.pdf (accessed June 5, 2017).

Table 13.4 HIV nonoccupational post-exposure prophylaxis (nPEP): general considerations

Initial nPEP evaluation

Obtain history of potential exposure event

HIV and HBV status of exposed person and source person, if available

Timing of most recent potential exposure

Type of exposure event and risk for HIV acquisition

Make determination if nPEP is indicated (see Figure 13.1)

If nPEP is indicated:

Conduct laboratory testing

HIV blood test (rapid combined Ag/Ab test, if available)

STIs (*Chlamydia, gonorrhea*, RPR), HBV, HCV, pregnancy, and CrCl and AST/ALT

Prescribe 28-day nPEP course

Educate patient about potential regimen-specific side effects and adverse events

Counsel patient about medication adherence

Provide patient with nPEP prescription or full 28-day nPEP course or nPEP starter pack and prescription

When necessary, assist patients with obtaining nPEP medication through a medication assistance program for the prescribed regimen

For all persons evaluated

Prescribe prophylaxis for STIs and HBV infection, if indicated

Provide counseling related to HIV prevention strategies, as appropriate

Document sexual assault findings and fulfill local reporting requirements

Conduct confidential reporting of newly diagnosed STIs and HIV infection to health department

Link HIV-infected persons to relevant medical and psychosocial support services

Follow-up evaluations for persons prescribed nPEP

Follow-up with local focused clinic or PMD with specific instructions to conduct HIV and any other indicated laboratory testing (see above)

Consider changing nPEP regimen if indicated by side effects or results of initial testing

Provide additional counseling and support for medication adherence and HIV prevention, if indicated

Other considerations

Forensic evidence collection

Emergency contraception

Wound care, assessment of tetanus immunization status

Psychosocial counseling (social worker or psychiatric nurse familiar with crisis)

Establish outpatient follow-up within minimum of 2–3 days for support

Abbreviations. ALT: alanine transaminase; AST: aspartate transaminase; CrCl: creatinine clearance; HBV: hepatitis B virus; HCV: hepatitis C virus; RPR: rapid plasma reagin; STIs: sexually transmitted infections;
Adapted from www.cdc.gov/hiv/pdf/programresources/cdc-hiv-npep-guidelines.pdf.

Table 13.5 PEP following nonoccupational exposure including sexual assault*

≥13 years of age and CrCl ≥60 mL/min	A three-drug regimen consisting of tenofovir DF 300 mg *and* fixed dose combination emtricitabine 200 mg (Truvada) once daily *with either* raltegravir 400 mg twice daily *or* dolutegravir 50 mg once daily
≥13 years of age and CrCl <59 mL/min	A three-drug regimen consisting of zidovudine *and* lamivudine, with both doses adjusted to degree of renal function *with either* raltegravir 400 mg twice daily *or* dolutegravir 50 mg once daily

2–12 years of age: A three-drug regimen consisting of the drugs listed below

Tenofovir DF	Emtricitabine	Raltegravir
Powder	Oral solution	Tablet
8 mg/kg q day (300 mg maximum)	6 mg/kg qday (240 mg maximum)	6–12 years of age and >25 kg: 400 mg tablet bid
or	*or*	*or*
Tablet	Tablet	Chewable tablets
17 to <22 kg: 150 mg tablet q day	≥33 kg: 200 mg tablet qday	2–12 years of age
22 to <28 kg, 200 mg tablet q day		11 to <14 kg: 75 mg bid
28 to <35 kg, 250 mg tablet q day		14 to <20 kg: 100 mg bid
≥35 kg: 300 mg tablet q day		20 to <28 kg: 150 mg bid
		28 to <40 kg: 200 mg bid
		≥40 kg: 300 mg bid

* There are multiple alternate regimens that are listed by the CDC and may be recommended by HIV specialists depending upon local epidemiology and experience.
Adapted from Centers for Disease Control. Updated guidelines for antiretroviral post-exposure prophylaxis after sexual, injection drug use, or other nonoccupational exposure to HIV – United States, 2016, pp. 321–327. www.cdc.gov/hiv/pdf/programresources/cdc-hiv-npep-guidelines.pdf.

Department of Health and Human Services, Panel on Antiretroviral Therapy and Medical Management of HIV-Infected Children. Guidelines for the use of antiretroviral agents in pediatric HIV infection. http://aidsinfo.nih.gov/contentfiles/lvguidelines/pediatricguidelines.pdf (accessed June 5, 2017).

Department of Health and Human Services, Panel on Opportunistic Infections in HIV-Exposed and HIV-Infected Children. Guidelines for the prevention and treatment of opportunistic infections in HIV-exposed and HIV-infected children. http://aidsinfo.nih.gov/contentfiles/lvguidelines/oi_guideli nes_pediatrics.pdf (accessed June 5, 2017).

Siberry GK. Preventing and managing HIV infection in infants, children, and adolescents in the United States. *Pediatr Rev.* 2014;35(7):268–286.

Infectious Diarrhea

Most infectious etiologies of diarrhea in children are self-limited and do not require specific diagnosis or therapy beyond supportive care. Even when specific agents are found, antibiotic therapy is often not indicated or may potentially be harmful. The most common bacterial pathogens are *Escherichia Coli*, *Shigella* spp., non-typhoidal *Salmonella* serovars, and *Campylobacter* spp.

Enteric *E. coli* infections can be subdivided into five major pathotypes, but the most important delineation is between shiga toxin-producing *E. coli* (STEC), which can be associated with hemolytic-uremic syndrome, and non-shiga toxin-producing strains.

Clostridium difficile-associated diarrhea is an increasing problem in children. It may be healthcare- or community-acquired and can occur without prior antibiotic exposure.

Parasites such as *Giardia intestinalis* and *Cryptosporidium* spp. cause a more protracted non-inflammatory diarrhea. Other parasitic causes of diarrhea are uncommon in the United States unless the patient has traveled to an endemic area.

"Routine" viral diarrhea (pp. 255–260) and diarrhea in the returned traveler (pp. 431–432) are discussed elsewhere.

Clinical Presentation

Bacterial Enteritis

Dysentery, defined as acute grossly bloody diarrhea with fever and abdominal pain, is more common with a bacterial enteritis than a viral etiology, but there is some overlap. The presence of fever is not specific for bacterial causes of diarrhea, and some bacterial causes may not be bloody. Fecal leukocytes or elevated fecal calprotectin generally, but not always, indicates the presence of a bacterial enteritis.

Hemolytic-uremic syndrome (HUS; pp. 681–683) is a severe sequelae of STEC infection, with up to a 5% mortality rate. It is characterized by the triad of microangiopathic hemolytic anemia, thrombocytopenia, and acute kidney injury that occurs about one week (range up to three weeks) after onset of diarrhea with STEC. It occurs in 6% of patients with O157:H7 STEC infection and 1% of non-O157:H7 STEC strains. Children younger than five years of age are at the highest risk of this complication.

Clostridium Difficile-Associated Diarrhea

Patients usually present with protracted watery and/or mucousy nonbloody diarrhea. Rarely, there can be a fulminant colitis with an ileus and signs of septic shock. Risk factors include antibiotic exposure in the past three months, gastric acid suppression, recent hospitalization, inflammatory bowel disease, immunodeficiencies (including malignancy, solid organ transplant, hematopoietic stem cell transplant), and Hirschsprung's disease.

Parasitic Enteritis

Giardia intestinalis and *Cryptosporidium* spp. are protozoal pathogens that present similarly with GI symptoms, but without systemic symptoms or eosinophilia. Outbreaks of both have been associated with recreational water activities, drinking unfiltered and untreated freshwater, and daycare center attendance. Disease can range from asymptomatic passage of cysts to chronic diarrhea, malabsorption, and weight loss. Most symptomatic patients experience a fairly characteristic syndrome of diarrhea with foul-smelling stools and gas, bloating, and abdominal cramps. Eosinophilia does not occur, fever is uncommon, and symptoms usually persist for days but can linger for months. A syndrome of chronic malabsorption can occur with weight loss, protuberance of the abdomen, and anemia.

Diagnosis

Specific diagnostics are usually not indicated for children presenting with acute diarrheal illness. Indications for bacterial stool cultures include severe acute bloody diarrhea, prolonged diarrhea (≥ 1 week), contact with a known outbreak of a potentially treatable etiology, or an immunocompromised state.

Order antigen detection tests for the diagnosis of suspected *Giardia intestinalis* and *Cryptosporidium* spp. infections. Stool ova and parasite examination is rarely necessary for most children with acute diarrhea. Indications include protracted diarrhea if other tests have been negative, history of travel to endemic areas, "worms" have been seen in the patient's stool, or if the child has unexplained peripheral eosinophilia. Note that some parasites (such as *Cystoisospora* and *Cyclospora*) may require special staining.

Many young children can have asymptomatic *C. difficile* colonization, which does not represent disease. Do not routinely test for *C. difficile* in otherwise healthy children under three years of age presenting with diarrhea unless they have had prolonged illness with other causes excluded. The specimen for *C. difficile* must be loose or liquid stool. Importantly, no clinically available test can differentiate between *C. difficile* colonization and disease.

ED Management

Empiric therapy is generally not indicated for any of the above infections prior to definitive microbiologic diagnosis, with the potential exception of critically ill children in whom *C. difficile* disease is suspected. The results of most laboratory tests will return after discharge or admission, although newer rapid multiplex PCR panels may change this. Indications for hospitalization and empiric antibiotic treatment are patients with higher risk of invasive disease, such as infants below three months of age and patients with hemoglobinopathies, malignancies, HIV, or other immunosuppressed conditions. Place patients with dysentery or concern for *C. difficile* on contact precautions.

E. Coli

Most enteritis is self-limited so that antibiotics are not indicated. Do not give antibiotics for proven or suspected STEC infection, due to potentially increased risk of progression to the hemolytic-uremic syndrome. If STEC is confirmed, obtain a CBC, BUN, and creatinine. If these are normal three days after diarrhea has resolved, the risk of developing hemolytic-uremic syndrome is very low.

Nontyphoidal *Salmonella*

Antibiotics are generally not indicated for asymptomatic patients or healthy patients with gastroenteritis because it does not hasten resolution of uncomplicated disease and may prolong shedding. Prescribe antibiotics if the patient has severe disease (ill enough for hospitalization) or is at higher risk of invasive disease, including infants under three months of age, or children with hemoglobinopathies, malignancies, HIV, or other immunosuppressed conditions. Empiric choices, before antibiotic susceptibilities are known, include ceftriaxone (50 mg/kg/day), azithromycin (10 mg/kg/day PO), or ciprofloxacin (20–30 mg/kg/day PO div q 12h, or 15–20 mg/kg/day IV div q 12h). Give a 3–7-day course for non-immunosuppressed patients, but consult an infectious disease specialist for immunocompromised patients.

Shigella spp.

Antibiotics are generally not indicated except for severe disease or immunocompromised patients. Treatment options include ceftriaxone (50 mg/kg/day IV for three days), azithromycin (10 mg/kg/day PO for three days), or ciprofloxacin (20–30 mg/kg/day PO div q 12h or 15–20 mg/kg/day IV div q 12h for three days).

C. Difficile

Prescribe metronidazole 30 mg/kg/day PO div q 6h for 10–14 days. Use vancomycin 40 mg/kg/day PO div q 6h for 10–14 days for severe disease, second recurrence, or in immunocompromised patients. Tests of cure is not necessary.

Campylobacter spp.

Treat with azithromycin (10 mg/kg/day PO for three days) or erythromycin (40 mg/kg/day div q 6h for five days).

Giardia

Use metronidazole (15 mg/kg/day PO div q 8h for five days), tinidazole (≥3 years of age only: 50 mg/kg PO once), or nitazoxanide (1–3 years: 100 mg q 12h for three days; ≥4–11 years of age: 200 mg q 12h for three days; ≥12 years: 500 mg q 12h for three days).

Cryptosporidium

Antiprotozoal therapy is generally not needed for immunocompetent individuals. If diarrhea is severe or has not resolved in two weeks, treat with nitazoxanide (1–3 years: 100 mg q 12h for three days; ≥4–11 years: 200 mg q 12h for three days; ≥12 years: 500 mg q 12h for three days). Consult an infectious disease specialist for immunosuppressed patients, as prolonged therapy may be indicated.

Follow-up

- Primary care within one week
- Patients with known STEC infection: in 2–3 days to monitor for developing HUS

Indications for Admission

- Inability to maintain hydration status orally
- Severe dysentery or severe *C. difficile*-associated diarrhea
- Concern for hemolytic-uremic syndrome
- Febrile dysentery in a patient who is <3 months of age, and/or has hemoglobinopathies, malignancy, HIV, or other immunosuppressed conditions

Bibliography

American Academy of Pediatrics Committee on Infectious Diseases. *Clostridium difficile* infection in infants and children. *Pediatrics*. 2013;**131**(1):196–200.

American Academy of Pediatrics. *Red Book: 2015 Report of the Committee on Infectious Diseases*. Elk Grove Village, IL, American Academy of Pediatrics, 2015; 273–275; 312–315; 343–347; 353–355; 695–702; 706–709.

Dekate P, Jayashree M, Singhi SC. Management of acute diarrhea in emergency room. *Indian J Pediatr.* 2013;80(3):235–246.

Ochoa TJ, Zambruni M, Chea-woo E. Approach to patients with gastrointestinal tract infections and food poisoning. In Cherry JD, Harrison GJ, Kaplan SL, Steinbach WJ, Hotez PJ (eds.) *Feigin and Cherry's Textbook of Pediatric Infectious Diseases* (7th edn.). Philadelphia, PA: Elsevier, 2014; 598–632.

Zella GC, Israel EJ. Chronic diarrhea in children. *Pediatr Rev.* 2012;33(5):207–217

Infectious Disease Associated With Exanthems

Illnesses with cutaneous manifestations are caused by a variety of agents including viruses, Chlamydiae, Rickettsiae, *Mycoplasma*, bacteria, fungi, and protozoa. Today, enteroviruses are the leading cause of exanthematous diseases. Although most exanthematous illnesses are benign, the differential diagnosis is important because skin involvement may be an early sign of potentially fatal bacterial and rickettsial diseases, emerging viruses (West Nile, dengue), and reemerging vaccine-preventable viral infections (measles, mumps), or diseases in returning travelers.

Clinical Presentation

Nonspecific Viral Exanthems

The most common etiologies of nonspecific viral exanthems are enteroviruses (coxsackieviruses, echovirus, enterovirus) and respiratory viruses (adenovirus, rhinovirus, parainfluenza virus, respiratory syncytial virus, influenza virus). Most summertime exanthems are due to enteroviruses, while the respiratory viruses predominate during the colder months. The typical nonspecific viral exanthem presents as blanching erythematous macules and papules, distributed diffusely on the trunk and extremities, with occasional facial involvement. Associated symptoms can include fever, headache, upper respiratory tract or gastrointestinal symptoms, myalgias and fatigue. Viral exanthems are also commonly seen in febrile returned travelers (pp. 431–432)

Enteroviruses: Coxsackieviruses, Enterovirus, and Echoviruses

Group A coxsackieviruses can cause fever and herpangina (1–5 mm vesicles and ulcers of the posterior pharynx), as well as an erythematous, maculopapular exanthem that may start on the face and spread to the trunk and neck, after the patient defervesces. Coxsackie A16 virus causes hand–foot–mouth syndrome which presents with a mild fever, anorexia, malaise, and a sore mouth, followed by a vesicular eruption on the hands and/or feet associated with herpangina-like intraoral lesions. Of note, not all patients have lesions in all three locations, and some also have an eruption in the diaper area. Echoviruses can cause nonspecific cold symptoms, but are known to be associated with aseptic meningitis, particularly echovirus 11 during the summer and autumn.

Measles (Rubeola)

Although vaccination has greatly reduced the incidence of measles in the United States, outbreaks continue to occur, primarily during the winter and spring, and are increasingly linked to contact with returning travelers and communities with a large number of unvaccinated individuals. Measles is spread by direct contact with infectious droplets or by airborne spread, with a subsequent incubation period of 8–12 days. Measles classically presents with the "three Cs": cough, coryza, and conjunctivitis, usually associated with a high fever (up to 40 °C/104 °F). During the prodrome, pathognomonic Koplik's spots appear. They consist of small white spots with a red background on the buccal mucosa. Koplik's spots usually disappear within 48 hours of the onset of the exanthem, which typically appears on the fourth day of the illness. Nonpruritic erythematous macules and papules appear first on the face and spread to the trunk and extremities. The rash fades in the same order as it appeared. Complications include pneumonia, otitis, bronchitis, encephalitis, and myocarditis.

Erythema Infectiosum (Fifth Disease)

This infection is caused by parvovirus B19. It is most common in the spring, primarily affecting 4–10-year-olds. Transmission is by respiratory droplets, followed by an incubation period of 6–14 days. Some patients have a mild prodrome of headache, low-grade fever, malaise, pharyngitis, joint pain, and gastrointestinal symptoms before the onset of the rash. The eruption begins with the sudden appearance of "slapped cheeks" (erythematous patches on the cheeks). It then progresses to the trunk and extremities, where it appears as erythematous macules and papules, before developing into a lacy reticular pattern. Arthralgia and arthritis can be present in 10% of patients. Parvovirus can suppress the bone marrow, so that patients with shortened RBC life spans (sickle cell disease, thalassemia, hereditary spherocytosis, pyruvate kinase deficiency) are at risk for a transient aplastic crisis. Parvovirus infection during pregnancy can cause fetal hydrops and death

Roseola Infantum

Roseola, caused by human herpesvirus-6, is transmitted by respiratory droplets. It affects children between six months and two years of age, with a peak incidence at 6–7 months. It is generally a self-limited, benign illness characterized by 3–5 days of high fever up to 40.5 °C (104.9 °F), which peaks in the evening. Other symptoms are rare, but can include mild respiratory symptoms, irritability, and malaise. The fever ends abruptly, followed by the rash within 24–48 hours. The eruption is characterized by pink, blanching, discrete macules and papules over the trunk. The rash is rarely pruritic and usually fades over 1–2 days.

Varicella Zoster Virus (VZV; Chicken Pox)

Once an exceedingly common childhood disease, varicella is now seen rarely, as a result of vaccination. It is a highly contagious disease with an incubation period of 11–21 days. The patient presents with fever, malaise, headache, anorexia, and abdominal pain. After 24–48 hours the intensely pruritic rash appears on the face, scalp, or trunk, and spreads peripherally. It begins as erythematous macules, which evolve into papules, and then vesicles containing serous fluid. The vesicles spontaneously rupture and develop into crusts, before resolving. Subsequent crops of lesions develop over 4–6 days, so that the presence of lesions in different stages is characteristic of varicella. The patient is infectious from the beginning of the prodromal illness (about two days before the rash erupts) until each pox has a crust, about 7–10 days. Complications include bacterial superinfection of the skin (which may rarely progress to necrotizing fasciitis), pneumonia, thrombocytopenia, arthritis, hepatitis, cerebellar ataxia, encephalitis, meningitis, and glomerulonephritis. The virus establishes latency in the dorsal root ganglia during primary infection, and reactivation results in herpes zoster (shingles).

Herpes Zoster

Herpes zoster is caused by reactivation of the varicella virus. Pain and tenderness along a dermatome precede the eruption of classic chicken pox lesions clustered within 1–3 continuous dermatomes. Pain, tenderness, and localized lymphadenopathy persist while the skin lesions are present (1–2 weeks). Patients with lesions near the eye are at risk for sight-threatening keratitis, uveitis, or acute retinal necrosis. Other complications include meningitis, encephalitis, and motor neuropathies, while immunocompromised hosts are at risk for disseminated disease.

Herpes Simplex

Primary HSV gingivostomatitis (pp. 124–126) causes fever, irritability, and lesions involving the gingival and mucous membranes of the mouth. Genital herpes (p. 332), characterized by vesicular lesions, is most common in adolescents. Consider sexual abuse if genital herpes is seen in a prepubertal child. Reactivation of the latent virus causes "cold sores," single or grouped vesicles in the perioral region, but not inside the mouth, or as lesions on the external genitalia. Neonatal HSV can present as a focal or systemic infection (p. 124), presenting any time from the day of birth until 4–6 weeks of life.

Bacterial Infections

Toxic Shock Syndrome

Staphylococcal toxic shock syndrome (SaTSS) and *Streptococcal* toxic shock syndrome (SpTSS) are clinically overlapping acute febrile illnesses caused by a group of specific toxins (superantigens) produced by *Staphylococcus aureus* and invasive group A *Streptococci*, respectively.

Initially SaTSS was almost exclusively seen with high-absorbency tampon use during menses. Non-menstrual cases are more common, however, associated with surgical and postpartum wound infections, cutaneous and subcutaneous lesions (especially of the extremities, perianal area, and axillae), and respiratory infections following influenza. The onset of the illness is usually abrupt, with headache, fever, chills, malaise, conjunctival hyperemia, sore throat, myalgias, muscle tenderness, fatigue, vomiting, diarrhea, abdominal pain, orthostatic dizziness, and syncope. In the first 1–2 days, diffuse erythroderma, severe watery diarrhea, decreased urine output, and cyanosis and edema of the extremities may be present. Somnolence, confusion, irritability, agitation, and hallucinations may occur as a result of cerebral ischemia or edema or toxin-mediated CNS effects. Progression to multiple organ involvement and shock can occur.

The clinical characteristics of SpTSS (fever, profound hypotension, shock, and multiorgan failure) are similar to those found with SaTSS, although the onset of SpTSS often spans several days and there is no vomiting, diarrhea, or significant encephalopathy. Skin involvement is variable, and presents as an extremely painful sandpaper-like rash, rather than erythroderma.

Meningococcemia

N. meningitides is a gram-negative diplococcus which is carried in the upper respiratory tract in up to 25% of adolescents. Disease occurs more commonly in the winter and early spring, and the majority of cases are seen in children under two years of age, adolescents, and patients living in dormitories. The disease can progress extremely rapidly, presenting with a range of severity from self-resolving bacteremia to meningitis to septic shock and coma. The rash usually presents with nonblanching petechiae and purpura, classically described as asymmetric gunmetal-gray palpable purpura of the extremities. Maculopapular, bullous, and pustular lesions can also occur. This rapidly progressive disease must be considered in any child presenting with fever and petechiae.

Scarlet Fever

Scarlet fever is caused by group A beta-hemolytic *Streptococci*. After an incubation period of 1–7 days, the illness presents with fever, vomiting, abdominal pain, headache, and pharyngitis. The tonsils are hyperemic and edematous and may be covered with exudates, there may be palatal petechiae, and the tongue may have a strawberry appearance (pp. 164–165). The rash is usually erythematous, punctate or finely papular, with the texture of sandpaper. It appears in the axillae, groin, and neck first and generalizes within 24 hours. Accentuation in the flexion creases (Pastia's lines) and circumoral pallor are common. Desquamation begins on the face at the end of the first week and proceeds over the trunk and then to the hands and feet.

Diagnosis

The diagnosis of most viral exanthems is made clinically, as confirmation will usually not change the treatment. An assessment of possible exposure, season of the year, and travel history, along with an awareness of the incubation period of various infections, are important in diagnosing patients with a rash. Inquire about exposure to a similar illness, immunization, and medication histories. The appearance, progression, and distribution of the rash can be very helpful, as can the time elapsed between the exposure and the current illness. Certain diseases occur more commonly in particular age groups. For example, roseola infantum occurs primarily in 6–24-month-olds, erythema infectiosum in 2–12-year-olds, and scarlet fever in school-age children. Some diseases have seasonal predilection, such as scarlet fever in the late winter and early spring and enteroviruses during the summer and fall.

Maculopapular rashes are the most common and are usually associated with enteroviral infections. Vesicular exanthems present either as single or localized lesions (herpes simplex, herpes zoster), generalized lesions (varicella), or in a peripheral distribution (hand–foot–mouth disease).

Pertinent physical findings include the patient's appearance, presence of regional or generalized lymphadenopathy, conjunctivitis, hepatomegaly, or gastrointestinal involvement. Children who are very ill-appearing may have meningococcemia, SaTSS or SpTSS, Rocky Mountain spotted fever, Kawasaki disease, dengue fever, or measles. Meningococcemia is confirmed with a positive blood culture. The diagnosis of TSS is made on the basis of clinical criteria and presentation, although blood cultures are frequently positive in SpTSS (60%), but negative in SaTSS (95%).

Other considerations include a drug allergy or amoxicillin rash, bullous impetigo and insect bites (resembling varicella), although these lesions do not erupt in crops or go through a series of stages; and contact dermatitis (resembling zoster), in which pruritus is more common than pain. The rash of meningococcemia can appear similar to other etiologies of bacterial sepsis, thrombocytopenia (idiopathic thrombocytopenic purpura), and Rocky Mountain spotted fever.

ED Management

There is no specific treatment for many of these diseases. Therapy consists largely of reassurance and supportive care. Treat fever with acetaminophen (15 mg/kg q 4h) or ibuprofen (10 mg/kg q 6h). Assess the hydration status and give intravenous fluids when appropriate. In general, blood tests and cultures are not necessary unless the patient appears seriously ill.

Measles

Overall, treatment is supportive. Admit a patient with pneumonia (for antibiotic therapy), and perform a lumbar puncture if the child presents with lethargy, excessive irritability, or nuchal rigidity. Notify public health officials of any suspected case of measles so that appropriate community measures can be instituted. Vitamin A decreases the morbidity and mortality of measles in children with vitamin A deficiency. Give vitamin A once daily for two days (≤6 months: 50,000 international units; 6–11 months: 100,000 international units; ≥12 months: 200,000 international units). Institute appropriate prophylaxis to contacts, with either measles vaccination (within 72 hours) to incompletely or unvaccinated children 6–11 months of age or intramuscular immune globulin (0.5 mL/kg, once within six days, 15 mL maximum) for unvaccinated or immunosuppressed contacts. Advise the parents that an unvaccinated child should not return to daycare or school from days 5 to 21 post-exposure.

Varicella

Treat pruritus with antihistamines, such as diphenhydramine (1 mg/kg q 6–8h, 50 mg/dose maximum), hydroxyzine (2 mg/kg/day div tid), or one dose/day of cetirizine (2–5 years: 2.5–5 mg; ≥6 years: 5–10 mg). Do not use aspirin due to an increased risk of Reye's syndrome. Do not prescribe acyclovir routinely in otherwise healthy children with varicella. Possible indications include exposed patients >12 years of age who do not have a history of varicella, have chronic cutaneous or pulmonary disorders, are receiving long-term salicylate therapy, or are presently taking glucocorticoids (including short, intermittent, or aerosolized courses). Give acyclovir 80 mg/kg/day orally div qid for five days (3200 mg/day maximum). Give a post-exposure immunization to a susceptible patient within 72 hours and possibly up to 120 hours after varicella exposure.

A newborn whose mother develops varicella within five days before delivery or up to 48 hours after delivery, a patient with varicella pneumonia, or an immunocompromised patient with zoster has a serious risk of overwhelming infection. Admit these patients and consult an infectious disease specialist regarding antiviral therapy.

Consult a pediatric infectious disease specialist to determine the need for prophylaxis with either varicella zoster immune globulin (VZIG) or immune globulin intravenous (IGIV). Potential candidates include significant exposure (5–60 minutes of face-to-face play, residing in the same household) of an immunocompromised patient who does not have a history of chicken pox, susceptible pregnant women, and newborns whose mothers develop chicken pox within five days before or up to 48 hours after delivery.

Herpes Zoster

Treatment is supportive, but effective analgesia (pp. 715–720) is a priority. Immunocompromised patients are at risk for disseminated disease. Consult with a pediatric infectious disease specialist to determine the need for antiviral therapy.

Herpes Simplex

The treatment of herpes is summarized on pp. 125–126. Consult an ophthalmologist emergently if there is any concern for ocular involvement.

Toxic Shock Syndrome

If TSS is suspected, provide oxygen, assist with ventilation as needed, and establish IV access with a large-bore cannula. Begin volume replacement and vasopressors, if necessary. Give 20 mL/kg of NS or lactated Ringer's solution immediately, and repeat the fluid bolus as needed until the vital signs return to normal (see Shock, pp. 28–35).

Treat empirically as soon as possible with the combination of ceftriaxone (100 mg/kg/day div q 12h), vancomycin (60 mg/kg/day div q 6h), and clindamycin (40 mg/kg/day IV div q 6h) to reduce toxin production. Refine the antibiotic regimen once the sensitivity of the organism is known. For documented SpTSS, use the combination of penicillin (400,000 units/kg/day div q 4–6h) and clindamycin (40 mg/kg/day div q 6–8h, 4.8 g/day maximum). Obtaining blood cultures prior to antibiotic treatment is preferable, but should not delay antibiotic administration.

Given the widespread involvement of TSS, evaluate for systemic infection and end-organ involvement by obtaining blood cultures, CBC with differential, electrolytes, BUN, creatinine, liver transaminases, PT and PTT, CPK, and blood cultures. Order a urinalysis and obtain cultures of the throat, stool, and urine. If there is an alteration in the level of consciousness, perform a lumbar puncture (if the patient can tolerate the procedure).

Remove any vaginal tampons or wound packing immediately. Explore and drain infected wounds. Immediate surgical consultation may be required for more extensive infections such as necrotizing fasciitis. Obtain cultures of the cervix, vagina, or incisional wounds.

Meningococcemia

If meningococcemia is suspected, immediately obtain a blood culture and initiate antibiotic therapy with IV cefotaxime (200 mg/kg/day IV div q 6h) or ceftriaxone (50 mg/kg IV q 12h, maximum 2000 mg/dose). Perform a lumbar puncture if there are meningeal signs or altered consciousness (see Meningitis, pp. 422–425). If meningococcemia is confirmed, treat with IV penicillin or cefotaxime (as above). Give prophylaxis with oral rifampin for 2 days (<1 month old: 5 mg/kg/dose bid; ≥1 month old: 10 mg/kg/dose bid; 600 mg/day maximum), or IM ceftriaxone (< 12 years: 125 mg IV once; ≥12 years: 250 mg IV once), or oral ciprofloxacin (500 mg once) to household, daycare, and nursery school contacts, persons having direct contact with the patient's secretions (kissing, shared toothbrush, eating utensils), as well as any medical provider who has had close contact with the patient's secretions (unprotected mouth-to-mouth resuscitation, intubation, suctioning).

Scarlet Fever

The treatment is the same as for streptococcal pharyngitis (pp. 164–165)

The most common regimen is oral amoxicillin as a single daily dose (50 mg/kg; maximum, 1000–1200 mg) for ten days.

Follow-up

- Return immediately to ED for altered consciousness, respiratory distress, inability to take adequate fluids
- Possibly susceptible pregnant patient in the third trimester exposed to varicella: obstetrical follow-up immediately
- Possibly susceptible pregnant patient in the first trimester exposed to parvovirus: obstetrical follow-up within 2–3 days
- Herpes zoster: 2–3 days

Indications for Admission

- Measles, pneumonia or encephalitis
- Immunocompromised patient or newborn with varicella, zoster, or suspected HSV
- Suspected meningococcemia, TSS
- Dehydrated patients requiring IV fluid therapy
- Toxic appearance or unstable vital signs

Bibliography

American Academy of Pediatrics. Human herpesvirus 6 (including roseola) and 7. In Kimberlin DW, Brady MT, Jackson MA, Long SS (eds.) *Red Book: 2015 Report of the Committee on Infectious Diseases* (30th edn.). Elk Grove Village, IL: American Academy of Pediatrics, 2015; 449–452.

American Academy of Pediatrics. Staphylococcal infections. In Kimberlin DW, Brady MT, Jackson MA, Long SS (eds.) *Red Book: 2015 Report of the Committee on Infectious Diseases* (30th edn.). Elk Grove Village, IL: American Academy of Pediatrics, 2015; 715–732.

Centers for Disease Control and Prevention. Post-exposure varicella vaccination. www.cdc.gov/vaccines/vpd-vac/varicella/hcp-post-exposure.htm (accessed June 5, 2017).

Centers for Disease Control and Prevention. Toxic shock syndrome (other than streptococcal) (TSS) 2011 case definition. wwwn.cdc.gov/nndss/conditions/toxic-shock-syndrome-other-than-streptococcal/case-definition/2011 (accessed June 5, 2017).

Centers for Disease Control and Prevention. Streptococcal toxic shock syndrome (STSS) 2010 case definition. wwwn.cdc.gov/nndss/conditions/streptococcal-toxic-shock-syndrome/case-definition/2010 (accessed June 5, 2017)

Murray PR, Rosenthal KS, Pfaller MA. Picornaviruses. In *Medical Microbiology* (8th edn.). Philadelphia, PA: Elsevier, 2015; 458–468.

Influenza

In the United States, flu season lasts from November to May and peaks between January and March. Transmission is via direct contact with respiratory droplets, usually caused by coughing or sneezing. It is highly contagious, and patients may be infectious up to 24 hours prior to onset of symptoms. Viral shedding peaks in three days and typically ceases by seven days. During an outbreak, the highest incidence of influenza infection is among school-aged children. Immunocompromised patients and patients with chronic illnesses are particularly susceptible to more severe disease, although nearly half of pediatric deaths associated with influenza are in previously healthy children.

Clinical Presentation

Influenza is characterized by the abrupt onset of fever, myalgia, chills, and malaise, followed by upper respiratory symptoms, including cough, rhinitis, and pharyngitis. Upper respiratory manifestations may progress to lower respiratory tract illness, resulting in pneumonia and bronchiolitis. The incubation period is 1–4 days, the usual duration of febrile illness is up to four days, and the entire illness lasts about one week.

Complications include otitis media and pneumonia, which may be either viral or a secondary bacterial infection due to *Streptococcus pneumoniae* or *Staphylococcus aureus* (including MRSA). Febrile seizures, encephalopathy, and encephalitis can occur, and myocarditis is a rare but potentially lethal complication. Reye's syndrome may result in patients who have influenza B and are exposed to salicylates.

Diagnosis

The diagnosis of influenza requires careful consideration of clinical symptoms, epidemiological context, and laboratory testing. The clinical presentation of influenza is often very similar to other viral illnesses, but during an epidemic may be diagnosed with some clinical certainty. Importantly, in patients who do not warrant treatment (see CDC recommendations below), diagnostic testing is of little value. For those who may benefit, treatment does not necessarily need to await laboratory confirmation, especially in high-risk populations. Availability of testing varies by institution, but the sensitivity/specificity is prevalence-dependent and is indicated only during the local influenza season. Depending on the test, rapid influenza diagnostic tests may be obtained on nasopharyngeal swabs or aspirates (throat swabs are occasionally acceptable but tend to be inferior), and they have a quick turnaround of less than 30 minutes. These tests vary widely in sensitivity, especially when a novel strain occurs. Therefore, a negative rapid test should not preclude treatment if suspicion is high and the patient is experiencing or at risk of severe complications.

The direct immunofluorescence test provides results in 1–4 hours, but it requires specific laboratory expertise and personnel and may not be as widely available. Sensitivity is high for the RT-PCR test, and it is preferable when available.

ED Management

In the acute setting, evaluate for and manage complications of influenza, including pneumonia, otitis media, febrile seizure, and encephalitis. Otherwise, for mild to moderate illness, supportive care is all that is necessary. Avoid salicylates due to risk of Reye's syndrome. Suspect possible myocarditis (p. 65) and obtain an ECG and troponins if the patient has persistent tachycardia or chest pain.

Antiviral medications administered early in the course of illness, ideally within 48 hours of symptom onset, may reduce the risk of complications and shorten the duration of symptoms. Early treatment of hospitalized patients may reduce mortality and shortens the length of hospitalization. The CDC recommends antiviral treatment for previously healthy patients if they present within 48 hours of symptom onset. Also prescribe antiviral treatment to patients with confirmed or suspected influenza who are at high risk of complications. This includes all patients being admitted, children under two years of age, or those with chronic pulmonary illness (including asthma), sickle cell disease, diabetes mellitus, neurodevelopmental conditions, metabolic disorders, congenital heart disease, immunosuppression, or are pregnant or within two weeks postpartum, or on long-term aspirin therapy, and if the patient is American-Indian or an Alaskan native.

Oseltamivir is the drug of choice for children. The dose is:

<1 year of age:

3 mg/kg bid for five days.

≥1 year of age:

<15 kg: 30 mg bid for five days;

≥15–23 kg: 45 mg bid for five days;

≥23–40 kg: 60 mg bid for five days;

≥40 kg: 75 mg bid for five days.

Follow-up
- Mild illness or minor complication (otitis media): 2–3 days
- Moderate illness or complication (pneumonia, febrile seizure, etc.): one day

Indications for Admission
- Respiratory compromise
- Severe complications, such as encephalitis, status epilepticus, myocarditis
- Inability to maintain hydration

Bibliography

American Academy of Pediatrics. Influenza. In Kimberlin DW, Brady MT, Jackson MA, Long SA (eds.) *Red Book: 2015 Report of the Committee on Infectious Diseases* (30th edn.). Elk Grove Village, IL: American Academy of Pediatrics, 2015; 476–493.

Centers for Disease Control and Prevention. Influenza (flu). www.cdc.gov/flu/index.htm (accessed June 5, 2017).

Esposito S, Principi N. Oseltamivir for influenza infection in children: risks and benefits. *Expert Rev Respir Med*. 2016;**10**(1):79–87.

Fox TG, Christenson JC. Influenza and parainfluenza viral infections in children. *Pediatr Rev*. 2014;**35**(6):217–227.

Kawasaki Disease

Kawasaki disease (KD) is an acute, self-limited, multiorgan vasculitis affecting approximately 3000 children per year in the United States. It predominately affects young children, three months to eight years. The etiology of KD is unknown, but believed to be due to an infectious agent with immune system activation playing a role in its pathogenesis. Prompt recognition and treatment is critical, as up to 25% of untreated children develop coronary artery aneurysms or ectasia that may lead to ischemic heart disease and/or sudden death.

Clinical Presentation

There are three distinct stages of the illness. The acute stage (days 1–10) is characterized by an abrupt (no prodrome) onset of high fever, typically >40 °C (104 °F), for at least five days. The fever persists for a mean of 12 days if untreated. Within 2–5 days of the onset of fever, the patient develops some, or all, of the other characteristic features of the illness, including conjunctival injection without exudate; erythema of the mouth and pharynx, a strawberry tongue, and cracked, red lips; erythematous rash of almost any pattern; induration of the hands and feet with erythematous palms and soles; and isolated, unilateral cervical lymphadenopathy (>1.5 cm), typically seen on the first day of fever.

Cardiac manifestations in the first stage may include tachycardia (60%), myocarditis with associated pericardial effusion (30%), and ECG changes such as prolongation of the PR interval (first-degree heart block).

In the subacute stage (days 11–24), the fever, rash, and lymphadenopathy resolve, and periungual and perineal desquamation occur during the second to third week of the illness. Patients may remain irritable and anorectic after defervescence. Cardiac complications, including coronary artery aneurysms, coronary obstruction and thrombosis, and myocardial and endocardial inflammation occur in as many as 20–25% of patients. Males and infants are at highest risk.

In the final stage (after day 24) there is resolution of the external findings. The cardiovascular complications either resolve or progress to myocardial infarction or chronic myocardial ischemia.

Other clinical features of KD include arthralgias and arthritis, involving the small joints during the acute phase and later the large, weight-bearing joints. Myringitis, urethritis with sterile pyuria, aseptic meningitis, and rarely, hydrops of the gallbladder may be present. Other features include diarrhea, vomiting, abdominal pain, cranial nerve palsies, and thrombosis.

Atypical presentations, often termed incomplete Kawasaki disease, are increasingly common, especially among infants <12 months of age. Patients may have fever and fewer than four of the principle diagnostic features.

Cardiac sequelae occur in up to 25% of patients with untreated KD. Males under six months of age are at greatest risk of coronary involvement, emphasizing the importance of timely diagnosis and treatment.

Diagnosis

The diagnosis of KD is summarized in Table 13.6.

In addition to clinical characteristics, there are typical laboratory abnormalities with KD, and these can persist for up to 6–10 weeks, including elevated inflammatory markers (ESR ≥40 mm/h CRP ≥3.0 mg/dL); CBC abnormalities (WBC > 15,000/mm^3; anemia; platelets >450,000/mm^3 after the first week); hyponatremia (<130 mmol/L); hypoalbuminemia (<3 g/dL); elevated alanine aminotransferase and aspartate aminotransferase (>60 units/L); and sterile pyuria (>10 WBC/HPF).

Table 13.6 Clinical diagnostic criteria for Kawasaki disease

Complete Kawasaki disease[a]

Fever for more than five days

Presence of at least four principle criteria:

    Bilateral limbic sparing or bulbar, non-exudative conjunctivitis

    Oropharyngeal mucous membrane changes
        Erythematous/fissured lips
        Strawberry tongue
        Injected pharynx

    Peripheral extremity changes
        Acute: erythema palms and soles, edema of hands or feet
        Convalescent: periungual desquamation

    Polymorphous rash, primarily truncal (non-vesicular)

    Cervical lymphadenopathy ≥1.5 cm in diameter, usually unilateral

Exclusion of other diseases with similar signs/symptoms, such as adenovirus, infectious mononucleosis, scarlet fever, staphylococcal exotoxin disease, drug reaction, and systemic juvenile idiopathic arthritis

Incomplete Kawasaki disease

Fever for more than five days and two or three of the above diagnostic criteria

Infant ≤6 months of age with fever for seven or more days, without another explanation *even if there are no clinical criteria for KD*

Additional patient characteristics consistent with KD

Hepatomegaly or jaundice

Hydrops of the gallbladder

Irritability

Multi-joint arthritis/ arthralgias (large and small joints)

Myocarditis

Sterile pyuria

Vomiting, diarrhea, abdominal pain

[a] Diagnose complete KD if a patient has only four days of fever, but all five other criteria in the absence of another explanation.

ED Management

The goals of acute phase management are reducing inflammation in the myocardium and coronary artery wall and preventing thrombosis. The mainstays of therapy are aspirin (80–100 mg/kg/day div q 6h) plus high-dose IV immunoglobulin (2 g/kg IVSS over 10–12 hours), but defer initiating treatment to the inpatient setting. The American Heart Association has created a detailed algorithm with indications for echocardiography and intravenous gamma globulin (IVIG) treatment. Admit the patient because of the high rate of cardiac complications during the subacute stage and consult a pediatric cardiologist for an echocardiogram within 24 hours.

Indications for Admission
- Suspected KD

Bibliography

McCrindle BW, Rowley AH, Newburger JW, et al. Diagnosis, treatment, and long-term management of Kawasaki disease: a scientific statement for health professionals from the American Heart Association. *Circulation*. 2017;**135**(17):e927–e999.

Saguil A, Fargo M, Grogan S. Diagnosis and management of Kawasaki disease. *Am Fam Physician*. 2015;**91**(6):365–371.

Sánchez-Manubens J, Bou R, Anton J. Diagnosis and classification of Kawasaki disease. *J Autoimmun*. 2014;**48–49**:113–117.

Son MB, Newburger JW. Kawasaki disease. *Pediatr Rev*. 2013;**34**(4):151–162.

Zhu FH, Ang JY. The clinical diagnosis and management of Kawasaki disease: a review and update. *Curr Infect Dis Rep*. 2016;**18**(10):32.

Lyme Disease

Lyme disease, caused by the spirochete *B. burgdorferi*, is the most common vector-borne illness in the United States. The most important vector is the *Ixodes* (deer) tick, which has a two-year lifecycle, including larval, nymph, and adult forms. The tiny nymphs are most prevalent in the spring and summer and feed on white-footed mice. White-tailed deer are the preferred hosts of mature ticks, which feed throughout the fall, winter, and early spring. Both nymphs and mature ticks may attach to humans and transmit the spirochete if they are attached for >24 hours.

Cases have been reported from all parts of the country, but most occur in the Northeast, some Mid-Atlantic states, and parts of Minnesota and Wisconsin.

Early Lyme disease occurs primarily during the late spring and early summer when nymphal ticks are active. In contrast, Lyme arthritis or more disseminated disease may begin in any season, weeks to months after initial infection.

Clinical Presentation

The disease is categorized into three stages: early localized disease, early disseminated disease, and late disseminated disease.

Early Localized Disease

Early localized disease occurs 1–2 weeks after the tick bite. The classic erythema migrans rash is present in 70–80% of patients with Lyme disease and begins as a red papule at the bite site that slowly expands to >5 cm in diameter. The lesion is annular, with a raised red border and central clearing, and is often described as having a bull's eye appearance. They often occur at the scalp margin, the groin, or extremities in older children. Nonspecific symptoms may accompany early localized disease, including low-grade fever (<39 °C; 102.2 °F), fatigue, headache, neck pain, arthralgias, and myalgias. These symptoms overlap with many viral illnesses and are not an indication for Lyme testing.

Early Disseminated Disease

Early disseminated disease occurs in the days to weeks following primary infection. There may or may not be a history of tick bite or rash. Approximately 15% of patients develop multiple erythema migrans lesions, 10% have neurologic involvement, and 5% develop Lyme carditis. Neurologic involvement may include cranial nerve palsies (especially peripheral VIIth, which may be bilateral), meningitis, and pseudotumor cerebri/papilledema. Lyme carditis can occur in both the early and late disseminated stage, and has a varied morphology that includes different forms of AV block, myocarditis and pericarditis, presenting as presyncope, syncope, chest pain, and sudden cardiac death, although some patients are asymptomatic.

Late Disseminated Disease

Late disseminated disease typically occurs months following initial infection. Lyme arthritis is the most common manifestation (50–60%) and is characterized by a swollen tender joint without warmth or erythema; fever is uncommon. Lyme arthritis is the presenting symptom in 7% of children and affects mono/oligo large joints, especially the knee (90%). Other symptoms of late disseminated disease include fatigue, acrodermatitis, chronic meningoencephalitis, recurrent flares of large-joint arthritis, and peripheral neuropathies.

Diagnosis

A history of a tick bite or travel to an endemic area is helpful, but the absence of this information does not eliminate the possibility of Lyme disease.

EM can resemble an insect bite reaction, nummular eczema, tinea corporis, cellulitis, and rarely erythema marginatum or erythema multiforme. However, erythema migrans typically is asymptomatic and macular without scaling, and it enlarges over days or weeks into a ring-like lesion (see Table 5.7 for the differential diagnosis of annular lesions; p. 123).

The diagnosis of early localized disease is made *clinically* by the presence of EM rash alone. Do not send Lyme serologies at this stage, as they will not yet be positive. Treat empirically to prevent later disease.

If early or late disseminated Lyme disease is suspected, but there is no history of EM, use a two-tiered approach for serologic testing by obtaining a sensitive ELISA screening test followed by a confirmatory Western immunoblot. For patients early in the disease (<4 weeks' duration of symptoms) interpret both the IgM and IgG tests, but use only the IgG for later disease (appears at 6–8 weeks, peaks at 4–6 months.), since false-positive results may occur with the IgM immunoblot.

If the patient has a flu-like illness, other etiologies (e.g., EBV, influenza) are more likely than Lyme disease. Obtain Lyme serology if the patient has a VIIth nerve palsy, but a lumbar puncture is not necessary unless there is a strong clinical suspicion of meningitis (e.g., nuchal rigidity, prolonged headache).

Lyme meningitis can be differentiated from aseptic meningitis by a clinical decision rule called the "Rule of 7s," pending Lyme testing. Patients with <7 days of headache, the absence a cranial nerve VII or other palsy, and <70% CSF mononuclear cells are consistent with a low risk for Lyme meningitis, which classically shows a low-grade pleocytosis (CSF WBC <100 cells/mm^3 with a mononuclear (mononuclear and lymphocyte) predominance of ≥70%), normal glucose, and a mild protein elevation. The diagnosis of Lyme meningitis is confirmed by positive serologies in the setting of a CSF mononuclear pleocytosis, but do not send Lyme PCR from the CSF, as it is not sensitive.

Septic arthritis, trauma, transient synovitis, and rheumatologic diseases (ARF, JRA, SLE) can all present with a swollen joint. In addition, acute joint swelling with fever always raises the concern of septic arthritis, which presents with a hot, red, tender joint. With Lyme arthritis, however, the joint may be swollen and tender, but warmth and erythema are absent. If a patient in an endemic area presents with a non-erythematous swollen joint (especially the knee) and there is no concern for septic joint, the diagnosis of Lyme arthritis can be made with serologic testing and does not require an arthrocentesis.

An ECG is indicated for every patient who is suspected of having early or late disseminated disease. There may be any degree of AV block, ST–T-wave changes, transient prolongation of the QTc interval, or it may be suspicious for myo/pericarditis.

ED Management

Lyme disease tends to have more of an indolent onset, and patients rarely present in extremis. Recommend supportive care with NSAIDS and hydration as needed.

Ticks attach themselves by secreting a chemical and screwing themselves into the skin in a clockwise direction. To remove an attached tick intact, rub a cotton ball or gauze soaked in a warm soapy water solution directly over the tick, in a counterclockwise circular motion to dissolve the chemical attachment and "unscrew" them from the skin.

If the patient has only an EM rash or a cranial nerve palsy (without meningitis), treat with either doxycycline (≥8 years of age: 100 mg PO bid) or amoxicillin (<8 years of age: 50 mg/kg/day div q 8h; 1.5 g/day maximum) for 14–21 days. Cefuroxime (30 mg/kg/day div q 8h; 1 g/day maximum) is an acceptable alternative. Treat Lyme arthritis with the same oral antibiotics for a longer, 28-day course. Macrolides, including erythromycin and azithromycin, are not as effective and are indicated only for patients who have type-1 allergy to amoxicillin, doxycycline, and cefuroxime.

Admit a patient with Lyme carditis for IV antibiotics and telemetry if the child is (1) symptomatic with chest pain, dyspnea, or syncope; (2) has second- or third-degree AV block; or (3) has first-degree AV block with a markedly prolonged PR interval (≥300 ms). Treat IV with either ceftriaxone (50–75 mg/kg q day, 2 g/day maximum) or penicillin G (200–400,000 units/kg/day div q 4h, 18–24 million units/day maximum). If the patient has ECG changes, but meets none of the above criteria, treated with oral antibiotics with the same regimen as for early disease.

Treat Lyme meningitis with IV ceftriaxone or penicillin G (doses as for carditis): 200,000–400,000 units/kg/day div q 4h for 14 days.

Routine prophylaxis to prevent Lyme disease following known tick bites is not recommended in children. However, a patient ≥8 years of age may benefit from a single dose of doxycycline (4 mg/kg, 200 mg maximum) only if the following criteria are met:

- an engorged adult or nymphal *I. scapularis* tick has been attached for ≥36 hours;
- prophylaxis can be given within 72 hours of tick removal;
- the local rate of tick infection with *B. burgdorferi* is ≥20%;
- doxycycline is not contraindicated.

Follow-up

- Patients discharged on oral antibiotics: 2–3 days

Indications for Admission

- Lyme meningitis
- Lyme carditis requiring telemetry (symptomatic patients with chest pain, dyspnea, or syncope; second- or third-degree AV block; first-degree AV block with a markedly prolonged PR interval ≥300 ms)
- Refractory Lyme arthritis requiring IV therapy

Bibliography

American Academy of Pediatrics. Lyme disease. In Kimberlin DW, Brady MT, Jackson MA, Long SA (eds.) *Red Book: 2015 Report of the Committee on Infectious Diseases* (30th edn.). Elk Grove Village, IL: American Academy of Pediatrics, 2015; 516–525.

Centers for Disease Control and Prevention. Lyme disease. www.cdc.gov/lyme (accessed June 6, 2017).

Koedel U, Pfister HW. Lyme neuroborreliosis. *Curr Opin Infect Dis.* 2017;**30**(1):101–107.

O'Connell S, Wolfs TF. Lyme borreliosis. *Pediatr Infect Dis J.* 2014;**33**(4):407–409.

Sood SK. Lyme disease in children. *Infect Dis Clin North Am.* 2015;**29**(2):281–294.

Malaria

Malaria is an acute systemic illness caused by *Plasmodium falciparum, P. vivax, P. ovale, P. malariae, or P. Knowlesi*. The infection is most commonly transmitted by the *Anopheles* mosquito, although transfusion-related and congenital infections can occur. The incubation period is 6–30 days, depending on the species. Acquisition in the United States is possible, but most infections occur in travelers returning from endemic areas, particularly those who have not received adequate prophylaxis.

Clinical Presentation

Malaria presents with nonspecific symptoms, including malaise, headache, fatigue, abdominal pain, and myalgias, which are then followed by fever. In uncomplicated infections, the physical and laboratory findings may be limited to fever, mild jaundice, palpable hepatosplenomegaly, and/or mild anemia. Severe malaria causes end-organ dysfunction, including altered mental status, respiratory distress related to lactic acidosis and/or pulmonary edema, liver dysfunction, renal impairment, splenomegaly, metabolic acidosis, severe anemia, and/or bleeding diathesis. Severe malaria is also defined as a parasitemia of >5%. Cerebral malaria, a diffuse symmetric encephalopathy, may present with a range of neurological signs, including seizures, and progresses to coma.

 P. falciparum is the most common cause of imported malaria in the United States and is the most likely to cause severe malaria, although *P. vivax and P. knowlesi* can also cause severe disease. *P. malariae* infection can persist subclinically for more than 30 years with periodic recrudescence. *P. knowlesi* is a nonhuman primate malaria found mainly in South East Asia that can also infect humans.

Malarial paroxysms, in which fever spikes, chills, and rigors occur at regular intervals, suggest prolonged infection with *P. vivax* and *P. ovale*. These species persist in a dormant stage (hypnozoites) in the liver for several months to up to five years and may cause periodic relapses.

Diagnosis

Suspect malaria in any febrile patient returning from an endemic area, regardless of whether prophylaxis was taken. Thick and thin blood smears are the gold standard for the diagnosis of malaria. The microscopist will determine the presence of *Plasmodium* on the thick smear and then identify the species and parasite density on the thin smear. Rapid diagnostic tests (RDTs) exist that are simple, extremely sensitive, specific antibody-based tests that provide results within 15 minutes. However, RDTs are not available in all hospitals, may not test for all *Plasmodium* species, and may miss malarial infections with very low parasitemia.

ED Management

Rapid diagnosis and prompt initiation of treatment is important to prevent complicated malaria, as even well-appearing children may decompensate quickly. The CDC (www.cdc.gov/malaria/resources/pdf/treatmenttable.pdf) and the American Academy of Pediatrics *Red Book: 2015 Report of the Committee on Infectious Diseases* provide detailed recommendations for drug treatment. Also consult with an infectious disease specialist, if available. The CDC Malaria Hotline provides assistance with suspected cases and is available during business hours at 855-856-4713 and any time after-hours at 770-488-7100.

Screen all patients for glucose-6-phosphate dehydrogenase deficiency as primaquine can trigger hemolysis. If severe malaria is suspected but the results of diagnostic tests are not immediately available, initiate empiric parenteral treatment. Quinidine can cause hypoglycemia, hypotension, and QTc or QRS prolongation. Therefore, before administration, obtain a glucose and an EKG. Admit the patient to an ICU or telemetry setting.

Supportive care for complications of anemia, multiorgan dysfunction, metabolic acidosis, and shock include intubation, judicious use of isotonic fluid resuscitation, early initiation of vasopressors, blood transfusions (for hemoglobin <7 mg/dL or hemodynamic instability), and hemodialysis. Exchange transfusion is no longer recommended by the CDC. Aggressive fluid overload may result in pulmonary edema.

Follow-up

- If initial blood smears for *Plasmodium* species are negative but malaria remains on the differential diagnosis, repeat the smear every 12–24 hours during a 72-hour period
- Primary care or infectious disease at the completion of therapy

Indications for Admission

- Severe malaria
- Parasitemia >5%

- Suspected or confirmed *P. falciparum* malaria, given the high risk for rapid decompensation; patients who are well enough to take oral medications can be observed overnight on a general inpatient service

Bibliography

Centers for Disease Control and Prevention. Malaria. www.cdc.gov/malaria (accessed June 2, 2017).

American Academy of Pediatrics. Malaria. In Kimberlin DW, Brady MT, Jackson MA, Long SA (eds.) *Red Book: 2015 Report of the Committee on Infectious Diseases* (30th edn.). Elk Grove. Village, IL: American Academy of Pediatrics, 2015; 528–535.

American Academy of Pediatrics. Drugs for parasitic infections. In Kimberlin DW, Brady MT, Jackson MA, Long SA (eds.) *Red Book: 2015 Report of the Committee on Infectious Diseases* (30th edn.). Elk Grove. Village, IL: American Academy of Pediatrics, 2015; 927–956.

Dyer E, Waterfield T, Eisenhut M. How to interpret malaria tests. *Arch Dis Child Educ Pract Ed.* 2016;**101**(2):96–101.

Hahn WO, Pottinger PS. Malaria in the traveler: how to manage before departure and evaluate upon return. *Med Clin North Am.* 2016;**100**(2):289–302.

Meningitis

Meningitis is an inflammation of the membranes surrounding the brain and spinal cord. It is caused by a wide variety of agents, most commonly bacteria and viruses. Widespread use of the *Haemophilus influenza* type B conjugate vaccine has virtually eliminated this pathogen in the United States. Similarly, since the introduction of routine pneumococcal vaccination (PCV7 and then PCV 13), the incidence of all invasive pneumococcal infections has decreased by more than 80% for children under two years of age.

The most common etiology of viral meningitis are the enteroviruses. Herpes simplex virus, cytomegaloviruses, and arboviruses may also be implicated. Other viral etiologies are similar to those described for encephalitis (pp. 383–385).

Bacterial causes of meningitis vary by age group. In infants under one month of age, group B Streptococcus, *Escherichia coli*, and *Listeria monocytogenes* cause most cases. Throughout the remainder of infancy, childhood, and adolescence, *Streptococcus pneumoniae* is the most common etiology, while *Neisseria meningitides* occurs far less frequently. Immunocompromised patients (including patients with cancer undergoing systemic or intrathecal chemotherapy, brain surgery, and/or bone marrow transplantation) are also susceptible to meningitis caused by a variety of pathogens including *Cryptococcus* and other fungi, *Toxoplasma gondii*, and tuberculosis, among others.

Clinical Presentation

Meningitis presents with fever, headache, neck pain and stiffness, nausea, vomiting, photophobia, and irritability. However, these signs and symptoms are often absent in immunocompromised patients. Young infants may exhibit irritability, somnolence, bulging fontanel, and low-grade fever, or may have only isolated fever. Nuchal rigidity in older children may be elicited by a positive Kernig's sign (while the hip and knee are flexed 90°, passive knee extension produces spasm and/or pain) and Brudzinski's sign (passive neck flexion causes hip flexion). Seizures occur in up to 20–30% of patients and the syndrome of inappropriate antidiuretic hormone (SIADH) occurs in 30–60%.

Table 13.7 Typical cerebrospinal fluid findings

WBC/mm³	%PMN	Protein mg/dL	Glucose mg/dL	RBC/mm³
Infant <2 weeks				
0–30	<60	<170	30–115	0–2
Child				
0–6	0	20–30	40–80	0–2
Bacterial meningitis				
>1000	>50	>100	<30	0–10
Viral meningitis				
100–500	<40	50–100	>30	0–2
Herpes meningitis				
10–1000	<50	>75	>30	10–500
Tuberculous meningitis				
100–500	<30	50–80	<40	0–2

Viral meningitis can mimic bacterial meningitis. During summertime enterovirus epidemics, older children with viral meningitis may present with fever, headache, photophobia, myalgias, meningeal signs, and an exanthem (that can be petechial)

Herpes simplex virus can cause meningitis or encephalitis, particularly in newborns up to six weeks of life (most are <21 days of age), many of whom do not have skin lesions and usually do not have fever (or may be hypothermic). It can present with irritability, seizures, and skin vesicles or mucosal lesions. In the majority of cases there is no history of maternal HSV lesions. In older infants and children, HSV meningitis has milder, self-limited findings, usually associated with HSV-2. There may be an associated Bell's palsy, atypical pain syndromes, or trigeminal neuralgia.

Diagnosis

In bacterial meningitis, the CSF has a pleocytosis with a polymorphonuclear leukocyte (PMN) predominance, decreased glucose, and elevated protein (Table 13.7). Immunocompromised individuals often have a muted CSF inflammatory response. Gram stain and culture of the CSF are the standards for establishing the etiologic diagnosis of bacterial meningitis, although latex agglutination and immunoelectrophoresis may help identify the etiologic agent, particularly if the patient has received antibiotics before the lumbar puncture. In viral meningitis, the spinal fluid has a normal glucose, slightly elevated protein, and a mononuclear predominance, although early in the course there can be a predominance of PMNs.

ED Management

If meningitis is suspected, perform a lumbar puncture. The only contradictions are increased intracranial pressure, impending respiratory failure, or extreme toxicity with

Table 13.8 Empiric antibiotic therapy for suspected bacterial meningitis

0–1 weeks of age

<2 kg	Ampicillin 100 mg/kg/day div q 12h
	plus
	Cefotaxime 100 mg/kg/day div q 12h
≥2 kg	Ampicillin 150 mg/kg/day div q 8h
	plus
	Cefotaxime 150 mg/kg/day div q 8h

≥1–4 weeks of age

	Ampicillin 200 mg/kg/day div q 6h
	plus
	Cefotaxime 150 mg/kg/day div q 6h

≥4–8 weeks of age

	Ampicillin 200 mg/kg/day div q 6h
	plus
	Ceftriaxone 100 mg/kg/day div q 12h
	or
	Cefotaxime 200 mg/kg/day div q 6h

≥8 weeks

	Vancomycin (60 mg/kg/day div q 6h, 1 g/day maximum)
	plus
	Ceftriaxone 100 mg/kg/day div q 12h
	or
	Cefotaxime 200 mg/kg/day div q 6h

inability to tolerate the procedure. Obtain a CT scan prior to lumbar puncture in the presence of papilledema, focal neurologic signs, or if frontal sinusitis is suspected (to exclude intracranial empyema or brain abscess with mass effect), but treat empirically with antibiotics (Table 13.8) before obtaining the CT scan.

CSF analysis must include a Gram stain, protein, glucose, cell count with differential, and culture. A Gram stain of a CSF smear can be performed quickly and may guide initial management. Other important diagnostic tests include blood cultures, CBC, platelet count, electrolytes, liver enzymes, and urine for urinalysis and culture. If viral meningitis is suspected, send CSF and throat and fecal swabs for viral culture and CSF for viral PCRs (especially HSV), if available.

Start empiric treatment for HSV acyclovir (≤14 days of age: 20 mg/kg every 12 hours; >14 days of age: 20 mg/kg every 8 hours) in infants under six weeks of age who are ill-appearing, or present with abnormal neurological status, a vesicular rash, hepatitis, and/or a maternal history of primary HSV infection.

Monitor the patient for SIADH (pp. 198–200), which is characterized by hyponatremia, low serum osmolality, and high urine specific gravity. If the patient is not in shock or dehydrated, restrict IV fluids to two-thirds maintenance. However, give sufficient IV fluids to maintain a normal systolic blood pressure in order to preserve cerebral perfusion pressure.

Indications for Admission
- Severely ill patients with meningitis of any etiology, including altered mental status or respiratory compromise
- Suspected bacterial meningitis
- Dehydration, inability to take oral fluids

Bibliography

Bonadio W. Pediatric lumbar puncture and cerebrospinal fluid analysis. *J Emerg Med.* 2014;**46** (1):141–150.

Centers for Disease Control and Prevention. Meningitis. www.cdc.gov/meningitis/index.html www.cdc.gov/meningitis/index.html (accessed June 6, 2017).

Nigrovic LE, Kuppermann N, Macias CG, et al. Clinical prediction rule for identifying children with cerebrospinal fluid pleocytosis at very low risk of bacterial meningitis. *JAMA.* 2007;**297**:52–60.

Nigrovic LE, Malley R, Kuppermann N. Meta-analysis of bacterial meningitis score validation studies. *Arch Dis Child.* 2012;**97**(9):799–805.

Safdieh JE, Mead PA, Sepkowitz KA, Kiehn TE, Abrey LE. Bacterial and fungal meningitis in patients with cancer. *Neurology.* 2008;**70**:943–947.

Swanson D. Meningitis. *Pediatr Rev.* 2015;**36**(12):514–524.

Mononucleosis and Mononucleosis-Like Illnesses

Infectious mononucleosis (IM) is a clinical syndrome consisting of prolonged fever, pharyngitis, and lymphadenopathy. Epstein–Barr virus (EBV) causes approximately 90% of cases of IM. Other pathogens that can cause a mononucleosis-like syndrome include, in the order of their frequency, human herpes virus 6 (HHV-6), CMV, HSV-1, group A strep, *Toxoplasma gondii*, HIV, and adenovirus. Additional diseases that present with similar clinical pictures include connective tissue disorders (sarcoidosis, SLE), malignancies (Hodgkin's disease, non-Hodgkin's lymphoma), infections (diphtheria, enteroviruses, hepatitis A or B virus, rubella), and drug reactions (carbamazepine, minocycline, phenytoin).

EBV is a ubiquitous herpes virus that replicates in epithelial cells and B-lymphocytes. It primarily infects children and young adults. By adulthood, 90% of people worldwide have serologic evidence of prior EBV infection. The incidence of symptomatic disease is 30 times higher in whites than in African-Americans, with no known gender differences. There is no obvious seasonal pattern of EBV infection.

Transmission occurs primarily through exposure to oropharyngeal secretions, although transmission via blood products can occur. Despite the fact that the virus has been found to be present in cervical mucosa and semen, sexual transmission has not been demonstrated. Like other herpes viruses, EBV remains in the body for life.

Clinical Presentation

Clinical manifestations of IM are age-related. After an incubation period that can range from 30 to 50 days, a young child (under four years old) is usually asymptomatic or has mild nonspecific symptoms, such as a URI, tonsillopharyngitis (without exudate), or a prolonged febrile illness with or without lymphadenopathy. This age group has a higher frequency of organomegaly. The older child or teenager is more likely to develop the classic triad of fever, sore throat, and lymphadenopathy. The patient may have a prodromal illness consisting of 1–2 days of malaise, anorexia, fatigue, headache, and high fever (40 °C, 104 °F), before the onset of sore throat and lymphadenopathy. Pharyngitis is often most severe in the first 3–5 days, and 30% of patients have exudative pharyngitis. There may also be palatal petechiae.

An enlarged spleen is palpated in about 20% of patients, but splenomegaly has been documented on ultrasound in all patients. Bilateral, nontender, posterior and anterior cervical lymphadenopathy often occurs. Less common clinical features include: abdominal pain, hepatomegaly, jaundice, and periorbital edema. Rash occurs in 5% and may be macular, petechial, scarlatiniform, urticarial or erythema multiforme-like. In about 90% of patients, a non-allergic maculopapular, pruritic rash develops 7–10 days after starting a beta-lactam antibiotic. Symptoms peak at seven days after onset and fade over the next 1–3 weeks. Fever can last 1–2 weeks, splenomegaly usually resolves within four weeks of the onset of symptoms, but fatigue can persist for months.

Complications include thrombocytopenia (25–50%), upper airway obstruction due to tonsillar enlargement (<5%), hemolytic anemia (3%), and splenic rupture (<0.5%). Neurologic complications occur in 1–5% of cases, and include meningoencephalitis, Guillain-Barré syndrome, transverse myelitis, encephalitis, and cranial nerve palsies. An "Alice in Wonderland" syndrome, characterized by metamorphopsia (distortion of sizes, shapes, and spatial relations of objects), can rarely occur.

Diagnosis

Although the diagnosis of IM is clinical, laboratory testing is useful for confirmation, especially when the presentation is atypical. While the heterophile antibody (monospot) test can be clinically helpful when positive in typical cases of IM (specificity >96%), it does have a relatively low sensitivity (70–90%). False-negatives are common early in illness and in children under four years of age. In addition, there is a variable timeline for seroconversion during the course of illness. When it is necessary to confirm the diagnosis of IM, obtain IgG and IgM antibodies to viral capsid antigen (VCA), IgG to early antigen (EA), and antibody to EBV nuclear antigen (EBNA). See Table 13.9 for the interpretation of EBV serology.

Associated lab abnormalities include: elevated white blood cell count with relative lymphocytosis (≥50%), atypical lymphocytes (≥10%), neutropenia, elevated hepatic transaminases, and proteinuria, pyuria, and/or microscopic hematuria.

For non-EBV causes of IM, send a PCR or serology for HHV-6, CMV, HSV-1, *Toxoplasma gondii*, and adenovirus. Obtain HIV testing for sexually active adolescents as acute HIV is an IM-like illness.

Table 13.9 Interpretation of Epstein–Barr antibodies

Infection status	VCA IgG	VCA IgM	EBNA
No current or prior infection	−	−	−
Acute primary infection	+	+	−
Recent (<6 months ago) infection	+	+/−	+/−
Past infection	+	−	+

VCA: viral capsid antigen; EBNA: EBV nuclear antigen.

ED Management

Treatment for IM is supportive. For patients with an exudative or erythematous pharyngitis and anterior cervical lymphadenopathy, perform a rapid strep test. Encourage rest and fluids and recommend acetaminophen (15 mg/kg q 4h) or ibuprofen (10 mg/kg q 6h) for symptomatic relief from sore throat or headache.

Admit a patient with significant upper airway obstruction (stridor). Continuously monitor the oxygen saturation and treat with elevation of the head of the bed, IV hydration, and humidified air. If it is certain that the patient does not have an oncologic disease, such as leukemia or lymphoma, give systemic corticosteroids (dexamethasone 0.25–0.5 mg/kg, 10 mg maximum) or prednisone 2 mg/kg (60 mg/day maximum).

Advise the patient to avoid contact sports or strenuous activities for four weeks, as splenic rupture may occur even without palpable splenomegaly. If the patient has left upper quadrant or left shoulder pain, evaluate for splenic rupture with an abdominal ultrasound or CT with contrast. If splenic rupture occurs, surgical consultation for splenectomy and transfusions for severe anemia and thrombocytopenia are indicated.

Follow-up

- Primary care follow-up in 2–4 weeks. Instruct the family to return immediately for stridor or inability to swallow (persistent drooling)

Indications for Admission

- Upper airway obstruction
- Inadequate fluid intake
- Neurologic complications

Bibliography

Balfour HH Jr, Dunmire SK, Hogquist KA. Infectious mononucleosis. *Clin Transl Immunology*. 2015;4 (2):e33.

Centers for Disease Control and Prevention. Epstein–Barr virus and infectious mononucleosis. www.cdc.gov/epstein-barr/index.html (accessed June 5, 2017).

Lennon P, Crotty M, Fenton JE. Infectious mononucleosis. *BMJ*. 2015;**350**:h1825.

McCulloh R. Mononucleosis. In Ferri F (ed.) *Ferri's Clinical Advisor*. Philadelphia, PA: Elsevier, 2018; 846–846e.2.

Womack J, Jimenez M. Common questions about infectious mononucleosis. *Am Fam Phys.* 2015;**91**:372–376.

Nontuberculous Mycobacteria Diseases

Nontuberculous mycobacteria (NTM) species are ubiquitous in nature and are found in soil, food, water, and animals. NTM species that most commonly cause infection in children in the United States are *Mycobacterium avium* complex or MAC (includes *Mycobacterium avium* and *Mycobacterium avium-intracellulare*), *Mycobacterium fortuitum*, *Mycobacterium abscessus*, and *Mycobacterium marinum*. There is no human-to-human transmission of NTM.

Clinical Presentation

The most common manifestation of NTM in otherwise healthy patients is a chronic cervical lymphadenitis. It usually presents in young children as a subacute or chronic unilateral, violaceous, painless, swollen cervical or preauricular node that has not responded to treatment with the antibiotics typically used for cervical lymphadenitis. Over time the node may become fluctuant and form a sinus tract. NTM pulmonary disease is rare in children who do not have underlying chronic lung diseases, such as a cystic fibrosis, while disseminated disease occurs in the setting of a primary immunodeficiency or HIV/AIDS.

Diagnosis

Definitive diagnosis of NTM lymphadenitis requires culture of the organism. Because the purified protein derivative preparation (derived from *M. tuberculosis*) shares certain antigens with some NTM species, patients with NTM infection can have a positive tuberculin skin test (TST) result, usually ≤10 mm of induration. Interferon gamma release assays (IGRAs) can cross-react, most notably with *M. kansassi* and *M. marinum*.

ED Management

Refer an otherwise healthy patient with suspected NTM lymphadenitis to an otolaryngologist for possible complete surgical excision. Simple incision and drainage is relatively contraindicated, as there is a substantial risk of developing a sinus tract. For suspected pulmonary or disseminated NTM infection, consult with an infectious disease specialist.

Follow-up

- Suspected NTM adenitis: with ENT and/or ID specialist

Indications for Admission

- Severe pulmonary or disseminated NTM infections

Bibliography

American Academy of Pediatrics. Diseases caused by nontuberculous mycobacteria. In Kimberlin DW, Brady MT, Jackson MA, Long SS (eds.) *Red Book: 2015 Report of the Committee on Infectious Diseases* (30th edn). Elk Grove Village, IL: American Academy of Pediatrics, 2015; 831–839.

Linam MW. Jacobs RF. Other mycobacteria. In Cherry JD, Harrison GJ, Kaplan SL, Steinbach WJ, Hotez PJ (eds.) *Feigin and Cherry's Textbook of Pediatric Infectious Diseases* (7th edn.). Philadelphia, PA: Elsevier, 2014; 1381–1391.

Pertussis

Pertussis (whooping cough) is a highly communicable disease of the respiratory tract caused by *Bordetella pertussis*, for which humans are the only known host. The disease occurs worldwide and affects all age groups, but is recognized primarily in children and is most serious in young infants. Pertussis has become increasingly prevalent as a result of vaccine noncompliance and waning vaccine-induced immunity.

Transmission occurs by droplets from a coughing patient and is most likely early in the illness. Pertussis is most common in the summer and fall and epidemics occur in 2–5-year intervals, suggesting that early childhood immunization does not prevent transmission of the organism. Unrecognized infection in adults (commonly manifested as a cough persisting for more than two weeks) is an important reservoir of infection for susceptible unimmunized or partially immunized child household contacts, in whom attack rates range from 70% to 100%. The Tdap vaccine has proven to be both safe and efficacious in patients from adolescence through age 64.

Clinical Presentation

The clinical presentation of pertussis varies by age. In older children, adolescents, and adults symptoms are milder, so that the diagnosis of pertussis is often not entertained.

After an incubation period of 7–10 days, the classic illness occurs in children 1–10 years old and consists of three stages: catarrhal, paroxysmal, and convalescent. The catarrhal stage lasts two weeks and resembles a URI with rhinorrhea, conjunctival injection, low grade or no fever, and a mild cough that gradually worsens. In the paroxysmal stage, coughing increases in frequency and severity over a 2–4-week period. Repetitive, forceful coughs in a series of 5–10 occur during a single exhalation. These paroxysms are followed by a massive inspiratory effort producing the characteristic whoop, as air is inhaled forcefully through a narrowed glottis. Most young infants are unable to generate sufficient respiratory effort to whoop, so they are mistakenly diagnosed with a respiratory virus. Posttussive emesis, cyanosis, and apnea early in the disease course may occur. The paroxysms are exhausting and the patient may appear dazed and apathetic. The convalescent stage is characterized by less frequent coughing spells and decreased severity of episodes over a 1–2-week period.

Common complications associated with pertussis include pneumonia and otitis media. Others include seizures, activation of latent tuberculosis, subconjunctival hemorrhages, umbilical or inguinal hernia, rectal prolapse, and dehydration. The most important, but rare, systemic complication of pertussis is encephalopathy, the cause of which is not known but is likely explained by hypoxia associated with coughing paroxysms.

Diagnosis

Suspect pertussis in any patient with coughing spasms and vomiting (especially posttussive), especially if the primary DTaP vaccination series has not been completed. The gold standard laboratory test is a nasopharyngeal culture obtained on Dacron or calcium alginate swab, but a PCR assay is much faster. The PCR assay is most sensitive during the first three weeks of cough and requires a nasopharyngeal aspirate or wash. False-negatives may occur if the patient has received antibiotics. A CBC may show an elevated WBC count with lymphocytosis. The chest radiograph is usually normal, but may have some perihilar, lobar, and diffuse or patchy infiltrates.

A pertussoid illness can be caused by adenovirus and *B. parapertussis*, but confirming an etiologic diagnosis is not crucial to proper management. *Chlamydia pneumonia* presents with a staccato cough in an afebrile, tachypneic infant younger than 12 weeks of age (pp. 648–651). Rhinorrhea is usually absent, but eosinophilia and bilateral infiltrates on chest x-ray are characteristic. Also consider bronchiolitis (pp. 633–635), bacterial pneumonia (pp. 648–652), cystic fibrosis, tuberculosis (pp. 435–439), and an airway foreign body.

ED Management

Prompt isolation with droplet precautions of infants presumed to have pertussis may decrease the transmission of pertussis to other patients and hospital staff. Treatment consists of supportive therapy, avoidance of stimuli that trigger coughing attacks, maintenance of hydration and nutritional needs, and antibiotics.

Erythromycin (40–50 mg/kg/day div q 6h for 14 days) or azithromycin (10 mg/kg [maximum 500 mg] on day 1; 5 mg/kg [maximum 250 mg] daily on days 2–5) reduces infectivity and, if started during the catarrhal stage, may reduce the severity of the illness. Note that infants under one month who receive *any* macrolide are at increased risk for developing pyloric stenosis.

Provide post-exposure prophylaxis (PEP) with a five-day course of azithromycin (dosing as above) to all household contacts of a pertussis case and to infants and pregnant women in their third trimester who are in close contact with the index case. Details on the most up-to-date recommendations for PEP are on the Centers for Disease Control and Prevention website (see below).

Follow-up

- Young child >6 months of age: every 1–2 days with primary care physician until improving

Indications for Admission

- Cyanosis, respiratory distress, dehydration, or feeding difficulties
- Suspected pertussis in any infant less than 3–6 months old due to high risk of morbidity and mortality

Bibliography

American Academy of Pediatrics. Pertussis. In Kimberlin DW, Brady MT, Jackson MA, Long SA (eds.) *Red Book: 2015 Report of the Committee on Infectious Diseases* (30th ed). Elk Grove Village, IL: American Academy of Pediatrics, 2015; 608–621.

Centers for Disease Control and Prevention. Pertussis. www.cdc.gov/pertussis/index.html (accessed June 5, 2017).

Hale S, Quinn HE, Kesson A, Wood NJ, McIntyre PB. Changing patterns of pertussis in a children's hospital in the polymerase chain reaction diagnostic era. *J Pediatr.* 2016;**170**:161–165.

Leber AL. Pertussis: relevant species and diagnostic update. *Clin Lab Med*. 2014;34(2):237–255.

McMahon M, Kulasingam S, Kenyon C, Miller C, Ehresmann K. Predictors of pertussis polymerase chain reaction positive results in Minnesota, 2005–2009. *Pediatr Infect Dis J*. 2015;34(11):1271–1273.

Returned Traveler With Diarrhea

Diarrhea, with or without fever, is a common complaint in returned travelers. When a patient presents within 1–2 weeks of return, 70–80% of pathogens are likely to be bacterial, with viral and parasitic infections less likely. The most common bacterial cause is entero-toxigenic *E. coli* (ETEC), along with enteroaggregative *E. coli* (EAEC), *Salmonella*, *Campylobacter*, *Shigella*, and *Aeromonas*. Shiga toxin-producing *E. coli*, which is associated with hemolytic-uremic syndrome, is an unusual cause of acute traveler's diarrhea. Parasitic causes are more likely in chronic diarrhea, with *Giardia lamblia* being the most common, along with *Cryptosporidium* species, *Entamoeba histolytica*, and *Microsporidium*.

Clinical Presentation

The patient will have ≥3 loose stools per 24 hours (or two-fold increase in the number of loose stools in a young child), often associated with abdominal cramps, tenesmus, nausea, and vomiting. The patient may have dysentery, a systemic illness that includes fever and bloody stools. Children under two years of age with dysentery are at higher risk for complications, including septic or hypovolemic shock.

Diagnosis

If traveler's diarrhea is suspected, obtain stool samples for bacterial culture, as well as ova and parasites (fresh specimen on three consecutive days.) In addition, direct fluorescent antibody (DFA) or enzyme immunoassay (EIA) tests may increase the yield of microscopy, and can be sent for *Giardia lamblia*, *Cryptosporidium* spp., and *Entamoeba histolytica*. *C. difficile* testing is indicated if the patient has recently taken antibiotics. See pp. 432–433 for the evaluation of a returned traveler with fever. The evaluation and management of a patient with diarrhea is summarized on pp. 255–260.

ED Management

For most children, supportive care suffices while awaiting the results of stool studies. For empiric treatment of moderate to severe or bloody suspected bacterial traveler's diarrhea, the antibiotic of choice is azithromycin 10 mg/kg as a single daily dose, for three days. Alternatives include ciprofloxacin 20–30 mg/mg/day div bid for 3–5 days. If the patient requires admission, treat empirically with IV ceftriaxone 50 mg/kg/day, pending cultures.

The empiric treatment of *Giardia* is either metronidazole (15 mg/kg/day div q 8h; 250 mg/dose maximum) for 5–7 days or tinidazole (over three years of age; 50 mg/kg once; 2 g maximum). For *Entamoeba histolytica* use either metronidazole (50 mg/kg/day div q 8h for 7–10 days; 750 mg/dose maximum) or tinidazole (50 mg/kg/day for three days; 2 g/ day maximum). In addition, add a luminal amebicide, either iodoquinol (40 mg/kg/day div q h9 for 20 days; 1.95 g/day maximum) or, in absence of intestinal obstruction, paromo-mycin 30 mg/kg/day div q 8h for seven days).

Follow-up

- Primary care or travel clinic in 24–48 hours

Indications for Admission

- Fever and/or dysentery in a patient ≤2 years of age
- Inability to maintain hydration status via oral intake

Bibliography

Ashkenazi S, Schwartz E, O'Ryan M. Travelers' diarrhea in children: what have we learnt? *Pediatr Infect Dis J.* 2016;**35**(6):698–700.

CaJacob, NJ, Cohen, MB. Update on diarrhea. *Pediatr Rev.* 2016; **37** (8): 313–322.

Centers for Disease Control and Prevention. Persistent travelers diarrhea. wwwnc.cdc.gov/travel/yellowbook/2016/post-travel-evaluation/persistent-travelers-diarrhea (accessed June 2, 2017).

Steffen R, Hill DR, DuPont HL. Traveler's diarrhea: a clinical review. *JAMA.* 2015;**313**(1):71–80.

Zaidi D, Wine E. An update on travelers' diarrhea. *Curr Opin Gastroenterol.* 2015;**31**(1):7–13.

Returned Traveler With Fever

A febrile patient who has recently returned from international travel most likely has a "cosmopolitan" (non-travel related) etiology of the illness. Malaria is the most commonly imported tropical disease in returned travelers, followed by afebrile diarrheal illness, and dengue. Typhoid, hepatitis, rickettsial infections, and HIV conversion occur in <1–2% of travelers. Risk factors for imported tropical disease include presentation within six weeks of travel, visiting friends and relatives (VFR), travel duration >30 days, traveling for missionary/volunteer work, and adventure travel. Children under five years of age are at higher risk because about half of those traveling to the developing world are visiting friends and relatives.

Return from certain geographic areas suggests the more likely diagnoses, although many common illnesses occur in all tropical/developing regions. Malaria is most often imported from Africa and Central America; dengue from Asia, South America, and the Caribbean; rickettsial infections from Africa; and typhoid from South Central Asia. In general, the rarer the tropical disease, the more likely it is geographically related.

Diagnosis and ED Management

Use the following resources to assess and manage a febrile (fever ≥38.5 °C; 101.3 °F) patient without a source, who has returned sometime during the previous 30 days from an area of endemic disease:

wwwnc.cdc.gov/travel/yellowbook/2018/post-travel-evaluation/fever-in-returned-travelers; or a site of a recent disease outbreak: wwwnc.cdc.gov/travel/notices.

Assess whether there were any preventative measures prescribed and the compliance with them, including vaccinations and prophylactic medications. Inquire about any unusual exposures during travel, including bites, animals (including rodents), food/water source (including unpasteurized dairy), swimming in freshwater, high-risk sexual activity, and tattoos/injections received.

Determine whether additional isolation precautions are required, based on the suspected infection(s). However, most common diagnoses do not specifically require additional precautions, and universal precautions are appropriate.

Choose specific laboratory testing based on the infections that are suspected. But, in general, obtain the following for every patient: CBC with differential, comprehensive metabolic panel, blood culture (especially if typhoid fever is a concern), malaria testing (thin/thick smear and/or rapid malaria test) if the patient traveled to an endemic area, stool culture (typhoid, *E. coli*), and a urinalysis. Based on the countries visited, the clinical picture, and the results of these first tests, other studies that may be indicated include: a chest radiograph, monospot/EBV titers, HIV testing, PT/INR and PTT (concern for sepsis/DIC/ hemorrhagic fever, and lumbar puncture (altered mental status).

Order other testing based on the patient's identified risk factors (schistosomiasis if history of swimming in freshwater, etc.).

Follow-up
- Primary care, infectious diseases, or travel medicine clinic within 24 hours
- If dengue is a concern, daily follow-up with CBCs until afebrile, looking for signs of dengue hemorrhagic fever (hemoconcentration as defined by >20% increase in hematocrit; >20% post-volume fall in hematocrit if IV fluids given; thrombocytopenia <100,000/mm^3)

Indications for Admission
- Suspicion of malaria, particularly if severe
- Suspicion of dengue hemorrhagic fever

Bibliography

Centers for Disease Control and Prevention. Travelers' health: destinations. wwwn.cdc.gov/travel/d efault.aspx (accessed June 2, 2017).

Centers for Disease Control and Prevention. Travelers' health: fever in returned travelers. wwwnc.cdc .gov/travel/yellowbook/2016/post-travel-evaluation/fever-in-returned-travelers#4829 (accessed June 2, 2017).

Feder HM Jr, Mansilla-Rivera K. Fever in returning travelers: a case-based approach. *Am Fam Physician*. 2013;**88**(8):524–530.

Kotlyar S, Rice BT. Fever in the returning traveler. *Emerg Med Clin North Am*. 2013;**31**(4):927–944.

Thwaites GE, Day NP. Approach to fever in the returning traveler. *N Engl J Med*. 2017;**376**(6):548–560.

Tickborne Diseases

The most clinically significant tickborne diseases in children in the United States, aside from Lyme disease (pp. 417–420), include *Rickettsia rickettsia* (Rocky Mountain spotted fever [RMSF]), *Ehrlichia chaffeensis* (human monocytic ehrlichiosis), and *Anaplasma phagocytophilum* (human granulocytic anaplasmosis). For all three, the majority of cases occur between April and September, but seasonality can shift depending upon the local climate and tick activity. The clinical manifestations and geographic distributions of these diseases overlap, so that it can be very difficult to differentiate among them. The incubation periods vary slightly but are generally within two weeks of a tick bite, although the absence of a history of a tick bite does not rule-out these diagnoses. A firm diagnosis in the ED is unlikely, but early empiric therapy is warranted when a spotted fever rickettsiosis is being considered.

Clinical Presentation

Rocky Mountain Spotted Fever

RMSF is the most prevalent rickettsial disease in the United States. The principal vectors are the Rocky Mountain wood tick in the western United States, the American dog tick in the east, and the brown dog tick throughout the country. Most cases occur in Arkansas, Delaware, Missouri, North Carolina, Oklahoma, and Tennessee, although the disease has been reported throughout the continental United States.

R. rickettsii infection causes a systemic, small vessel vasculitis characterized by a rash, headache, and myalgias. The rash develops 2–4 days after fever onset, although it may not be present at the time of evaluation. Blanching erythematous macules progress to become maculopapular and petechial, which in untreated patients may become hemorrhagic and confluent. The rash appears peripherally first and then spreads to the trunk, with characteristic involvement of the palms and soles. Rarely, the rash may be absent. Symptoms of meningoencephalitis as well as focal cranial nerve or peripheral neuropathies can occur, while signs of septic shock and acute respiratory distress syndrome can develop very rapidly. The WBC may be normal or slightly elevated and thrombocytopenia, transaminitis, and mild hyponatremia may develop later on in the illness.

Ehrlichiosis

E. chaffeensis is transmitted by the lone star tick, whose range includes the entire East Coast and the Midwest. It infects monocytes and macrophages, but does not cause a systemic vasculitis like *R. rickettsii*. The presentation may be similar to RMSF, except a rash is less common (60%) and gastrointestinal (GI) symptoms, including vomiting, are more prominent, particularly in children. Although thrombocytopenia, transaminitis, and hyponatremia can occur, leukopenia is more common with ehrlichiosis than with RMSF.

Anaplasmosis

A. phagocytophilum is transmitted by the blacklegged (deer) and western blacklegged ticks, with most cases reported in the northeast and upper Midwestern states. These ticks can also transmit *Borrelia burgdorferi* (Lyme disease) and *Babesia microti* (Babesiosis). Patients present with fever, headache, and myalgias, while rash and GI symptoms are rare. The laboratory values are similar to those in ehrlichiosis. Anaplasmosis is generally more mild and self-limiting than RMSF and ehrlichiosis, but patients must be managed as if they could have the latter two illnesses, as there are no absolute differentiating symptoms or laboratory values.

Diagnosis

Rickettsial diseases are a possibility in patients with a fever and rash residing in, or having traveled to, one of the endemic areas during spring and summer. Consider all three of these pathogens, given the difficulty reliably differentiating them at the time of presentation. The one exception is potential co-infection with anaplasmosis in a patient with known or suspected Lyme disease who has cytopenias.

Antibodies are rarely positive during the first week of illness. To confirm the diagnosis, send IgG IFA titers at presentation and then repeat 2–4 weeks later, looking for a four-fold titer rise. Because *Ehrlichia* spp. and *A. phagocytophilum* infect circulating leukocytes, they can be reliably and rapidly detected by PCR from whole blood, obtained prior to the initiation of antibiotics. In the ED setting, it may be helpful to send a blood smear to look for morulae for *Ehrlichia* spp. or anaplasmosis. Contact the hospital hematology laboratory to be sure they can perform such an evaluation. A negative smear, however, does not rule-out disease; therefore confirmation by PCR or titers is required. Although these diagnostic assays may not provide timely information to affect patient management, they are important to validate the diagnosis and provide crucial public health information.

ED Management
Rickettsial infections may be severe or fatal in untreated patients and initiation of therapy early in the disease course minimizes complications. Patient outcome is best if therapy is started before day five of illness. If the presumptive diagnosis is a rickettsial disease, treat all patients, regardless of age, with doxycycline (4 mg/kg/day div q 12 hours, 100 mg bid maximum) until three days after fever subsides (5–7 days minimum). Tooth staining and enamel hypoplasia does not occur with doxycycline.

Indication for Admission
• Suspected rickettsial disease

Bibliography
Biggs HM, Behravesh CB, Bradley KK, et al. Diagnosis and management of tickborne rickettsial diseases: Rocky Mountain spotted fever and other spotted fever group rickettsioses, ehrlichioses, and anaplasmosis – United States. MMWR Recomm Rep. 2016;**65**(2):1–44

Centers for Disease Control and Prevention. *Tickborne Diseases of the United States: A Reference Manual for Health Care Providers* (3rd edn.). Atlanta, CA: CDC, 2015. www.cdc.gov/lyme/resources/TickborneDiseases.pdf (accessed May 15, 2017).

Choi E, Pyzocha NJ, Maurer DM. Tick-borne illnesses. *Curr Sports Med Rep.* 2016;**15**(2):98–104.

Mukkada S, Buckingham SC. Recognition of and prompt treatment for tick-borne infections in children. *Infect Dis Clin North Am.* 2015;**29**(3):539–555.

Woods CR. Rocky Mountain spotted fever in children. *Pediatr Clin North Am.* 2013;**60**(2):455–470.

Tuberculosis
Tuberculosis (TB) is caused by *Mycobacterium tuberculosis* complex, which contains both *Mycobacterium tuberculosis* and *Mycobacterium bovis*. *M. tuberculosis* is the dominant cause of TB and is primarily spread through prolonged respiratory contact with other infected humans. Risk factors for infection include immigration from or prolonged travel to endemic countries, lower socioeconomic status, HIV infection, illicit drug use, homelessness, history of incarceration, and employment in healthcare facilities. For children, foreign birth or household contacts with the above risk factors are the most likely causes of infection.

Mycobacterium bovis is a zoonotic pathogen usually acquired from consuming unpasteurized dairy products, particularly those imported from or consumed in other countries.

With *latent tuberculosis infection* (LTBI), tubercle bacilli establish an infection, usually in the lung, but there is no clinical or radiological evidence of disease, despite a positive tuberculin skin test (TST) or interferon gamma release assay (IGRA). These individuals are not contagious.

Between 5% and 10% of patients with latent tuberculosis infection will progress to *tuberculosis disease* during their lifetimes. Tuberculosis disease is usually manifested by clinical symptoms and/or radiological findings, most often (75%) pulmonary in children. Extrapulmonary disease may occur in any part of the body, with 70% of cases presenting as lymphatic disease. Infants and immunocompromised individuals may progress directly from infection to disease without a latent period.

Clinical Presentation

Primary Tuberculosis

Most childhood TB disease is primary. The hallmark is the Ghon complex, consisting of a primary pulmonary focus (site of initial seeding), lymphangitis, and regional (hilar or paratracheal) lymphadenopathy. There is no typical clinical presentation of primary TB, which is most often subtle despite significant radiographic changes. When symptoms do occur, there may be low-grade fever, cough, anorexia, weight loss, irritability, malaise, or fatigue. The cough in childhood TB is typically mild and nonproductive. Infrequently, primary TB may progress rapidly and mimic bacterial pneumonia, with sudden onset of high fever, cough, and respiratory distress, with or without pleural effusions. Infants may have wheezing and respiratory distress, or develop a purulent pneumonia from bronchial obstruction secondary to enlarged hilar nodes.

Chronic Pulmonary Tuberculosis

Reactivation disease results from activation of dormant bacilli in untreated individuals with latent tuberculosis infection. It rarely occurs before adolescence. Manifestations include a cough that may become productive with blood-streaked sputum, fever, weight loss, night sweats, and malaise.

Meningitis

Most cases of TB meningitis occur within six months of the onset of pulmonary disease, particularly in children four months to six years of age. Unlike bacterial meningitis, the initial course is indolent, with nonspecific symptoms such as headache, poor feeding, and low-grade fever. The CSF has a mononuclear predominance with a markedly elevated protein and low glucose. If untreated, signs of increased intracranial pressure develop later in the course. In about 50% of cases the chest radiograph is abnormal.

Miliary Tuberculosis

The patient initially is febrile and may appear toxic, although there may be no localizing signs. Later, diffuse lymphadenopathy and hepatosplenomegaly develop. The chest radiograph, which may initially be negative, displays mottling within 1–3 weeks of presentation.

Other Infections

TB lymphadenitis presents with chronic, unilateral, discrete, painless cervical lymph node enlargement. In the United States, TB lymphadenitis is much less common than nontuberculous mycobacterial lymphadenitis. When TB is suspected, aspiration or incision and drainage is absolutely contraindicated. Tuberculosis can also involve bones, eyes, ears, skin, kidneys, adrenals, or the genitourinary or gastrointestinal tracts. Congenital disease occurs rarely and only in infants whose mothers have disseminated tuberculosis

Diagnosis

Asymptomatic patients can be evaluated for LTBI with either a tuberculin skin test (TST) or, in children of five years or older, an interferon gamma release assay (IGRA), such as the QuantiFERON-TB Gold In-Tube assay or T-SPOT. Both types of tests have similar sensitivity and neither can distinguish between LTBI and TB disease. IGRAs are more expensive, but do not require a second visit for interpretation, and are not affected (no false-positives) by previous BCG vaccination or most pathogenic nontuberculous mycobacteria. However, if active TB disease is suspected, also arrange for the collection of appropriate specimens for culture, as well as possible nucleic acid amplification tests (NAATs), as discussed below.

A negative TST result does not exclude latent tuberculosis infection or tuberculosis disease. TST reactivity cannot be demonstrated initially in approximately 10–15% of immunocompetent children with culture-documented disease. Factors, such as young age, poor nutrition, immunosuppression, HIV, certain viral infections (especially measles, varicella, and influenza), recent tuberculosis infection, and disseminated tuberculosis disease can diminish TST reactivity. Measles vaccination causes suppression of the skin test reaction 48–72 hours after vaccination, but the vaccine may be given at the same time as the skin test. The same limitations may exist for IGRAs. Interpret TST results *regardless* of prior receipt of BCG vaccine, but note that IGRAs are preferred in such patients.

Consider a TST to be Positive, If:

>5 mm. Consider positive in patients with suspected TB disease, immunocompromised (including HIV), taking immunosuppressive medication (systemic steroids, TNF-alpha inhibitors), or have close contact with known case of active TB.

>10 mm. Consider positive in patients under four years of age, those born in or having traveled to TB endemic regions, and if there is frequent exposure to high-risk adults (HIV-infected, homeless, illicit drug users, nursing home or institution residents, incarcerated).

>15 mm. Consider positive in children of four years and older without any risk factors.

False-positive reactions to TST may occur in patients sensitized to nontuberculous mycobacteria and in patients previously vaccinated with BCG. These reactions tend to be <10 mm, and can be useful in diagnosing atypical mycobacterial infections. Individuals with a true positive TST will remain reactive for life, so do not administer repeat TSTs.

Obtain a chest x-ray for all patients with a positive TST or IGRA. Children with latent tuberculosis infection have no findings, while in active disease hilar or paratracheal adenopathy, perihilar hazy densities, and/or pleural thickening are often noted. Alveolar densities, atelectasis, and effusion may be present. Apical lesions and, rarely, cavitation may be present in individuals with chronic TB.

If the patient is able to produce sputum, obtain culture specimens sent on three consecutive mornings to identify *Mycobacterium tuberculosis* and to determine drug susceptibility. In infants and young children, gastric aspirates are most commonly used, although there are safe and effective procedures for hypertonic saline-induced sputum collection in this age group that have increased diagnostic yield. Most children have smear and culture negative disease, reflecting the relatively paucibacillary nature of TB in children.

Children younger than 12 months of age suspected of having any manifestation of tuberculosis disease require a lumbar puncture with glucose, protein, cell counts, and culture for *Mycobacterium*. This should be done regardless of the presence of neurologic symptoms, given the potential for disseminated disease in this age group.

ED Management

If an asymptomatic patient with a positive TST or IGRA has a normal chest x-ray, they arrange for follow-up as an outpatient for initiation and management of therapy for LTBI. Otherwise, admit patients with suspected tuberculosis *disease*, because of the specialized procedures needed for diagnosis. Because tuberculosis disease is usually a subacute/chronic infection, specific therapy for TB can usually be delayed until after admission while the evaluation is ongoing. Consult with an infectious disease specialist as well as the local public health department.

If empiric therapy is started, begin four-drug therapy with isoniazid (10–15 mg/kg/day, 300 mg maximum), rifampin (10–20 mg/kg/day, 600 mg maximum), pyrazinamide (30–40 mg/kg/day, 2 g maximum), and ethambutol (15–25 mg/kg/day, 1 g maximum). If meningitis is suspected, substitute ethionamide (15–20 mg/kg/day, 1 g maximum) for the ethambutol, and add prednisone (2 mg/kg/day, 60 mg maximum).

Children younger than ten years with tuberculosis disease are generally not contagious, because they tend to have paucibacillary disease and lack the adult tussive force to expel infectious droplets. Therefore, airborne precautions are usually unnecessary for children with suspected TB unless they have cavitary disease, are sputum positive (which is uncommon), have laryngeal involvement, or are undergoing intubation or other aerosolizing procedures. However, given that they likely acquired the disease from a close contact with an actively infectious adult, instruct all accompanying adults with respiratory symptoms to wear surgical masks until they can be evaluated. Consult with your hospital's infection prevention and control department for specific institutional policies.

Recent Contacts of a Known Case

Place a TST or obtain an IGRA and obtain a chest radiograph. If both are known to be negative and the child is under four years old or immunocompromised, they should be treated empirically for presumptive LTBI and have the TST or IGRA repeated in 8–10 weeks after last exposure to the source case to confirm possible infection. Therapy can be stopped at that time if the follow-up testing is negative and the child is immunocompetent.

Follow-up

- LTBI: primary care, infectious disease, or department of health follow-up in 1–2 weeks

Indications for Admission

- Suspected active TB disease

Bibliography

American Academy of Pediatrics. Tuberculosis. In Kimberlin DW, Brady MT, Jackson MA, Long SS (eds.) *Red Book: 2015 Report of the Committee on Infectious Diseases.* Elk Grove, IL: American Academy of Pediatrics, 2015; 805–831.

Centers for Disease Control and Prevention. Tools for health care providers: tuberculosis. www.cdc .gov/tb/education/provider_edmaterials.htm (accessed June 5, 2017).

Chiappini E, Lo Vecchio A, Garazzino S, et al. Recommendations for the diagnosis of pediatric tuberculosis. *Eur J Clin Microbiol Infect Dis.* 2016;**35**(1):1–18.

Dunn JJ, Starke JR, Revell PA. Laboratory diagnosis of *Mycobacterium tuberculosis* infection and disease in children. *J Clin Microbiol.* 2016;**54**(6):1434–1441.

Starke JR. Interferon-γ release assays for diagnosis of tuberculosis infection and disease in children. *Pediatrics.* 2014;**134**(6):e1763–e1773.

Viral Hemorrhagic Fever

Viral hemorrhagic fevers (VHF) are caused by five distinct viral families, all of which have an animal or insect host that serves as the natural reservoir. Examples include Lassa fever (Arenaviridae), sin nombre virus (Bunyaviridae), *Ebola* virus and Marburg virus (Filoviridae), and yellow fever and dengue fever (Flaviviridae). Humans are incidental hosts, but human-to-human spread is possible in some VHFs, including Lassa virus, Crimean–Congo hemorrhagic fever, *Ebola* virus and Marburg virus. Others, such as yellow fever, require an insect vector.

Clinical Presentation

The incubation period for the different infections varies from three days to three weeks. Initial presentation of VHF may be vague and include fever, chills, myalgia, and rash. Bleeding dyscrasias develop as the disease progresses.

Diagnosis

Suspect VHF in febrile travelers returning from areas of epidemic or endemic transmission. Outbreaks are reported by the CDC Special Pathogens Branch (www.cdc.gov/ncezid/dhcp p/vspb/outbreaks.html). Laboratory diagnosis varies by infection.

ED Management

Depending on the suspected VHF, rapid isolation of the case and use of appropriate personal protective gear is critically important for interrupting transmission. Contact your hospital's infectious disease and infection control departments, as well as the local public health department, regarding proper management and mandatory reporting for any suspected cases. Laboratory specimens may require special handling. Lassa fever, hemorrhagic fever with renal syndrome (an Old World hantavirus in the Bunyavirdiae family), and hendra virus (*Paramyxoviridae*) may be treated with ribavirin. The management of other VHFs is generally supportive care.

Follow-up

- Varies by disease; as per consultation with infectious disease

Indications for Admission

- Concern for VHF with human-to-human spread: institute appropriate infection precautions and notify hospital infection control and the public health department
- Ill-appearing patient with a non-person-to-person transmitted VHF

Bibliography

Broadhurst MJ, Brooks TJ, Pollock NR. Diagnosis of *Ebola* virus disease: past, present, and future. Clin Microbiol Rev. 2016;**29**(4):773–793.

Centers for Disease Control and Prevention. Viral special pathogens branch (VSPB). www.cdc.gov/ncezid/dhcpp/vspb/outbreaks.html (accessed June 2, 2017).

Centers for Disease Control and Prevention. Viral hemorrhagic fevers (VHFs). www.cdc.gov/vhf/index.html (accessed June 2, 2017).

Dahl BA, Kinzer MH, Raghunathan PL, et al.. CDC's response to the 2014–2016 *Ebola* epidemic: Guinea, Liberia, and Sierra Leone. *MMWR Suppl.* 2016;**65**(3):12–20.

DuPont HL. Emerging infectious diseases, animals, and future epidemics. *Tex Med.* 2017;**113**(2):31–36.

Zika Virus

The Zika virus was first identified in 1947, but was not detected in the Americas until March 2015, during an outbreak of an exanthematous illness in Brazil. In February 2016, the World Health Organization declared this outbreak a "Public Health Emergency of International Concern." Zika has now spread to 33 countries and territories in the Americas. Zika is transmitted from human to human by the *Aedes* mosquito. Sexual transmission has been reported, and an infected pregnant mother may also transmit it to her fetus.

Clinical Presentation

The incubation period is 3–12 days and asymptomatic infection is common. Symptoms include low-grade fever, a pruritic macular or papular rash, nonpurulent conjunctivitis, myalgias or arthralgia or arthritis, headache, retro-orbital pain, edema of the hands and ankles, and vomiting. Neurological complications include meningoencephalitis, acute myelitis, and Guillain-Barré syndrome. Congenital infection may result in early fetal loss, microcephaly, and ocular abnormalities.

Diagnosis

Include Zika virus on the differential diagnosis for a patient with classic symptoms returning from an area with active transmission. Laboratory detection by RT-PCR is definitive, but the viremia is often transient. As the viremia wanes, IgM antibodies appear and persist for several months.

ED Management

Treatment for Zika virus is supportive. Advise an actively infected patient or anyone traveling to or returning from areas of Zika transmission to use barrier protection during sexual activity to avoid transmission to partners.

Follow-up
- Pregnant women: obstetrics within one week

Indications for Admission
- Neurological complications (Guillain-Barré syndrome, meningoencephalitis)

Bibliography

Basarab M, Bowman C, Aarons EJ, Cropley I. Zika virus. *BMJ*. 2016;**352**;i1049.

Centers for Disease Control and Prevention. Zika virus. www.cdc.gov/zika (accessed June 2, 2017).

He A, Brasil P, Siqueira AM, Calvet GA, Kwatra SG. The emerging Zika virus threat: a guide for dermatologists. *Am J Clin Dermatol*. 2017;**18**(2):231–236.

Patterson J, Sammon M, Garg M. Dengue, Zika and chikungunya: emerging arboviruses in the New World. *West J Emerg Med*. 2016;**17**(6):671–679.

Petersen LR, Jamieson DJ, Powers AM, Honein MA. Zika virus. *N Engl J Med*. 2016;**374** (16):1552–1563.

Ingestions

Stephen M. Blumberg, Vincent Nguyen, and Katherine J. Chou

Evaluation of the Poisoned Patient

Acute pediatric poisonings generally present in preschool-aged children or in adolescents. Children under five years of age typically ingest a household product or medication unintentionally, while adolescents may ingest medications or illicit substances recreationally or in the context of a suicide attempt.

Clinical Presentation

Young children often present to the emergency department without symptoms, so it is important to differentiate an exposure (e.g., found in an area with pills available) from an actual ingestion, which in this age group usually involves a single medication or household product. With liquids, the parents may report that the child ingested a single or multiple swallows of a substance before spitting it out. In adolescents, the ingestion may be impulsive, whether stemming from recreational use or psychiatric disorders (mood disorders, schizophrenia, substance abuse), and the history may be unclear at the time of presentation. These ingestions can involve multiple medications, illicit drugs and alcohol, and frequently result in symptoms. If the ingestant is known, assess the likelihood of toxicity. Most household products and plants are nontoxic, although some common plants are toxic. A continuously updated reference, which includes a listing of poisonous and non-poisonous plants and household products, can be found on the National Capital Poison Center website: www.poison.org. Several medications can be fatal to infants in very small amounts (Table 14.1) and certain medications may cause delayed toxicity (Table 14.2).

Symptoms can also develop from toxins that are ingested, inhaled, or absorbed through the skin. This is especially important when evaluating neonates or infants due to their relatively large body surface area to mass ratio.

Diagnosis

In most instances, the diagnosis can be made based on history. Estimate the volume of a swallow to be approximately 0.25 mL/kg. In adolescents, and occasionally in toddlers, the parent or child may intentionally conceal the ingestant or it may not be known. Consider an ingestion in any previously well child with a change in mental status, lethargy, hallucinations, delirium, seizures, dysrhythmia, or coma.

In the critically ill child, the first priority is the ABCs, including, intravenous/intraosseous (IV/IO) access and monitoring. Empiric therapy for common disorders,

Table 14.1 One pill can kill: highly toxic drugs and poisons

Drug/poison	Potentially fatal dose	Toxic dose for a 10 kg child	Toxicity
Benzocaine	20 mg/kg	2 mL of 10% gel	Methemoglobinemia, seizures
Calcium antagonists (verapamil)	40 mg/kg	1–2 tabs	Bradycardia, hypotension, seizures, hypoglycemia
Camphor	100 mg/kg	5 mL of 20% solution	Seizures, CNS and respiratory depression
Chloroquine	30 mg/kg	1 tab	Seizures, arrhythmias, hypokalemia
Codeine	20 mg/kg	3 tabs	CNS and respiratory depression, bradycardia
Clonidine		1 tab or 1 patch	CNS and respiratory depression, bradycardia
Diphenoxylate	1.2 mg/kg	2 tabs	CNS and respiratory depression
Hydrocarbons (aspiration)	One swallow		Pneumonitis, CNS depression
Lindane	6 mg/kg	2 tsp of 1% lotion	CNS depression, seizures,
Methyl salicylate (oil of wintergreen)	200 mg/kg	½ tsp	CNS depression, seizures, hypotension
Phenothiazines	20 mg/kg	1 tab	CNS depression, seizures, arrhythmias
Quinidine	50 mg/kg	2 tabs	CNS depression, seizures, arrhythmias
Selenious acid (gun bluing agent)	20 mL	One swallow	CNS depression, seizures, arrhythmias
Sulfonylureas (glyburide)	1 mg/kg	2 tabs	Hypoglycemia
Theophylline	50 mg/kg	1 tab	Seizures, arrhythmias
Tricyclic anti-depressants	15 mg/kg	1 tab	Seizures, arrhythmias, hypotension

such as dextrose for hypoglycemia and naloxone for opioid toxicity, can then be considered. After assessment of vital signs and initiation of therapy, the specific toxin may be determined by history, physical findings, and/or laboratory data, and specific care may be rendered.

Table 14.2 Delayed toxicity

Drug	Onset	Toxicity
Acetaminophen	24–72 h	Hepatic necrosis
Acetonitrile (acrylic nail remover)	12–24 h	Cyanide toxicity
Aspirin (enteric coated)	Up to 8–12 h	Acidosis, hyperthermia, hypotension, seizures
Astemizole	Up to 24 h	Ventricular arrhythmias
Calcium channel blockers (sustained release)	6–12 h	Bradycardia, hypotension, cardiovascular collapse
Diphenoxylate/atropine (Lomotil)	Up to 12–24 h	Respiratory depression
Lithium	6–14 h	Seizures, bradycardia, asystole
MAO inhibitors	Up to 12 h	Cardiovascular collapse
Methanol	12–24 h	Acidosis, blindness
Mushrooms		
Amanita, Glaerina	6–24 h	Hepatic necrosis
Lepiota	6–24 h	Hepatic necrosis
Gyromitra	6–12 h	Hepatic necrosis, seizures
Cortinarius	2–17 days	Renal failure
Napthalene	1–5 days	Hemolytic anemia
Organophosphates (sulfur-containing)	Days[a]	Cholinergic toxidrome, seizures, cardiac arrest
Sulfonylureas		
Chlorpropamide	Up to 48 h	Hypoglycemia
Glipizide/glyburide	Up to 24 h	Hypoglycemia
Thyroid hormone	6 h to 11 days	Adrenergic symptoms
Tricyclic antidepressants	Up to 6–24 h[b]	Arrhythmias, cardiovascular collapse, seizures

[a] Delayed toxicity with sulfur-containing organophosphates (e.g., parathion, chlorpyriphos) occurs because the compound is stored in adipose tissue and slowly released. Most patients with delayed toxicity have at least mild symptoms within the first six hours after ingestion.

[b] Severe arrhythmias and cardiovascular collapse may occur several days after ingestion if the patient becomes symptomatic. An asymptomatic patient with a normal heart rate at six hours is unlikely to develop toxicity.

In addition, delayed symptoms may occur when: medications form concretions (e.g., theophylline, aspirin, iron, meprobamate, bromides); are packaged in sustained-release formulations (calcium channel blockers, theophylline, acetaminophen, lithium); or are ingested with medications that slow gastrointestinal motility (anticholinergics, opioids).

In less acute situations, or after stabilization, a thorough physical examination focusing on vital signs, mental status, pupillary responses, bowel sounds, and skin and mucosal findings may lead to identification of a specific exposure.

The Unconscious Patient

1. Assess the airway, breathing and circulation (ABCs), provide continuous cardiorespiratory monitoring, and secure (IV) or (IO) access.
2. If there are clinical signs of hypoperfusion (delayed capillary refill, poor pulse quality, pallor, cool extremities), give a rapid bolus (20 mL/kg) of normal saline or Ringer's lactate (may be repeated twice), and if possible place the patient in the Trendelenburg position.
3. Obtain an ECG.
4. Assess the level of alertness, pupillary responses, gag reflex, muscle tone, deep tendon reflexes, and examine the head and neck carefully for evidence of injury while maintaining the cervical spine in neutral position.
5. Remove the patient's clothing to facilitate the examination, to look for signs of trauma, and to search for pills and other substances.
6. Measure the temperature and, if possible, weigh the patient.
7. Obtain an ABG to assess the adequacy of ventilation and the acid–base status.
8. Obtain blood specimens for rapid blood glucose, CBC, liver function tests, serum electrolytes, carboxyhemoglobin (if CO poisoning cannot be ruled out by history), and methemoglobin (if cyanosis is present). Also, draw and hold tubes for type and screen and further serum tests as indicated.
9. Give 0.5 g/kg of glucose to any unresponsive patient either empirically or in response to a low bedside measured glucose.
10. Give naloxone 0.1 mg/kg, maximum 2.0 mg (preferably IV, but can be given IM, SC, or ET) either empirically or to correct respiratory depression of opioid toxicity. If there is no response within 1–2 minutes, give a second dose. A positive response may last only 30 minutes, so if resedation occurs either give repeated doses or start a continuous IV infusion at two-thirds the effective dose, infused every hour (e.g., if a total of 0.6 mg was initially required, start the infusion at 0.4 mg/h). If habitual use is suspected in an adolescent, lower the initial dose to 0.05–0.1 mg, increasing to 0.4 mg, and then to 2.0 mg, in order to avoid acute withdrawal. Separate repeated dosing of IV naloxone by 1–2 minutes, as the onset of action for naloxone administered IV is 1–2 minutes.
11. Obtain urine by catheter for dipstick examination, urine toxicology, and, in adolescent females, a pregnancy test.
12. Consider gastrointestinal decontamination as indicated if the airway is maintainable and bowel sounds are present (see pp. 451–452).

If the ingestion was witnessed, determine the specific substance, amount, and time of the ingestion. It may be important to contact someone at the home to check information on pharmaceuticals, or to contact the pharmacy where prescriptions are typically filled. Refer to Table 14.3 for information to include in the history.

Perform a thorough physical examination (Table 14.4), including assessment of the pupils, mucosal membranes, heart, lungs, abdomen, skin, and a thorough neurologic examination (level of consciousness, pupils, motor, reflexes, and gag reflex). Certain poisons

Table 14.3 Important history

Where was the patient found?

Who has the patient visited recently?

Who has visited the patient's home recently?

Is anyone in the home taking any medications or herbals?

Is anyone else in the home suffering from headaches, seizures, fevers, or other illnesses?

Are there any pills, pill bottles, or other open containers in the house (including the garbage), or were any unusual odors noticed?

Does anyone in the house use any unusual chemicals for work or hobbies?

Was a suspect substance or pharmaceutical in the original container, or was it transferred into another one?

Was there more than one suspect substance in a container?

Was the patient given milk, clear liquids, syrup of ipecac, or food prior to arrival?

Has the patient vomited since the suspected ingestion?

Table 14.4 Physical examination findings

Finding	Drugs/toxins
Vital signs	
Hyperthermia	Amphetamines, anticholinergics, cocaine, phencyclidine salicylates, theophylline, tricyclics
Hypothermia	Barbiturates, ethanol, gamma-hydroxybutyric acid, opioids, phenothiazines Hypotension
Tachycardia	Amphetamines, anticholinergics, caffeine, cannabis, cocaine, ethanol, iron, opioid withdrawal, phenothiazines, theophylline Hypoglycemia or hypotension
Bradycardia	Barbiturates, β-blockers, calcium channel blockers, clonidine, digoxin, gamma-hydroxybutyric acid, opioids Hypoglycemia or hypotension Increased intracranial pressure
Tachypnea	Amphetamines, salicylates, theophylline Metabolic acidosis,
Depressed respirations	Botulism, clonidine (early) CNS depressants (ethanol, barbiturates, opioids, sedative-hypnotics)
Hypotension	Barbiturates, β-blockers, calcium channel blockers, cardiac glycosides, clonidine, ethanol, iron, opioids, tricyclic antidepressants
Hypertension	Clonidine, MAO inhibitors, SSRIs Anticholinergics (antihistamines, atropine, phenothiazines, scopolamine, tricyclic antidepressants) Sympathomimetics (amphetamines, cocaine, phencyclidine, theophylline)

Table 14.4 (cont.)

Finding	Drugs/toxins
Skin	
Cyanosis	Methemoglobinemia Hypoxia
Flushing	Amphetamines, anticholinergics
Diaphoresis	Amphetamines, anticholinesterase pesticides, cocaine, salicylates
Hot, dry skin	Anticholinergics
Piloerection	Opioid withdrawal
Bullae	Barbiturates, carbon monoxide,
Pruritus	Vitamin A
Eyes	
Miosis	Clonidine, ethanol, opioids, organophosphates, phenothiazines, sedative-hypnotics
Mydriasis	Amphetamines, anticholinergics, antihistamines, cannabis, cocaine, dextromethorphan, ethanol, LSD, opioid withdrawal, phenylephrine, phencyclidine, psilocybin Hypoglycemia
Conjunctival injection	Cannabis, direct irritants
Nystagmus	Alcohols, carbamazepine, ketamine, phencyclidine, phenytoin
Visual disturbances	Botulism, digitalis, methanol, parathion, vitamin A
Neck	
Rigidity	Phencyclidine, strychnine Dystonia from phenothiazines and haloperidol
Breath sounds	
Rhonchi, wheezes	β-blockers, cholinesterase-inhibitor pesticides, petroleum distillate aspiration, toxic inhalants
Abdomen	
Distention, ↓bowel sounds	Anticholinergics, CNS depressants (many), tricyclics
↑ Bowel sounds	Amphetamines, cholinesterase-inhibitor pesticides, cocaine, drug withdrawal Food poisoning
Tenderness	Acetaminophen, alcoholic gastritis, corrosives, iron, salicylates
Distended bladder	Anticholinergics, tricyclics
Neurologic	
Ataxia	Alcohols, benzodiazepines, carbon monoxide, phenytoin, sedative-hypnotics, solvents

Table 14.4 (cont.)

Finding	Drugs/toxins
Coma	Anticholinergics, alcohols, anticonvulsants, antipsychotics, carbon monoxide, clonidine, opioids, organophosphates, salicylates
Delirium	Anticholinergics, drugs of abuse, heavy metals, phenothiazines, sympathomimetics,
Focal signs	Alcohols Hypoglycemia Increased intracranial pressure due to a mass lesion
Tremor	Arsenic, carbon monoxide, ethanol, lithium, mercury, parathion, phenothiazines, solvents

Table 14.5 Toxidromes

Sympathomimetic

Findings: Hyperthermia, tachycardia, hypertension, mydriasis (reactive), warm/moist skin, agitated/delirium

Causes: Amphetamines, cocaine, phencyclidine, theophylline, ethanol withdrawal

Anticholinergic

Findings: hyperthermia, tachycardia, hypertension, hot/red/dry skin, mydriasis (unreactive), urinary retention, absent bowel sounds, confusion/hallucinations

Causes: Antihistamines, atropine, phenothiazines, scopolamine, tricyclic antidepressants

Cholinergic

Findings: SLUDGE (Salivation, Lacrimation, Urinary incontinence, Diarrhea/Diaphoresis, GI upset/hyperactive bowel sounds, Emesis), miosis, bradycardia, bronchial secretions, seizures, altered mental status, paralysis

Causes: Carbamates, chemical warfare agents (VX, Soman, Sarin), organophosphates, pilocarpine eye drops

Opioid (narcotic)

Findings: Miosis, respiratory depression, depressed mental status, hypothermia, bradycardia, hypotension

manifest consistent and unique sets of vital signs and physical examination findings, grouped into "toxidromes" (Table 14.5).

Distinctive odors may also help make the diagnosis (Table 14.6).

Routine urine or blood toxicology screens are rarely helpful in the poisoned patient and each institution's screen detects different drugs. Specific levels are available for several medications and may assist in making treatment decisions (Table 14.7). Obtain an acetaminophen level after an oral ingestion or if the patient is comatose, as it is a common co-ingestant.

Table 14.6 Odors

Odor	Toxin
Acetone	Aspirin, chloroform, isopropanol, ketoacidosis, methanol
Bitter almonds	Cyanide (silver polish)
Eggs (rotten)	Disulfiram, hydrogen sulfide, mercaptans
Fish or raw liver (musty)	Hepatic failure, zinc phosphide
Fruit-like	Amyl nitrite, ethanol, isopropanol, ketoacidosis
Garlic	Arsenic, dimethylsulfoxide (DMSO), organophosphates, phosphorus, selenium, thallium
Mothballs	Camphor
Peanuts	N-pyridylmethylurea (Vacor), other rodenticides
Pear-like (acrid)	Chloral hydrate, paraldehyde
Petroleum	Petroleum distillates
Shoe polish	Chlorinated hydrocarbons, nitrobenzene
Violets (urine)	Turpentine
Wintergreen	Methylsalicylate

Table 14.7 Important drug levels

Drug	Level	Intervention
Acetaminophen	Nomogram	N-acetylcysteine
Carbamazepine	40 mg/L	Activated charcoal + hemodialysis
Carboxyhemoglobin	25% (any if pregnant)	Hyperbaric oxygen
Digoxin	15 ng/mL[1]	Digoxin-specific Fab fragments
Ethanol	Low level	Necessitates search for other toxins
Ethylene glycol	25 mg/dL	Ethanol or fomepizole or hemodialysis
Iron	500 mcg/dL	Deferoxamine
Lithium	4 mEq/L[2] (acute)	Hemodialysis
Methanol	25 mg/dL	Ethanol or fomepizole or hemodialysis
Methemoglobin	25%	Methylene blue
Phenobarbital	100 mcg/mL	Hemodialysis ± activated charcoal
Salicylate	100 mg/dL (acute)	Bicarbonate, hemodialysis
Theophylline	100 mg/L	Activated charcoal + hemodialysis
Valproic acid	1000 mg/L	Hemodialysis

[1] Treatment with digoxin-specific Fab fragments is based on symptoms and an elevated potassium (>5.0 mEq/L). However, if the digoxin level is >10 ng/mL in an overdose, give Fab fragments, regardless of symptoms.
[2] Treatment with hemodialysis is based on symptoms (severely altered mental status, seizures, arrhythmias). However, a lithium level >4 mEq/L is indicative of severe toxicity and hemodialysis is indicated.

Table 14.8 Causes of increased anion gap metabolic acidosis (Mudpiles CAT)

Methanol or **m**etformin	**C**yanide
Uremia	**A**lcohols or **a**cids (valproic)
Diabetic ketoacidosis	**T**oluene or bheophylline
Paraldehyde or **p**henformin	
Iron, **i**soniazid, or **i**buprofen	
Lactic acidosis	
Ethylene glycol	
Salicylates	

Acid–base status can be determined from arterial blood gas and chemistry panels. The mnemonic "MUDPILES CAT" represents the list of toxins that produce an elevated anion gap with a metabolic acidosis (Table 14.8). The anion gap is calculated by: $[Na^+] - ([HCO3^-] + [Cl^-])$

The normal anion gap is typically <12, but use the upper limit of normal set by each laboratory, since this reflects differences in the methods used to calculate the electrolytes.

Order a serum osmolality in cases of suspected poisoning due to ethylene glycol, methanol, or isopropanol. To calculate the osmolar gap, subtract the calculated osmolality from the measured osmolality:

Osmol gap $=$ measured osmolality–calculated osmolality

Calculated osmolality $= (2 \times Na^+) + (BUN/2.8) + (glucose/18) + (ethanol/4.6)$

Including ethanol in the calculated gap increases the likelihood of correctly identifying gaps attributable to methanol, ethylene glycol, or isopropanol. A normal osmol gap is ±10, while an elevated osmol gap (>40 mOsm/L) is consistent with the presence of a toxic alcohol ingestion. However, a normal osmol gap cannot be used to exclude the diagnosis of a toxic alcohol ingestion.

Assess ECG for conduction delays, as they may precede significant rhythm disturbances. Additionally, as is the case with tricyclic antidepressant ingestions, abnormalities on the ECG may predict the development of seizures or other toxic effects.

Radiographic evaluation of the poisoned patient is generally unnecessary; however, the mnemonic CHIPES refers to tablets that may be seen on abdominal x-ray: chloral hydrate, heavy metals (lead, iron, arsenic), iodides, phenothiazines, enteric-coated medications, and sodium and other elements (calcium, potassium, bismuth). In practice, only the heavy metals are readily visible on abdominal x-rays. "Body packers" who are intentionally transporting illicit drugs wrapped in packages in their intestines will often have visible oblong densities on x-ray. A chest x-ray, including the upper airway, is indicated if there is possibility of aspiration or if the patient ingested a button battery or mini-magnets.

Decontamination

If the patient has been exposed to the toxin on the skin, remove all of the patient's clothing, using gloves, and place it in bags. Thoroughly cleanse the skin with copious amounts of water; a shower is the most effective method. Wear personal protective equipment including a face mask until the chemical is identified.

In the case of ocular exposure to chemicals, thoroughly irrigate the eyes with a minimum of one liter of saline using a Morgan lens (p. 553). Check the pH of the corneal surface with pH paper prior to and after irrigation. Continue irrigation until the pH is approximately 7.0. Most ocular exposures cause an irritant conjunctivitis; however, substances which are acid or alkali may cause chemical ocular burns. These require specific therapy and ophthalmologic consultation.

Recommendations regarding the use of various modalities of gastrointestinal (GI) decontamination have continued to evolve. Determining the indications and appropriate methods for GI decontamination requires review of the risk versus benefits of the technique, as well as the toxicity of the substance ingested. The majority of pediatric ingestions are not life-threatening and therefore do not merit aggressive GI decontamination. Factors which need to be considered before administering any GI decontamination are: the length of time since the ingestion, the likelihood the decontamination method will decrease toxin absorption, the potential adverse effects of the decontamination, the toxicity of the substance ingested, the amount of the substance ingested, and the availability of an antidote.

Do not use syrup of ipecac in the emergency department. Its use is limited to the prehospital setting in the case of a life-threatening ingestion where there may be a significant delay in transport to a medical center.

Gastric lavage involves aspiration of pill fragments from the stomach using a large-bore orogastric tube (size 32–40 Fr). Routine use is not indicated except for an adolescent who has taken a potentially life-threatening dose of a substance without a known antidote less than one hour prior. Lavage can be performed only if the patient possesses a gag reflex and has an easily maintainable airway or if the patient is intubated. Place the patient in the left lateral decubitus position with the neck flexed 20 degrees. The appropriate tube length is the distance from the mouth to the epigastrium, allowing for a curve in the pharynx. After placement, confirm the position by auscultation of air bolused into the stomach. Then, instill 200 mL boluses of water or normal saline into the tube and aspirate by suction. Repeat until the effluent is clear.

Activated charcoal (AC) acts as an adsorbent to bind toxins and prevent their absorption into the systemic circulation. AC binds to most substances except heavy metals, alcohols, caustics, hydrocarbons, and large ions such as lithium. Limit the use of AC to patients presenting within 1–2 hours of ingestion of a potentially life-threatening substance. The dose is 1 g/kg up to 50 g. Use a slurry made with a flavored beverage (cherry syrup, cola, chocolate syrup) to improve palatability. Serve the slurry in a covered opaque container to disguise the color. Do not insert a nasogastric tube solely for charcoal instillation. Multiple doses of charcoal every 2–4 hours are useful for ingestions of delayed release preparations or large amounts of life-threatening toxins. In addition, administer multiple doses of AC in cases of salicylate, theophylline, carbamazepine, and phenobarbital poisoning as the charcoal interrupts enterohepatic and enteroenteric circulation. Use sorbitol only with the first dose of charcoal.

Whole-bowel irrigation may be useful for an ingestion of a sustained release or enteric-coated product, for substances which are slowly absorbed from the GI tract, and for patients in whom charcoal is not indicated. This technique involves instillation of large volumes of polyethylene glycol, which decreases GI transit time, in order to decrease absorption. Instill small quantities at first (toddler: 50 mL; adolescent: 250 mL) and increase the rate to

500 mL/h in children nine months to six years of age, 1 L/h in children up to 12 years old, and 2 L/h in older patients. Continue until the patient's effluent is clear.

Antidote

Most poisoned patients require supportive care and not specific antidote therapy (Table 14.9). If an antidote is available it may be indicated in certain situations in

Table 14.9 Antidotes

Poison	Antidote	Dose
Acetaminophen	N-acetylcysteine	PO: 140 mg/kg load
		IV: 150 mg/kg load over 1 h
Anticholinergic (not tricyclic)	Physostigmine	0.02 mg/kg IV (adult 2 mg)
Calcium channel blocker	Calcium gluconate	60–100 mg/kg (3 g maximum)
Cholinergic	Atropine	0.05–0.01 mg/kg (minimum 0.1 mg, adult 2–5 mg)
Clonidine	Naloxone	1–2 mg IV/IM
Cyanide	Cyanide antidote kit	70 mg/kg
Digoxin	Digibind	Based on amount ingested
Ethylene glycol	Fomepizole	15 mg/kg IV load, then
		10 mg/kg q 12h
	Thiamine	0.5 mg/kg (adult 100 mg)
Hypoglycemia	Dextrose	0.5–1 g/kg IV
Iron	Deferoxamine	50 mg/kg IM q 6h or 15 mg/kg/h IV
Isoniazid	Pyridoxine	Gram for gram, 70 mg/kg if amount is unknown (adult 5 g)
Methanol	Fomepizole	15 mg/kg IV load, then
	(4-Methylpyrazole)	10 mg/kg q 12h
	Folate	1–2 mg/kg IV q 6h
Methemoglobinemia	Methylene blue 1%	1–2 mg/kg
Opioid	Naloxone	1–2 mg IV/IM
Oral hypoglycemic	Octreotide	1 mcg/kg q 6h SC
Organophosphate	Pralidoxine (2-PAM)	25 mg/kg IV, adult 1–2 g
Phenothiazine	Benztropine	0.02–0.05 mg/kg
(dystonic reaction)	Diphenhydramine	1–2 mg/kg IM, IV
Sodium channel blocker	Sodium bicarbonate	1–2 mEq/kg IV
Tricyclic antidepressant	Sodium bicarbonate	1–2 mEq/kg IV
Warfarin (rat poison)	Vitamin K1	1–10 mg SC/IM/IV

which the ingestion has the potential to cause serious toxic effects. It is important to remember that antidotes may have different pharmacokinetics than the drugs they are treating. For instance, in the case of naloxone for opioid intoxication, the antidote effects last for a shorter time than the effects of the opioid and therefore the antidote may need to be repeatedly administered.

Bibliography

Albertson TE, Owen KP, Sutter ME, Chan AL. Gastrointestinal decontamination in the acutely poisoned patient. *Int J Emerg Med*. 2011;**12**(4):65.

Barrueto Jr. F, Gattu R, Mazer-Amirshahi M. Updates in the general approach to the pediatric poisoned patient. *Pediatr Clin North Am*. 2013;**60**(5):1203–1220.

Calello DP, Henretig FM. Pediatric toxicology: specialized approach to the poisoned child. *Emerg Med Clin North Am*. 2014;**32**(1):29–52.

Marraffa JM, Cohen V, Howland MA. Antidotes for toxicological emergencies: a practical review. *Am J Health Syst Pharm*. 2012;**69**(3):199–212.

Mowry JB, Spyker DA, Cantilena LR Jr, McMillan N, Ford M. 2013 annual report of the American Association of Poison Control Centers' National Poison Data System (NPDS): 31st annual report. *Clin Toxicol (Phila)*. 2014;**52**(10):1032–1283.

Acetaminophen

Acetaminophen is the most common oral ingestant in the United States and a common co-ingestant. It is found in many over-the-counter preparations, particularly cough, cold, and pain relief medicines. Acetaminophen overdose is a leading cause of poisoning related deaths and it is the most common cause of acute liver failure in children in the United States.

Acetaminophen is normally metabolized in the liver by sulfation and glucuronidation. In the overdose setting, these metabolic pathways are saturated and the excess acetaminophen is metabolized by the P450 enzymes to a toxic metabolite called N-acetyl-p-benzoquinonimine (NAPQI) that causes centrilobular hepatic necrosis. Rapid diagnosis is necessary, as an antidote N-acetylcysteine (NAC; Mucomyst) effectively prevents toxicity.

Acetaminophen usually reaches peak serum levels within 60 minutes, but this may be delayed to up to two hours if extended-release preparations are ingested. In addition, peak serum levels may be delayed by food and co-ingestions of opioids or anticholinergics.

Clinical Presentation

In the first hours after an ingestion of acetaminophen, symptoms may be absent or mild and may include nausea, vomiting, and anorexia, but these are not predictive of the subsequent course. Liver function tests (LFTs) are normal during this stage. Between 24 and 48 hours after ingestion, subclinical hepatotoxicity occurs and is evidenced by mild right upper quadrant (RUQ) abdominal pain, nausea, and vomiting, with elevations of AST (SGOT), ALT (SGPT), bilirubin, and prothrombin time. Over the next several days, fulminant hepatic failure may develop with jaundice, renal failure, cerebral edema, and hypotension. A patient who survives the stage of maximum hepatotoxicity will recover due to hepatic regeneration.

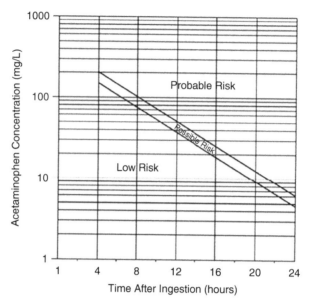

Figure 14.1 Acetaminophen nomogram.
Adapted from Rumack BH, Matthew H. Acetaminophen poisoning and toxicity. *Pediatrics* 1975;55:871–876

Diagnosis

The potential for an acetaminophen ingestion to cause hepatotoxicity may be predicted by obtaining a serum level four or more hours after the ingestion. Plot the serum level on the acetaminophen nomogram (Figure 14.1). If the level appears above the "possible hepato-toxicity" line, treat with NAC. A patient whose level falls below this line does not need treatment, including those who ingested a sustained-release product.

Toxicity may be predicted less reliably by calculating whether the ingested dose is greater than 150 mg/kg. Toxicity is less common in toddlers since they generally ingest smaller quantities and have a larger relative liver size as compared with adults. In addition, young children can metabolize via the sulfation pathway at a faster rate, limiting the production of NAPQI, and they may have greater glutathione stores. Toxicity is unlikely in a child under six years of age unless >200 mg/kg was ingested.

ED Management

Immediately administer 1 g/kg of activated charcoal if the ingestion was less than two hours prior to arrival. Although charcoal does adsorb some acetaminophen, it is not the treatment of choice, so in a case of an isolated acetaminophen ingestion, do not force the patient to accept a nasogastric tube simply to instill charcoal.

NAC is indicated if the serum level is on or above the "possibly hepatotoxic" line on the nomogram. It is 100% effective in preventing hepatotoxicity if given within eight hours of ingestion. Both oral and intravenous routes are approved for use and are equally efficacious and available in the United States. IV administration has more side effects, including a risk of an anaphylactoid reaction, but it is preferred if the patient presents with fulminant hepatic failure or is unable to tolerate the oral formulation.

The oral loading dose is 140 mg/kg, followed by 70 mg/kg q 4h for 17 more doses. Oral NAC is foul-smelling and often causes emesis, so dilute it 1:4 in juice to increase its palatability. In addition, give an antiemetic, such as metoclopramide (1–2 mg/kg/dose IV, IM, PO) or ondansetron (8–15 kg: 2 mg PO; 15–30 kg: 4 mg PO; >30 kg: 8 mg PO). Giving IV NAC decreases the treatment time to 21 hours versus 72 hours for oral NAC. Give a 150 mg/kg IV loading dose over 60 minutes, followed by 50 mg/kg over the next four hours, then 100 mg/kg over the final 16 hours.

If the acetaminophen level will not be available until more than eight hours after ingestion, give a single oral loading dose of NAC while waiting for the result. Treat a patient who arrives for care >24 hours post-ingestion, or one in whom the time of ingestion cannot be determined, with a course of NAC if the acetaminophen level is detectable or the AST is elevated.

Obtain a CBC, electrolytes, creatinine, liver function tests, and PT and INR in a patient who meets criteria for treatment.

Indications for Admission
- Possible acetaminophen toxicity requiring antidotal therapy
- Evidence of hepatotoxicity
- Suicide attempt or gesture without psychiatric clearance and appropriate follow-up arranged

Bibliography
Blackford MG, Felter T, Gothard MD, Reed MD. Assessment of the clinical use of intravenous and oral N-acetylcysteine in the treatment of acute acetaminophen poisoning in children: a retrospective review. *Clin Ther.* 2011;**33**(9):1322–1330.

Lancaster EM, Hiatt JR, Zarrinpar A. Acetaminophen hepatotoxicity: an updated review. *Arch Toxicol.* 2015;**89**(2):193–199.

Rumack BH, Bateman DN. Acetaminophen and acetylcysteine dose and duration: past, present and future. *Clin Toxicol.* 2012;**50**(2):91–98.

Seifert SA, Kirschner RI, Martin TG, et al. Acetaminophen concentrations prior to 4 hours of ingestion: impact on diagnostic decision-making and treatment. *Clin Toxicol (Phila).* 2015;**53**(7):618–623.

Shastri N. Intravenous acetaminophen use in pediatrics. *Pediatr Emerg Care.* 2015;**31**(6):444–448.

ADHD Medications
A variety of medication subclasses are used to treat ADHD, including drugs that are stimulants, atypical antidepressants, tricyclic antidepressants (see pp. 491–492), and alpha-adrenergic agonists. Stimulants include amphetamines, dextroamphetamines, methylphenidate, dexmethethylphenidate, atomoxetine, and pemoline. Atypical antidepressants include bupropion, which inhibit CNS dopamine and norepinephrine reuptake, and venlafaxine, which is a serotonin and norepinephrine reuptake inhibitor (SNRI). The centrally acting antihypertensives inhibit release of norepinephrine in the brain and include clonidine (pp. 470–471) and guanfacine.

Clinical Presentation

Amphetamine and other stimulant toxicity consist of a typical sympathomimetic toxidrome (hyperthermia, tachycardia, hypertension, dilated but reactive pupils, and diaphoresis). Clonidine toxicity resembles an opioid overdose and includes miosis, sedation, coma, hypothermia, hypotension, respiratory depression, and bradycardia. Paradoxical hypertension may develop because, early in overdose, these medications have a preponderance of peripheral alpha stimulation, prior to entry of the drug into the central nervous system. This paradoxical hypertension is then followed by hypotension. Bupropion toxicity can cause a hyperadrenergic state with agitation and seizures, although seizures can occur with normal therapeutic doses.

Diagnosis

Diagnosis is generally made by history as well as by identifying the signs and symptoms consistent with the appropriate toxidrome.

ED Management

Assess the ABCs and vital signs. Check the glucose level and obtain an ECG. Administer activated charcoal (1 g/kg PO) to a patient who arrives in the ED within two hours of ingestion. Treat agitation quickly with benzodiazepines such as midazolam (0.1–0.3 mg/kg IV, 0.2–0.4 mg/kg IM, or 0.4–0.9 mg/kg PO), as it may lead to acidosis, hyperthermia, and rhabdomyolysis. Aggressively treat severe hyperthermia (>40 °C; 104 °F) by covering the patient with a wet sheet and applying ice packs to the groin and axillae. The cardiovascular manifestations generally respond to benzodiazepines; also use benzodiazepines for seizures. Treat sustained tachycardia and hypertension, despite adequate sedation and cooling, with phentolamine (0.02–0.1 mg/kg IV q 10 min).

Naloxone (0.1 mg/kg IV, 2 mg maximum) is variably effective in reversing the sedation caused by clonidine toxicity. Give up to 10 mg before considering the intervention ineffective.

Indications for Admission

- Abnormal vital signs or mental status
- Suicide attempt or gesture without psychiatric clearance and appropriate follow-up arranged

Bibliography

Cooper WO, Habel LA, Sox CM, et al. ADHD drugs and serious cardiovascular events in children and young adults. *N Engl J Med*. 2011;365:1896–1904.

Cortese S, Holtmann M, Banaschewski T, et al. Practitioner review: current best practice in the management of adverse events during treatment with ADHD medications in children and adolescents. *J Child Psychol Psychiatry*. 2013;54(3):227–246.

Spiller HA, Hays HL, Aleguas, A. Overdose of drugs for attention-deficit hyperactivity disorder: clinical presentation, mechanisms of toxicity, and management. *CNS Drugs*. 2013;27:531–543.

Anticholinergics

Anticholinergic poisoning in children may be caused by ingestion of antihistamines (H_1 receptor antagonists), atropine, scopolamine, phenothiazines, antiparkinsonians, mydriatics, jimson weed (*Datura stramonium*), and tricyclic antidepressants.

Clinical Presentation

The anticholinergic toxidrome must be diagnosed clinically since laboratory tests are typically not helpful. Symptoms result from peripheral blockade of acetylcholine at the muscarinic receptors and include dry mucous membranes, flushed dry skin, mydriatic and unreactive pupils, blurred vision (loss of accommodation), constipation, urinary retention, and tachycardia. Central muscarinic blockade causes temperature elevation, delirium, hallucinations, seizures, and coma.

Symptoms can be described by the mnemonic, "Dry as a bone, mad as a hatter, red as a beet, hot as Hades and blind as a bat."

Diagnosis

Suspect an anticholinergic ingestion in any patient with a change in mental status, hallucinations, coma, sinus tachycardia, seizures, or a wide QRS/prolonged QTc on ECG. On examination, the pupils are usually dilated and nonreactive to light and accommodation. Absent bowel sounds, dry mucous membranes, urinary retention, and dry flushed skin also suggest the diagnosis. Obtain blood for a CBC, electrolytes, acetaminophen level (co-ingestion in many cold preparations or attempted suicides), pregnancy test (if indicated), and fingerstick glucose determination. Also order an ECG and urine toxicology if cocaine, amphetamine, or tricyclic ingestion is a possibility.

It is important to differentiate the anticholinergic toxidrome from the *sympathomimetic toxidrome*, as therapy is quite different. Both the anticholinergics and sympathomimetics can cause confusion, agitation, mydriasis, and tachycardia. The pupil, skin, and abdominal examination findings may differentiate these toxidromes. Sympathomimetics cause large yet reactive pupils, with normal or increased bowel sounds, and cool, diaphoretic skin.

ED Management

Initiate supportive care and cardiac monitoring. Administer activated charcoal if the ingestion is likely to have been within the previous two hours, as anticholinergics delay gastric emptying and increase the efficacy of activated charcoal. The treatment of coma is supportive. Treat seizures with lorazepam (0.05–0.1 mg/kg slow IV) or diazepam (0.1–0.3 mg/kg slow IV). If seizures recur give phenobarbital (loading dose 20 mg/kg IV), although propofol or general anesthesia may be necessary for intractable status epilepticus. Treat wide complex tachycardias with sodium bicarbonate (1–2 mEq/kg IV).

Physostigmine can be used in pure anticholinergic poisonings such as atropine, scopolamine, diphenhydramine, and jimson weed. Continued seizures, hemodynamic compromise, or severe agitation or hallucinations are indications for its use. Do not use physostigmine merely to arouse a comatose patient. Give a dose of 0.02 mg/kg *slowly* over five minutes (1–2 mg for adults). This may be repeated every ten minutes until a satisfactory endpoint is achieved. Rapid administration may cause seizures or bradycardia, and an overdose can precipitate a cholinergic crisis (salivation, lacrimation, bradycardia, hypotension, or asystole). Do not use physostigmine in a patient suspected of having tricyclic antidepressant toxicity (QRS >100 ms, PR >200 ms), as it may precipitate terminal cardiotoxicity. Also, in a patient with gamma-hydroxybutyrate toxicity, physostigmine may precipitate fasciculations and seizure activity. Always be prepared to give atropine (one-half the physostigmine dose) to a patient with physostigmine side effects.

Agitation may be reversed entirely with small doses of physostigmine. This reversal allows confirmation of the diagnosis as well as eliminating the need for further invasive diagnostic studies (i.e., CT and lumbar puncture). Repeated dosing of physostigmine at 30–60 minute intervals may be necessary. Sedation with benzodiazepines may be effective, although large doses are often necessary.

Indications for Admission
- Lethargy or persistent signs of toxicity (tachycardia, confusion, sedation)
- Coma, arrhythmia, or seizures
- Suicide attempt or gesture without psychiatric clearance and appropriate follow-up arranged

Bibliography

Dawson AH, Buckley NA. Pharmacological management of anticholinergic delirium: theory, evidence and practice. *Br J Clin Pharmacol.* 2016;**81**(3):516–524.

Glatstein MM, Alabdulrazzaq F, Garcia-Bournissen F, Scolnik D. Use of physostigmine for hallucinogenic plant poisoning in a teenager: case report and review of the literature. *Am J Ther.* 2012;**19**(5):384–388.

Glatstein M, Alabdulrazzaq F, Scolnik D. Belladonna alkaloid intoxication: the 10-year experience of a large tertiary care pediatric hospital. *Am J Ther.* 2016;**23**(1):e74–e77.

Antidepressants

Antidepressants include the tricyclic antidepressants, monoamine oxidase (MAO) inhibitors, selective serotonin reuptake inhibitors (SSRI), serotonin-norepinephrine reuptake inhibitors (SNRIs), and the atypical antidepressants. Tricyclic antidepressants have a unique toxicity and are discussed on pp. 491–492.

MAO inhibitors include tranylcypromine (Parnate), phenelzine (Nardil), isocarboxazid (Marplan), and selegeline (Emsam). The enzyme MAO degrades catecholamines in the CNS, liver, and intestine, as well as tyramine. Toxicity is related to enhanced catecholamine release.

SSRIs include citalopram (Celexa), escitalopram (Lexapro), fluoxetine (Prozac), sertraline (Zoloft), fluvoxamine (Luvox), and paroxetine (Paxil). Receptor binding is relatively specific for the serotonin reuptake mechanism and not adrenergic receptors, and therefore SSRIs have less toxicity than their predecessors.

Atypical antidepressants include amoxapine (Ascendin), bupropion (Wellbutrin, Budeprion, Zyban), duloxetine (Cymbalta), mirtazapine (Remeron), nefazodone (Serzone), trazodone (Desyrel), and venlafaxine (Effexor). These newer medications have varying mechanisms of action, but generally block reuptake of serotonin and catecholamines.

Clinical Presentation

Acute overdose of MAO inhibitors leads to a sympathomimetic toxidrome, consisting of tachycardia, tachypnea, hyperthermia, anxiety, flushing, tremor, hyperreflexia, diaphoresis, agitated delirium, and severe hypertension. The initial hyperadrenergic crisis may be followed by cardiovascular collapse and multisystem failure. These toxic effects may be delayed up to 24 hours after ingestion, so an asymptomatic patient is still at risk.

MAO inhibitors may lead to a hypertensive reaction when tyramine-rich foods (aged cheese, smoked or pickled meat, and red wine) are consumed, since MAO normally degrades tyramine in the intestine. Hypertensive reactions can also occur when additional sympathomimetic drugs are ingested. The hallmarks of such hypertensive reactions are extreme elevations in blood pressure and severe headaches.

The serotonin syndrome may develop in patients who ingest MAO inhibitors with other medications that increase serotonin in the synapse (e.g., SSRIs, meperidine, dextromethorphan). Serotonin syndrome is characterized by the triad of neuromuscular hyperactivity (hyperreflexia, clonus, rigidity, shivering), autonomic instability (tachycardia, hypertension, diaphoresis, mydriasis, tremor), and mental status changes (agitation, anxiety, confusion).

SSRI overdose can cause nausea, vomiting, sedation, and very rarely seizures. Citalopram and escitalopram cause delayed-onset QTc interval prolongation and seizures in a dose-related manner. The newer, atypical antidepressants also cause sedation and ataxia. Bupropion may initiate seizures and/or QRS prolongation. Overdose also causes tachycardia, agitation, and hallucinations. Trazodone may cause priapism, as well as hypotension secondary to alpha-blockade.

Diagnosis

A provisional diagnosis sufficient to initiate treatment can be made when the appropriate clinical presentation is identified.

ED Management

Assess the ABCs and vital signs and obtain an ECG. Treat severe hypertension secondary to MAO inhibitor toxicity with phentolamine (0.02–0.1 mg/kg IV bolus, repeat q 10 min) or nitroprusside. Treat hypotension with multiple fluid boluses (20 mL/kg each), followed by a norepinephrine infusion. Begin with 0.1 mcg/kg/min and increase every five minutes (add a 4 mg ampule to 1 L of D_5 W to make a 4 mcg/mL solution). Give activated charcoal (1 g/kg PO) to a patient who arrives within two hours of ingestion. Admit any patient with MAO inhibitor, citalopram/escitalopram, and bupropion ingestions to a monitored setting for 24 hours, because toxicity may be delayed.

Treat serotonin syndrome with aggressive cooling for hyperthermia and benzodiazepines for muscle rigidity and agitation.

Indications for Admission

- Signs of severe toxicity (seizures, vital sign abnormalities)
- All ingestions of MAO inhibitors, citalopram/escitalopram, and bupropion
- Serotonin syndrome

- Suicide attempt or gesture without psychiatric clearance and appropriate follow-up arranged

Bibliography

Bruccoleri RE, Burns MM. A literature review of the use of sodium bicarbonate for the treatment of QRS widening. *J Med Toxicol.* 2016;**12**(1):121–129.

Kant S, Liebelt E. Recognizing serotonin toxicity in the pediatric emergency department. *Pediatr Emerg Care.* 2012;**28**(8):817–821.

Stork CM. Serotonin reuptake inhibitors and atypical antidepressants. In Hoffman RS, Howland MA, Lewin NA, Nelson LS, Goldfrank LR (eds.) *Goldfrank's Toxicologic Emergencies* (10th edn.). New York: McGraw-Hill, 2015; 1018–1028.

Wang RZ, Vashistha V, Kaur S, Houchens NW. Serotonin syndrome: preventing, recognizing, and treating it. *Cleve Clin J Med.* 2016;**83**(11):810–817.

Antipsychotics

Antipsychotic medications are widely used for the treatment of psychosis and are now being prescribed for other conditions, such as migraine headaches, control of emesis, chemical restraint, and movement disorders. Although overdose may be common, severe toxicity is rare.

Antipsychotics are divided into typical and atypical classes. Typical antipsychotics are older medications, including chlorpromazine (Thorazine), thioridazine (Mellaril), pro-chlorperazine (Compazine), and haloperidol (Haldol). Their mechanism of action is via dopamine and serotonin receptor blocking in the central nervous system. In addition, they also have alpha-adrenergic blockade, anticholinergic and antimuscarinic effects which may become more pronounced in overdose.

The newer, atypical antipsychotics include clozapine (Clozaril), olanzapine (Zyprexa), quetiapine (Seroquel), risperidone (Risperdal), and ziprasidone (Geodon). In general the atypicals are more active at serotonin receptors than dopamine receptors and therefore less likely to have (extrapyramidal) adverse effects at therapeutic doses.

Clinical Presentation

Toxicity from antipsychotics is manifested in the CNS and the cardiovascular system, although tolerance to the sedating effects of antipsychotics can be seen in a patient on chronic therapy. The most common toxicity, at both therapeutic levels and in the overdose setting, is an acute dystonic reaction that includes torticollis, opisthotonos, difficulty speaking, facial grimacing, and oculogyric crisis. Onset can be delayed for up to three days after ingestion and the spasm may wax and wane. Postural hypotension and an anticholinergic toxidrome may also occur. In an overdose, antipsychotics commonly cause impaired consciousness ranging from somnolence to coma. In addition, antipsychotics may also lower the seizure threshold.

Cardiotoxicity from antipsychotics results in tachycardia (anticholinergic effect), and hypotension, especially postural (alpha-blockade). Many of the antipsychotics may also cause QTc prolongation and a rightward deviation or widening of the QRS complex.

Neuroleptic malignant syndrome is an extremely rare reaction that can be life-threatening. It is characterized by altered mental status, hyperthermia, muscular rigidity, and autonomic instability. The reaction can occur at any time following initiation of antipsychotic medications.

Diagnosis

A provisional diagnosis, which is sufficient to initiate treatment, can be made when a consistent clinical presentation is identified. It is important to obtain a thorough history by contacting family, friends, and paramedics.

ED Management

Provide supportive care as indicated, obtain an ECG, and administer activated charcoal (1 g/kg) if the ingestion has occurred within 1–2 hours. Treat a dystonic reaction with diphenhydramine (1 mg/kg IM or IV, 50 mg maximum) and/or benztropine mesylate (0.05 mg/kg IV or IM, 2 mg maximum). Prescribe a two-day course of diphenhydramine (5 mg/kg/day div qid, 200 mg/day maximum) or benztropine mesylate (toddler: 0.5 mg bid; child or adolescent: 1.0 mg bid) to prevent a recurrence of the symptoms.

Treat seizures with lorazepam (0.05–0.1 mg/kg slow IV) or diazepam (0.1–0.3 mg/kg slow IV). Treat orthostatic hypotension with 20 mL/kg of isotonic IV fluid, but do not treat sinus tachycardia unless it is associated with ischemia. QTc prolongation requires no specific treatment other than monitoring and correction of potential causes such as hypokalemia and hypomagnesemia. The management of an anticholinergic syndrome is detailed on pp. 457–458.

Treat neuroleptic malignant syndrome with aggressive cooling, sedation with benzodiazepines, fluid resuscitation, and potentially a dopamine agonist such as bromocriptine.

Follow-up

- Dystonic reaction: next day

Indications for Admission

- Decreased level of consciousness
- Neuroleptic malignant syndrome
- Seizures or persistent hypotension
- ECG changes
- Suicide attempt or gesture without psychiatric clearance and appropriate follow-up arranged

Bibliography

Meli M, Rauber-Lüthy C, Hoffmann-Walbeck P, et al. Atypical antipsychotic poisoning in young children: a multicentre analysis of poisons centres data. *Eur J Pediatr.* 2014;**173**:743–750.

Pileggi DJ, Cook AM. Neuroleptic malignant syndrome. *Ann Pharmacother.* 2016;**50**(11):973–981.

Rasimas JJ, Liebelt EL. Adverse effects and toxicity of the atypical antipsychotics: what is important for the pediatric emergency medicine practitioner. *Clin Pediatr Emerg Med.* 2012;**13**(4):300–310.

Tse L, Barr AM, Scarapicchia V, Vila-Rodriguez F. Neuroleptic malignant syndrome: a review from a clinically oriented perspective. *Curr Neuropharmacol.* 2015;**13**(3):395–406.

Beta-Blockers

Beta-adrenergic blocking drugs are widely used for the treatment of hypertension, angina, arrhythmias, migraine headaches, and various other conditions. Members of this group include propranolol, atenolol, betaxolol, bisoprolol, penbutol, carvedilol, metoprolol, nadolol, sotalol, timolol, pindolol, and acebutolol. Sustained-release preparations are also available. The primary beta-blocker effect is slowing the rate of sinoatrial (SA) node discharge and conduction through the atria and atrioventricular (AV) node. Sotalol will also cause potassium channel blockade.

Clinical Presentation

Unintentional ingestions in children rarely result in significant toxicity. Symptoms and signs occur within six hours of overdose, unless a sustained-release preparation or sotalol has been ingested. The most common finding is bradycardia. Abnormalities on ECG may include an increased PR interval, bundle branch block, and, in massive intoxications, a widened QRS interval. Sotalol causes prolongation of the QTc, which predisposes to ventricular dysrhythmias, such as torsades de pointes. Other possible ventricular arrhythmias include various escape rhythms and ventricular tachycardia.

Hypotension and cardiogenic shock can occur, but are very unlikely in younger children who have had an unintentional ingestion. Patients with propranolol overdose are at particular risk for CNS manifestations, including depressed level of consciousness, delirium, coma, and seizures. Other findings may include hyperkalemia, bronchospasm in patients with asthma, and hypoglycemia in younger children.

Diagnosis

Consider beta-blocker poisoning in a patient presenting with bradycardia and hypotension or seizure. Other cardiotoxic medications, such as calcium channel blockers, digitalis glycosides, and central alpha-agonists (clonidine) may also cause bradycardia and hypotension. Serum levels are rarely necessary.

ED Management

Initiate supportive care and administer a dose of activated charcoal if less than 1–2 hours has elapsed since the ingestion. Continuously monitor the ECG and blood pressure. Obtain blood for electrolytes and glucose and treat hypotension with 20 mL/kg boluses of an isotonic fluid (normal saline or Ringer's lactate). If there is no response to 2–3 boluses, consult a toxicologist and pediatric cardiologist, and arrange admission to a pediatric intensive care unit.

Glucagon (50 mcg/kg, 5 mg maximum) is the drug of choice for severe beta-blocker toxicity. Calcium will treat hypotension but has little effect on the heart rate. Give calcium gluconate 10% (60 mg/kg, 3 g maximum) slowly IV through a peripheral or central venous line, or calcium chloride 10% (20 mg/kg), slowly IV, through a central venous line. If calcium and glucagon are not effective, begin a norepinephrine or isoproterenol infusion. The combination of high-dose insulin and glucose has also been shown to improve cardiac function (bolus regular insulin 1 unit/kg with 0.5 g/kg of dextrose [2 mL/kg of D_{25}]), followed by an infusion of insulin 0.5–1 units/kg/h with 1 g/kg/h glucose). Monitor capillary blood glucose q 10 min until stable, then q 30–60 min while infusing insulin. Cardiac pacing may be necessary in refractory bradycardia.

Hypoglycemia (pp. 194–197) is a particular risk in children. Treat with supplemental glucose (2–4 mL/kg of D_{25} W or 5–10 mL/kg of D_{10}). Correct significant hyperkalemia (pp. 186–188). Treat seizures with lorazepam (0.05–0.1 mg/kg slow IV) or diazepam (0.1–0.3 mg/kg slow IV). Treat bronchospasm with nebulized bronchodilators (p. 625).

Indications for Admission
- History of beta-blocker overdose, unless the patient remains asymptomatic for six hours after ingestion and the product is not sustained-release or sotalol
- Suicide attempt or gesture without psychiatric clearance and appropriate follow-up arranged

Bibliography
Graudins A, Lee HM, Druda D. Calcium channel antagonist and beta-blocker overdose: antidotes and adjunct therapies. *Br J Clin Pharmacol.* 2016;**81**(3):453–461.

Jang DH, Spyres MB, Fox L, Manini AF. Toxin-induced cardiovascular failure. *Emerg Med Clin North Am.* 2014;**32**(1):79–102.

Palatnick W, Jelic T. Emergency department management of calcium-channel blocker, beta blocker, and digoxin toxicity. *Emerg Med Pract.* 2014;**16**(2):1–19.

Truitt CA, Brooks DE, Dommer P, LoVecchio F. Outcomes of unintentional beta-blocker or calcium channel blocker overdoses: a retrospective review of poison center data. *J Med Toxicol.* 2012;**8**(2):135–139.

Caffeine
Caffeine is a methylxanthine which is widely available in beverages, food, over-the-counter drugs, prescription medications, herbals, and dietary supplements. In addition, bulk bags of pure powdered caffeine can be easily obtained over the internet. It acts as an antagonist to the inhibitory function of adenosine, and as such produces CNS stimulant effects. At higher doses it is a cardiac, respiratory, and neuropsychiatric stimulant.

A typical cup of coffee contains approximately 100 mg of caffeine and over-the-counter supplements usually contain 100–200 mg; a teaspoon of pure caffeine powder is roughly equal to 28 cups of coffee. A dose of 50–200 mg causes mild stimulation, but the lethal dose is unclear, estimated to be 150–200 mg/kg in children and adults and higher in neonates.

Clinical Presentation
Most patients with caffeine ingestions will display mild CNS stimulant effects. At a sufficient dose, however, there may be nausea, vomiting, headache, anxiety, agitation, insomnia, tremor and irritability, hallucinations, and seizures. Patients may also have symptoms similar to other adrenergic ingestants, including hypokalemia, hyperglycemia, and metabolic acidosis. Caffeine also has both positive inotropic and chronotropic effects. In an overdose, it can cause SVT, VPCs, ventricular tachycardia, and hypertension. Beta-2-mediated vasodilation may result in hypotension.

Diagnosis

Caffeine levels are not commonly available except in hospitals where neonates are routinely treated with caffeine for apnea.

ED Management

Provide supportive care as needed and continuously monitor the heart rate and rhythm. Give activated charcoal (1 g/kg PO) if there are active bowel sounds. Repeat-dose activated charcoal may enhance elimination. If the patient is vomiting, give an antiemetic such as ondansetron (0.1–0.5 mg/kg/dose IV, 4 mg maximum). SVT may be refractory to adenosine (or its effect may be transient), thus treat hypertension and tachydysrhythmias with IV propranolol or esmolol. Treat hypotension with multiple IV NS boluses and, if necessary, a pure alpha-agonist such as phenylephrine (5–20 mcg/kg/dose q 10–15 min PRN; 5 mg maximum cumulative dose). Give a benzodiazepine (diazepam 0.1–0.3 mg/kg/dose q 15–30 min, <5 years 5 mg maximum; ≥5 years, 10 mg maximum) for agitation, seizures, and muscle fasciculations. Seriously intoxicated patients may require hemodialysis.

Indications for Admission

- Coma, seizures, tachydysrhythmias
- Suicide attempt or gesture without psychiatric clearance and appropriate follow-up arranged

Bibliography

Beauchamp GA, Johnson AR, Crouch BI, et al. A retrospective study of clinical effects of powdered caffeine exposures reported to three US poison control centers. *J Med Toxicol.* 2016;**12**(3):295–300.

Jabbar SB, Hanly MG. Fatal caffeine overdose: a case report and review of literature. *Am J Forensic Med Pathol.* 2013;**34**(4):321–324.

Seifert SM, Schaechter JL, Hershorin ER, Lipshultz SE. Health effects of energy drinks on children, adolescents, and young adults. *Pediatrics.* 2011;**127**(3):511–528.

Calcium Channel Blockers

Calcium channel blocking (CCB) drugs are widely used for the treatment of angina, hypertension, and supraventricular cardiac arrhythmias. The dihydropyridines (nifedipine, amlodipine, felodipine, nicardipine, isradipine) primarily affect peripheral blood vessels, whereas the non-dihydropyridines (verapamil, diltiazem) act on the heart. Several CCBs are available in sustained-release formulations (Calan SR, Covera HS, Cardizem CD, Carizem SR, Cartia XT, Adalat CC, Procardia XL). More recently, preparations combined with angiotensin-converting enzyme inhibitors (Lexxel, Lotrel, Tarka) or with angiotensin II receptor antagonists (Exforge) have been marketed. These may cause more profound hypotension. Another recent combination is with an HMG-CoA reductase agent or statin (Caduet).

Clinical Presentation

As little as one tablet can be potentially life-threatening to a small child. Toxicity reflects the distribution of calcium channels in the cardiovascular system, including the sinus and atrioventricular nodes, vascular smooth muscle, and myocardium. Overdose may cause sinus bradycardia, AV block, and hypotension. Variable degrees of CNS depression, ranging from drowsiness to coma, may occur. Metabolic effects include hyperglycemia and lactic acidosis. Adynamic ileus can manifest as hypoactive bowel sounds. Effects may be delayed 6–8 hours following ingestion of a sustained-release preparation, but have occurred as late as 12–18 hours.

Diagnosis
Consider a calcium channel blocker overdose in a patient presenting with hypotension, bradycardia, syncope, or cardiogenic shock.

ED Management
Initiate supportive care and administer a dose of activated charcoal if under two hours have elapsed since the ingestion. Gastrointestinal decontamination is paramount and orogastric lavage may alter the outcome in a life-threatening ingestion presenting within the first hour. If a sustained-release preparation was ingested, give multiple doses of activated charcoal or initiate whole-bowel irrigation. Continuously monitor the ECG and blood pressure, and obtain blood for electrolytes, glucose, CBC, ABG, and for a patient with an unknown toxic bradycardia, a digoxin level.

If the patient has bradycardia or hypotension, initiate treatment immediately as these symptoms are often refractory to therapy and are an ominous sign. Obtain large-bore IV access and give 20 mL/kg bolus of isotonic fluid and atropine (0.02 mg/kg) for bradycardia. Glucagon (50 mcg/kg, adult dose 3–5 mg) and cardiac pacing have shown variable success. Administer calcium gluconate 10% (60 mg/kg, 3 g maximum) slowly IV through a peripheral or central venous line or calcium chloride 10% (20 mg/kg), slowly IV, through a central venous line. If there is no response, start a high-dose dopamine or norepinephrine infusion (pp. 23–25). The combination of high-dose insulin and glucose can improve cardiac function (regular insulin 1 unit/kg bolus with 0.5 g/kg of D_{25}, followed by an infusion of insulin 0.5–1 units/kg/h with 1 g/kg/h glucose). Consult with a toxicologist and pediatric cardiologist and arrange pediatric intensive care unit admission.

Indications for Admission
- Symptomatic calcium channel blocker ingestion (hypotension, bradyarrhythmias, altered mental status)
- History of calcium channel blocker overdose, unless the patient remains asymptomatic for six hours after the ingestion
- History of sustained-release calcium channel blocker overdose
- Suicide attempt or gesture without psychiatric clearance and appropriate follow-up arranged

Bibliography
Graudins A, Lee HM, Druda D. Calcium channel antagonist and beta-blocker overdose: antidotes and adjunct therapies. *Br J Clin Pharmacol.* 2016;**81**(3):453–461.

Palatnick W, Jelic T. Emergency department management of calcium-channel blocker, beta blocker, and digoxin toxicity. *Emerg Med Pract.* 2014;**16**(2):1–19.

Shenoy S, Lankala S, Adigopula S. Management of calcium channel blocker overdoses. *J Hosp Med.* 2014;9(10):663–668.

St-Onge M, Dubé PA, Gosselin S, et al. Treatment for calcium channel blocker poisoning: a systematic review. *Clin Toxicol (Phila).* 2014; 52:926–944.

Carbon Monoxide

Carbon monoxide (CO) is a colorless, odorless, tasteless gas found in exhaust from combustion engines (automobiles, space heaters, portable generators), and in smoke from fires or tobacco products. CO competitively binds to hemoglobin 250 times more avidly than oxygen, thereby shifting the oxygen/hemoglobin dissociation curve to the left. This effect impairs delivery of oxygen to peripheral tissues and puts ischemic stress on the heart and CNS. In addition, carbon monoxide binds to myoglobin (potentiating myocardial ischemia), and mitochondrial cytochrome oxidase, and causes glutamate release and lipid peroxidation in the central nervous system.

Clinical Presentation

Symptoms of carbon monoxide intoxication are nonspecific and often misdiagnosed. Suspect CO if multiple patients from the same environment or family are displaying similar symptoms. At low levels, headache, nausea, vomiting, and weakness occur. At higher CO levels, patients develop tachycardia, respiratory distress, lethargy, coma, seizures, and death. Severely CO poisoned patients may present with cherry-red colored skin (and blood) and/or cutaneous bullae.

Diagnosis

Obtain a serum carboxyhemoglobin (COHb) level from a venous blood gas (arterial puncture is not necessary). Pulse co-oximetry does not provide an accurate COHb level. If symptoms are severe, obtain serum electrolytes, CBC, urine or serum βhCG, and an ECG. Serum levels correlate poorly with symptoms, but may indicate a significant exposure and therefore guide therapy. Ascertain the interval between the end of the exposure and when the level is obtained. If the interval is long (more than four hours) or the patient was treated with oxygen before arrival in the ED, he or she may be more severely affected than the COHb level indicates. Normal COHb level ranges from 1% to 3% in nonsmokers from catabolism of hemoglobin and exogenous exposure. Cigarette smokers may have levels as high as 10–15%. Blood samples from neonates can have falsely higher COHb levels (up to 8%) because fetal hemoglobin interferes with spectroscopy, which reads the percentage of hemoglobin saturated with CO.

ED Management

As increasing the partial pressure of inspired oxygen significantly reduces the half-life of CO, give all patients 100% oxygen via a tight-fitting nonrebreathing mask upon arrival in the ED while awaiting the COHb level. Indications for hyperbaric oxygen therapy (HBO) (pp. 221–224) include a history of unconsciousness after exposure to CO regardless of COHb level, a history of or continued mental status change or other neurologic deficit, cardiac dysfunction or ischemia, a COHb level >25% regardless of symptoms, and pregnancy with a history of CO exposure (regardless of COHb level). The only absolute contraindication to HBO is an untreated pneumothorax.

Follow-up

- Patient treated for CO poisoning: next day

Indications for Admission

- Initial COHb >25%
- Any patient requiring treatment for CO poisoning who has not returned to baseline status

Bibliography

Bleecker ML. Carbon monoxide intoxication. *Handb Clin Neurol.* 2015;**131**:191–203.

Cho CH, Chiu NC, Ho CS, Peng CC. Carbon monoxide poisoning in children. *Pediatr Neonatol.* 2008;**49**:121–125.

Macnow TE, Waltzman ML. Carbon monoxide poisoning in children: diagnosis and management in the emergency department. *Pediatr Emerg Med Pract.* 2016;**13**(9):1–24.

Tomaszewski C: Carbon monoxide. In Hoffman RS, Howland MA, Lewin NA, Nelson LS, Goldfrank LR (eds.) *Goldfrank's Toxicologic Emergencies* (10th edn.). New York: McGraw-Hill Education, 2015; 1581–1593.

Weaver LK. Carbon monoxide poisoning. *N Engl J Med.* 2009;**360**:1217–1225.

Caustics

Most caustic ingestions involve alkalis, such as lye, ammonia, oven or drain cleaners, Clinitest tablets, and dishwasher detergents. Non-industrial strength household bleach (5% sodium hypochlorite) is not a strong caustic and does not cause significant injury. Some ingestions involve acids such as toilet bowl and drain cleaners, battery fluid, metal cleaners, de-greasers, and industrial acids. Esophageal injury occurs in approximately 10% of cases of acid ingestion, usually in association with serious gastric damage.

Alkalis frequently cause oropharyngeal injury and serious esophageal ulcerations due to liquefaction necrosis on contact, while acids cause a coagulation necrosis, typically affecting both the esophagus and the stomach. Consequences include esophageal perforation with mediastinitis, gastro–intestinal bleeding, gastric ulceration, and strictures. Liquid products are more likely than powdered caustics to cause esophageal and stomach burns with minimal oral burns.

Clinical Presentation

Oropharyngeal pain and drooling are common, and vomiting occasionally occurs. Findings may also include perioral burns, vomiting, stridor, and dyspnea. Chest pain, abdominal pain, hematemesis, or shock suggest a perforation and mediastinitis

Diagnosis

The presence (or absence) of oropharyngeal burns does not correlate with esophageal injury, but a serious esophageal injury after an alkali ingestion is unlikely in the absence of stridor, vomiting, drooling, or other serious signs.

ED Management

A patient with vomiting, drooling, or stridor is at risk for airway compromise and serious esophageal injury. For a symptomatic patient, obtain IV access, send blood for CBC, type and cross-match, and obtain a chest x-ray (mediastinal widening indicates mediastinitis). Make the patient NPO, and begin maintenance IV hydration. Obtain prompt visualization of the hypopharynx, vocal chords, and epiglottis, and intubate patients with evidence of burns or swelling. *Do not* induce emesis, insert a nasogastric tube, try to neutralize the caustic, or administer activated charcoal or steroids. A patient with a history of possible alkali ingestion, with or without oropharyngeal burns, but without vomiting, drooling, or stridor is at low risk of serious esophageal injury. If the chest x-ray is normal and the patient is comfortable and can drink readily, he or she can be sent home if telephone contact is possible. Arrange for immediate endoscopy if a patient who has ingested an acid is symptomatic or has oropharyngeal burns.

Indications for Admission

- History of alkali ingestion and vomiting, drooling, or stridor
- History of acid ingestion with oropharyngeal burns, abdominal pain, or other symptoms
- Symptoms of intestinal injury
- Suicide attempt or gesture without psychiatric clearance and appropriate follow-up arranged

Bibliography

Arevalo-Silva C, Eliashar R, Wohlgelernter J, Elidan J, Gross M. Ingestion of caustic substances: a 15 year experience. *Laryngoscope.* 2006;**116**:1422–1426.

Shub MD. Therapy of caustic ingestion: new treatment considerations. *Curr Opin Pediatr.* 2015;**27** (5):609–613.

Uygun I. Caustic oesophagitis in children: prevalence, the corrosive agents involved, and management from primary care through to surgery. *Curr Opin Otolaryngol Head Neck Surg.* 2015;**23**(6):423–432.

Valdez AL, Casavant MJ, Spiller HA, et al. Pediatric exposure to laundry detergent pods. *Pediatrics.* 2014;**134**:1127–1135.

Wightman RS, Read KB, Hoffman RS. Evidence-based management of caustic exposures in the emergency department. *Emerg Med Pract.* 2016;**18**(5):1–17.

Cholinergics

Cholinergic toxicity may be the result of a variety of agents, most notably insecticides and gases used in bioterrorism, but also products containing nicotine and plants such as hemlock. Poisoning from organophosphate insecticides and bioterror agents is life-threatening, and specific life-saving antidotal therapy is available.

Organophosphate (malathion, parathion) and carbamate (aldi–carb, propoxur) insecticides block acetylcholinesterase. The subsequent elevation of acetylcholine in the CNS and peripheral nervous system is responsible for the signs and symptoms. Toxicity is usually associated with products formulated for outdoor, industrial, or bioterror settings; household "bug bombs" rarely cause significant toxicity as they contain pyrethrins/pyrethroids, which do not affect cholinesterase. Plant alkaloid and nicotine excess cause symptomatology via nicotinic cholinergic receptor stimulation.

Clinical Presentation and Diagnosis
Carbamates and organophosphates produce a clinical state of cholinergic excess. Findings include the muscarinic symptoms of salivation, lacrimation, bronchorrhea, bronchospasm, diaphoresis, diarrhea, and miosis, and the typical pesticide odor may be apparent. A useful mnemonic is DUMBELS: Diarrhea, Urination, Miosis, Bronchorrhea, Bronchospasm, Bradycardia, Emesis, Lacrimation, and Salivation.

Nicotinic signs and symptoms such as muscle fasciculations, weakness, and paralysis are present, as are CNS effects such as confusion, seizures, and coma. Due to the competing muscarinic and nicotinic effects, heart rate may be increased or decreased, and pupils may be miotic or mydriatic. Death is usually due to respiratory failure because of respiratory muscle paralysis, increased pulmonary secretions, and bronchoconstriction. Occasionally the patient may develop hydrocarbon aspiration pneumonitis, as some pesticides are commonly formulated in hydrocarbon suspensions.

ED Management
For a cutaneous exposure, remove and double-bag all clothing, and thoroughly wash the patient with soap and water. The ED staff must protect themselves by wearing impervious gloves and aprons made with butyl rubber, as most hospital gloves do not prevent the penetration of these agents.

Provide supportive care, and secure a stable airway. Start an IV and attach an ECG and pulse oximeter. Meticulous respiratory support is critical, and intubation and ventilation are often required.

High-dose atropine therapy is the antidote for cholinergic toxicity. Titrate the dose against the patient's response, which varies with the specific exposure. The endpoint is clear lungs and the reversal of the muscarinic toxic syndrome. Start with 0.02 mg/kg (0.5 mg IV for a toddler; 1–2 mg IV for an adolescent) and double the dose q 5 min until improvement has begun. A severely affected patient may require a constant atropine infusion in the ICU setting.

Pralidoxime is an adjunctive antidote for organophosphate poisonings and is indicated when multiple doses of atropine are required or for nicotinic symptoms, especially muscle weakness. Use pralidoxime in conjunction with atropine, and never as a sole therapeutic agent. The IV bolus dose is 25–50 mg/kg IV for a child and 1–2 g for an adolescent. Pralidoxime and atropine are also packaged together in autoinjector kits, carried by first responders. The autoinjectors contain 600 mg pralidoxime and 2 mg atropine. The dose is one kit for children 3–7 years of age, two kits for 8–14-year-olds, and three kits for patients 15 years and older.

Indications for Admission
- Presence of any cholinergic clinical findings
- Suicide attempt or gesture without psychiatric clearance and appropriate follow-up arranged

Bibliography
Eddleston M, Chowdhury FR. Pharmacological treatment of organophosphorus insecticide poisoning: the old and the (possible) new. *Br J Clin Pharmacol*. 2016;**81**(3):462–470.

Eddleston M, Clark RF. Insecticides: organic phosphorus compounds and carbamates. In Hoffman RS, Howland MA, Lewin NA, Nelson LS, Goldfrank LR (eds.) *Goldfrank's Toxicologic Emergencies* (10th edn.). New York: McGraw-Hill, 2015; 1409–1424.

King AM, Aaron CK. Organophosphate and carbamate poisoning. *Emerg Med Clin North Am.* 2015;**33**(1):133–151.

Vale A, Lotti M. Organophosphorus and carbamate insecticide poisoning. *Handb Clin Neurol.* 2015;**131**:149–168.

Clonidine

Clonidine is both a peripheral and a central alpha-agonist. It causes central inhibition of sympathetic output and, to a lesser extent, peripheral vasoconstriction. Clonidine is often used as an antihypertensive, but it is frequently prescribed for children with significant behavior disorders, including ADHD. Small children are extremely sensitive to clonidine and toxicity has been reported after ingestion of a single tablet. It is also available as transdermal patches, which present a unique danger for toddlers, as a used patch when ingested can contain the equivalent of more than 50 tablets.

Clinical Presentation and Diagnosis

A patient may present with symptoms mimicking the classic opiate triad of *coma, respiratory depression, and miosis.* Onset of symptoms can occur shortly after ingestion. Occasionally, a young child is asymptomatic at presentation and suddenly develops apnea. Hypotension is usual, but transient hypertension is occasionally seen early in the course. Hypothermia and bradycardia also occur frequently. There are no specific diagnostic findings or rapidly available tests.

ED Management

Institute supportive care and administer activated charcoal within two hours of ingestion. Treat clinically significant bradycardia with atropine (0.02 mg/kg). Hypertension is usually transient and followed by hypotension, so do *not* give antihypertensive therapy. Treat hypotension with a fluid challenge of 20 mL/kg of isotonic crystalloid. If this fails, administer a vasopressor such as dopamine, and titrate against the patient's response. Naloxone (0.1 mg/kg) is variably effective, but it may prevent the need for endotracheal intubation in a patient with respiratory depression. Use a maximum dose of 10 mg before considering it ineffective.

Monitor asymptomatic patients with known or suspected clonidine ingestion for four hours in the ED prior to discharge.

Indications for Admission

- Coma, respiratory depression, or altered vital signs
- Suicide attempt or gesture without psychiatric clearance and appropriate follow-up arranged

Bibliography

Ahmad SA, Scolnik D, Snehal V, Glatstein M. Use of naloxone for clonidine intoxication in the pediatric age group: case report and review of the literature. *Am J Ther.* 2015;**22**(1):e14–e16.

Spiller HA, Hays HL, Aleguas A Jr. Overdose of drugs for attention-deficit hyperactivity disorder: clinical presentation, mechanisms of toxicity, and management. *CNS Drugs.* 2013;27(7):531–543.

Wang GS, Le Lait MC, Heard K. Unintentional pediatric exposures to central alpha-2 agonists reported to the National Poison Data System. *J Pediatr.* 2014;164(1):149–152.

Cough and Cold Medications

Ingestion of cold preparations is common among children because the products are in most households and are available in flavored elixirs. Cold medicines may include any combination of the following: antihistamines, sympathomimetics, acetaminophen, ibuprofen, aspirin, dextromethorphan, and guaifenesin. Resultant symptoms depend on the specific contents of the ingested product. Adolescents seeking the euphoric effects of dextromethorphan and anticholinergics may knowingly ingest cold preparations.

Clinical Presentation

Antihistamines such as diphenhydramine, chlorpheniramine, brompheniramine, and triprolidine produce sedation and anticholinergic effects, including tachycardia, dilated unreactive pupils, warm, dry and red skin, decreased bowel sounds, and urinary retention. In contrast, newer "non-sedating" antihistamines such as loratadine and cetirizine cause almost no toxicity.

Sympathomimetics include pseudoephedrine and phenylephrine. Phenylephrine is a selective α-agonist and may cause severe hypertension. Pseudoephedrine (an isomer of ephedrine) is an α- and β-agonist and causes a sympathomimetic toxidrome with tachycardia, hypertension, dilated but reactive pupils, and diaphoresis. Of note, pseudoephedrine-containing products are often sought in large quantities for the illicit synthesis of methamphetamine.

Diagnosis

Diagnosis is made by history. Suspect dextromethorphan ingestion in a patient with mild mental status changes and hallucinations. Additionally, dextromethorphan may produce a false-positive result on PCP immunoassays.

ED Management

Severe toxicity is rare. Administer activated charcoal to a patient arriving within two hours of ingestion, or longer if the preparation contains an anticholinergic agent (delays stomach emptying). While sinus tachycardia may result from either anticholinergic or sympathomimetic mechanisms, generally no therapy is needed. Treat severe hypertension associated with stimulants with phentolamine (0.05–0.1 mg/kg IV, repeat q 10 min as needed; 5 mg/dose maximum). Psychomotor agitation may be alleviated with benzodiazepines or haloperidol. See pp. 457–458 for the use of physostigmine to reverse anticholinergic symptoms.

Always consider occult acetaminophen poisoning, as many preparations contain this drug. Obtain an acetaminophen level when the preparation is unknown or to confirm and estimate an ingestion if the timing is known.

Give a patient with suspected dextromethorphan ingestion and significant respiratory depression intravenous naloxone. Start with 0.1 mg/kg (initial dose 2.0 mg maximum), but larger dosages may be required.

Indications for Admission

- Severe symptoms (hypotension, seizure, sedation)
- Suicide attempt or gesture without psychiatric clearance and appropriate follow-up arranged

Bibliography

Isbister GK, Prior F, Kilham HA. Restricting cough and cold medicines in children. *J Paediatr Child Health*. 2012;**48**(2):91–98.

Paul IM, Reynolds KM, Kauffman RE, et al. Adverse events associated with pediatric exposures to dextromethorphan. *Clin Toxicol (Phila)*. 2017;**55**(1):25–32.

Digoxin and Cardiac Glycosides

Ingestion of digoxin in children is uncommon and generally occurs when a patient has access to an adult relative's medications. Digoxin inhibits the function of the sodium–potassium–ATPase pump, resulting in hyperkalemia and increased intracellular calcium. The minimum toxic dose is about 0.1 mg/kg. Children are more resistant to the effects of digoxin than adults, so the lethal dose may be up to 20–50 times the daily maintenance dose. Cardiac glycosides, and related substances, are also found in several plants (rhododendron, foxglove, oleander, lily of the valley, and red squill) and toad venom (bufotoxin), but ingestion of these is very rare.

Clinical Presentation

Acute ingestion almost always results in nausea and vomiting. Headache, weakness, and confusion may occur, and seizures are rare. Severe ingestions may lead to hyperkalemia, bradycardia, hypotension, and dysrhythmias. Digoxin causes an increase in automaticity and AV blockade, which leads to bradycardia, and ventricular escape rhythms. Cardiac toxicity may be more profound in the setting of hypokalemia, hypercalcemia, or hypomagnesemia.

Diagnosis

Suspect digoxin overdose when either a previously well patient who lives with someone maintained on digoxin presents with an arrhythmia or a patient already taking digoxin presents with nausea, vomiting, or abdominal pain, and a new arrhythmia, hyperkalemia, hypotension, or CNS depression.

ED Management

Consult a toxicologist for all cases of digoxin exposure. Give activated charcoal if less than two hours have elapsed since ingestion and obtain blood for electrolytes, calcium, and magnesium. Wait until six hours post-ingestion to obtain a digoxin level in order to avoid overtreating a predistribution level, which may be high but nontoxic. Assess the ECG for arrhythmias or a prolonged PR interval, and attach a cardiac monitor to follow changes in the rhythm. The classic digoxin-induced dysrhythmias are paroxysmal atrial tachycardia with block or ventricular bigeminy. Other common digoxin dysrhythmias are ventricular ectopy, AV blocks, and sinus bradycardia.

Treat clinically significant bradycardia with atropine, 0.02 mg/kg IV (minimum dose 0.1 mg, maximum 0.5 mg). Avoid pacemaker placement, if possible, because of an increased risk of ventricular arrhythmias. Avoid calcium products in treating hyperkalemia secondary to digoxin toxicity because of concern for a theoretical increase in cardiotoxicity.

A life-threatening arrhythmia or a potassium concentration >5 mEq/L are indications for Fab antibody fragments (Digibind/DigiFab). Acute ingestion of 4 mg in a child, a serum digoxin concentration >15 ng/mL at any time, or >10 ng/mL six hours post-ingestion, are other indications for treatment with Fab antibody fragments. Be cautious treating a patient who uses digoxin therapeutically, as eliminating the therapeutic effect of the drug by treating only mild elevations of the digoxin level may not be warranted. The dose of Fab antibody fragments is:

$$\text{of vials of Fab} = \text{mg ingested} \times 1.6$$

However, if the serum level is known, the dose is:

$$\text{of vials of Fab} = (\text{digoxin level in ng/mL} \times \text{weight in kg})/100$$

If neither the dose nor the level is known, give ten vials empirically. If both are known, treat the level.

Indications for Admission

- Ingestion of >0.1 mg/kg
- New arrhythmia, visual disturbance, headache, CNS depression, hypotension
- Suicide attempt or gesture without psychiatric clearance and appropriate follow-up arranged

Bibliography

Chan BS, Buckley NA. Digoxin-specific antibody fragments in the treatment of digoxin toxicity. *Clin Toxicol (Phila)*. 2014;**52**(8):824–836.

Moffett BS, Garner A, Zapata T, et al. Serum digoxin concentrations and clinical signs and symptoms of digoxin toxicity in the paediatric population. *Cardiol Young*. 2016;**26**(3):493–498.

Palatnick W, Jelic T. Emergency department management of calcium-channel blocker, beta blocker, and digoxin toxicity. *Emerg Med Pract*. 2014;**16**(2):1–19.

Pincus M. Management of digoxin toxicity. *Aust Prescr*. 2016;**39**(1):18–20.

Drugs of Abuse

Adolescents frequently overdose on drugs of abuse such as cocaine, marijuana, amphetamines, and heroin. In addition, teenagers use a unique group of drugs that are quite rare in other age groups, such as 3,4-methylenedioxymethamphetamine (MDMA, "Ecstasy," "Molly"), diphenhydramine, gamma-hydroxybutyrate (GHB), ketamine, and cold medicines. Additionally, synthetic cannabinoids (K2, Spice), bath salts, and synthetic opioids have emerged as consequential drugs of abuse. Suicidal ideation and attempt are always a concern, so that appropriate counseling and psychiatric evaluation are necessary.

Clinical Presentation

Many adolescents who present with intoxication have taken multiple substances, and thus may not exhibit a clear toxidrome. Furthermore, drugs of abuse may be adulterated with unknown substances, resulting in a mixed, or more severe, presentation.

Sedatives/Hypnotics

Sedatives/hypnotics include the benzodiazepines, barbiturates, chloral hydrate, and GHB. These agents cause CNS depression, nystagmus, ataxia, hypotension, and possible respiratory depression. Pupils are generally normal or small and vital signs often remain normal. These drugs may be used to facilitate sexual assault (commonly GHB or flunitrazepam/Rohypnol/roofies).

CNS Stimulants

CNS stimulants include cocaine, amphetamines, phenylephrine, pseudoephedrine, and ephedrine. They are commonly found in weight loss medications, cold preparations, and herbal products (Ma Huang). These produce tachycardia, hypertension, hyperthermia, dilated but reactive pupils, diaphoresis, and agitated delirium (agitation, confusion, and paranoia). Seizures, coma, arrhythmias, and myocardial infarction may occur in severe intoxications.

Cannabis

Cannabis, or marijuana, is one of the most commonly abused drugs in the United States. Most commonly smoked in "joints" or cigarettes, marijuana causes euphoria, conjunctival injection, orthostatic hypotension, xerostomia, and tachycardia. Uncommonly, patients may experience palpitations, anxiety, paranoia, and hallucinations.

Synthetic Cannabinoids and Bath Salts

Synthetic cannabinoids and bath salts can be relatively easily obtained at small retail shops or over the internet. Both classes of drugs are referred to by various common names, can be consumed by various routes, and cause unpredictable effects depending on the type and amount of synthetic compound. Unlike cannabis use, patients who take synthetic cannabinoids may present either in severe agitation with stimulant effects, or in deep sedation. Patients who have ingested bath salts will usually present with hallucinogenic/psychotic and stimulant effects, similar to PCP.

Opioids

Opioids include heroin, morphine, codeine, meperidine, hydromorphone, fentanyl, oxycodone, hydrocodone, methadone, and buprenorphine. New synthetic opioids have emerged as contaminants/adulterants in conventional opioids, or as new, novel substances of abuse. Small doses of these potent synthetics may lead to severe intoxication. Opioids bind to specific opiate receptors in the CNS and cause euphoria, sedation, miosis, respiratory depression, and bradycardia. Severe intoxication may lead to coma, respiratory depression, pulmonary edema, and aspiration.

Hallucinogens

Hallucinogens include lysergic acid diethylamide (LSD), phencyclidine (PCP), MDMA, mescaline (peyote), and psilocybin (hallucinogenic mushrooms or "shrooms"). Several other methamphetamine derivatives are commonly abused by teenagers, such as "Eve," MDA, and PMA. These products bind to central serotonin and dopamine receptors and produce hallucinations and sympathomimetic effects. Patients seek medical care when unusual behavior is noted or when the patient complains of a "bad trip." PCP may cause aggressive behavior as well as seizures. MDMA leads to destruction of serotoninergic neurons and may result in severe depression and memory loss for weeks or permanently. MDMA users may also develop a severe dilutional hyponatremia secondary to an intense thirst along with inappropriate ADH secretion.

Diagnosis

The diagnosis is often made through information obtained from friends, family members, and the patient. If this is not possible or not helpful, ask the paramedics if there was drug paraphernalia at the scene, as patients from a rave party or club are more likely to ingest MDMA, GHB, ketamine, or cold preparations. Urine drug screens are unlikely to affect management, and are generally unhelpful due to poor sensitivities and specificities.

A thorough physical examination will provide enough information to direct therapy and disposition. The patient must be fully undressed and the clothes checked for drugs or paraphernalia. Note the presence of "track marks," or fresh needlesticks. Lethargy implies a CNS depressant or an opioid, whereas agitation suggests a CNS stimulant. Large, reactive pupils and diaphoresis imply sympathomimetic drugs. Small pupils may be seen with sedatives/hypnotics, opioids, and PCP. Paranoia and tachycardia may be seen with hallucinogens.

ED Management

The priorities in severe intoxications are of the airway, breathing, and circulation, followed by treatment of grossly abnormal vital signs. Initially, treat hypertension with agitation from stimulants with benzodiazepines such as diazepam (0.1–0.3 mg/kg/dose), but use phentolamine (0.02–0.1 mg/kg/dose, maximum 5 mg) or nitroprusside (continuous IV, start with 0.3–0.5 mcg/kg/min; titrate to effect) for hypertensive urgencies. Do not use beta-blockers in suspected cocaine intoxication as they may result in unopposed alpha-adrenergic-mediated hypertension.

Treat severe hyperthermia (>40 °C, 104 °F.) with aggressive cooling measures (pp. 219–221) until the core temperature is <38.3 °C (101 °F). Drug-related hyperthermia, in contrast to environmental hyperthermia, can continue in the hospital and must be treated immediately. Hyperthermia may lead to rhabdomyolysis, myoglobinuria, renal failure, and death.

If the patient has respiratory depression or is in coma, obtain a bedside glucose evaluation and give naloxone, preferably IV (up to 0.1 mg/kg, maximum 2.0 mg), either empirically, or to correct the coma and respiratory depression seen in opioid toxicity. If there is no response within 1–2 minutes, give a second dose. A positive response may last only 30 minutes, so repeated doses or a continuous IV infusion at two-thirds the effective dose infused every hour are indicated if resedation occurs. For example, if a total of 0.6 mg was required to correct the initial respiratory depression, give the patient another bolus and start on an infusion of 0.4 mg/h. If habitual use is suspected in an adolescent, give an initial dose of 0.04 mg, increasing to 0.4 mg, and then to 2 mg, so as not to precipitate acute withdrawal.

Although flumazenil is a GABA antagonist, it is not recommended in the overdose of benzodiazepines because it may induce seizures in patients who co-ingest epileptogenic medications or are chronic benzodiazepine abusers. Safer therapy is careful observation and endotracheal intubation, if necessary. Infants and children are less likely to be habituated to benzodiazepines, and flumazenil may be used more safely in the setting of a confirmed benzodiazepine overdose in this population.

Treat seizures with lorazepam (0.05–0.1 mg/kg IV slow IV, 4 mg maximum) or diazepam (0.1–0.3 mg/kg IV slow IV, 10 mg maximum). If necessary, sedate the agitated patient with benzodiazepines (diazepam, lorazepam, or midazolam, pp. 717–720). Haloperidol (5 mg IM) is a useful adjunct in PCP ingestions.

Treat serotonin syndrome (mydriasis, hypertension, psychomotor agitation, altered mental status) secondary to MDMA with cyproheptidine when supportive care fails (see Antidepressants, pp. 458–460).

Indications for Admission
- Continued CNS or respiratory depression
- Ventricular arrhythmia
- Serotonin syndrome
- Suspected opioid or CNS depressant withdrawal
- Suicide attempt or gesture without psychiatric clearance and appropriate follow-up arranged

Bibliography

Huestis MA, Tyndale RF. Designer drugs 2.0. *Clin Pharmacol Ther.* 2017;**101**(2):152–157.

Nelson ME, Bryant SM, Aks SE. Emerging drugs of abuse. *Emerg Med Clin North Am.* 2014;**32**:1–28.

Richards JR, Garber D, Laurin EG, et al. Treatment of cocaine cardiovascular toxicity: a systematic review. *Clin Toxicol (Phila).* 2016;**54**(5):345–364.

Tenenbein M. Do you really need that emergency drug screen? *Clin Toxicol (Phila).* 2009;**47**:286–291.

Ethanol

Ethanol is a selective CNS depressant at low doses and a general depressant at higher doses. It is probably the most frequently abused drug and is the most common co-ingestant in suicide attempts. Ethanol is found in alcoholic beverages, as well as colognes, after-shave, food flavorings (vanilla extract), mouthwash, hand sanitizers, medicinal preparations, and many other products. A standard alcoholic beverage (1 oz of 100 proof liquor, 4 oz glass of wine, 10 oz bottle of beer) will generally result in an ethanol level of about 40 mg/dL in a patient weighing 70 kg.

Clinical Presentation

Mild intoxication, which occurs at levels of 50 mg/dL, causes euphoria, ataxia, nystagmus, nausea, emotional lability, and impaired judgment. Moderately intoxicated patients may have aggressive behavior, vomiting, and slurred speech. With severe intoxication (serum level ≥250 mg/dL), patients may develop respiratory depression, aspiration, hypotension, hypothermia, and coma. Young children are at high risk of hypoglycemia with resultant seizures.

Diagnosis

The diagnosis is usually made by history. The presence or absence of an ethanol odor is not indicative of whether a person recently consumed ethanol or is intoxicated. Clinical signs of intoxication will be more obvious in adolescents but may be altered by co-ingestions. Infants and children with ethanol intoxication may present with hypoglycemia, repeated emesis, and altered mental status.

Obtain an ethanol level if alcohol toxicity is suspected. Ethanol levels usually correlate with intoxication, although experienced drinkers can tolerate higher levels of ethanol without symptoms. An anion gap acidosis, as well as an osmolar gap, may be present.

Ethanol withdrawal may present within six hours of abstinence, but delirium tremens (DT) rarely occurs before 48–96 hours. Typical symptoms include tremors, hypertension, tachycardia, and psychomotor agitation. Progression to visual auditory and tactile hallucinations may ensue until frank psychosis, or DT, presents. Alcohol withdrawal seizures may take place during this continuum.

ED Management

Management of the intoxicated patient depends on the severity of intoxication. If there is CNS depression, protect the airway (if necessary), obtain IV access, obtain a CBC, electrolytes, ethanol level, and fingerstick glucose, and give a dextrose-containing fluid. Gastric decontamination is generally ineffective.

A patient who is mildly intoxicated requires an ethanol level for confirmation, a careful physical examination to rule-out organic causes of confusion (such as head injury), and observation, with frequent reassessments, until the mental status has returned to baseline. The mental status of an intoxicated patient gradually and consistently improves. A CT scan of the head is indicated, however, if the mental status does not improve, the ethanol level is inconsistent with the mental status, there are signs of head trauma, or asymmetry of the EOMs or pupillary response or motor responses. An intoxicated patient is at higher risk for risky behavior and falls, so mental status changes that are attributed to alcohol may actually represent intracranial pathology. Observation may be performed at home if the parents are reliable and the patient is alert and ambulatory.

Pediatric patients rarely chronically abuse alcohol. If there is a suspicion that the patient is withdrawing from ethanol, give thiamine 100 mg, folate 1 mg, and magnesium 2 mg IV in addition to the glucose-containing IV fluid. Treat associated agitation and tachycardia with lorazepam (0.05 mg, 4 mg maximum) or diazepam (0.1 mg/kg PO, 10 mg maximum). Also, arrange for psychiatric consultation.

Indications for Admission

- Intoxicated preadolescent with an unstable home environment
- Severe intoxication (persistent coma, altered mental status, alcohol level >250 mg/dL)
- Suicide attempt or gesture without psychiatric clearance and appropriate follow-up arranged

Bibliography

Minera G, Robinson E. Accidental acute alcohol intoxication in infants: review and case report. *J Emerg Med.* 2014;**47**(5):524–526.

Rayar P, Ratnapalan S. Pediatric ingestions of house hold products containing ethanol: a review. *Clin Pediatr (Phila).* 2013;**52**:203–209.

Yip L. Ethanol. In Hoffman RS, Howland MA, Lewin NA, Nelson LS, Goldfrank LR (eds.) *Goldfrank's Toxicologic Emergencies* (10th edn.). New York: McGraw-Hill, 2015; 1082–1093.

Foreign Body Ingestion

The frequency of button battery and mini-magnet ingestions is rising among younger children. Button batteries are used for watches, calculators, hearing aids, and some small electronic toys. Most ingestions have an uneventful course, although serious complications can occur if the battery lodges in the esophagus. In contrast, the ingestion of one magnet is usually harmless, but if a child swallows multiple magnets they may attract each other, increasing the risk of GI complications such as pressure necrosis, perforation, fistula formation, or intestinal obstruction.

Clinical Presentation

Most patients will present to the ED usually soon after the suspected or witnessed ingestion. The majority are asymptomatic, but if the magnet or battery is lodged in the esophagus, the child may have drooling, dysphagia, or substernal pain. Patients presenting late with GI complications of multiple-magnet ingestion may have abdominal pain, vomiting, fever, hematemesis, diarrhea, and hematochezia.

Diagnosis

The diagnosis of an ingested battery or magnet is made by obtaining a single AP radiograph of the neck, chest, and abdomen. If the foreign body is seen in the esophagus or airway, a lateral radiograph is also needed.

ED Management

Emergent endoscopic removal is required for any button battery lodged in the esophagus. However, spontaneous passage generally occurs if it has passed into the stomach. If the battery is <12 mm in diameter and the patient is asymptomatic, discharge the patient who can resume normal activity. Instruct the family to confirm passage by inspecting the stools. If the battery is >12 mm, there is an increased chance for lodgment in the GI tract. Repeat the radiograph in 1–2 weeks if the family cannot confirm passage in the stool. Specific instructions are available through the Button Battery Ingestion Hotline, which is operated by the National Capital Poison Center in Washington, DC at 202-625-3333 or www.poison.org.

If a patient swallows multiple magnets or a combination of button battery and magnets, endoscopy is also required. If the patient has evidence of GI obstruction or perforation, immediate surgical intervention is necessary.

Indications for Admission

- Evidence of intestinal obstruction, perforation
- Multiple mini-magnet ingestion
- Lodgment in esophagus

Bibliography

Hussain SZ, Bousvaros, A, Gilger M, et al. Management of ingested magnets in children. *J Pediatr Gastroenterol Nutr.* 2012;55(3):239–242.

Jayachandra S, Eslick GD. A systematic review of paediatric foreign body ingestion: presentation, complications, and management. *Int J Pediatr Otorhinolaryngol.* 2013;77(3):311–317.

Kramer RE, Lerner DG, Lin T, Manfredi M, et al. Management of ingested foreign bodies in children: a clinical report of the NASPGHAN Endoscopy Committee. *J Pediatr Gastroenterol Nutr.* 2015;**60**(4):562–574.

Litovitz T, Whitaker N, Clark L, White NC, Marsolek M. Emerging battery ingestion hazard: clinical implications. *Pediatrics.* 2010;**125**(6):1168–1177.

Wright CC, Closson FT. Updates in pediatric gastrointestinal foreign bodies. *Pediatr Clin North Am.* 2013;**60**(5):1221–1239.

Hydrocarbons

Hydrocarbons are organic compounds such as camphor, motor oil, gasoline, kerosene, mineral seal oil, pine oil, phenol, carbon tetrachloride, and naphthalene. The main toxicity of hydrocarbons is aspiration pneumonitis, which occurs most often from products with low viscosity, low surface tension, and high volatility (gasoline, lighter fluid, turpentine). The halogenated and aromatic hydrocarbons can have systemic toxicity.

Clinical Presentation

Two populations of pediatric patients are at highest risk for hydrocarbon exposures: small children who unintentionally ingest, and may aspirate, hydrocarbons, and adolescents who intentionally abuse inhalants. Most patients who ingest simple hydrocarbons are asymptomatic, although pulmonary aspiration may lead to chemical pneumonitis. These patients may present with acute pulmonary symptoms, including cough, tachypnea, hypoxia, and dyspnea, or the onset may be delayed for up to 4–6 hours.

Ingestion of, or vapor exposure to, complex hydrocarbons (halogenated, aromatic, substituted) can cause systemic symptoms including coma, seizures, and arrhythmias. For example, pine oil may produce severe CNS depression, camphor may cause seizures, and carbon tetrachloride may cause cardiac arrhythmias.

Diagnosis

Determine the type of hydrocarbon ingested. Have a family member return home and bring the container to the ED. Call the Poison Control Center or the manufacturer for assistance.

ED Management

In general, GI decontamination with gastric lavage or activated charcoal is not indicated in pediatric hydrocarbon ingestions if the hydrocarbon does not have significant systemic toxicity. The serious risk of aspiration chemical pneumonitis outweighs the potential benefits.

The type of hydrocarbon ingested is a useful determinant in predicting toxicity. Wood-derived hydrocarbons such as pine oil are absorbed by the GI tract and may cause pulmonary edema and CNS toxicity without aspiration. In contrast, do not attempt to remove petroleum-derived hydrocarbons, such as gasoline or kerosene, as they must be aspirated to cause toxicity, and therefore are best left in the GI tract.

Observe the patient for CNS depression, seizures, and respiratory complaints for 4–6 hours. If symptoms occur, admit the patient. Obtain a chest radiograph only if the patient develops respiratory symptoms; a baseline, empiric chest radiograph is not necessary for an asymptomatic patient. Do not use steroids or prophylactic antibiotics.

Inhalation or ingestion of hydrocarbons with systemic toxicity may lead to a sensitization of myocardial cells to catecholamines. Therefore, place all patients on a cardiac monitor and avoid catecholamines, such as epinephrine, if possible.

Indications for Admission
- Ingestion of hydrocarbons with significant systemic toxicity
- Pulmonary signs or symptoms
- Suicide attempt or gesture without psychiatric clearance and appropriate follow-up arranged

Bibliography
Beuhler MC, Gala PK, Wolfe HA, Meaney PA, Henretig FM. Laundry detergent "pod" ingestions: a case series and discussion of recent literature. *Pediatr Emerg Care*. 2013;**29**(6):743–747

Makrygianni EA, Palamidou F, Kaditis AG. Respiratory complications following hydrocarbon aspiration in children. *Pediatr Pulmonol*. 2016;**51**(6):560–569.

Niaz K, Bahadar H, Maqbool F, Abdollahi M. A review of environmental and occupational exposure to xylene and its health concerns. *EXCLI J*. 2015;**14**:1167–1186.

Tormoehlen LM, Tekulve KJ, Nañagas KA. Hydrocarbon toxicity: a review. *Clin Toxicol (Phila)*. 2014;**52**(5):479–489.

Iron

Iron is readily available for the treatment of anemia and in prenatal vitamins and multivitamins. Most adult iron formulations contain 60–90 mg of elemental iron per tablet and children's formulations generally contain 15 mg per tablet or 10–20 mg/mL. Ferrous gluconate is 12% elemental iron (32 mg Fe per 325 mg tablet), ferrous fumarate is 33% (100 mg Fe per 325 mg tablet), and ferrous sulfate is 20% (65 mg Fe per 325 mg tablet). Most chewable multivitamins have 10–18 mg of elemental iron per tablet.

The minimal toxic dose is 20 mg/kg of elemental iron. Ingestion of 20–60 mg/kg is associated with mild to moderate toxicity and >60 mg/kg causes severe toxicity.

Clinical Presentation

Iron toxicity results from both direct gastrointestinal injury and diffuse cellular toxicity; it presents in five stages. The initial stages are localized to the GI tract and the later stages include systemic toxicity. In the initial phase (first six hours), GI symptoms predominate, with vomiting, hematemesis, abdominal pain, diarrhea, and hematochezia. During the next few hours, there may be a period in which the GI symptoms abate; however, patients in this second stage generally have lethargy, tachycardia, and metabolic acidosis. During the third stage, at 6–24 hours after ingestion, the patient develops hypotension, hepatic failure, shock, seizures, coma, metabolic acidosis, coagulopathy, and hyperglycemia. The fourth stage occurs 2–5 days post-ingestion and is characterized by hepatic failure. Stage V is gastric outlet or intestinal stricture, which may occur 2–8 weeks after the ingestion.

Diagnosis

The diagnosis of iron overdose is easily overlooked if the history does not suggest the possibility of ingestion. A high index of suspicion must be maintained in young children presenting with blood in the vomit or stools or whose mother is taking prenatal vitamins. Older siblings of a newborn are at particularly high risk.

Clinically significant iron toxicity is possible if the history suggests that more than 20 mg/kg of elemental iron was ingested or the patient is symptomatic (abdominal pain, vomiting, or diarrhea). It is extremely uncommon for a child to develop iron toxicity in the absence of vomiting. Obtain a serum iron concentration at the expected peak, 4–6 hours after ingestion. The peak iron level predicts toxicity, but the total iron-binding capacity is not a reliable marker. A level <300 mcg/dL is nontoxic, 300–500 mcg/dL correlates with localized GI symptoms and possible systemic effects, and a level >500 mcg/dL correlates with severe toxicity

Elevation of the white blood cell count >15,000/mm^3 and glucose >150 mg/dL often occur in patients who are iron toxic, but normal results cannot be used to rule-out toxicity. Abdominal radiographs may help identify pills that are radiopaque; however, x-rays will be normal in a patient who ingested liquid or children's formulations.

ED Management

Calculate the amount of elemental iron ingested. Discharge a patient who has ingested <20 mg/kg of elemental iron and is asymptomatic. For all other patients, obtain an abdominal radiograph and serum iron level.

If a significant number of tablets are seen on the radiograph, decontaminate the gut by whole-bowel irrigation (WBI) with polyethylene glycol electrolyte lavage solution (COLYTE, GoLYTELY) using a nasogastric tube (pp. 451–452). Contraindications to WBI include an unprotected airway in a comatose patient, ileus, GI obstruction, perforation, or significant hemorrhage. Activated charcoal does not adsorb iron significantly and is recommended only if there is a significant co-ingestant.

Provide supportive care as indicated. Start an IV, and pay special attention to perfusion and acid–base status. Large amounts of fluid and bicarbonate are frequently required.

Obtain a serum iron level 4–6 hours after ingestion; if it is >500 mcg/dL, initiate deferoxamine therapy (15 mg/kg/h IV, 6 g/day maximum; start infusion at 5 mg/kg/h to prevent hypotension). Deferoxamine chelates free iron into a water-soluble complex, which is excreted in the urine and makes the urine a vin-rosé color. Other indications for deferoxamine therapy are shock, intractable vomiting, or severe acidosis. Correct intravascular volume deficits before instituting chelation therapy because deferoxamine in the presence of decreased renal blood flow can lead to acute renal failure. Continue deferoxamine until the patient appears well, the acidosis has improved, and the urine color has returned to normal. Deferoxamine side effects include hypotension, which can be minimized by starting the infusion at a slower rate, and anaphylactoid reactions. Obtain blood for a CBC, electrolytes, coagulation profile, BUN, creatinine, liver function tests, and type and hold and a urinalysis before instituting chelation therapy.

Indications for Admission
- Serum iron >500 mcg/dL
- Signs or symptoms of iron toxicity
- Suicide attempt or gesture without psychiatric clearance and appropriate follow-up arranged

Bibliography

Chang TP, Rangan C. Iron poisoning: a literature-based review of epidemiology, diagnosis, and management. *Pediatr Emerg Care.* 2011;**27**(10):978–985.

Gumber MR, Kute VB, Shah PR, et al. Successful treatment of severe iron intoxication with gastrointestinal decontamination, deferoxamine, and hemodialysis. *Ren Fail.* 2013;**35**(5):729–731.

Madiwale T, Liebelt E. Iron: not a benign therapeutic drug. *Curr Opin Pediatr.* 2006;**18**:174–179.

Thanacoody R, Caravati EM, Troutman B, et al. Position paper update: whole bowel irrigation for gastrointestinal decontamination of overdose patients. *Clin Toxicol (Phila).* 2015;**53**:5–12.

Mothballs

Most mothballs in the United States contain paradichlorobenzene, which is a relatively nontoxic substance. Older mothballs, however, may be composed of naphthalene or, less commonly, camphor. Naphthalene can cause sedation, seizures, and methemoglobinemia, as well as severe hemolysis in patients with G-6-PD deficiency. Camphor, which is also available as an oil in herbal preparations and ointments, also predominantly causes CNS effects such as seizures.

Clinical Presentation

In most cases the patient is asymptomatic. Hemolysis in a G-6-PD deficient patient typically does not present until 24–72 hours post-exposure, when weakness, pallor or jaundice, dark urine, and oliguria may occur. A patient who ingests naphthalene or camphor may develop lethargy, sedation, and seizures within hours of ingestion.

Diagnosis

When the chemical nature of the mothball is unknown, an x-ray of the mothball can differentiate the two: paradichlorobenzene is radiopaque whereas naphthalene is not. Another method for identifying the type of mothball is to get a large amount of salt and make a concentrated salt solution (about one tablespoon of salt in 4 oz of water). Naphthalene mothballs float in this solution, but paradichlorobenzene does not. Mothballs containing camphor are oilier than the other two types of mothballs.

Hemolysis can be documented with serial hematocrit determinations (decreasing), the peripheral smear (fragmented red cells), and a urinalysis (dipstick positive for blood and bilirubin, but no RBCs seen). If the patient is symptomatic, a low level on a G-6-PD quantitative assay (not a qualitative screen) confirms that the child is at risk.

ED Management

Most patients who unintentionally ingest one naphthalene or paradichlorobenzene moth-ball do not require medical intervention or GI decontamination. If a large number of mothballs are ingested, give activated charcoal. If the mothball contains naphthalene, determine the patient's G-6-PD status. For an asymptomatic patient no further work-up is necessary. Instruct the family to return at once if pallor, jaundice, lethargy, or dark urine is noticed. If sedation or seizures occur, admit the patient to a monitored setting for supportive care and close observation. If camphor was ingested, observe the patient for 2–4 hours, as most seizures will occur within 1–2 hours post-ingestion.

If the patient is symptomatic, obtain a CBC, type and cross-match, urinalysis, electrolytes, BUN, and creatinine. Give small transfusions (5 mL/kg) of packed red cells to maintain the hematocrit at about 80% of normal.

Treat symptomatic methemoglobinemia with IV methylene blue (1–2 mg/kg).

Treat seizures with lorazepam (0.05–0.10 mg/kg slow IV) or diazepam (0.1–0.3 mg/kg slow IV).

Indications for Admission
- Suspected naphthalene ingestion in a patient known to be G-6-PD deficient
- Significant sedation
- Seizures
- Evidence of intravascular hemolysis
- Suicide attempt or gesture without psychiatric clearance and appropriate follow-up arranged

Bibliography

Chauhan V, Sharma R, Sharma K, et al. Naphthalene poisoning manifesting as hemoglobinuria. *Toxicol Int.* 2014;21(3):314–315.

Kovacic P, Somanathan R. Nitroaromatic compounds: environmental toxicity, carcinogenicity, mutagenicity, therapy and mechanism. *J Appl Toxicol.* 2014;34(8):810–824.

MacKinney TG, Soti KR, Shrestha P, Basnyat B. Camphor: an herbal medicine causing grand mal seizures. *BMJ Case Rep.* 2015 11;2015.

Sudakin DL, Stone DL, Power L. Naphthalene mothballs: emerging and recurring issues and their relevance to environmental health. *Curr Top Toxicol.* 2011;7:13–19.

Nonsteroidal Anti-Inflammatory Drugs

Nonsteroidal anti-inflammatory drugs (NSAIDs) are widely used for the treatment of pain, arthritis, and dysmenorrhea. Among the many agents in this category, ibuprofen and naproxen are nonprescription, and ibuprofen is readily available as a pleasant-tasting liquid. These medications are rapidly absorbed, with peak levels occurring within two hours. Sustained-release preparations require 2–5 hours to reach peak level.

NSAIDS inhibit cyclooxygenase (COX), thereby decreasing prostaglandin synthesis. The most common side effects is gastrointestinal, which is due to disruption of the mucosal protective effects of prostaglandin. Overdose may also cause decreased renal blood flow or CNS effects. Nonetheless, overdoses of NSAIDs rarely produce serious consequences. COX-2 inhibitors (rofecoxib, celecoxib) lose their selectivity for the COX-2 enzyme when ingested in overdose and display a toxicity that is similar to all other NSAIDS.

Clinical Presentation

Mild GI distress, such as epigastric pain, nausea, and vomiting are the rule, although lethargy and drowsiness sometimes occur. Very large overdoses of ibuprofen can cause metabolic acidosis. Some NSDAIDS can cause more severe toxicity, such as mefenamic acid (seizures, muscle twitching, apnea, cardiovascular collapse), diflunisal (can resemble salicylate poisoning), and phenylbutazone (aplastic anemia).

Diagnosis

The history suggests the diagnosis. Serum ibuprofen levels do not correlate well with outcomes. Elevation of liver transaminases, metabolic acidosis, and hypoprothrombinemia may occur in massive overdoses.

ED Management

Typically, no interventions are required unless very large amounts (>400 mg/kg for ibuprofen) have been ingested. In such a case, administer activated charcoal, monitor the level of consciousness, and obtain an ABG. Treat seizures with lorazepam (0.05–0.10 mg/kg slow IV) or diazepam (0.1–0.3 mg/kg slow IV). Manage minor GI distress with magnesium hydroxide/aluminum hydroxide PO (Maalox 1 mL/kg, 30 mL maximum) and an oral or IV H_2 antagonist such as ranitidine (2–4 mg/kg/24 h PO div q 12h, 150 mg/dose maximum).

Indications for Admission

- Decreased level of consciousness or metabolic acidosis or seizures
- Suicide attempt or gesture without psychiatric clearance and appropriate follow-up arranged

Bibliography

Argentieri J, Morrone K, Pollack Y. Acetaminophen and ibuprofen overdosage. *Pediatr Rev.* 2012;**33** (4):188–189.

Hunter LJ, Wood DM, Dargan PI. The patterns of toxicity and management of acute nonsteroidal anti-inflammatory drug (NSAID) overdose. *Open Access Emerg Med.* 2011;3:39–48.

Lodise M, De-Giorgio F, Rossi R, d'Aloja E, Fucci N. Acute ibuprofen intoxication: report on a case and review of the literature. *Am J Forensic Med Pathol.* 2012;33(3):242–246.

Unzueta A, Vargas HE. Nonsteroidal anti-inflammatory drug-induced hepatoxicity. *Clin Liver Dis.* 2013;**17**(4):643–656

Oral Hypoglycemics

Oral hypoglycemic agents include the sulfonylureas (acetohexamide, chlorpropamide, glipizide, glyburide, tolazamide, and tolbutamide) and meglitinides (repaglinide, nateglinide, and mitiglinide). These two classes of drugs cause hypoglycemia by stimulating pancreatic insulin release as well as enhancing peripheral insulin receptor sensitivity and inhibiting gluconeogenesis. Ingestion of a single pill may cause hypoglycemia in a small child.

Biguanides are unlikely to cause severe, persistent hypoglycemia, but have been implicated in severe, and potentially fatal, lactic acidosis. The glitazones (rosiglitazone and pioglitazone), alpha-glucosidase inhibitors, and dipeptidyl peptidase-4 (DDP-4) inhibitors are also unlikely to produce hypoglycemia because they do not increase insulin release.

Clinical Presentation

Signs and symptoms of hypoglycemia include pallor, diaphoresis, tachycardia, depressed level of consciousness, seizures, and coma.

Diagnosis

Consider an oral hypoglycemic ingestion in any patient with hypoglycemia. The differential diagnosis of hypoglycemia is discussed on pp. 194–196.

ED Management

Immediately obtain a blood sugar (bedside and venipuncture) if there is a history of possible oral hypoglycemic ingestion. Administer activated charcoal if the ingestion occurred less than two hours prior to arrival, and start an IV.

Treat hypoglycemia with 0.5 g/kg of dextrose (children and adolescents: 2 mL/kg of D_{25}; infants and toddlers: 5 mL/kg of D_{10}), then repeat the blood sugar. If hypoglycemia persists, give another bolus of dextrose and titrate maintenance fluids with D_{10} ½ NS to maintain euglycemia. Once the patient is awake, start PO feeds.

If this is unsuccessful, give octreotide to inhibit insulin secretion (25–50 mcg SC). The response may take 30 minutes, and a repeat dose may be required in 6–12 hours because the oral hypoglycemics have longer half-lives than octreotide. Glucagon has a limited effect in young children as glycogen stores are minimal and it may aggravate the emesis. Urine alkalinization to a pH of 7.0–8.0 with sodium bicarbonate (1–2 mEq/kg bolus followed by 0.5 mEq/kg/h) is effective in chlorpropamide ingestions.

Do not give prophylactic IV glucose as it complicates discharge decisions. The patient must be euglycemic without sugar supplementation. Discharge normoglycemic patients with a history of ingestion of a biguanide or other antidiabetic agents after four hours of observation.

Indications for Admission

- Hypoglycemia
- History of oral sulfonylurea agent ingestion
- Suicide attempt or gesture without psychiatric clearance and appropriate follow-up arranged

Bibliography

Dougherty PP, Lee SC, Lung D, Klein-Schwartz W. Evaluation of the use and safety of octreotide as antidotal therapy for sulfonylurea overdose in children. *Pediatr Emerg Care*. 2013;**29**(3):292–295.

Glatstein M, Scolnik D, Bentur Y. Octreotide for the treatment of sulfonylurea poisoning. *Clin Toxicol (Phila)*. 2012;**50**:795–804.

Klein-Schwartz W, Stassinos GL, Isbister GK. Treatment of sulfonylurea and insulin overdose. *Br J Clin Pharmacol*. 2016;**81**(3):496–504.

Lung DD, Olson KR. Hypoglycemia in pediatric sulfonylurea poisoning: an 8-year poison center retrospective study. *Pediatrics*. 2011;**127**:e1558–e1564.

Rat Poison

The vast majority of commercial rodenticides are superwarfarins, profoundly long-acting anticoagulants. Included in this group are brodifacoum, bromadiolone, difenacoum, valone, and diphacinone. Historically, rat poisons have been made of arsenic, thallium, strychnine, PNU, ANTU, norbormide, and red squill. These preparations are no longer manufactured in the United States, but exposure to these and others such as tetramine and aldicarb may be possible as there have been reports of these products being imported from Asia or Latin America. In view of the varied toxicity of this eclectic group of compounds, it is crucial to identify the rat poison ingested when evaluating a poisoned patient.

The superwarfarin products inhibit hepatic synthesis of the vitamin K-dependent coagulation factors (II, VII, IX, and X). Anticoagulation occurs approximately two days after ingestion, as new synthesis is impaired but existing functional factors remain. As the existing factors are consumed, elevation of the prothrombin time (PT) and international normalized ratio (INR) occur. Anticoagulation may continue for weeks to months after a single small ingestion.

Clinical Presentation

Most patients who ingest one of the superwarfarin products are asymptomatic on presentation and remain so. However, if the ingestion was large and occurred days prior to presentation, there may be evidence of coagulopathy, such as ecchymoses, bleeding gums, melena, hematemesis, hematuria, or intracranial hemorrhage.

Diagnosis

The diagnosis is generally made by history. Send a family member to retrieve the product, as identification of the product is absolutely necessary.

ED Management

It is not necessary to routinely measure PT and INR post-ingestion in a small child with unintentional ingestion of a superwarfarin, unless it is known that a large quantity was consumed. The patient can be safely discharged but instruct the family to return for any bleeding problems. Have all patients return to measure the PT and INR 36–48 hours post-ingestion. Do not give prophylactic vitamin K1, as this will affect the interpretation of future coagulation studies.

At time of repeat evaluation, if the INR is normal, no further management is required. If the INR is elevated or if the patient develops small, nuisance bleeding, give oral vitamin K1, 10 mg/day PO div q 6–8h. Adjust the dose of vitamin K1 as needed to maintain a satisfactory INR. If there is evidence of severe bleeding, consult with a hematologist, give intravenous vitamin K1 (0.3 mg/kg, 10 mg maximum), fresh frozen plasma (15 mg/kg), or prothrombin complex concentrates, and transfuse packed RBCs as needed.

Follow-up

- 36–48 hours, for coagulation studies

Indications for Admission
- Coagulopathy
- Suicide attempt or gesture without psychiatric clearance and appropriate follow-up arranged

Bibliography

Card DJ, Francis S, Deuchande K, Harrington DJ. Superwarfarin poisoning and its management. *BMJ Case Rep.* 2014;2014. DOI: 10.1136/bcr-2014-206360.

Fang Y, Ye D, Tu C, et al. Superwarfarin rodent poisons and hemorrhagic disease. *Epidemiology.* 2012;**23**(6):932–934.

King N, Tran MH. Long-acting anticoagulant rodenticide (superwarfarin) poisoning: a review of its historical development, epidemiology, and clinical management. *Transfus Med Rev.* 2015;**29** (4):250–258

Schulman S, Furie B. How I treat poisoning with vitamin K antagonists. *Blood.* 2015;**125**(3):438–442.

Salicylates

Salicylates are widely used because of their antipyretic, anti-inflammatory, and antiplatelet actions. Aspirin (acetylsalicylic acid) is in many nonprescription analgesics and cold preparations. Methylsalicylate is the active ingredient in some nonprescription topical creams such as Icy Hot, Ben Gay, and Tiger Balm (30% methylsalicylate), and oil of wintergreen (98% methyl salicylate). One teaspoon of oil of wintergreen is equivalent to 7000 mg of aspirin.

The toxicity of salicylates is due to direct stimulation of the CNS respiratory center, which causes an initial hyperventilation and respiratory alkalosis. This is followed by an uncoupling of oxidative phosphorylation with a subsequent increased anion gap metabolic acidosis. The result is a characteristic mixed acid–base presentation.

The potentially acute toxic dose is 150 mg/kg, or about 20 tabs of baby aspirin in a 10 kg child. Serious toxicity is possible if >300 mg/kg is ingested.

Clinical Presentation

Mild poisoning causes tinnitus, abdominal pain, vomiting, and hyperpnea (respiratory alkalosis). The early signs of respiratory alkalosis are more common in adults as children tend to present with a metabolic acidosis. With larger doses, marked hyperpnea, hyperthermia, lethargy, dehydration, metabolic acidosis, and hypo- or hyperglycemia occur. Severe poisoning leads to coma, seizures, severe metabolic acidosis, oliguria, pulmonary edema, and death. An unusual presentation is acute behavior change, including confusion, agitation, hallucinations, or psychosis.

Diagnosis

Obtain serum salicylate levels and pH at presentation and every 2–4 hours. In general, levels between 15–30 mg/dL are therapeutic, >30 mg/dL may be associated with signs of toxicity, and >100 mg/dL are very serious and may require hemodialysis. More important than the patient's serum level is the patient's clinical and acid–base status. The Dome nomogram correlates poorly with serum levels and is no longer used. A VBG and serum electrolytes will demonstrate a respiratory alkalosis early after overdose. An increased anion gap acidosis may develop at the same time or slightly later, and hypo- or hyperglycemia may occur.

Salicylate toxicity may mimic other clinical presentations. For example, the mixed acid–base disturbance (pH 7.40; pCO_2 25 mmHg) may resemble a septic presentation. Patients may have both elevated serum ketones and elevated lactates, suggesting a ketoacidosis, infection, or other intoxications. Universal salicylate screening is not indicated for all patients, but obtain a salicylate level on patients who are tachypneic/hyperpneic, or present with an otherwise unexplained acid–base disturbance.

ED Management

Provide supportive care as needed, administer activated charcoal (under two hours post-ingestion or anytime for a symptomatic patient who may have delayed gastric emptying of the salicylate), secure an IV, and obtain blood for electrolytes, glucose, PT, and CBC. Also obtain a salicylate level and VBG at the time of presentation and every two hours thereafter. Consider the possibility of co-ingestion of acetaminophen, and obtain a level at four hours post-ingestion (pp. 453–455). Fluid losses can be significant secondary to the hypermetabolic state; treat aggressively with 20 mL/kg normal saline or Ringer's lactate boluses.

If the patient has an altered mental status, give 0.5 g/kg of dextrose IV and maintain the serum glucose level at approximately 150 mg/dL. Once there is satisfactory urine output, initiate urinary alkalization for any patient who manifests signs and symptoms of salicylate toxicity or has a serum level >40 mg/dL. Infuse D_5 W with 132 mEq bicarbonate and 40 mEq/L of potassium chloride (add three 50 mL ampules of sodium bicarbonate solution to 1 L of D_5 W) at twice the maintenance rate. The goal is a urine pH ≥7.5. Carefully monitor the serum potassium, since it is lowered by both sodium bicarbonate administration and hyperventilation; serum potassium in the high normal range is desired. Discontinue alkalization when the serum level is below 40 mg/dL and the patient has clinically improved and has a normal acid–base status.

Hemodialysis is indicated for an acute salicylate level >100 mg/dL, severe acidosis, oliguria or anuria, pulmonary edema, coagulopathy, intractable seizures, or progressive deterioration despite appropriate therapy regardless of the salicylate level. Hemodialysis may be indicated for chronic toxicity with a serum level >60 mg/dL in association with lethargy, mental status changes, or acidosis. Multiple doses of activated charcoal (1 g/kg q 3h × 4) may decrease serum half-life, but is not as effective as hemodialysis.

Avoid mechanical ventilation if possible. A salicylate-toxic patient compensates for metabolic acidosis with significant tachypnea. Decreasing the respiratory rate to "normal" with mechanical ventilation may lead to severe acute acidosis, seizures, arrest, and death. If intubation is necessary, pretreat with boluses of bicarbonate and set the ventilator to a high respiratory rate.

Indications for Admission
- Salicylate level >45 mg/dL
- Signs and symptoms of salicylism in a patient taking salicylates
- Suicide attempt or gesture without psychiatric clearance and appropriate follow-up arranged

Bibliography

Calello DP, Henretig FM. Pediatric toxicology: specialized approach to the poisoned child. *Emerg Med Clin North Am.* 2014;**32**(1):29–52.

Flomenbaum NE. Salicylates. In Hoffman RS, Howland MA, Lewin NA, Nelson LS, Goldfrank LR (eds.) *Goldfrank's Toxicologic Emergencies* (10th edn.). New York: McGraw-Hill, 2015; 516–527.

Juurlink DN, Gosselin S, Kielstein JT, et al. Extracorporeal treatment for salicylate poisoning: systematic review and recommendations from the EXTRIP workgroup. *Ann Emerg Med.* 2015;**66** (2):165–181.

Robinson K, Rauch A, Hannan L. Salicylate poisoning following topical administration of methylsalicylate. *Emerg Med Australas.* 2015;**27**(4):374–375.

Shively RM, Hoffman RS, Manini AF. Acute salicylate poisoning: risk factors for severe outcome. *Clin Toxicol (Phila).* 2017;**55**(3):175–180.

Toxic Alcohols (Ethylene Glycol, Methanol, and Isopropanol)

The toxic alcohols include ethylene glycol, methanol, and isopropanol, as well as benzyl alcohol and propylene glycol. Ethylene glycol can be found in antifreeze (up to 95%) and is generally ingested unintentionally by children because of its sweet taste. Methanol is found in solvents, windshield-wiper fluid, and duplicating fluids. Isopropanol is the main ingredient in rubbing alcohol (70%) and is also found in solvents and disinfectants.

These alcohols may be ingested unintentionally by children or as an alcohol substitute by adolescents. All three cause intoxication similar to ethanol, as well as gastritis. Isopropanol is metabolized to acetone, producing a "ketosis without acidosis" with a toxic picture similar to that of ethanol. Methanol is metabolized to formic acid and ethylene glycol is metabolized to glycolic, glyoxylic, and oxalic acids. These "toxic metabolites" produce an anion gap metabolic acidosis and may lead to death

Clinical Presentation and Diagnosis

Ethylene Glycol

Ethylene glycol toxicity occurs in two distinct stages. Within the first 3–4 hours, there is inebriation, with ataxia, nystagmus, nausea, and euphoria. At this stage, the ethylene glycol level is high, the osmol gap is elevated, but there is no acidosis. As the ethylene glycol is metabolized into toxic metabolites, the patient develops an anion gap metabolic acidosis leading to tachypnea, tachycardia, hypotension, renal failure from crystalline deposits in renal tubules, cerebral and pulmonary edema, and seizures. In this acidemic stage, the ethylene glycol levels may be lower, osmol gap may be lower, but acidosis is present.

Methanol

Methanol produces a similar two-stage toxicity (high osmol gap, followed by high anion gap). The initial intoxication is not as pronounced as with ethylene glycol or ethanol. As the methanol is metabolized, an anion gap metabolic acidosis develops with tachypnea, tachycardia, visual changes, blindness, seizures, and death.

Isopropyl Alcohol

Isopropyl alcohol produces inebriation that is more pronounced than ethanol. In the first few hours, euphoria, nausea, and vomiting predominate. Laboratory studies reveal an elevated osmol gap without metabolic acidosis. Metabolism of isopropanol to acetone leads to CNS depression and a distinctive ketone odor. Because the predominant metabolite is acetone without further acidic byproducts, the hallmark of isopropanol toxicity is ketosis without acidosis.

ED Management

Lethal oral doses of ethylene glycol and methanol containing compounds are very small, approximately 1.5 mL/kg. For any potential ingestion, obtain a CBC, electrolytes, VBG, lactate, ethanol, serum osmolality and, if possible, a specific alcohol level. Calculate the osmolality and subtract it from the measured osmolality to determine the osmol gap (p. 450). Osmol gaps are imperfect and nonspecific, but may hint at a cause. Illness in general may cause a low-level rise in the osmol gap (<20 mOsm/L), but a gap >30–40 mOsm/L is more specific for exposure to an osmotically active agent, namely toxic alcohols (or ethanol, mannitol, IV contrast).

If the laboratory is unable to perform levels of the specific toxic alcohols, approximate them by multiplying the osmol gap by the following conversion factors: ethylene glycol (6.2), isopropyl alcohol (6.0), and methanol (3.2). For example, if the osmol gap is 20 mOsm/L, then the estimated ethylene glycol level is 124 mg/dL. Slight increases in lactate may be seen in toxic alcohol exposures, but a significant hyperlactatemia represents a false-elevation due to the laboratory assay mistaking the ethylene glycol metabolite (glyoxylic acid) for lactate.

The treatment of methanol and ethylene glycol poisoning involves blocking the production and enhancing the clearance of toxic metabolites. This can be accomplished by competitively inhibiting the enzyme alcohol dehydrogenase with either ethanol or fomepizole, which is FDA-approved for the treatment of both methanol and ethylene glycol ingestions in adults. The advantages of fomepizole over ethanol are that there are no levels to monitor and it does not cause gastritis or hypoglycemia. After the enzyme has been blocked, hemodialysis is the mainstay of therapy, allowing both clearance of the alcohol and the acidosis. Gastric decontamination is generally not beneficial because alcohols are rapidly absorbed.

Indications for ethanol or fomepizole are suspicion of methanol or ethylene glycol ingestion with one of the following: methanol >25 mg/dL or ethylene glycol >25 mg/dL; or a suspected poisoning with an osmol gap >10 mOsm/L or a metabolic acidosis. The loading dose of fomepizole is 15 mg/kg IV over 30 minutes, followed by 10 mg/kg q 12h for four doses. Since the endogenous clearance of toxic alcohols in the setting of fomepizole is significantly lengthened (methanol half-life = 54 h, ethylene glycol half-life = 17 h), hemodialysis is necessary. Also, adjust the fomepizole dose if hemodialysis is initiated to allow for clearance of fomepizole.

The loading dose of ethanol (10% solution) is 10 mL/kg IV, followed by 1–2 mL/kg/h. An ethanol level of 100 mg/dL is sufficient to block most of the metabolite production. Serum ethanol levels and bedside glucose checks must be performed frequently. Ethanol may also be given via nasogastric tube, but this can cause a severe gastritis.

Indications for Admission
- Toxic levels of ethylene glycol, methanol, or isopropanol
- CNS depression, nausea, hypoglycemia, tachycardia, or other symptoms of alcohol ingestion
- Suicide attempt or gesture without psychiatric clearance and appropriate follow-up arranged

Bibliography

Jammalamadaka D, Raissi S. Ethylene glycol, methanol, and isopropyl alcohol intoxication. *Am J Med Sci.* 2010;**339**:276–281.

Kraut JA. Diagnosis of toxic alcohols: limitations of present methods. *Clin Toxicol (Phila).* 2015;**53** (7):589–595.

Kruse JA. Methanol and ethylene glycol intoxication. *Crit Care Clin.* 2012;**28**(4):661–711.

McMartin K, Jacobsen D, Hovda KE. Antidotes for poisoning by alcohols that form toxic metabolites. *Br J Clin Pharmacol.* 2016;**81**(3):505–515.

Tricyclic Antidepressants

Tricyclic antidepressants (TCAs) are used for the treatment of depression, migraines, enuresis, OCD, ADD, and chronic pain. Common TCAs include amitriptyline, amoxapine, clomipramine, desipramine, doxepin, imipramine, nortryptyline, protriptyline, and trim-pramine. Clinical toxicity results from anticholinergic effects, peripheral α-blockade, sodium channel blockade, GABA inhibition, direct myocardial (quinidine-like) depression, and acidosis. Toxic doses vary with specific drugs but all TCAs have similar side effects. The lethality of these drugs in overdose is secondary to cardiovascular and CNS effects.

Clinical Presentation

The central anticholinergic effect causes hyperthermia, as well as mental status changes ranging from combativeness, delirium, and hallucinations to lethargy and coma. Peripheral anticholinergic effects include tachycardia, decreased bowel sounds, flushed skin, and urinary retention (see Anticholinergics, pp. 457–458). Transient hypertension may occur early after ingestion due to increased catecholamines, but hypotension is more frequent and is predominantly due to the alpha-blockade. Sodium channel blockade slows ventricular depolarization, causing a prolonged QRS and contributing to the hypotension; GABA inhibition leads to seizures. Refractory hypotension is the most common cause of death.

Diagnosis

Suspect a TCA overdose in a patient presenting with an acute change of mental status, seizures, abnormal vital signs, or an arrhythmia. Attach a cardiac monitor and obtain an ECG. All patients who are exposed to TCAs (therapeutically or in overdose) have an R-wave in AVR, and a rightward shift of the terminal 40 msec QRS axis deviation (absence of these findings essentially rules-out a significant exposure). Since TCAs are potent sodium channel blockers, toxicity can be predicted by the QRS interval. One-third of patients with QRS >100 msec will develop seizures, and one-half of patients with QRS >160 msec will develop ventricular dysrhythmias.

ED Management

Initiate supportive care and place the patient on a continuous ECG monitor. Perform gastric lavage if a potentially lethal dose of a TCA was taken within 1–2 hours of presentation; administer activated charcoal if ingestion was within two hours of presentation. If the QRS interval is >100 msec, give 1–2 mEq/kg of sodium bicarbonate IV over two minutes and repeat every five minutes until the QRS narrows to <100 msec. Start a bicarbonate drip and titrate the serum pH to 7.45–7.55. Do not treat hypertension, which is usually transient, since hypotension frequently follows. Treat hypotension with sodium bicarbonate (as above) and a 20 mL/kg bolus of an isotonic crystalloid (normal saline, Ringer's lactate). If fluids and bicarbonate are unsuccessful, norepinephrine (0.1–0.2 mcg/kg/min IV, 2 mcg/kg/min maximum) is the preferred pressor; titrate the dose against the patient's response. Treat seizures with lorazepam (0.05–0.1 mg/kg IV) or diazepam (0.1–0.3 mg/kg slow IV) or phenobarbital. It is not necessary to treat supraventricular arrhythmias, but give lidocaine (1 mg/kg IV) for life-threatening ventricular arrhythmias. Overdrive pacing may be needed. Do not use physostigmine, as asystole has been reported.

Consult a toxicologist and cardiologist, and admit a symptomatic patient to an ICU, where continuous cardiac monitoring and close nursing supervision can be provided, until the patient is symptom-free for 12 hours. Patients who do not develop any symptoms within six hours and have a normal ECG can be discharged from the ED.

Indications for Admission

- Any signs or symptoms of tricyclic overdose
- History of possible tricyclic overdose, unless six hours has elapsed and the patient has remained asymptomatic with normal vital signs, a normal mental status, and no changes on ECG monitoring
- Suicide attempt or gesture without psychiatric clearance or appropriate follow-up arranged

Bibliography

Body R, Bartram T, Azam F, Mackway-Jones K. Guidelines in Emergency Medicine Network (GEMNet): guideline for the management of tricyclic antidepressant overdose. *Emerg Med J*. 2011;**28** (4):347–368.

Bruccoleri RE, Burns MM. A literature review of the use of sodium bicarbonate for the treatment of QRS widening. *J Med Toxicol*. 2016;**12**(1):121–129.

Carvalho AF, Sharma MS, Brunoni AR, Vieta E, Fava GA. The safety, tolerability and risks associated with the use of newer generation antidepressant drugs: a critical review of the literature. *Psychother Psychosom*. 2016;**85**(5):270–288.

O'Sullivan JC, Johnson AD, Waterman MA. Comparative resuscitation measures for the treatment of desipramine overdose. *Mil Med*. 2014;**179**(11):1266–1272.

Chapter 15

Neurologic Emergencies

Stephanie Morris, Soe Mar, and Shannon Liang

Acute Ataxia

While the common etiologies of acute ataxia are benign, some diagnoses require emergent intervention. Acute ataxia is usually the result of cerebellar dysfunction, but may also be due to conditions affecting vestibular function, motor output, and/or sensory input. The most common causes (Table 15.1) are intoxications (alcohol, benzodiazepines, anticonvulsant medications) and parainfectious viral infections. However, serious concerns include a mass lesion (posterior fossa, brainstem, spinal cord), hydrocephalus, head trauma, meningitis, encephalitis, post-ictal state, and a metabolic or vascular etiology.

Table 15.1 Etiologies of acute ataxia

Infection

Abscess

Encephalitis

Meningitis

Ischemic or vascular events

Arteriovenous malformation

Sickle cell anemia

Vasculitis

Vertebrobasilar dissection

Metabolic disorders

Hypoglycemia (pseudoataxia)

Inborn errors of metabolism

Parainfectious

Acute disseminated encephalomyelitis

Cytomegalovirus

Enteroviruses

Epstein–Barr virus

Herpes simplex

Table 15.1 (cont.)

Measles

Mumps

Mycoplasma pneumoniae

Varicella

Paraneoplastic

Opsoclonus–myoclonus syndrome

Paretic ataxia

Corticospinal lesions

Myasthenia syndromes

Spinal cord lesion/compression

Transverse myelitis

Sensory ataxia

Guillain-Barré syndrome

Miller-Fisher syndrome

Toxic ingestions

Anticonvulsants

Antihistamines

Benzodiazepines

Ethanol

Marijuana

Trauma

Extra-axial (subdural or epidural)

Intra-axial (cerebellar)

Posterior fossa hemorrhage

Tumors with/without hydrocephalus

Brainstem

Posterior fossa

Clinical Presentation

Ataxia is the impaired coordination of movements, usually manifested as unsteady, wide-based gait or truncal instability (titubation). More subtle signs of ataxia include dysmetria (undershoot/overshoot), intention tremor, dysdiadochokinesia (impaired rapid alternating movements), dysrhythmic "scanning" speech, and nystagmus. In general, acute ataxia evolves over <72 hours.

Parainfectious Acute Cerebellar Ataxia

Acute cerebellar ataxia most often occurs days to weeks after a viral infection (before or after an exanthem), such as varicella or Epstein–Barr virus (EBV), but it can also follow an immunization. Typically, a preschool-aged child presents with a short history (hours to days) of incoordination, unsteady gait, tremor, speech abnormalities, titubation, and/or nystagmus). The mental status and the remainder of the neurologic examination are normal. The well appearance of the child helps distinguish this entity from encephalitis and meningitis. The CSF may be normal, or there may be a mild pleocytosis or protein elevation.

Acute Cerebellitis

Acute cerebellitis is a potentially worrisome process, which can occur during or after a systemic infection, such as with EBV, varicella, rotavirus, *Mycoplasma*, or HHV-6. In contrast to a pure cerebellar syndrome, there are more global neurologic features, including headache, vomiting, and altered mental status. The clinical presentation is related to cerebellar edema and brainstem compression, with potential fourth ventricular outflow obstruction and resultant hydrocephalus. Neuroimaging abnormalities are confined to the cerebellum.

Acute Disseminated Encephalomyelitis

Acute disseminated encephalomyelitis (ADEM) is an immune-mediated, inflammatory demyelinating disease of the CNS that often presents with ataxia two days to four weeks after a viral infection or vaccination. In contrast to acute cerebellar ataxia, by definition patients with ADEM have encephalopathy. This may present as lethargy or behavioral changes, often associated with multifocal neurologic findings on examination. The brain MRI reveals diffuse, patchy T2 signal abnormalities, usually involving the white matter more than gray matter.

Toxic Ingestion

Toxic ingestions are the second most frequent cause of acute ataxia, affecting both toddlers (accidental) and adolescents (intentional). The most common agents implicated are anti-convulsants (e.g., benzodiazepines, phenytoin, carbamazepine), ethanol, marijuana, tricyclic antidepressants, and dextromethorphan. Associated symptoms may include decreased consciousness, vomiting, or seizures.

Meningitis

Ataxia, with or without fever, may be the first sign of bacterial or viral meningitis (pp. 422–425). Other meningeal signs, such as nuchal rigidity and Kernig's and Brudzinski's signs, may also be present.

Encephalitis

A viral infection affecting the brainstem can present with ataxia and cranial nerve abnor-malities (pp. 383–386). There is minimal effect on the level of consciousness unless higher cortical structures are also involved. Common agents are varicella, enterovirus, echovirus, adenovirus, and coxsackievirus. CSF findings are consistent with viral meningitis (pleocy-tosis without significant protein elevation or hypoglycorrhachia).

Posterior Fossa Tumor

A posterior fossa tumor usually presents with an insidious onset of headaches and vomiting, with slowly progressive ataxia. Acute ataxia can occur as the result of obstructive hydro-cephalus, hemorrhage into the lesion, or edema.

Stroke

Sickle cell disease, congenital heart disease, and hypercoagulable states can cause vertebro-basilar disease or hemorrhagic strokes, presenting with ataxia (pp. 493–498). Trauma may be associated with vertebral artery dissection and stroke.

Paraneoplastic Syndrome

Oposoclonus–myoclonus syndrome is a paraneoplastic process, most often associated with neuroblastoma. It presents with ataxia, opsoclonus (chaotic "dancing eye movements"), and irritability.

Transverse Myelitis

Transverse myelitis is a presumed parainfectious inflammation at a specific level of the spinal cord. It may initially present with ataxia, back or neck pain, and paresthesias, followed by the rapid development of weakness at and below the level of the lesion.

Guillain-Barré Syndrome

In the Miller-Fisher variant of Guillain-Barré syndrome, ataxia is accompanied by ophthalmoplegia (usually diplopia). This may be followed by areflexia, an ascending weakness, and autonomic symptoms (flushing, pulse and blood pressure changes, gastrointestinal symptoms). Classically, the CSF demonstrates cytoalbuminologic dissociation (elevated protein without pleocytosis).

Migraine Syndrome

Basilar migraines and hemiplegic migraines can present with ataxia, dizziness, and diplopia. In addition, patients with migraine may have benign paroxysmal vertigo, which can be difficult to differentiate from ataxia.

Seizure Disorder

Ictal or post-ictal phases of a seizure may present as ataxia.

Diagnosis

Determine the time of onset, progression of the symptoms (chronic ataxia usually results from tumors, metabolic disorders, or hereditary ataxias), associated symptoms, and whether there was any antecedent trauma, viral illness, rash, or toxin exposure. Inquire about the possibility of recreational drug use, ingestion (including ethanol), or overuse of prescription (anticonvulsants, sedatives, TCAs) and over-the-counter medications (dextromethorphan, topical diphenhydramine applied over a large surface area).

Pertinent general physical examination findings include fever, meningeal signs, viral exanthem (varicella, measles), and an ethanol or marijuana odor.

A careful neurologic examination is necessary to confirm the presence of ataxia (truncal, appendicular, and/or gait), and to identify associated findings (encephalopathy, headache, opthalmoplegia, opsoclonus). Abnormal mental status suggests a toxic ingestion, ADEM, meningitis, encephalitis, or stroke.

A posterior fossa mass can be associated with intracranial hypertension, bulging anterior fontanelle, papilledema with absence of spontaneous venous pulsations, cranial nerve palsies (head tilt, lateral gaze palsy, facial weakness), or long-tract findings (hemiparesis, spasticity, extensor plantar responses).

Consider Guillain-Barré syndrome if the patient is hyporeflexic or areflexic. Check for a sensory level, suggestive of a spinal cord lesion (transverse myelitis, tumor).

Acute Cerebellar Ataxia

In acute cerebellar ataxia, mental status is preserved, there are no meningeal signs, the sensory examination is normal, and there is no focal weakness. For most of the disorders listed in Table 15.1, the associated lethargy helps to distinguish these entities from acute cerebellar ataxia.

Vertigo

It can be difficult to distinguish an unsteady stance or gait secondary to vertigo (acute labyrinthitis, migrainous vertigo, benign positional vertigo) from ataxia. This is particularly true in children who are unable to articulate a sense of motion or spinning. Nausea, vomiting, and nystagmus usually accompany vertigo, which can be provoked or worsened by changes in head position.

ED Management

If the child is lethargic, immediately assess the airway, breathing, and cardiovascular functions, give oxygen if necessary, and obtain intravascular access. If there is papilledema, focal neurologic findings, bradycardia, or hypertension, begin treatment for increased intracranial pressure (pp. 527–529) and arrange for an emergent noncontrast head CT scan to rule-out a posterior fossa lesion. If meningitis is suspected, obtain a blood culture and give meningitic doses of IV antibiotics (pp. 422–425) before obtaining the head CT.

If the head CT reveals no evidence of increased intracranial pressure or mass effect, perform a lumbar puncture, including a measurement of the opening pressure (with the patient's legs extended). To evaluate for a toxic ingestion, check serum osmolality (increased with ethanol), and blood level of the suspected drug (e.g., ethanol, phenobarbital, phenytoin, or carbamazepine). If there is encephalopathy, arrange for a brain MRI, to evaluate for ADEM and cerebellitis.

An evaluation for an inborn error of metabolism is necessary only if the patient has a past history of recurrent episodic ataxia, mental status changes, or a family history of metabolic disorders. Obtain liver function tests, serum amino acids, urine organic acids, lactate, pyruvate, and ammonia. These tests are most valuable if they are obtained before IV fluids and dextrose are given.

Indications for Admission

- All patients with acute ataxia until the cause has been established and the course stabilized.

Bibliography

Caffarelli M, Kimia AA, Torres AR: acute ataxia in children – a review of the differential diagnosis and evaluation in the emergency department. *Pediatr Neurol.* 2016;**65**:14–30.

Poretti A, Benson JE, Huisman TA, et al. Acute ataxia in children: approach to clinical presentation and role of additional investigations. *Neuropediatrics.* 2013;**44**:127–141.

Sivaswamy L. Approach to acute ataxia in childhood: diagnosis and evaluation. *Pediatr Ann.* 2014;**43** (4):153–159.

Whelan HT, Verma S, Guo Y, et al. Evaluation of the child with acute ataxia: a systematic review. *Pediatr Neurol.* 2013;**49**:15–24.

Acute Hemiparesis and Stroke

Acute hemiparesis in children can be difficult to recognize due to subtle motor signs, sometimes confounded by encephalopathy or pain. Thus, there can be a delay in the recognition of a potentially emergent medical situation. The most common etiologies of acute hemiparesis are ischemic or hemorrhagic stroke, prolonged focal seizures or post-ictal period (Todd's paralysis), acute disseminated encephalomyelitis, meningitis, encephalitis, brain abscess, mass lesions, and hemiplegic migraine. While serious bacterial infections such as sepsis, endocarditis, and meningitis have well-established associations with arterial ischemic stroke in children, minor infections (such as a viral URI) in the week prior to presentation are more common. Other etiologies of acute hemiparesis include blood dyscrasias, vasculopathies, vascular malformations, and trauma (Table 15.2).

Table 15.2 Etiologies of acute hemiparesis in childhood

Embolic events

Atrial myxoma

Congenital heart disease

Posttraumatic (fat or air embolus)

Prosthetic valves

Subacute bacterial endocarditis

Hematologic disorders

Anticardiolipin antibodies

Antithrombin III deficiency

Factor V Leiden mutation

Leukemia or other neoplasms

Lipoprotein abnormalities

Lupus anticoagulant

MTHF deficiency mutation

Plasminogen deficiency

Polycythemia vera

Pregnancy or puerperium

Protein S or C deficiency

Sickle cell disease

Ischemic events

Arterial thrombosis

Table 15.2 (cont.)

(carotid or vertebral circulations)

Inflammatory arterial occlusion

Penetrating oral trauma

Posttraumatic dissection

Vasculitis/vasculopathy

Infections

Encephalitis

Mastoiditis

Meningitis

Sinusitis

Intracranial hemorrhage

Aneurysm (rare in prepubertal children)

Arteriovenous malformation rupture

Hemorrhagic tumor or stroke

Venous angioma

Mass lesion

Abscess

Neurofibroma

Neoplasm

Vascular disease

Moyamoya disease

Polyarteritis nodosa

Systemic lupus erythematosus

Venous thrombosis

Cyanotic heart disease with polycythemia

Dehydration

Paraneoplastic

Other

Fabry disease

Metabolic strokes

Mitochondrial disease

Posterior reversible encephalopathy

Prolonged post-ictal state

Note: hemiplegic migraine and acute infantile hemiplegia are diagnoses of exclusion

Clinical Presentation

The clinical presentation of acute ischemic stroke varies by age, and size and location of the injury. An infant may have an asymmetric startle response or absent grasp reflex on the affected side. Toddlers can demonstrate subtle hemiparesis as a refusal to reach with the weaker side, or an asymmetric gait. A larger stroke typically presents with decreased level of consciousness, hypertension, apnea, seizures, or hypotonia. Older children may present like adults, with visual field deficits, gaze deviation, aphasia, dysphagia, or other neurological deficits accompanying the hemiparesis. Alteration of consciousness and seizures can occur with a large ischemic or hemorrhagic stroke, meningitis, and encephalitis. Initially, there will be flaccid weakness of the involved arm or leg, which may evolve over days to weeks to a decorticate posture (shoulder adduction, flexion of the elbow, wrist, and fingers; pronation of the hand; extension of the knee; and eversion and plantar flexion of the foot). Subacute to chronic hemiparesis is associated with hyperreflexia, spasticity, and extensor plantar reflexes (corticospinal tract signs).

Arterial Ischemic Stroke (AIS)

AIS is defined as an acute focal neurological deficit lasting >24 hours, associated with neuroradiological evidence of cerebral infarction (diffusion changes on MRI). The most common risk factors are congenital heart disease, preceding infection, red blood cell disorders such as sickle cell disease, and genetic or acquired coagulopathies. Non-inflammatory arteriopathies include arterial dissection, Moyamoya syndrome, and transient cerebral vasculopathy. Infectious conditions include bacterial meningitis, encephalitis, brain abscess, sepsis, and viral infections such as varicella, influenza, HIV, and parvovirus B19.

Intracranial Hemorrhage

An intracranial hemorrhage typically has a sudden onset and rapid evolution. Headache, vomiting, and obtundation are common, and there may be other signs of increased intracranial pressure, such as hypertension, bradycardia, and papilledema (pp. 527–529). Seizures may also occur early in the course.

Hemiplegic Migraine

Hemiplegic migraine is a rare form of migraine. It can be sporadic or familial, with onset often in childhood. It is a stroke mimic, and may be associated with impaired consciousness, inability to speak, and typical migraine features like headache, nausea, and photophobia.

Acute Alternating Hemiplegia of Childhood

Acute alternating hemiplegia of childhood is a rare disorder presenting with episodic sudden weakness and altered mental status. The motor deficit persists for minutes to days and is often followed by seizures and slowed mentation. The typical patient is under three years of age and previously well. Repeated episodes can affect one or both sides of the body, but the child is well in between and neuroimaging studies are all normal.

Diagnosis

Although the etiology may not be definitively determined in the ED, inquire about the onset of the weakness, progression of symptoms, and occurrence of seizures, fever, trauma, infections (URI, sinusitis, mastoiditis), or change in mental status. Determine past medical history (sickle cell disease, congenital heart disease, coagulopathies, lupus, neurofibromatosis, epilepsy, prior hemiparetic episode). Consider non-accidental trauma, particularly in an infant or toddler.

On physical examination, check for hypertension and a bulging fontanelle, which may indicate increased intracranial pressure, and nuchal rigidity suggesting an infectious process (meningitis, encephalitis). Examine the skin for neurofibromas and café-au-lait spots, check for cyanosis, and look for signs of head or neck trauma. Auscultate the head and neck for a bruit and the chest for a cardiac murmur.

Perform a thorough neurologic exam, with special attention to mental status, strength, and reflexes. A unilateral, nonexpanding, hemispheric lesion does not necessarily cause a change in mental status. If the patient is lethargic, consider a brainstem stroke, bihemispheric stroke, hemorrhage, infection, metabolic derangement, or postictal state.

ED Management

Management takes priority over etiologic diagnosis. Perform a quick survey to assess the adequacy of the airway, breathing, and cardiovascular function, and obtain a complete set of vital signs. Check the extraocular movements (EOMs), pupil size and reactivity, and the fundi for papilledema, and assess the level of consciousness. See pp. 527–529 for the management of increased intracranial pressure, but allow for permissive hypertension (avoid iatrogenic hypotension, which can worsen the cerebral hypoperfusion in children with acute stroke). Secure an IV and obtain blood for a CBC, platelet count, PT and PTT, sickle cell testing (if patient's status is unknown), focused drug/toxin testing, inflammatory markers (ESR and/or CRP), Dextrostix, comprehensive metabolic panel, VBG or ABG, and a blood culture if the patient is febrile or has meningeal signs.

Immediately consult a pediatric neurologist and/or neurosurgeon, and arrange for a noncontrast CT scan to rule-out hemorrhage or an emergent brain MRI to evaluate for ischemic stroke. If there is no evidence of mass effect (tumor, acute infarct, hematoma) or increased intracranial pressure, perform a lumbar puncture (including opening pressure) and obtain specimens for cell count, protein and glucose, Gram stain, and culture. Save an additional tube of CSF in the event that testing for varicella zoster virus, herpes simplex virus, or enterovirus is indicated (elevated CSF WBC or protein).

For patients with AIS, thrombolytic therapy is warranted if symptom onset is within three hours for treatment with IV tPA and within 3–6 hours for intra-arterial tPA. However, most children present too late (>24 hours) for these therapies to be beneficial. If arterial thrombosis is discovered in a large vessel, consult with neurointerventional radiology to determine if emergent clot retrieval is indicated.

If the patient has fever and altered mental status, empirically treat with broad-spectrum antibiotics and acyclovir until cultures and herpes PCR are negative. The management of sickle cell disease (pp. 370–375), encephalitis (pp. 383–386), meningitis (pp. 422–425), and headache (pp. 515–521) is discussed elsewhere.

Indications for Admission

- Acute hemiparesis for evaluation of etiology and management.

Bibliography

Bhate S, Ganesan V. A practical approach to acute hemiparesis in children. *Dev Med Child Neurol.* 2015;**57**:689–697.

Fullerton HJ, Hills NK, Elkind MSV, et al. Infection, vaccination, and childhood arterial ischemic stroke: results of the VIPS study. *Neurology.* 2015;**85**:1459–1466.

Mirsky DM, Beslow LA, Amlie-Lefond C, et al. International Paediatric Stroke Study Neuroimaging Consortium and the Paediatric Stroke Neuroimaging Consortium: pathways for neuroimaging of childhood stroke. *Pediatr Neurol.* 2017;**69**:11–23.

Rivkin MJ, Bernard TJ, Dowling MM, et al. Guidelines for urgent management of stroke in children. *Pediatr Neurol.* 2016;**56**:8–17.

Acute Weakness

Although acute weakness is uncommon in childhood, it usually indicates a significant neurologic disorder. The possibility of rapid progression to respiratory failure makes the onset of acute weakness a true neurologic emergency until the cause and course are established.

Clinical Presentation and Diagnosis

The history is vital to defining the underlying process. Determine the time of onset, progression, pattern of weakness (unilateral, bilateral, hemi-, di-, para-, or quadriparetic; flaccid versus spastic), fluctuation of weakness with time, shortness of breath (respiratory muscle involvement), difficulty swallowing or choking, and associated systemic features. Always inquire about associated sensory changes, muscle or extremity pain, and bladder or bowel incontinence. It is also important to differentiate weakness from ataxia, which can be challenging in young children. A history of fever or viral prodrome suggests an infectious or parainfectious process.

Guillain-Barré Syndrome (GBS)

GBS, or acute demyelinating polyneuropathy, is the most common cause of acute flaccid paralysis in otherwise healthy children. It is usually a post-vaccination or post-infectious phenomenon; about two-thirds of patients have a history of an antecedent respiratory tract or gastrointestinal (*Campylobacter* most frequent) infection. GBS is characterized by premonitory sensory changes or pain, ascending motor weakness, and depressed or absent deep tendon reflexes, with intact bowel and bladder sphincter function. There may be associated cranial nerve involvement (bilateral facial weakness is most common). The weakness is often asymmetric at the onset, but becomes symmetrical as the disease progresses. About 10% of patients have serious respiratory, cardiac, and/or autonomic dysfunction, which may progress rapidly and be unrelated to the degree of motor weakness.

Examination of the CSF early in the course may show a mild pleocytosis, but later the classic finding is cytoalbuminologic dissociation: marked elevation of protein without pleocytosis.

Miller-Fisher Syndrome (MFS)

Patients with this GBS variant have external ophthalmoplegia, ataxia, and muscle weakness with areflexia. These children may also have other cranial nerves palsies. Most of these patients have cross-reacting antibodies to GQ1b ganglioside.

Myasthenia Gravis

Myasthenia gravis (MG) is a rare autoimmune disorder that causes weakness by impeding postsynaptic neuromuscular transmission, typically related to blocking the acetylcholine receptor. Weakness develops subacutely (over weeks to months), and commonly presents as ptosis, diplopia, or blurry vision due to extraocular muscle weakness, with or without generalized muscle weakness. Patients with bulbar weakness may present with difficulty in chewing and swallowing, drooling, nasal voice, or poor cough. Fluctuation of the weakness and fatigability are hallmarks of MG, as the symptoms are least prominent on awakening, and become more obvious through the day. Rarely, there may be a severe acute presentation with life-threatening weakness of the respiratory musculature (myasthenic crisis). Patients typically have normal mental status, pupillary reflexes, deep tendon reflexes, sensation, and coordination. Ptosis becomes evident with sustained upward eye gaze (at least 30 seconds). The diagnosis is confirmed by a therapeutic challenge with edrophonium.

Acute Flaccid Myelitis

Although poliomyelitis is very rare in the United States, it may occur in a patient with a history of incomplete or inadequate immunization. Clusters of cases of polio-like myelitis have emerged in the summer/fall months recently. The leading identified viral cause is enterovirus D68, and possibly other enteroviruses (echovirus, Coxsackievirus). It typically presents with a history of a mild febrile illness, with headache, sore throat, vomiting, and fatigue, followed by a few days of recovery. Then the patient has recurrent fever accompanied by weakness, lethargy, and irritability, which may be associated with meningeal signs. There is selective destruction of motor neurons (anterior horn cells), characterized by motor weakness, as well as severe back, neck, and muscle pain. The disease tends to preferentially affect proximal muscles and the legs, but bulbar involvement may also occur, causing dysphagia, dysarthria, and difficulty managing secretions. Reflexes are decreased or absent, but the sensory examination is normal. The CSF shows a pleocytosis with protein elevation.

Transverse Myelitis

Transverse myelitis is an inflammatory, demyelinating process that develops over hours to days in patients without evidence of a compressive lesion. Transverse myelitis can occur alone (known as clinically isolated syndrome) or as part of other demyelinating diseases, including neuromyelitis optica, acute disseminated encephalomyelitis, or multiple sclerosis. Patients usually present with acute paraparesis, paresthesia (bilateral segmental sensory loss below the level of inflammation), sphincter dysfunction, absent deep tendon reflexes, and extensor plantar responses.

Spinal Cord Pathology

Spinal cord lesions can produce acute weakness with either paraplegia or quadriplegia. Trauma is the most likely cause. Patients with Down syndrome or rheumatoid arthritis are particularly susceptible to C1 to C2 subluxation, which can result in quadriparesis. The presence of fever and vertebral tenderness strongly suggests a spinal epidural abscess, which is a neurosurgical emergency. Weakness can also be caused by paraspinal or spinal cord tumor with acute cord compression, spinal cord infarction (most common in the thoracic levels), or hemorrhage secondary to arteriovenous malformation.

Infantile Botulism

Botulism (pp. 379–380) causes a fairly rapid progression of cranial nerve dysfunction (diplopia, ptosis, pupillary dilation, dysarthria, dysphagia) and weakness. With infantile botulism there is a history of constipation, followed by a subacute progression of bulbar and extremity weakness, presenting as a symmetric ascending paralysis, inability to suck and swallow, and ptosis, which may progress to generalized flaccidity and respiratory compromise.

Tick Paralysis

A toxin released by dog and wood ticks prevents the release of acetylcholine at nerve endings, causing a rapidly progressive (12–48 hours), ascending, generalized paralysis. Deep tendon reflexes are depressed or absent and there may also be mild facial muscle weakness, dysarthria, dysphagia, ptosis, double vision, and respiratory compromise.

Tick paralysis must be considered in the differential diagnosis of any child presenting with acute ataxia, which is quickly followed by acute ascending paralysis, especially during the late spring and summer seasons. In contrast to Guillain-Barré syndrome, there is no elevation of the CSF protein. A high index of suspicion is imperative as any delay of diagnosis and treatment may result in life-threatening respiratory failure.

Metabolic Causes

Metabolic causes (hypokalemia, hypo- and hypercalcemia, hypo- and hyperthyroidism) typically have associated systemic manifestations. Episodic paralysis, particularly during rest after exercise, suggests periodic paralysis, especially if there is a positive family history.

Other Causes

Acute or subacute weakness with a rash, fever, and myalgias suggests an inflammatory process such as dermatomyositis, polymyositis, or systemic lupus erythematosus. Certain toxins, especially the anticholinesterase-inhibiting insecticides (organophosphates, carbamates), cause acute weakness.

Psychogenic Causes

Consider psychogenic causes when the history and physical examination fail to suggest an organic etiology or the neurologic examination shows neurophysiologic inconsistencies. There may be a history of a stressful precipitating event or situation.

ED Management

Ask about change in voice (nasal voice), dysphagia, shortness of breath, bladder fullness, constipation, or incontinence of urine or stool. Perform a careful neurologic examination to define the extent, pattern, fluctuation, and fatigability of the weakness, and document any associated sensory findings (particularly a sensory level). Neck flexion/extension weakness may be a sign of impending respiratory compromise, as C3–C5 also innervate the diaphragm. Check the rectal tone and percuss or obtain an ultrasound of the bladder for fullness secondary to urinary retention. Examine the skin for a rash or a tick (often found hidden in hairy areas) and palpate muscles for pain. Evaluate for signs of respiratory distress, like paradoxical breathing. Ask the patient to count aloud as high as they can, after maximal inspiration, in one breath – each number equals about 100 mL in vital capacity. To assess the respiratory status, obtain an ABG, pulse oximetry, negative inspiratory force (<20 cm H_2O indicates respiratory weakness), and forced vital capacity (<20–25 mL/kg is worrisome).

Obtain a CBC, electrolytes, glucose, and urinalysis. If the patient is febrile, also check a blood culture and ESR. A lumbar puncture is indicated, particularly if Guillain-Barré syndrome is suspected, but it can be delayed until after consulting a pediatric neurologist. Obtain an MRI of the spine, with contrast, if the patient has signs and symptoms suggestive of spinal cord pathology. Potentially life-threatening spinal cord lesions are located in the upper cervical cord, which can affect the nerves innervating the pharyngeal muscles and diaphragm, and upper thoracic lesions above T6, which can result in autonomic dysreflexia and lead to hypertension, bradycardia, diaphoresis, and urinary retention.

Admit a patient with Guillain-Barré syndrome, myasthenic crisis, acute transverse myelitis, or acute flaccid myelitis to the intensive care unit, as respiratory compromise can occur acutely. Consult a neurologist, who may recommend plasmapheresis, high-dose IV gamma globulin (2 g/kg divided over 2–5 days), or IV methylprednisolone (30 mg/kg/day, 1 g/day maximum). However, during a myasthenic crisis, IV steroids can cause initial worsening of weakness, even though high-dose prednisone is used as a maintenance treatment.

To diagnose myasthenia gravis at bedside, perform a Tensilon (edrophonium chloride) test in consultation with a pediatric neurologist. Another diagnostic maneuver is to apply a cold pack to the eyelids. If the patient has myasthenia, the ptosis may improve.

The management of the trauma victim is detailed on pp. 749–758, but if there is any history of trauma, stabilize the patient in a neutral position. Obtain the appropriate spine films (cervical, areas of tenderness), and consult neurosurgery.

If a spinal epidural abscess or spinal cord compression is suspected, obtain an urgent neurosurgery and neurology consultation.

See pp. 379–380 for the treatment of botulism.

For tick paralysis, remove the tick, including the mouth parts; if these are left behind, toxin may continue to release into the host. Symptoms resolve quickly with treatment, estimated around 1.5 days.

Arrange for psychological counseling if the weakness is determined to be psychogenic.

Indications for Admission

- Acute weakness of any etiology, including suspected psychogenic weakness if unable to ambulate.

Bibliography

Messacar K, Schreiner TL, Van Haren K, et al. Acute flaccid myelitis: a clinical review of US cases 2012–2015. *Ann Neurol.* 2016;**80**:326–338.

Pecina CA. Tick paralysis. *Semin Neurol.* 2012;**32**:531–532.

Sieb JP. Myasthenia gravis: an update for the clinician. *Clin Exper Immunol.* 2014;**175**:425–438.

Willison HJ, Jacobs BC, van Doorn PA. Guillain-Barré syndrome. *Lancet.* 2016;**388**:717–727.

Wolf VL, Lupo PJ, Lotze TE. Pediatric acute transverse myelitis overview and differential diagnosis. *J Child Neurol.* 2012;**27**:1426–1436.

Anti-NMDA Receptor Encephalitis

The understanding of pediatric acute neuropsychiatric syndromes has expanded since the discovery of the N-methyl-D-aspartate (NMDA) receptor antibody and other antibody-mediated autoimmune encephalopathies. Although the differential diagnoses of acute neuropsychiatric disorders is broad, most of these diseases are reversible with proper treatment. Therefore, it is extremely important to expeditiously diagnose these disorders.

Clinical Presentation

Anti-NMDA receptor encephalitis presents with the rapid onset (less than three months) of the following major groups of symptoms:

- abnormal (psychiatric) behavior or cognitive dysfunction;
- speech dysfunction (pressured speech, verbal reduction, mutism);
- seizures, either focal or generalized;
- movement disorder, dyskinesias, or rigidity/abnormal postures;
- decreased level of consciousness;
- autonomic dysfunction or central hypoventilation.

Teenagers usually present with abnormal behavior (psychosis, delusions, hallucinations, agitations, aggression, catatonia) followed by sleep problems and movement disorders. Compared to the teenagers, young children more frequently present with seizures and abnormal movements.

Diagnosis

Consider anti-NMDA receptor encephalitis if the patient presents with the rapid onset (under three months) of a combination of abnormal (psychiatric) behavior or cognitive dysfunction, speech dysfunction, seizures, movement disorder, altered level of consciousness, and autonomic dysfunction. The definite diagnosis requires IgG anti-GluN1 antibodies and reasonable exclusion of other disorders such as meningitis and encephalitis.

ED Management

If an acute neuropsychiatric syndrome is suspected, consult a neurologist who will direct the evaluation. In general, an MRI with and without gadolinium is indicated, although it can sometimes be normal. Urgently obtain a head CT if the patient has focal weakness, cranial nerve palsy or ataxia. If the CT is normal, perform a lumbar puncture for cell count and differential, protein, glucose, bacterial culture, HSV PCR, autoimmune encephalopathy panel (which includes testing for NMDA receptor antibodies), oligoclonal bands, and IgG index, and save at least 2–3 mL of CSF to send for further investigations, based on MRI findings.

Once the studies are obtained, start antibiotics (meningitic doses) and acyclovir if there are white cells in the CSF.

Indications for Admission

- Altered mental status
- Autonomic dysfunction

- Psychosis
- CSF pleocytosis

Bibliography

Graus F, Titulaer MJ, Balu R, et al. A clinical approach to diagnosis of autoimmune encephalitis. *Lancet Neurol*. 2016;**15**(4):391–404.

Hacohen Y, Wright S, Waters P, et al. Paediatric autoimmune encephalopathies: clinical features, laboratory investigations and outcomes in patients with or without antibodies to known central nervous system autoantigens. *J Neurol Neurosurg Psychiatry*. 2013;**84**(7):748–755.

Suleiman J, Brilot F, Lang B, Vincent A, Dale RC. Autoimmune epilepsy in children: case series and proposed guidelines for identification. *Epilepsia*. 2013;**54**(6):1036–1045.

Van Mater H. Pediatric inflammatory brain diseases: a diagnostic approach. *Curr Opin Rheumatol*. 2014;**26**(5):553–561.

Breath-Holding Spells

Breath-holding spells are common (about 5% incidence) paroxysmal nonepileptic events of infancy, which typically begin at 6–18 months and disappear by six years in 90% of cases. Spell frequency can range from several per day, to once per year, but the majority have 1–6 spells per week. In 30% of cases, there is a positive family history of breath-holding. Although the physiologic basis of breath-holding is unclear, the episodes are not associated with an increased risk of epilepsy.

Clinical Presentation

The term breath-holding is a misnomer, as these episodes are involuntary and occur during expiration. Breath-holding spells are brief, lasting about 30 seconds. They are classified based on color change – cyanotic or pallid. A child generally has only one type of spell.

Cyanotic Spell

A cyanotic spell is often preceded by vigorous crying, which may be due to anger, frustration, fear, or pain. The child becomes silent and holds their breath in expiration, followed by a rapid onset of cyanosis and loss of consciousness, sometimes accompanied by limpness, rigid limbs, or opisthotonos.

Pallid Spell

A pallid spell is triggered by sudden fright, pain, or minor head trauma. The child may gasp or cry briefly, stops breathing, loses consciousness, and becomes pale and limp. Clonic jerks may be noted at the end of a more severe episode. Pallid breath-holding spells are due to an exaggerated vagal response, leading to cerebral hypoperfusion.

Diagnosis

The diagnosis is made from the history, as the patient usually appears well and back to baseline upon arrival in the ED. Breath-holding spells are often confused with seizures, but convulsions generally do not have an external precipitating factor, such as sustained crying or minor injury. Also, spells may be confused with syncopal episodes. Fainting is very unusual in young children, however, and is not usually associated with rigidity or opisthotonos.

ED Management

If the history of the event is typical and a thorough neurologic examination is normal, reassure the family about the benign, self-resolving nature of the episodes (no risk of epilepsy). Children with breath-holding spells have normal developmental and intellectual outcomes. Advise the parents to place the child in the lateral recumbent position during a spell. As iron-deficiency anemia has been associated with breath-holding spells, check CBC and ferritin level, and treat with iron as indicated. Spells resolve in 50% of patients on iron therapy. As these convulsive spells are nonepileptic, anticonvulsants are not indicated.

If the history is unusual or unclear, obtain a CBC, fingerstick glucose, basic chemistry panel, calcium, and perform an ECG with rhythm strip to rule-out a prolonged QT syndrome (see Syncope, pp. 79–82, and Cyanosis, pp. 70–71). If a seizure cannot be ruled out from the history, or there is a long post-ictal period, ask about a family history of epilepsy, inquire about developmental delay, examine for focal neurologic signs or neurocutaneous stigmata (café-au-lait macules or ash leaf spots), advise the family to take a video of further episodes, schedule a routine EEG, and refer to neurology.

Follow-up

- Suspicion for seizures, such as spells associated with a prolonged post-ictal period: pediatric neurology follow-up in 2–4 weeks

Indications for Admission

- Cyanotic episode that cannot be confidently diagnosed as a breath-holding spell

Bibliography

Goldman RD. Breath-holding spells in infants. *Can Fam Physician.* 2015;**61**(2):149–150.

Rathore G, Larsen P, Fernandez C, et al. Diverse presentation of breath holding spells: two case reports with literature review. *Case Rep Neurol Med.* 2013;**2013**:1–4.

Robinson JA, Bos JM, Etheridge SP, Ackerman MJ. Breath holding spells in children with long QT syndrome. *Congenit Heart Dis.* 2015;**10**(4):354–361.

Tieder JS, Bonkowsky JL, Etzel RA, et al. Brief resolved unexplained events (formerly apparent life-threatening events) and evaluation of lower-risk infants. *Pediatrics.* 2016;**137**:e1–32.

Coma

Terms describing mental status are often misused, with variable meanings to different medical providers. The neurologic definitions of these terms, in order of decreasing level of arousal, follow.

Lethargy

Lethargy is severe drowsiness, with difficulty maintaining an aroused state. The patient can be aroused by moderate stimuli and answers questions when addressed, but will drift to sleep without continual stimulation.

Obtundation

The obtunded patient can slowly respond to verbal or tactile stimuli and follow simple commands, but is never alert between sleep states.

Stupor

The stuporous patient responds only to vigorous/painful and repeated stimuli. When undisturbed, the patient lapses back into an unresponsive state.

Coma

Coma is a state of sustained pathologic unarousable unresponsiveness, with eyes closed, and with no response to noxious external or internal stimuli. This state must persist for at least one hour, and is due to dysfunction of the reticular activating system in the brainstem or bilateral cerebral hemispheres. Coma may result from medical (toxic-metabolic) causes or structural lesions. Distinguishing between metabolic causes and mass lesions is critical, as structural causes of coma may require emergent neurosurgical intervention, while metabolic coma can usually be managed medically.

Toxic-Metabolic

These derangements depress the cerebral hemispheres, and often brainstem structures as well. They may be due to endogenous substances (uremia, liver failure, respiratory failure, diabetic ketoacidosis), exogenous toxins (salicylates, tricyclics, sedatives, carbon monoxide, narcotics, anticonvulsants), cerebral hypoxia or hypoperfusion, hypoglycemia, or hyperammonemia. Also, subclinical seizures (nonconvulsive status epilepticus) may resemble coma.

Structural-Supratentorial

Supratentorial mass lesions exert compressive forces on the cerebral hemispheres as well as brainstem structures. Large lesions of the dominant hemisphere alone can induce coma. In children, the most common mass lesion leading to coma is intracranial bleeding and swelling due to head trauma. Tumors, spontaneous hemorrhages, and ischemic strokes are less common.

Structural-Infratentorial

These infiltrate or compress brainstem structures, such as the ascending reticular activating system. They may cause hydrocephalus and increased intracranial pressure due to obstruction of the fourth ventricle.

Infection

Meningitis, encephalitis, and septic shock may also present with coma.

Clinical Presentation and Diagnosis

Neurologic evaluation of the unconscious patient includes level of consciousness, brainstem reflexes, motor response, and breathing pattern.

Level of Consciousness

Level of consciousness can be evaluated by the Glasgow Coma Scale (GCS), which is widely used. The GCS has some limitations due to weighting toward motor scores and not including brainstem reflexes, which may indicate the severity of coma (see Head Trauma, pp. 521–527). To address these limitations, a new "Full Outline of UnResponsiveness" score includes eye responses, motor responses, brainstem reflexes, and respiration. In children, both of these scores are good predictors for in-hospital mortality and functional outcome, without a significant difference.

Cranial Nerves

Evaluation of the cranial nerves includes fundoscopy, pupillary size and responses, corneal reflex, oculocephalic reflex, gag, and cough reflex. Fundoscopy could reveal retinal hemorrhages or papilledema, suggestive of intracranial hypertension. Pinpoint pupils indicate pontine injury, usually from hemorrhage or infarction. An asymmetric fixed and dilated pupil suggests a focal structural lesion. Small, sluggish pupils can be seen in the earliest stage of central herniation, or also metabolic coma. A few medical states can produce nonreactive pupils (Table 15.3). Roving eye movements are seen in cortical depression, with an intact brainstem. Nystagmoid eye movements may indicate nonconvulsive status epilepticus. Depressed vestibulo-ocular reflexes may be the result of psychoactive or antiepileptic medications.

To test EOMs, perform the oculocephalic reflex (doll's eye maneuver) if no head or neck trauma is suspected. Intact doll's eyes are manifested by transient conjugate deviation away from the direction of rapid head rotation. Absent EOMs with the oculocephalic reflex can occur in an awake patient, while asymmetric EOMs suggests a structural lesion. To assess the vestibuloocular reflex in a trauma patient, ensure there is no trauma to the external auditory canal and tympanum before performing cold caloric testing. A normal response to cold-water vestibular stimulation is conjugate eye deviation toward the stimulated ear. Never perform cold calorics on a patient who is awake, as it causes severe vertigo, nausea, and vomiting.

Motor Function

Assess motor function by first observing any spontaneous movements or posturing. Next evaluate the response to verbal commands, gentle tactile stimulation, and then noxious stimulation (sternal rub or pressure to the nail bed, supraorbital ridge, or posterior

Table 15.3 Toxic-metabolic causes of fixed pupils

Cause	Pupils	Diagnosis/Characteristics
Anoxia	Fixed, dilated	Antecedent history of shock, cardiac or respiratory arrest
Anticholinergics (tricyclics, atropine)	Fixed, dilated	Tachycardia, QRS >0.12 seconds Warm, dry skin
Barbiturates, glutethimide	May be mid-sized or fixed and dilated	History of overdose
Cholinergics (organophosphates)	Small with barely perceptible reflex	Diaphoresis, vomiting, incontinence, lacrimation
Hypothermia	May be fixed	History of exposure
Opiates (heroin)	Very small with barely perceptible reflex	History of overdose, needle marks

mandibular ramus). Determine if responses are reflexic (triple flexion at leg, extensor posturing) or purposeful (move away from the noxious stimulus). Symmetric posturing in decorticate (arm flexion) or decerebrate (arm extension) positions may occur in structural and metabolic comas. Progression from purposeful motor responses to posturing and then to flaccidity suggests a structural lesion. Asymmetric posturing, motor responses, tone, or deep tendon reflexes are also suggestive of a structural etiology. However, focal neurologic findings may be seen in any metabolic encephalopathy (uremia, hypercalcemia, hepatic encephalopathy, and especially hypoglycemia), as these metabolic derangements may provoke signs and symptoms of previously subclinical lesions.

Breathing Pattern

Breathing patterns are challenging to interpret but may help localize the lesion. Pontine or midbrain lesions can cause neurogenic hyperventilation. Clustered breathing can be associated with injury to the pons, and ataxic or absence of spontaneous breathing is seen in medullary lesions.

Structural Versus Metabolic Coma

The *presence* of asymmetric (lateralizing) findings on examination helps to make the diagnosis of a structural lesion, but the *absence* of asymmetry does not rule-out a structural lesion, particularly in the case of midline lesions. If a metabolic cause of coma is not apparent from the history or initial examination, obtain a noncontrast head CT once the patient has been stabilized, even in the absence of lateralizing findings or history of trauma. If there is a history or suspicion of head trauma, assume that there has been cervical spine injury and immobilize the neck and treat appropriately until cervical trauma has been definitively ruled out (pp. 741–743).

Nonconvulsive status is suggested by subtle findings such as eye deviation, nystagmus, twitching, or changes in tone.

ED Management

The priority is evaluating the ABCs and stabilization of the vital signs, and protecting the airway, if necessary (intubation). Administer 100% oxygen, establish IV access, and give 20 mL/kg boluses of isotonic fluid to a hypotensive patient. If there are signs of focality on the neurologic examination (dilated unreactive pupil, asymmetric eye movements, asymmetric motor responses), obtain a head CT. If the CT is negative, consult a neurologist to evaluate for possible nonconvulsive seizures.

Initial blood tests include a CBC, electrolytes, BUN, fingerstick glucose, and an ABG. If the cause is unknown, also obtain a serum osmolality, PT, PTT, liver function tests, ammonia, urine drug screen, serum levels of toxins associated with altered mental status (barbiturates, ethanol, salicylates), and blood culture. Save an additional red-top tube for future analysis. Give all patients naloxone (0.1 mg/kg), and if the glucose is <80 mg/dL or unknown, give IV glucose (5 mL/kg D_{10} W or 2 mL/kg D_{25}) for diagnostic and therapeutic purposes.

If a structural coma is suspected, management is as described for head trauma (pp. 521–527), including an emergency CT scan to identify the lesion.

If a structural etiology is ruled out by head CT and meningitis is suspected (pp. 422–425), perform a lumbar puncture and administer appropriate antibiotics immediately. If the CT is delayed, give the antibiotics prior to obtaining CSF.

The general approach to a toxic-metabolic coma requires supporting the vital signs and correcting abnormalities in acid–base, electrolytes, and glucose. A toxic ingestion may require gastrointestinal decontamination and supportive therapy (pp. 450–452).

When the cause of the coma is unknown and the vital signs are stable, treatment can be directed by the results of the examination as outlined above. Consult a neurologist if there is concern for nonconvulsive status epilepticus.

Indications for Admission

- All comatose patients to the ICU

Bibliography

Kirkham FJ. Indications for the performance of neuroimaging in children. *Handb Clin Neurol.* 2016;**136**:1275–1290.

Kochar GS, Gulati S, Lodha R, et al. Full outline of UnResponsiveness score versus Glasgow Coma Scale in children with nontraumatic impairment of consciousness. *J Child Neurol.* 2014;**29**:1299–1304.

MacNeill EC, Vashist S. Approach to syncope and altered mental status. *Pediatr Clin North Am.* 2013;**60**(5):1083–1106.

Seshia SS, Bingham WT, Sadanand V. Nontraumatic coma in children and adolescents: diagnosis and management. *Neurol Clin.* 2011;**29**:1007–1043.

Stevens RD, Cadena RS, Pineda J. Emergency neurological life support: approach to the patient with coma. *Neurocrit Care.* 2015;**23**:S69–S75.

Facial Weakness

CN VII has the longest intraosseous course of any cranial nerve, thus is it the most susceptible to injury or infection. The most common presentation of CN VII dysfunction in children is a peripheral facial palsy. In such cases, the lesion is in the facial nerve nucleus or the peripheral nerve distal to the nucleus, so both the upper and lower halves of the face are affected (including the frontalis muscle). A peripheral CN VII palsy may be congenital, or caused by trauma, infections (Lyme disease, varicella, otitis, mastoiditis, parotitis, infectious mononucleosis), parainfectious phenomena (associated with Guillain-Barré syndrome), and neoplasms (neurofibromatosis, cerebellopontine angle tumors). A peripheral facial palsy of unknown origin is termed a Bell's palsy. Along with muscles of facial expression, CN VII is involved with taste on the anterior two-thirds of the tongue, salivary and lacrimal glands, and stapedius muscle in the inner ear.

A central facial palsy affects only the lower half of the face, sparing the frontalis muscle. It is secondary to a lesion in the contralateral cerebral hemisphere, most commonly caused by stroke, demyelinating disease, or tumor.

Clinical Presentation

Except for acute trauma, most peripheral facial palsies evolve over 24–48 hours, and may be preceded or accompanied by pain around or behind the ear, which can be severe and may be the presenting complaint. Along with asymmetry of the face, the patient may have other signs of CN VII involvement, including hyperacusis, decreased tearing of the ipsilateral eye, impaired taste, or difficulty eating or drinking. Often there is a feeling of numbness or tingling over the affected side of the face.

A central facial palsy is not accompanied by hyperacusis or alteration of taste. In contrast to a peripheral CN VII palsy, patients can wrinkle their forehead and elevate their eyebrow. With a vascular origin, the onset may be acute.

Diagnosis

Acute trauma and congenital causes of facial weakness can usually be excluded by findings from the history and examination. On general examination, check the external auditory canals and tympanic membranes for signs of infection (otitis, mastoiditis, or vesicular lesions associated with varicella or herpes simplex). Look for a rash (erythema migrans with Lyme disease, varicella, herpes) and café-au-lait macules (neurofibromatosis). Palpate for generalized adenopathy and splenomegaly (infectious mononucleosis), and evaluate the joints (particularly the knee in Lyme disease).

Perform a careful neurologic examination to rule-out other neurologic etiologies (Guillain-Barré syndrome). Test the cranial nerves, motor strength, and deep tendon reflexes. To determine if the weakness is peripheral or central, note whether the patient can wrinkle the forehead. If there is concern for a central facial palsy, examine for hemiparesis and aphasia (can manifest as mutism).

Lyme Disease

Most facial nerve palsies are unilateral; however, if bilateral facial weakness, suspect Lyme disease (pp. 417–420). Predictors of Lyme disease include symptoms in peak Lyme season, fever, headache, and absence of previous herpetic lesions. If the patient has a history of a recent tick bite or lives in an area where Lyme disease is endemic, obtain blood for a Lyme titer. Also perform a lumbar puncture if there is a history of headache, or if other cranial nerve deficits are noted. If there is CSF pleocytosis, administer IV ceftriaxone (100 mg/kg/day, maximum 4 g/day). The lumbar puncture may be deferred in the absence of headache, stiff neck, and other neurologic deficits.

Other Infectious Etiologies

Many patients with negative Lyme titers will have clinical evidence of HSV infection. Acute peripheral facial nerve palsy and vesicular lesion of the auricle or oropharyngeal mucosa defines Ramsay Hunt syndrome, attributed to varicella zoster virus. Other infections implicated in facial palsy include EBV, CMV, mumps, rubella, *M. pneumoniae*, and Coxsackievirus.

Bell's Palsy

Bell's palsy is a *diagnosis of exclusion* if no other cause of a peripheral CN VII palsy is evident.

ED Management

If the patient has eye pain or discomfort, perform a fluorescein dye test (p. 549) to rule-out a corneal abrasion. To prevent drying of the cornea of the affected eye, recommend artificial tears (1–2 drops qid, or as needed) during the day, and lubricating eye ointment and an eye patch to be worn at night. If the patient cannot cover the entire cornea with a blink, patch the eye and refer him or her to an ophthalmologist. Do not permit the patient to wear contact lenses.

If Lyme disease is suspected, obtain a Lyme titer and treat for three weeks with either amoxicillin (<8 years old; 40 mg/kg/day div tid) or doxycycline (≥8 years old; 100 mg bid). The management of otitis media (pp. 143–147), mastoiditis (pp. 154–155), Guillain-Barré syndrome (pp. 502–505), infectious mononucleosis (pp. 425–427), head trauma (pp. 521–527), and increased intracranial pressure (pp. 527–529) is discussed elsewhere. The presence of facial nerve weakness does not usually alter the treatment of the primary illness. If facial nerve palsy associated with an otitis media does not improve after two days of oral antibiotics, arrange for tympanocentesis, culture the middle ear fluid, and admit the patient for IV antibiotics (cefuroxime, 100 mg/kg/day div q 8h).

If the patient is seen within 48 hours of the onset of a peripheral facial weakness and the most likely diagnosis is idiopathic Bell's palsy, give a 5–7-day course of prednisone (2 mg/kg/day, 60 mg/day maximum). Ensure that the patient does not have other associated cranial nerve palsies or evidence of bacterial infection, as the steroids may mask a tumor or infection. Steroids have not been shown to affect the long-term prognosis of palsy resolution, but may hasten recovery and relieve associated pain. Treatment with antivirals is controversial, but administer valacyclovir or acyclovir if there is suspicion for HSV. If there is no improvement noted within three weeks (85% experience some recovery by this time), refer the patient to a neurologist for electromyography.

If the weakness is central and of new onset, consult a pediatric neurologist and obtain a head CT. Neuroimaging is indicated if facial palsy is slowly progressive or associated with other cranial nerve palsies.

The prognosis of peripheral facial weakness varies with the severity of the initial palsy; approximately 80% of patients recover completely, generally within two months, and improvement usually begins within 1–2 weeks of diagnosis.

Follow-up

- Peripheral facial weakness, including Lyme disease: 2–3 days, to check the affected eye and follow-up on laboratory tests

Indications for Admission

- Acute facial nerve palsy associated with progressive weakness, evidence of a mass lesion, CNS infection, intracranial hypertension, acute trauma, or other CNS signs

Bibliography

Lorch M, Teach SJ. Facial nerve palsy: etiology and approach to diagnosis and treatment. *Pediatr Emer Care*. 2010;**26**:763–772.

Malik V, Joshi V, Green KM, Bruce IA. 15 minute consultation: a structured approach to the management of facial paralysis in a child. *Arch Dis Child Educ Pract Ed*. 2012;**97**(3):82–85.

Özkale Y, Erol I, Saygi S, et al. Overview of pediatric peripheral facial nerve paralysis: analysis of 40 patients. *J Child Neurol*. 2015;**30**:193–199.

Vakharia K, Vakharia K. Bell's palsy. *Facial Plast Surg Clin N Am*. 2016;**24**:1–10.

Youshani AS, Mehta B, Davies K, et al. Management of Bell's palsy in children: an audit of current practice, review of the literature and a proposed management algorithm. *Emerg Med J.* 2015;**32**:274–280.

Headache

There are many causes of headache in childhood (Table 15.4). Fortunately, most are benign, such as migraine, tension-type, or chronic daily headache. However, many serious life-threatening illnesses can present with headache and must be considered before the patient is discharged from the ED.

Clinical Presentation

Although the following clinical entities are discussed individually, keep in mind that many patients have headaches that do not easily fit into one particular category and some have multiple different headache types (i.e., chronic tension-type headaches in patient who also has migraines).

Common Benign Causes of Headache

Migraine

Migraine is the most common type of headache in children of any age. In children, the incidence is equal between boys and girls, although females are generally more affected in adolescence. In 70–90% of cases, there is a family history of migraine in a first-degree relative. Migraine attacks may be triggered by stress, exercise, head trauma (which may be so insignificant that it is forgotten), skipping meals, particular foods, drugs, strong sunlight or odors, hormonal changes associated with the menstrual cycle and pregnancy, and possibly allergies. The duration of migraine headache is at least four hours in adolescents, but may be as short as 30 minutes in young children, and the frequency is widely variable ranging from one migraine per year to several per week. Patients with migraine are frequently treated with antibiotics for "sinus headache" before the diagnosis of migraine is finally considered.

Migraine Without Aura

Migraine without aura (previously common migraine) is not preceded by any visual, olfactory, or somatosensory aura and may be unilateral or bilateral. The headache is described as pulsating or throbbing, may be paroxysmal in onset or arise in the setting of a preexisting tension-type headache, and may be accompanied by photophobia, phonophobia, nausea, vomiting, and a desire to sleep or rest in a quiet, dark room.

Migraine With Aura

Migraine with aura (previously classic migraine) is characterized by recurrent attacks of fully reversible aura symptoms, which commonly entail scintillating lights, scotomata, blurry vision, visual hallucinations, or, rarely, an unusual alteration of body image known as the Alice-in-Wonderland syndrome. The accompanying headache is pulsatile and usually unilateral, although it may alternate sides. If the headache is always on the same side, there is greater concern about the possibility of an underlying intracranial lesion.

Table 15.4 Etiologies of headache

Benign causes of headache

Migraine

Migraine without aura (common)

Migraine with aura (classic)

Less common migraine syndromes

Acute confusional migraine

Basilar migraine

Cyclic vomiting

Hemiplegic migraine

Ophthalmoplegic migraine

Chronic tension-type headache

Stress-related

Posttraumatic headache

Visual abnormalities[1]

Exo-/esophoria causing alignment difficulty

Headache due to increased ICP

Brain abscess

Brain tumor

Carbon monoxide poisoning

Cerebral venous sinus thrombosis

Head trauma

Idiopathic intracranial hypertension

Ventriculoperitoneal shunt obstruction

Infection-related causes of headache

Bacterial meningitis

Dental infection

Group A *Streptococcus*

Influenza

Lyme disease

Mycoplasma pneumoniae

Sinusitis

Systemic infection

Viral ("aseptic") meningitis

---

[1] Not caused by uncorrected refractive errors.

Migraine Variants

Migraine variants may present with hemiplegia, ophthalmoplegia, ptosis, an acute confusional state, or recurrent vomiting. These manifestations may or may not be accompanied by headache and are diagnoses of exclusion. In most cases, the neurologic deficits are transient, so the presence of persistent neurologic impairment requires further investigation to exclude stroke.

Chronic Tension-Type Headache

This category of headache includes the headaches formerly known as "muscle contraction headache," "tension headache," and "psychogenic headache." The headaches are generally prolonged, may be waxing and waning in intensity, and are not preceded by an aura or accompanied by any neurologic deficits. The pain is described as dull, achy, or tight, and usually begins in the occipital region; however, it may move anteriorly to the vertex or the frontal region. The headaches typically occur in the late afternoon or evening and are relieved by mild analgesics such as acetaminophen. Unlike migraines, these headaches rarely interrupt normal activities. They may be triggered by a recent emotional or traumatic event and may be associated with personality changes, as evidenced by poor school performance, sleep disturbances, aggression, lack of energy, and self-deprecatory behavior.

Heterophorias

An exo- or esophoria that forces the patient to continually exert effort to align the eyes may cause headache. Typically, the onset is in the afternoon or evening after concentrated visual activity such as reading. Unlike heterotropia (constant misalignment of the eyes), heterophorias may be difficult to appreciate on physical exam without specific testing. Pure refractive errors such as myopia are usually not associated with headache.

Temporomandibular Joint Dysfunction (TMJD)

Disorders of TMJD may present with headache. Patients with bruxism and habitual gum chewers are at increased risk. The headache of TMJD may be associated with jaw or ear pain, locking of the jaw, or inability to open the mouth.

Posttraumatic Headache

Early-onset posttraumatic headache is common after minor head trauma. The headache may initially be isolated to the area of impact, but often becomes generalized, and may be associated with vomiting and/or somnolence. There are no focal neurologic deficits or signs of increased intracranial pressure (ICP), but the patient may have amnesia for the events surrounding the trauma. Headache with onset minutes to days after significant head trauma may be due to an epidural or subdural hematoma. Worrisome signs are a decreasing level of consciousness, projectile vomiting, and symptoms of increased ICP (bulging fontanelle, split sutures, unequal pupils, sixth nerve palsy, hypertension with bradycardia). Head trauma (pp. 521–527) and increased ICP (pp. 527–529) are discussed elsewhere.

Occasionally, posttraumatic headache may continue for prolonged periods (weeks to years), while migraines can be triggered by head trauma in a susceptible person. Psychogenic factors or the possibility of secondary gain may be involved.

Infection-Related Causes of Headache

Sinusitis

The headache of sinusitis (pp. 168–169) may be referred to the upper teeth, the cheek, or the frontal, or retro-orbital area. Associated symptoms include cough, mucopurulent nasal discharge, fever, and facial pain/tenderness. The pain typically occurs in the early morning and is accentuated by leaning forward.

Dental Infection

A dental infection (pp. 84–87) causes pain in the cheek or mandibular area as well as temporal headaches. The infected tooth or gum may be sensitive upon percussion or manipulation.

Systemic Infection

Systemic infections, such as group A *Streptococcus* infection, influenza, and *Mycoplasma* pneumonia, can cause a headache in addition to other symptoms (fever, sore throat, cough, coryza, conjunctivitis, or myalgias). Early Lyme disease (pp. 417–420) may present with headache, in addition to the distinctive rash, arthralgias, lethargy, and behavioral changes.

Meningitis

The headache of bacterial meningitis is generalized, constant, often described as "throbbing all over," and associated with fever, toxicity, nuchal rigidity (in older children), and other meningeal signs. Viral meningitis causes a similar presentation, usually during summertime epidemics. Even in older children, the absence of nuchal rigidity does not rule-out meningitis, particularly early in the course of infection.

Headache Caused by Increased ICP

Brain Abscess

A patient with a brain abscess may present with a nonspecific headache, usually accompanied by fever. Vomiting, diplopia, motor weakness, seizures (focal or generalized), and altered mental status may be present. Most intracranial abscesses are caused by direct extension from an adjacent infected focus such as ethmoid or frontal sinusitis or chronic otitis media. However, approximately one-third of cases are due to trauma to the head or face, or result from hematogenous spread of a distal infection.

Brain Tumor

The headache of a brain tumor is intermittent initially but very quickly increases in frequency and severity. It is often present in the very early-morning hours and may awaken the child from sleep, as lying supine slows the drainage of CSF, increasing ICP. There may be associated projectile vomiting in the absence of nausea. Localization may be difficult, especially in the case of midline lesions. Occipital headache may indicate a posterior fossa lesion, although the pain is frequently referred to a frontotemporal location. Thus, frontal headache may accompany either a supratentorial or a posterior fossa tumor.

Idiopathic Intracranial Hypertension
A patient with idiopathic intracranial hypertension (IIH; formerly pseudotumor cerebri) usually presents with intermittent headaches, vomiting, blurred vision, papilledema, and occasionally diplopia. Altered level of consciousness is rarely observed. Obesity and use of tetracycline antibiotics are well-known risk factors for development of IIH in adolescents and adults.

Ventriculoperitoneal Shunt Obstruction
See pp. 537–538.

Cerebral Venous Sinus Thrombosis (CVST)
Headache occurs in up to 90% of patients with CVST and is generally a consequence of increased ICP. The headache is diffuse, often progresses in severity over days to weeks, and may be associated with blurry vision due to papilledema, or diplopia due to sixth nerve palsy. Additional neurologic deficits including seizures (focal or generalized), hemiparesis, aphasia, or altered mental status may be indicative of acute focal cerebral injury due to venous infarction or hemorrhage.

Diagnosis
Despite the wide spectrum of causes, most headaches are due to one of the common benign causes listed in Table 15.4. With the exception of children whose headaches are accompanied by severe nausea and vomiting, these patients are afebrile; appear awake, alert, and nontoxic; and have normal physical and neurologic exams.

The minority of headaches in children are secondary to a serious intracranial process. However, consider one of these conditions if the patient complains of sudden onset of acute, severe headache; headaches which are severe, progressive, and persistent for less than six months duration; headaches which interfere with sleep or waken the patient during the night or early morning; headaches associated with persistent vomiting; a recent history of head trauma; or a change in personality or behavior. The new onset of headaches in an immunosuppressed patient is also concerning.

Obtain a complete description of the headaches, including onset, triggers, duration, location, quality, usual time of day they occur, exacerbating or alleviating factors, and trajectory of severity and frequency (improving, worsening, stable). This information may be difficult to elicit, especially in a young child. Avoid suggesting possible descriptive terms to the preschool child, who may agree that all apply, even if they are mutually exclusive. Ask about recent emotional stress, personality changes, head trauma, warning signs (aura), family history of migraines, medications, and associated symptoms, including fever, nausea or vomiting, photophobia or visual disturbances, rash, nasal discharge or cough, and possible tick or carbon monoxide (CO) exposure. CO poisoning (pp. 466–467) is rare, but commonly causes headache, fatigue, and irritability. It may affect several family or group members simultaneously.

Measure the blood pressure and perform a complete physical examination, looking for fever, split sutures, bulging fontanelle, facial tenderness, gingival swelling, dental caries and tooth percussion sensitivity, otitis media, nuchal rigidity and meningeal signs, and signs of a systemic infection. A thorough neurologic exam is necessary, including ophthalmoscopy. Asymmetry of the pupils, EOMs, or motor response suggests a structural abnormality such

Table 15.5 Indications for CT in patients with headache

Focal neurologic abnormality including seizures

Head trauma with focal neurologic signs or lethargy

Papilledema

Paroxysmal onset of excruciating headache

Persistent vomiting

Recurrent morning headache

as a brain tumor, abscess, or intracranial hemorrhage (see Coma, pp. 508–512). Finally, check the visual acuity and visual fields, as a visual field defect may be the only neurological abnormality in a patient with a pituitary tumor or craniopharyngioma.

ED Management

The priority is expeditious diagnosis and treatment of a CSF infection or increased ICP. The management of a suspected mass lesion, meningitis, head trauma, IIH, sinusitis, systemic infection, and dental infection is discussed elsewhere in the appropriate sections.

Indications for CT of the head are listed in Table 15.5. However, a normal CT does not rule-out subarachnoid hemorrhage or increased ICP. Perform a lumbar puncture with measurement of the opening pressure if a subarachnoid hemorrhage or increased ICP is suspected. A urinalysis, CBC, blood glucose, or carboxyhemoglobin level may be indicated, based on the clinical presentation. Obtain a shunt series, CT scan, and neurosurgical consultation for a child with a VP shunt and severe headache.

The ED treatment of chronic tension-type headaches is limited to oral analgesics (acetaminophen 15 mg/kg q 4h, ibuprofen 10 mg/kg q 6h) and reassurance that a serious disease process is not underway. Refer the patient to a primary care setting, where the stresses contributing to the headaches can be addressed.

Migraines

Migraines can be chronic and debilitating. For that reason, avoid treating with narcotics and other habit-forming drugs, and give only mild analgesics (as above). If ibuprofen does not help, prescribe sumatriptan nasal spray, 5–20 mg, for acute migraine in patients over 12 years old. In addition, aggressive IV hydration, IV ketorolac 0.5 mg/ kg (30 mg maximum), IV or PR metoclopramide (0.1 mg/kg by slow IV push, 10 mg maximum) can relieve the headache and associated vomiting. Dystonic reactions or akathisia, although rare, are possible at even minimal doses of metoclopramide. Consult a neurologist if the headache does not respond to these measures.

Refer a patient with frequent or intractable migraines to a primary care setting or a pediatric neurologist. The ED is not an appropriate site for instituting therapy with ergotamines or prophylactic agents such as propranolol, verapamil, or amitriptyline.

Ask the family or patient to keep a headache diary. For each headache, record the time of onset, duration, location, quality, exacerbating and remitting factors, and note any other associations that may help to identify the type of headache, its temporal pattern, and triggers. Have the parents of young children record any spontaneous complaints of headache, but advise them to avoid eliciting spurious complaints by asking the child if he or she has a headache. Have the patient or family take the diary to the follow-up appointment.

Follow-up
- Migraine requiring ED treatment (other than acetaminophen or ibuprofen): 2–3 days. Otherwise, primary care follow-up in 1–2 weeks.

Indications for Admission
- Focal neurologic findings
- Intracranial hypertension
- Meningitis
- Acute confusional state
- Frontal sinusitis
- Severe headache after head trauma

Bibliography

Blume HK. Pediatric headache: a review. *Pediatr Rev.* 2012;33(12):562–576.

Caviness V, Ebinger F. Headache in pediatric practice. *Handb Clin Neurol.* 2013;112:827–838.

Gofshteyn JS, Stephenson DJ. Diagnosis and management of childhood headache. *Curr Probl Pediatr Adolesc Health Care.* 2016;46:36–51

Hershey AD. Pediatric headache. *Continuum.* 2015:21:1132–1145.

Rothner AD, Parikh S. Migraine variants or episodic syndromes that may be associated with migraine and other unusual pediatric headache syndromes. *Headache.* 2016;56(1):206–214.

Head Trauma
Head trauma is a very common injury in childhood, accounting for three-quarters of trauma admissions and 70% of trauma deaths. Serious head trauma most often results from falls from height, sports injuries, and bicycle, motorcycle, and automobile accidents. Consider child abuse (shaking, whiplash injuries) in infants and young children. Always consider the possibility of associated cervical spine injury (pp. 741–743) in a patient with head trauma.

Clinical Presentation
Most pediatric head trauma victims do not suffer serious injury, although soft tissue swelling or laceration is common. The most common scenario is a toddler who runs into an object or falls from his/her own height. Occasionally the patient is sleepy but fully arousable, with a neurologic examination that is otherwise normal.

A less obvious presentation is the young afebrile infant with a full fontanelle who is lethargic or vomiting. This may represent abusive head trauma (previously called shaken baby), with or without other physical evidence of abuse (pp. 604–608).

Serious signs and symptoms include persistent headache, repeated episodes of vomiting, ataxia, blurred vision, altered level of consciousness, focal neurologic signs, seizures, a compound skull fracture, or evidence of increased ICP.

Contact seizures occur at the moment or within seconds of the head trauma. Although frightening to observers, contact seizures are of no clinical significance. In contrast, early posttraumatic seizures occur one minute to one week after the head trauma, whereas late posttraumatic seizures occur one week or more after the injury. About 25% of children with early posttraumatic seizures have late seizures, and nearly 75% of children with late posttraumatic seizures develop epilepsy. Nearly all patients with penetrating head trauma eventually have the diagnosis of epilepsy.

Specific brain injuries include the following.

Concussion

This is a brain injury that is not demonstrable by radiographic studies but may be associated with transient confusion or loss of consciousness.

Contusion

A cerebral contusion is an area of focal edema with or without hemorrhage that can be seen on CT scan. There is usually loss of consciousness, and there may be focal deficits.

Epidural Hematoma

An epidural hematoma results from a tear in one of the meningeal arteries (middle meningeal is the most common site) or meningeal or diploic veins. A temporoparietal skull fracture is present in up to 75% of children. The classic presentation is a concussion followed by a lucid interval and then loss of consciousness associated with signs of increased ICP. However, this classic presentation occurs in only about one-third of patients. With a large epidural hematoma there may be ipsilateral pupillary dilation and, less commonly, contralateral decerebrate posturing.

Subdural Hematoma

With a subdural hematoma, there is tearing of the bridging veins between the cerebral cortex and the dura, with compression of the underlying brain. They are often associated with more widespread shear injury to the brain, and have high morbidity and mortality rates. A subdural hematoma can present with coma or seizures, or it may develop more slowly and be associated with nonspecific signs and symptoms of increased ICP. They are most common in infancy; in young children, the presence of a subdural hematoma suggests child abuse.

Diffuse Axonal Injury

This serious injury is produced when shearing forces generated by rapid acceleration-deceleration cause disruption of myelin and tearing of long axonal fibers. Very young children can also exhibit visible tears in the white matter. A CT scan reveals diffuse brain swelling, which develops over 24–48 hours, but no mass lesions.

Basilar Skull Fracture

Common fractures of the base of the skull include longitudinal or transverse fractures of the petrous portion of the temporal bone and fractures of the cribriform plate. Suspect petrous fractures when there is hemotympanum, Battle's sign (retroauricular ecchymosis over the mastoid), CSF otorrhea, facial palsy, or hearing loss. Hemorrhage in the nose or nasopharynx, CSF rhinorrhea, or anosmia suggests fracture through the cribriform plate. Basilar skull fractures are rarely seen on plain film. If one is suspected, obtain a noncontrast CT with thin cuts through the area of interest.

Diagnosis

The treatment of a serious head injury takes priority over obtaining the history and performing a complete physical examination. Determine the nature of the trauma, including whether the patient lost consciousness or cried immediately. Ask about vomiting, seizures, recollection of the event, activities both before and after the injury, and past medical problems (seizure disorder, neurologic handicap). Once the patient is medically stabilized, obtain a developmental history. Many victims of severe head trauma have a history of behavioral or developmental problems.

Perform a complete physical examination, including vital signs. Look for scalp lacerations and hematomas, a depressed skull fracture, and evidence of a basilar skull fracture (retro-auricular or periorbital ecchymoses, hemotympanum, serous or serosanguineous rhinorrhea or otorrhea). Consider the possibility of cervical spine injury in all cases (pp. 741–743), and check for sources of bleeding and other major injuries (see Multiple Trauma, pp. 749–758).

Head trauma *per se* does not cause hypotension, except in very young infants or patients with serious scalp lacerations. Hypotension demands an immediate, thorough evaluation of

Table 15.6 Glasgow Coma Scale*

	Score
Eyes open	
Spontaneously	4
To speech	3
To pain	2
None	1
Best verbal response	
Oriented	5
Confused	4
Inappropriate words	3
Incomprehensible sound	2
None	1
Best motor response	
Obeys	6
Localizes	5
Withdraws	4
Abnormal flexion	3
Abnormal extension	2
None	1

* Total GCS is the sum of the scores of the three parts.

Table 15.7 Modified Glasgow Coma Scale*

	Score
Eyes open	
Spontaneously	4
To speech	3
To pain	2
None	1
Best verbal response	
Coos and babbles	5
Irritable cries	4
Cries to pain	3
Moans to pain	2
None	1
Best motor response	
Normal spontaneous movements	6
Withdraws to touch	5
Withdraws to pain	4
Abnormal flexion	3
Abnormal extension	2
None	1

* Total GCS is the sum of the scores of the three parts.

the rest of the body (particularly chest, abdomen, pelvis, and thighs) for sources of blood loss. Tachycardia, particularly in association with a narrowed pulse pressure, suggests impending shock (pp. 28–35).

Hypertension, followed by bradycardia and then slow or irregular respirations (Cushing's triad) indicate increased intracranial pressure, although very young children may not exhibit the full triad. Hypertension may not develop, or may be a late finding shortly before herniation. Treatment must be instituted immediately (see pp. 527–528).

Perform a careful neurologic examination, paying careful attention to the signs of structural coma (pp. 508–512): asymmetry of pupillary responses, EOMs, or motor response. Examine the cranial nerves, perform ophthalmoscopy (for papilledema, or loss of spontaneous venous pulsations, or retinal hemorrhage), and test the reflexes, strength, sensation, and coordination, comparing one side to the other.

Test fluid draining from the ear or nose for glucose. CSF has glucose in it, while mucus does not. If the fluid is bloody, touch it with a piece of filter paper. Formation of two concentric rings suggests that CSF is mixed with the blood.

Table 15.8 Risk assignment based on clinical examination

Low-risk injuries (GCS = 15)

> Asymptomatic
>
> Dizziness
>
> Mild headache
>
> Normal neurologic examination
>
> Short-term vomiting (duration <4 hours)

Moderate-risk injuries (GCS = 9–14)

> Altered mental status (including drug
>   or alcohol intoxication)
>
> Associated injuries (long-bone fracture,
>   contusion of internal organs)
>
> Basilar skull fracture
>
> Early posttraumatic seizure
>
> History of loss of consciousness
>
> Persistent vomiting (duration ≥4 hours)
>
> Progressive headache
>
> Suspected child abuse

High-risk injuries (GCS <9)

> Depressed level of consciousness
>
> Focal neurologic examination
>
> Penetrating injury to brain

The GCS indicates the initial severity of the head injury and facilitates monitoring of changes in the patient's status (Table 15.6). A modified GCS has been developed for preverbal children (Table 15.7).

The neurologic exam, the nature of the injury, and the age of the patient determine the need for skull x-rays. Since CT scans provide information about the skull and, more important, the underlying brain, skull radiographs are rarely needed. If a depressed skull fracture is suspected (trauma caused by a sharp, high-velocity object; large scalp hematoma preventing palpation of the skull below), obtain an x-ray tangential to the area in question. Skull x-rays are usually not needed to rule-out a linear compound fracture in a patient with a scalp laceration, since these wounds will be explored under local anesthesia.

Risk assignment may be helpful to guide further management (Table 15.8).

ED Management

Priorities are securing the airway, maintaining vital signs, stabilizing the cervical spine, and treating increased ICP. Serial examination of the patient, preferably by the same health care provider, is essential to the early detection of evolving injuries.

First, assess the airway and adequacy of ventilation and stabilize the cervical spine (if that was not done in the field) with a rigid neck collar. Since a patient with a depressed level of consciousness may have inadequate ventilation despite respiratory movements, obtain an ABG, monitor oxygen saturation, and give 100% oxygen if the patient is not fully awake and alert. Intubate any patient with a GCS ≤8, using in-line stabilization of the cervical spine and the jaw-thrust/chin-lift maneuver. Examine the chest for the presence of bilateral breath sounds and signs of respiratory distress.

Next, measure the vital signs at least every 15 minutes, more frequently in patients with severe head trauma or an abnormal pulse or blood pressure. Secure a large-bore IV in patients with hypotension or a GCS <15. The treatment of hypotension with 20 mL/kg boluses of isotonic crystalloid and packed red cell transfusions takes precedence over concerns about increased ICP. Once a normal BP is maintained, infuse D_5 ½ NS at a KVO rate.

A patient with a depressed skull fracture, penetrating head trauma, focal neurologic findings, or an early posttraumatic convulsion is at risk for the development of seizures. Give a loading dose of IV fosphenytoin (20 mg phenytoin equivalent/kg) slowly over 30 minutes. Give vancomycin 15–20 mg/kg/dose q 12h (1000 mg maximum) *plus* cefepime 50 mg/kg/dose q 12h (2000 mg/dose maximum) to a patient with a compound skull fracture before debridement, but do not give antibiotics routinely to a patient with a basilar skull fracture.

GCS <8 or GCS ≥8 but Worsening

Immediately intubate the patient and call for neurologic and neurosurgical consultations. Hyperventilate the patient to a pCO_2 of 30–35 mmHg, keep the head in the midline, the bed elevated to 30°, and restrict fluids to NS at a KVO rate. If there is pupillary asymmetry or decorticate posturing, give mannitol (0.5–1 g/kg) as an IV push. Arrange for an immediate CT scan (see Increased Intracranial Pressure, pp. 527–529).

GCS 9–14

Insert a large-bore IV for access, and repeat the GCS every 15 minutes. Arrange for an urgent CT. Admit the patient for close observation if the GCS remains <15 during the first hour in the ED.

GCS = 15

If the child has not vomited and has a normal examination, he or she may be discharged home if the parents can follow instructions and return immediately. If there is persistent vomiting or dizziness, arrange for a CT scan or admit for observation and serial neurologic examinations. Regardless of whether the CT is normal, if the parents are anxious, do not discharge a patient who is not back to baseline neurologic status.

Admit a patient with a basilar skull fracture if a CSF leak is suspected, there are associated neurologic findings, or the parents are apprehensive. If there is associated CSF leakage, elevate the head of the bed to 30° and consult with neurosurgery. A patient with CSF otorrhea or rhinorrhea is at risk for bacterial meningitis (10%); however, prophylactic antibiotics are not indicated. Most CSF leaks resolve spontaneously within 7–10 days.

Follow-up

- GCS = 15: next day. Instruct the parents to return immediately if the patient cannot be aroused, has diplopia, unsteady gait, recurrent episodes of vomiting, or a headache unresponsive to ibuprofen or acetaminophen

Indications for Admission

- GCS <15
- Early posttraumatic seizure (not a contact seizure)
- Compound or depressed skull fracture
- Persistent vomiting, dizziness, or abnormal neurologic findings in the ED
- Basilar skull fracture with associated neurologic findings or CSF leak

Bibliography

Atabaki SM. Updates in the general approach to pediatric head trauma and concussion. *Pediatr Clin North Am.* 2013;**60**(5):1107–1122.

Bharadwaj S, Rocker J. Minor head injury: limiting patient exposure to ionizing radiation, risk stratification, and concussion management. *Curr Opin Pediatr.* 2016;**28**(1):121–131.

Holmes JF, Borgialli DA, Nadel FM, et al. Do children with blunt head trauma and normal cranial computed tomography scan results require hospitalization for neurologic observation? *Ann Emerg Med.* 2011;**58**(4):315–322.

Huisman TA, Poretti A. Trauma. *Handb Clin Neurol.* 2016:**136**;1199–1220.

Piteau SJ, Ward MG, Barrowman NJ, Plint AC. Clinical and radiographic characteristics associated with abusive and nonabusive head trauma: a systematic review. *Pediatrics.* 2012;**130**(2):315–323.

Wing R, James C. Pediatric head injury and concussion. *Emerg Med Clin North Am.* 2013;**31**(3):653–675.

Increased ICP   *Neurosurgical Emergency*

An increase in the volume of any intracranial compartment (blood, CSF, or parenchyma) can cause an elevation in ICP, a true neurosurgical emergency. Head trauma is the most common cause of increased ICP in children. Although the onset of increased ICP is usually acute, onset may be delayed in patients with subdural or epidural hematomas. Other causes include brain tumor, meningitis, hemorrhage from a vascular malformation, intracerebral abscess, idiopathic intracranial hypertension (formerly pseudotumor cerebri), diffuse cerebral edema in the setting of fulminant liver failure, and shunt obstruction in a patient with hydrocephalus.

Clinical Presentation

Lethargy is an important finding in a patient with increased ICP. A patient with a GCS <9 or a falling GCS after head trauma requires an immediate evaluation for intracranial hypertension.

A patient with increased ICP may complain of early-morning headache, vomiting not associated with nausea, or headaches of recent onset that have become more frequent and severe. A verbal child may complain of blurry vision, frank diplopia, or intermittent loss of vision. Altered mental status, a change in personality (constant crying or irritability in an

Early morning Headache   ·Changes in Vision
Vomiting w/o nausea   or personality.
Head Tilt.

infant/toddler), neck pain, and a head tilt are also suggestive of increased ICP. Papilledema is a highly specific but insensitive finding within the first 24 hours of acutely raised ICP. In an infant, increased ICP may present with inconsolability, vomiting, widening of the sutures, rapidly increasing head circumference, a full or bulging fontanelle, and possibly, downward deviation or "sunsetting" of the eyes.

Clinical signs of imminent cerebral herniation include a deteriorating level of consciousness, unequal pupils (the dilated pupil is usually on the same side as the herniation), asymmetric EOMs, and decorticate (flexor-early) or decerebrate (extensor-late) posturing. Abnormal respirations, bradycardia, and hypertension (Cushing's triad) occur with severely increased ICP.

Diagnosis

A patient who has suffered significant head trauma is at risk for increased ICP. Always ask about persistent vomiting, and visual or behavioral changes. Check the level of consciousness, pupillary responses, and EOMs. Perform a careful ophthalmoscopic examination to evaluate for papilledema, and perform sensory and motor examinations, comparing one side of the body to the other. Coma can be due to metabolic causes (see pp. 508–512), but typically the pupils, EOMs, and motor response are symmetrical and there are no focal findings.

Congenital anisocoria, the use of mydriatic drops, or traumatic mydriasis or iritis can cause pupillary asymmetry. These are always diagnoses of exclusion in a patient with lethargy or any other signs suggesting increased ICP.

The evaluation of headaches is discussed on pp. 515–521. Morning headaches or headaches that are increasing in frequency and intensity are worrisome. However, headaches in an alert patient with no other abnormal neurologic findings are most likely to be migraines, tension-type, or psychogenic headaches.

ED Management

If increased ICP is suspected, immediately arrange for a CT scan and notify a neurosurgeon and a neurologist to assist in further management. See pp. 521–527 for the treatment of head trauma.

Continuously monitor the heart rate and blood pressure and assess the adequacy of ventilation with an ABG. Secure an IV with vascular access. If the patient is hypotensive, restoration of a normal BP with isotonic fluids takes priority over treatment of the increased ICP and is required in order to maintain adequate cerebral perfusion pressure. Avoid using hypotonic fluids. If there is concern for a cervical spine injury, keep the patient's head midline and, unless he or she is in shock, elevate the head of the bed 30°. Provide 100% oxygen, and intubate any patient who is hypoxic, hypercarbic (pCO_2 >40 mmHg), has a GCS <9, or is leaving the ED for diagnostic procedures (continuous monitoring will be difficult).

If the patient has signs of markedly increased ICP (unequal pupils, bradycardia and hypertension, abnormal posturing), employ all available modalities to lower the ICP while a neurologist and neurosurgeon are summoned. These include immediate intubation and hyperventilation to a pCO_2 of 30–35 mmHg (if the patient is intubated, increase the rate of ventilation) and, if a mass lesion is suspected, the administration of IV mannitol (0.5–1 g/kg) and dexamethasone (0.2 mg/kg, 16 mg maximum). When giving mannitol, insert a urinary bladder catheter. Limit the IV fluid rate to KVO unless the patient is in shock.

$PCO_2 > 40 mmHg$ – is Hypercarbia →
Hyper Ventilate – aim for < 30-35 mm Hg.

To avoid further increasing the ICP, it is preferable to perform intubation under controlled circumstances (see Rapid Sequence Intubation, pp. 14–18). As soon as intubation has been accomplished, insert a nasogastric tube (orogastric tube if the patient has sustained head trauma), aspirate the stomach contents, and connect the tube to suction.

Order a shunt survey if there is a suspected shunt obstruction. Arrange for a neurosurgeon to tap the reservoir to obtain CSF for culture, cell count, and chemistries if a shunt infection is suspected.

Indications for Admission
- Suspected or confirmed intracranial hypertension (to a pediatric ICU).

Bibliography

Kukreti V, Mohseni-Bod H, Drake J. Management of raised intracranial pressure in children with traumatic brain injury. *J Pediatr Neurosci*. 2014; **9**(3):207–215

Perez-Barcena J, Llompart-Pou JA, O'Phelan KH. Intracranial pressure monitoring and management of intracranial hypertension. *Crit Care Clin*. 2014;**30**(4):735–750.

Rogers DL. A review of pediatric idiopathic intracranial hypertension. *Pediatr Clin North Am*. 2014;**61**(3):579–590.

Victorio MC, Rothner AD. Diagnosis and treatment of idiopathic intracranial hypertension (IIH) in children and adolescents. *Curr Neurol Neurosci Rep*. 2013;**13**(3):336.

Seizures

Most pediatric seizures encountered in the ED will be either benign febrile convulsions or breakthrough seizures in the setting of known epilepsy. However, the priorities are to identify and treat status epilepticus and to rule-out life-threatening causes of seizures, such as meningitis, severe head trauma, intracranial bleeding, long QTc syndrome (LQTS), and metabolic derangements.

Clinical Presentation and Diagnosis

Some seizures, such as generalized convulsions, are easily recognized while other types are subtler in appearance and less familiar. Common features of seizures include rhythmic jerking of the head or extremities, changes in muscle tone, fixed staring with or without deviation of the eyes, myoclonic jerks, nystagmus, and/or unresponsiveness.

Infants, and neonates in particular, tend to have multifocal clonic seizures or subtle seizure activity such as tongue thrusting and lip smacking. In infants, posturing and unusual movements that are not otherwise accompanied by eye deviation or alteration in vital signs are usually not seizures.

Other paroxysmal events such as syncope, migraine, movement disorders, and "pseudoseizures," may be mistaken for seizures. These can usually be differentiated with a careful history. Syncope (pp. 79–82) is rare in very young children and is often preceded by a stressful event, giving rise to a vasovagal reaction. Syncope may be preceded by lightheadedness or nausea. However, a syncopal episode secondary to LQTS may present as a first afebrile seizure. Confusion or a decreased level of consciousness may accompany migraine, but headache is usually the most striking feature. Movement disorders disappear in sleep and are not associated with a decreased level of consciousness. In contrast, seizure

[handwritten annotations: Febrile Szr < 12mths LP — Indications and ① Lethargy, ② Irritable ③ Toxic appe ④ SE event a focus of infn]

activity frequently arises during sleep or shortly after awakening and often causes a change in level of alertness. Differentiating pseudoseizures or nonepileptic spells from true seizures is often difficult in the ED, unless the patient is known to have had previous nonepileptic spells. The patient may require extended monitoring with continuous EEG and closed circuit television.

For the purposes of evaluation and management in the ED, seizures are divided into status epilepticus, febrile seizures, first unprovoked seizure, and breakthrough seizures, without regard to the actual appearance of the seizure or its formal classification.

Status Epilepticus

Status epilepticus is defined as either a single seizure lasting longer than 15 minutes or a series of seizures without a return to baseline mental status between each episode. If the seizure started at home and has not stopped before arrival in the ED, the patient is most likely in status. The term *status epilepticus* refers only to the duration of the seizure and does not imply anything about the cause, prognosis, or type of seizure activity. Generalized tonic–clonic status, partial complex status, and febrile status are the most frequent types of status epilepticus.

The most common cause of status is low antiepileptic drug levels in a child with known epilepsy. Breakthrough seizures may also be triggered by fever, vomiting, and/or intercurrent infections. Less commonly, status is secondary to an acute encephalopathic process such as CNS infection (meningoencephalitis), metabolic disturbance (hypoxia, hypoglycemia, hyponatremia, hypocalcemia, hyperammonemia), intoxication or poisoning (cocaine, theophylline, tricyclic antidepressants, amphetamines, camphor), mass lesion (tumor, abscess, hemorrhage), or head trauma.

Children generally tolerate status epilepticus well, although there may be hypoxia and hypercarbia with metabolic and respiratory acidosis significant enough to require intubation and mechanical ventilation. Increased cerebral oxygen consumption and cerebral blood flow occur and may cause intracranial hypertension. This can lead to exacerbation of cerebral injury if the seizure is due to trauma or spontaneous intracranial hemorrhage. Physical injury and vomiting with aspiration are additional hazards. Therefore, treat status epilepticus as quickly as possible and prepare to provide advanced respiratory support to manage the respiratory depression and altered mental status which may occur with aggressive medical therapy.

Febrile Seizure   *[handwritten: 6 mths - 6 years.]*

Febrile seizures occur commonly (2–5%) in otherwise normal children between the ages of six months and six years. By definition, the seizure occurs during the course of a febrile illness that does not involve the CNS. The characteristics of febrile seizures are noted in Table 15.9.

When a seizure occurs with fever, meningitis or encephalitis must be ruled out. This is often possible during the history and physical examination of older children. However, young children can have meningitis without the typical signs: stiff neck, headache, Kernig's and Brudzinski's signs. Therefore, a lumbar puncture (LP) is indicated for any febrile patient less than 12 months of age unless he or she has an identified source of fever, appears well, and is functioning in a normal baseline fashion. Be particularly cautious with infants who are too young to sit, as clinical assessment may be difficult. For a patient less than 12 months of age, indications for an LP include lethargy, irritability, toxic appearance, and

FS = Neurologic deficit Chapter 15: Neurologic Emergencies | 531

get Neuroimaging before LP.

Table 15.9 Characteristics of febrile seizures

Family history in 10%

No prior CNS dysfunction or neurological disorder

Simple	Complex
Brief (<15 minutes)	Prolonged duration (including febrile status epilepticus)
Generalized	Focal (before, during, after)
Single event	More than one seizure within 24 hours

febrile status epilepticus, regardless of whether a possible source of infection is identified on clinical exam (e.g., otitis media). Have a low threshold for LP in a child who has been pretreated with oral antibiotics. In addition, neuroimaging prior to the LP is required to rule-out a mass lesion only if the child has focal neurological signs. *2/3 - once*

About two-thirds of patients have only one febrile seizure episode. Of patients who have a second episode, about one-half to two-thirds will have three or more febrile seizures. Recurrences are more likely in children less than 18 months old at the time of the first seizure and those who have febrile seizures with temperatures less than 40 °C (104 °F). Simple febrile seizures do not increase a child's lifetime risk of epilepsy; however, the risk of epilepsy is slightly higher than the general population for children with complex febrile seizures. Some children with an underlying epilepsy syndrome may initially present with seizures in the setting of febrile illnesses. *recurrence of FS*

① 1st episode < 18mths ② < 104°F.
First Unprovoked Seizure *i FS.*

An unprovoked seizure is one that is not associated with fever, infection, trauma, ingestion, metabolic abnormality, or any other identifiable cause. The first such episode can sometimes be the initial presentation of epilepsy, although the majority of patients never have another seizure.

Breakthrough Seizure

A breakthrough seizure occurs in a patient taking chronic antiepileptic medications. The most common cause is low antiepileptic drug level secondary to noncompliance (particularly common in teenagers), inability to obtain the medication(s), having outgrown the drug dose(s), or change in the patient's metabolism of the drug(s). Antibiotics, birth control pills, and other drugs metabolized through the hepatic P450 system may reduce antiepileptic drug levels. In contrast, erythromycin may lead to an increased carbamazepine level, and any new medication that is protein-bound may displace phenytoin from protein-binding sites and lead to transient toxicity. Adding a second antiepileptic agent can also change other drug levels. Also, a febrile illness or any other type of physiologic stress can lower the child's seizure threshold and result in a breakthrough seizure.

ED Management

The priorities are evaluation and stabilization of the patient's airway and vital signs, termination of ongoing seizure activity, prevention of recurrent seizures, and determination of the cause of the seizure. If the patient has seizure activity in the ED, document the features of the seizure, including any focal movements, gaze deviation, presence and direction of nystagmus, and alteration in autonomic function.

Obtain a complete history, including an accurate description of the seizure and how and where it started, any "aura" at the onset of the seizure, the time of day and the patient's activity at the time of the seizure (particularly whether the seizure had onset in sleep or early morning), and the post-ictal state. Inquire about medications taken, family history of epilepsy or other neurologic or neurocutaneous disorders, developmental history, and past medical history. On physical examination, check the skin for neuro-cutaneous stigmata, perform thorough general and neurologic examinations, including a complete mental status exam appropriate to the patient's age, and assess the patient's developmental status.

Once it is clear that the patient did have a seizure and is not in status epilepticus, the ED work-up and management are directed by the answers to the following questions:

1. Is this a first seizure, or is there a history of seizures? If there have been previous seizures, is this seizure similar with regard to type of activity, duration, and frequency?
2. Is the patient taking antiepileptic drugs? Has the child "outgrown" the dose, or has there been a problem with adherence to the drug regimen?
3. Is the patient febrile? Is this a febrile seizure in an otherwise normal child with a fever and an infection that does not involve the CNS? Is this a child with an underlying neurologic disorder who has seizures when febrile?
4. Is there evidence of meningitis?
5. Could the seizure have been provoked by something other than fever, such as hypoxia, hypoglycemia, ingestion of cocaine or another drug, electrolyte abnormality, or head trauma? Has the patient had previous syncopal episodes, raising the possibility of LQTS? *DD of Cause.*

Status Epilepticus

Assess the airway, breathing, and circulation before proceeding with treatment. Suction the oral cavity, apply a facemask with 100% oxygen over the nose and mouth, and monitor the vital signs and oxygen saturation. Secure an IV with D_5 NS (at KVO if the vital signs are stable), and obtain blood for laboratory tests as indicated by the history. These may include blood for antiepileptic drug levels, serum toxicology screen, CBC, electrolytes, glucose, calcium, and magnesium. If acute exposure to lead is a possibility, also obtain a lead level. Always obtain a rapid Dextrostix estimate of the serum glucose and an extra red-top tube for possible additional studies. If the child is febrile and appears toxic, obtain a blood culture. If the cause of the seizure is not clear, obtain a urine sample drug screen, including cocaine metabolites.

Protocol for Treatment of Status Epilepticus

While monitoring the blood pressure, ECG, and respiratory status, give:

1. Lorazepam 0.1 mg/kg (2–4 mg maximum) slow IV push over two minutes (preferred). Alternatives include diazepam 0.15–0.2 mg/kg (5–10 mg maximum) slow IV push over two minutes, and midazolam 5–10 mg (5 mg for 13–40 kg; 10 mg for >40 kg) single IM dose. If none of the above options are available, diazepam 0.2–0.5 mg/kg (20 mg maximum) rectally or intranasal midazolam. Respiratory depression and hypotension may occur. Lorazepam and diazepam may be given IO if no IV access is established. Do

not give lorazepam or diazepam IM because of erratic absorption. Repeat the dose if the seizure does not stop within five minutes.

2. Fosphenytoin 20 mg/kg phenytoin equivalents (1500 mg maximum) IV or IO given by slow push over 10–15 minutes (preferred). Alternatives include phenytoin 20 mg/kg IV given by slow push over 20–30 minutes, valproic acid 30–40 mg/kg (3000 mg maximum) IV over one hour, or levetiracetam 30–60 mg/kg (4500 mg maximum) IV over one hour, or phenobarbital 15 mg/kg IV over 10–15 minutes if no others available. If the seizure does not stop within five minutes after the dose is complete, proceed to step 3, and contact a pediatric neurologist. Fosphenytoin has significant advantages over phenytoin, since it can be given quickly with much less risk of cardiac arrhythmia or asystole, and is much less likely to cause extensive tissue necrosis in case of extravasation. Fosphenytoin can be diluted in NS or dextrose-containing fluids to concentrations from 1:2 to 1:25 as convenient, while phenytoin is only compatible with NS. However, do not give fosphenytoin IM for status epilepticus due to its slow absorption.

3. If seizure activity continues after administering first- and second-line medications, an alternative second-line medication or anesthetic doses of thiopental, midazolam, pentobarbital, or propofol may be given (with continuous EEG monitoring), in consultation with a pediatric intensivist or anesthesiologist. If there is any sign of respiratory depression or if the patient does not have adequate airway protection reflexes (gag and cough), intubate the patient prior to administration of these medications. If the seizure does not stop, consider steps 4 and 5.

4. Pentobarbital coma in an intensive care unit.

5. Continuous general anesthesia in an intensive care unit.

If the seizure activity is stopped by lorazepam, the patient usually needs no further antiepileptic medication. This includes febrile status and breakthrough seizures due to low antiepileptic drug levels. However, if a patient is unconsciousness, intubated, or has received paralytic agents, it is necessary to treat with IV fosphenytoin or phenobarbital as seizures may not be detectable clinically.

For the rare patient who does not have a history of epilepsy and does not respond to lorazepam or diazepam, check the electrolytes and obtain an ABG. A patient with a metabolic or hypoxic basis for status epilepticus usually does not require treatment with anticonvulsants, but rather a correction of the underlying problem. Treat hyponatremic seizures with water restriction and normal saline (see Hyponatremia, pp. 197–200). If needed, give hypertonic (3%) saline (2–4 mL/kg IV push). Correction of the sodium to 125 mEq/L is generally sufficient to stop seizures, but avoid a rapid correction to a normal sodium level. Treat hypertensive seizures with IV labetalol (0.25 mg/kg over ten minutes) or IV diazoxide miniboluses (1 mg/kg), which can be repeated up to five times at 10–15-minute intervals (see Hypertension, pp. 684–688).

Fever, irritability, or lethargy are indications for a blood culture and an LP, once the seizure has been terminated. It is essential that the child's respiratory status be stable before an LP is attempted. If there is apnea, hypoventilation, or signs of increased ICP such as papilledema or posturing, give antibiotics and delay the procedure. If the Dextrostix reading is low (<80 mg/dL), give an IV push of 0.5 g/kg glucose (2 mL/kg of D_{25}) after obtaining blood for glucose and insulin levels. Obtain urine to check for ketones, if the patient was hypoglycemic.

A patient with evidence of focality (except for known stable neurological deficits without new findings) or increased ICP on neurologic exam must undergo immediate CT scanning (see Increased ICP, pp. 527–529). However, a patient with generalized seizures with no residual defects does not require radiographic imaging in the ED. An EEG is indicated for a patient with new-onset status epilepticus with focal features, focal neurological deficits, or if the onset of seizure activity was unwitnessed, but it is more useful if deferred until after the immediate post-ictal period. An EEG is indicated in the ED when there is reason to suspect subclinical status epilepticus (subtle seizure activity that continues after convulsive status epilepticus has been treated).

Febrile Seizures

Treat a patient with a febrile seizure lasting more than 15–30 minutes as status epilepticus with the regimen described above. For most children with febrile seizures, vigorous anti-pyresis with acetaminophen (15 mg/kg q 4h) and/or ibuprofen (10 mg/kg q 6h) is commonly used to prevent recurrences, although there is no evidence that these measures are effective. Consult a neurologist to consider treatment with antiepileptic drugs or rectal diazepam for a patient whose seizures are unusually severe, frequent, or accompanied by aspiration or a need for intubation.

A patient with a febrile seizure without focality may be discharged from the ED when all infectious disease issues have been resolved, the neurologic status has returned to baseline, and the family has an adequate supply of antipyretics, with instructions for their use.

First Unprovoked Seizure

Long-term antiepileptic drug treatment for a first-time unprovoked seizure in an otherwise normal child may be postponed until the child has a second or third seizure. Defer these decisions to the primary medical provider or pediatric neurologist. Metabolic derangements are rare, although the likelihood increases in younger children and infants. For an older child who appears well and has returned to a normal neurological baseline following a seizure, routine electrolytes, calcium, and magnesium levels are seldom helpful. However, if the patient has a history of syncopal episodes or a family history of arrhythmia, syncope, sudden death, or deafness, obtain an ECG and rhythm strip to rule-out LQTS (see Syncope, pp. 79–82).

A patient with a new-onset unprovoked seizure without focality may be discharged from the ED when the neurologic status has returned to baseline, arrangements for appropriate follow-up have been made, and the immediate concerns of the child and family have been addressed.

Breakthrough Seizure

If the patient is known to have had a recent therapeutic anticonvulsant level, give an extra dose of that medication rather than a full loading dose. For example, give 5 mg/kg of either fosphenytoin, phenytoin, or phenobarbital IV over 15–20 minutes. Do not give either drug IM. If there are subsequent seizures, treat for status epilepticus, as described above. Valproic acid, but not carbamazepine, is now available in IV form. Use the same dose as for oral administration, over one hour.

A patient with a history of epilepsy and breakthrough seizures may be discharged from the ED when the neurologic status has returned to baseline, and the patient has an adequate supply of all necessary anticonvulsants. Obtaining anticonvulsant drug levels is rarely helpful in the ED, given the long turnaround time for most medications (exceptions are phenobarbital, phenytoin/fosphenytoin, valproic acid).

Follow-up
- Febrile or first unprovoked seizure: next day
- Breakthrough seizure: 2–3 days, to check anticonvulsant levels

Indications for Admission
- Status epilepticus
- Increasing number of breakthrough seizures or new types of seizures in a known epileptic
- Focality or evidence of increased intracranial pressure
- CNS infection
- Structural lesion (trauma, tumor, hemorrhage)
- Child who does not return to baseline mental status within 1–2 hours of the seizure

Bibliography

Abend N, Loddenkemper T. Management of pediatric status epilepticus. *Curr Treat Options Neurol.* 2014;**16**:301.

Freilich ER, Schreiber JM, Zelleke T, Gaillard WD. Pediatric status epilepticus: identification and evaluation. *Curr Opin Pediatr.* 2014;**26**(6):655–661.

Glauser T, Shinnar S, Gloss D, et al. Evidence-based guideline: treatment of convulsive status epilepticus in children and adults – report of the Guideline Committee of the American Epilepsy Society. *Epilepsy Curr.* 2016;**16**:48–61.

Kimia AA, Bachur RG, Torres A, Harper MB. Febrile seizures: emergency medicine perspective. *Curr Opin Pediatr.* 2015;**27**(3):292–297.

Subcommittee on Febrile Seizures, American Academy of Pediatrics. Neurodiagnostic evaluation of the child with a simple febrile seizure. *Pediatrics.* 2011;**127**:389–394.

Sleep Disorders
Nightmares, night terrors, and sleepwalking can occur with enough frequency to bring a patient to the ED.

Clinical Presentation and Diagnosis

Nightmares
Nightmares are frightening dreams that occur during rapid eye movement (REM) sleep. The child is easily arousable or awakens spontaneously, and typically has a good recall of the dream. Nightmares are fairly common in children beginning at about age 3, but it is important to obtain a careful medication history since withdrawal from minor tranquilizers, anticonvulsants, and sedative-hypnotics can be associated with nightmares.

Night Terrors
Night terrors are sleep disruptions that typically occur in children 3–8 years old. Episodes most often take place within 2–3 hours of falling asleep and are characterized by intense fear, screaming, and inconsolability. Signs of autonomic arousal are common, including increased heart rate, pupillary dilation, sweating, and even combativeness. In contrast to

nightmares, the child will be difficult to arouse during the episode and will have little, if any, recall of the episode after quickly falling back to sleep. A patient with night terrors frequently also has somnambulism (see below). Night terrors are easy to confuse with nightmares or nocturnal seizures. A thorough history is of primary importance in making the diagnosis.

Somnambulism

Somnambulism, or sleepwalking, occurs in 1–6% of the population (particularly boys), and there is often a positive family history. The child will be out of bed, often performing some sort of purposeful behavior, and may even respond somewhat to verbal commands. There is usually no recall for the event when the patient is fully awake. Somnambulism can be confused with psychomotor seizures, which do not occur exclusively at night.

Take a careful history of the event, and review the patient's general health status and medication history. Ask about recent stresses in the child's life.

ED Management

Nightmares

Occasional nightmares are of little concern. Recurrent episodes, especially if a particular dream occurs frequently, may be indicative of stress or emotional upset that requires further attention.

Night Terrors

Generally, a patient will "outgrow" night terrors, so reassurance is all that is needed. However, frequent recurrences suggest underlying stress. If nocturnal seizures cannot be ruled out (episodes also occur during the day or more than 2–3 hours after falling asleep), order a sleep-deprived EEG

Somnambulism

Sleepwalking is difficult to prevent and, once it begins, it may continue into adulthood. Advise the parents to secure the child's area to prevent injury during sleepwalking (protect stairways, doors, windows).

Follow-up

- Primary care follow-up in 2–4 weeks

Bibliography

Bhargava S. Diagnosis and management of common sleep problems in children. *Pediatr Rev.* 2011;**32** (3):91–98.

Hoban TF. Sleep disorders in children. *Ann N Y Acad Sci.* 2010;**1184**:1–14.

Honaker SM, Meltzer LJ. Bedtime problems and night wakings in young children: an update of the evidence. *Paediatr Respir Rev.* 2014;**15**(4):333–339.

Moreno MA. Sleep terrors and sleepwalking: common parasomnias of childhood. *JAMA Pediatr.* 2015;**169**(7):704.

Petit D, Pennestri MH, Paquet J, et al. Childhood sleepwalking and sleep terrors: a longitudinal study of prevalence and familial aggregation. *JAMA Pediatr.* 2015;**169**(7):653–658.

Ventriculoperitoneal Shunts

The survival of premature infants has led to a significant increase in the number of patients with ventriculoperitoneal (VP) shunts. A VP shunt places a patient at risk for increased ICP due to malfunction, infection, and in some cases, low-pressure headache due to over-draining of the CSF.

Clinical Presentation   *Parents may forget the V-P shunt.*

While the presentation may be dramatic, with signs of increased ICP or CNS infection, the parent may note only that the child "looked just like this the last time he/she had a shunt problem." Although most parents will mention that the patient has a shunt, occasionally this part of the patient's history may be forgotten, particularly if the shunt has been functioning well for a long time or if the presenting complaints are primarily referable to the abdomen.

Shunt Malfunction

Proximal (intracranial) obstruction can be caused by CSF protein, choroid plexus, or embedding of the tube in the brain parenchyma. Distal obstruction to CSF flow may result from the formation of an abdominal pseudocyst around the end of the shunt. Malfunction may also result from disconnection or kinking of elements of the shunt leading to symptoms of shunt obstruction. Proximal obstruction causes headache, vomiting, neck pain, lethargy, sixth nerve palsy, persistent downward gaze ("sunsetting" eyes), and feeding intolerance (see Increased ICP, pp. 527–529). If the obstruction is distal, the patient may also have nausea, abdominal pain, and a distended abdomen.   *6th CN -palsy*

Shunt Infection   *Sunsetting sign.*

Meningitis and ventriculitis present with fever, irritability or lethargy, meningismus, and signs of increased ICP. Infection is most likely to occur in the first three months after placement of the shunt, secondary to contamination at the time of the procedure. A late infection is due to hematogenous spread. Occasionally, a patient may develop peritonitis followed by an ascending infection of the shunt.   *Infection < 3 mths*

Low-Pressure Headache   *from surgical contamination.*

While newer shunts have anti-siphoning devices and may have programmable valves to allow for adjustment of the opening pressure, an older patient may have a shunt without these capabilities. The shunt may intermittently overdrain with subsequent tension on the dura and other pain-sensitive structures, causing nausea and severe headache. On CT scan, the ventricles appear slit-like. This syndrome is annoying but not life-threatening. Consult with the neurosurgeon.   *Infn > 3 mths is Hematogenous.*

Diagnosis

Perform a thorough evaluation for shunt problems if a patient with a VP shunt has headache, lethargy, vomiting, or abdominal pain. Inspect the overlying skin along the entire course of the shunt for erythema, erosions, or induration, which may suggest a source of infection. Evaluate for possible obstruction by depressing the subcutaneous reservoir. Inability to depress the reservoir suggests distal obstruction, while if the reservoir is depressible but does not refill within ten seconds, there may be obstruction proximal to

refill < 10 sec.

or within the one-way valve at the cranial end of the reservoir. If an obstruction is suspected, obtain a <u>noncontrast CT</u> of the brain and compare with previous studies to determine whether there has been an increase in the size of the ventricular system. However, an <u>unchanged CT does not rule-out obstruction</u>, particularly in cases where the patient has been shunted for a long time and the ventricles are no longer compliant. Also obtain a <u>shunt series</u> (a series of plain films that show the full extent of the shunt) to rule-out malfunction due to disconnection or kinking of the elements of the shunt.

If a <u>distal obstruction</u> is suspected, obtain an <u>abdominal ultrasound</u> to look for a <u>pseudocyst</u> or <u>fluid collection.</u>

If infection is suspected, consult a neurosurgeon to obtain a specimen of CSF for cell count and culture. Although a lumbar puncture can be attempted in any patient except those with meningomyelocele (in which case the location of spinal cord elements is unclear), the procedure is often unsuccessful because of alterations in CSF flow due to the presence of the shunt. Most shunts can be tapped directly by inserting a <u>butterfly needle</u> through the skin into the reservoir under sterile conditions.

ED Management

Assess the airway, breathing, and cardiovascular status, give oxygen, and obtain IV access, if necessary. Consult a neurosurgeon to assess shunt function and tap or externalize the shunt, if necessary. If there is papilledema, focal neurologic findings, bradycardia, or hypertension, begin treatment for increased ICP (pp. 527–529) while arranging for radiologic assessment of the shunt.

If the patient has Cushing's triad or asymmetry of the pupils suggesting that herniation is imminent, summon a neurosurgeon to insert a spinal needle through the bony defect along the track of the intracranial portion of the shunt catheter into the ventricle and allow CSF to drain out. Follow the neurological examination carefully before and during this procedure.

While waiting for neurosurgical intervention, assess airway, breathing, and circulation, and initiate prompt intubation for a patient with a GCS <8. Maintain normal oxygenation (PaO_2 >95%) and <u>initiate hyperventilation</u> with the goal of a $PaCO_2$ of 25–30 <u>mmHg.</u> Maintain the systolic blood pressure above the fifth percentile for age to ensure continued cerebral perfusion. Give aggressive fluid resuscitation with isotonic crystalloids, if appropriate, as hypotension during the initial resuscitation must be strictly avoided. Defer hyperosmolar therapy until after consulting with critical care or neurosurgical services. Treat seizures aggressively, but take care to avoid agents which may cause <u>transient hypotension,</u> such as <u>phenobarbital</u> and <u>fosphenytoin.</u> If a shunt infection is suspected, obtain appropriate blood and urine cultures and begin antibiotic treatment (<u>vancomycin</u> 60 mg/kg/day div q 6h, 4 g/day maximum) and IV <u>ceftriaxone</u> (50 mg/kg every 12 hours, 2 g/ dose maximum) *only* if the patient is unstable or the shunt cannot be tapped within a reasonable amount of time. *Staphylococcus epidermidis* and *Staphylococcus aureus* are the most common organisms. Vancomycin + ceftriaxone.

Indications for Admission

- All patients in whom there is evidence or strong clinical suspicion of shunt infection or malfunction

Bibliography

Kulkarni AV, Riva-Cambrin J, Butler J, et al. Outcomes of CSF shunting in children within a North American multicenter collaborative: results from the Hydrocephalus Clinical Research Network (HCRN) compared to historical controls. *JNS: Pediatrics*. 2013;**12**(4):334–338.

Riva-Cambrin J, Kestle JRW, Holubkov R, et al. Risk factors for shunt malfunction in pediatric hydrocephalus: a multi-center prospective cohort study. *JNS: Pediatrics*. 2015;**4**:1–9.

Simon TD, Butler J, Whitlock KB, et al. Risk factors for first cerebrospinal fluid shunt infection: findings from a multi-center prospective cohort study. *J Pediatr*. 2014;**164** (6):1462–1468.

Stone JJ, Walker CT, Jacobson M, Phillips V, Silberstein HJ. Revision rate of pediatric ventriculoperitoneal shunts after 15 years. *J Neurosurg Pediatr*. 2013;**11**(1):15–19.

Tamber MS, Klimo P Jr, Mazzola CA, Flannery AM, Pediatric Hydrocephalus Systematic Review and Evidence-Based Guidelines Task Force. Pediatric hydrocephalus: systematic literature review and evidence-based guidelines. Part 8: Management of cerebrospinal fluid shunt infection. *J Neurosurg Pediatr*. 2014;**14**(Suppl. 1):60–71.

Chapter 16

Ophthalmologic Emergencies

Carolyn Lederman and Martin Lederman

Anatomy

Knowledge of anatomy is required in order to evaluate the eye and related structures (refer to Figure 16.1).

The eye is protected by the lids and surrounding orbital bones. The most anterior part of the eye is the tear film layer covering the cornea (clear front portion of the eye). The corneal margin, where the cornea meets the sclera, is referred to as the limbus. The conjunctiva is a thin membrane covering both the white sclera (bulbar conjunctiva), and the inside of the lids (palpebral conjunctiva). Because the bulbar and palpebral conjunctivae join in the superior and inferior fornix (the area where they join is known also as a "cul-de-sac"), objects such as foreign bodies and contact lenses cannot slip behind the eye and be lost.

Behind the cornea is the anterior chamber, which is approximately 2–4 mm in depth and is filled with clear fluid, known as aqueous humor. The aqueous circulation begins in the ciliary body located behind the iris and flows through the pupil and out through the trabecular meshwork located in the angle between the iris and the peripheral cornea.

The iris contains a circular constrictor muscle and radial dilator muscles, each controlling the circular pupil.

Behind the iris plane is the crystalline lens, which functions as the focusing mechanism of the eye. It is kept in place and controlled by fine suspensory ligaments (zonules), which form an attachment from the lens to the ciliary body.

The inner volume of the eye is filled with a clear gel, the vitreous body. Lining the inner sclera is the retina, a fine network of blood vessels and photosensitive nerve cells which are the first receptors of the visual pathway.

The bony orbit surrounds, supports, and protects the globe. In addition to the globe, the contents of the orbit include connective tissue, blood vessels, fat, and the six extraocular muscles that control eye movement.

Evaluation

Except for chemical injury, when immediate flushing is indicated, the first part of an eye examination is the evaluation and recording of visual acuity. While parts of the following eye examination can be omitted when appropriate, always assess visual acuity.

The standard Snellen chart at 20 feet is best, but other distances may be used as long as that distance is noted. The numerator of the Snellen Fraction denotes the distance from the chart and the denominator is a number given to each line. A smaller denominator refers to a smaller letter (optotype) – i.e., a letter on the "20" line is half the size of a letter on the "40" line, and ten

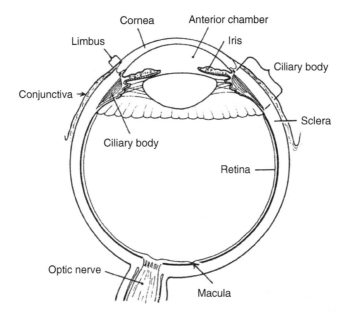

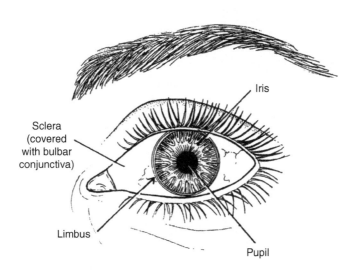

Figure 16.1 Anatomy of the eye.

times smaller than a letter on the "200" line. Thus, 20/200 means that a letter on the "200" line was correctly identified at 20 feet and 4/40 (its equivalent) means that the "40" line letter (five times smaller) was correctly identified at four feet (five times closer).

Charts using other symbols have been constructed for preliterate children but other methods can be used if a chart is not available, such as counting fingers at a specified distance, hand motions at a specified distance, observed eye closure when a light is directed in the eye (light rejection), or reading a newspaper headline at some distance. It is important to check each eye separately. Use a sterile gauze pad to occlude the non-tested eye without pressing on the globe. For children who wear corrective glasses, test visual acuity with and without the glasses. Test the "good" eye first in order to reduce anxiety. For infants and preverbal children, test visual acuity by assessing whether the child can fix on and follow an object.

Assuming that there are no other life-threatening or organ-threatening injuries, evaluate the eyes in a systematic manner, starting from the most anterior aspect of the eye to the most posterior. Look first at the lids and surrounding structures, palpate the bony orbital rim, assess the tears, look at the anterior aspect of the eye including the conjunctiva, cornea, and sclera, and assess ocular mobility by having the patient follow a finger (not a bright light, which may cause photophobia) moving in all positions of gaze (up, down, left, right). Note the depth and clarity of the anterior chamber, and observe pupillary reactivity to light. In a semi-darkened room, at a distance of 1–2 feet, dial the ophthalmoscope to sharply define iris markings (usually black or plus 1 or 2) and assess the clarity and symmetrical color of the pupils. Use the ophthalmoscope to evaluate the retina, which should be uniformly red, and note any hemorrhages or deposits. Look for the foveal reflex of the macula, which is temporal to the optic nerve and appears darker than the surrounding retina. If the macula is white or cherry-red, suspect blunt trauma, ischemia, or metabolic abnormalities. Finally, palpate the globes gently with your two index fingers if a ruptured globe is not suspected. If one eye is firmer than the other, suspect elevated intraocular pressure.

Decreased Vision

Decreased vision can be caused by life-threatening intraocular or intracranial tumors, eye-threatening diseases (trauma, iridocyclitis, idiopathic intracranial hypertension, glaucoma, retinal detachment), or minor conditions (corneal foreign body, conjunctivitis, tearing). In addition, decreased vision may be a functional complaint.

Clinical Presentation

The most common cause of an acute decrease in vision is ocular trauma, particularly a corneal abrasion. The priority is to rule-out a life-threatening or eye-threatening condition.

Diagnosis

Unless there is an obvious ruptured globe or chemical injury, the evaluation of the eyes (pp. 550–551) starts with a determination of visual acuity, preferably Snellen activity or the equivalent.

For infants and preverbal children, first note the vision in both eyes, then in each eye separately. The sleeping infant reacts to bright light directed into each eye with further eyelid closure ("light rejection") if the eye and vision sense are intact. Absence of light rejection or asymmetric light rejection suggests vision loss in one or both eyes.

The preverbal child follows objects of interest, such as toys (avoid shining a bright light in the awake child's eyes), by fixing centrally on the object and following it. Test each eye separately, using the examiner's or parent's thumb as an occluder. For an older child, use a Snellen chart that has been calibrated at 20 feet (p. 551). Testing can be done at a distance of 5–10 feet, although using shorter testing distances may miss subtle differences between the eyes. In the absence of a Snellen chart, ask the patient to count fingers held a few feet away or check the ability to read a newspaper headline at a set distance. The testing distance must be noted.

ED Management

Treat the chief complaint or primary illness. Indications for immediate ophthalmologic evaluation include a sleeping infant who does not reject light, an awake infant who does not follow with either or both eyes, and asymmetric vision, particularly if there has been ocular trauma.

Bibliography

Alley CL. Preschool vision screening: update on guidelines and techniques. *Curr Opin Ophthalmol.* 2013;**24**(5):415–420.

Bell AL, Rodes ME, Collier Kellar L. Childhood eye examination. *Am Fam Physician.* 2013;**88** (4):241–248.

Binenbaum G, Forbes BJ. The eye in child abuse: key points on retinal hemorrhages and abusive head trauma. *Pediatr Radiol.* 2014;**44**(Suppl. 4):S571–S577.

Nye C. A child's vision. *Pediatr Clin North Am.* 2014;**61**(3):495–503.

Excessive Tearing

Tears are produced immediately after birth, but the volume increases after the sixth week. Excess tearing is very common and is secondary to either excess production or insufficient drainage. Excess production is usually due to irritation, infection, foreign body, trauma, iritis, or glaucoma. Insufficient drainage is caused by a stenotic or blocked lacrimal system, usually at the level of the nasolacrimal duct, which conducts tears from the lacrimal sac into the nose.

Clinical Presentation

Excess Production

Tearing due to excess production is often accompanied by conjunctival injection in older children, but injection is usually absent in the newborn. Lid swelling and nasal discharge are common.

Congenital Glaucoma (Elevated Intraocular Pressure)

Congenital glaucoma is accompanied by excess growth of the eye (buphthalmos), photophobia, loss of vision, and tearing, with discharge at the nares. The clarity of the cornea may be reduced with obscuration of the iris markings. It may be unilateral or bilateral, and there may be a positive family history.

Iritis

Iritis is accompanied by photophobia, ciliary flush (conjunctival injection at the limbus), a small pupil with diminished response, and decreased visual acuity. It is uncommon in infancy, except after eye trauma.

Insufficient Drainage

Dacryostenosis (Nasolacrimal Duct Obstruction)

Dacryostenosis is the most common ophthalmologic cause of excess tearing in infancy, usually presenting in the first three months of life. A persistent mucoid or mucopurulent discharge is usually present, in addition to recurrent conjunctivitis. Nasolacrimal duct obstruction may be accompanied by dermatitis of the lids due to the chronic tearing, but there is no nasal discharge or photophobia (to distinguish dacryostenosis from congenital glaucoma).

Hydrops (Amniotocele)

Hydrops of the nasolacrimal sac is usually present at or shortly after birth and is secondary to blockage of the proximal and distal portions of the nasolacrimal sac. It presents as a bluish discoloration medially at the location of the lacrimal sac and can be confused with a meningocele. Secondary infection is common.

Dacryocystitis

Acute dacryocystitis is a suppurative infection of the nasolacrimal sac. It presents with tenderness and swelling of the nasolacrimal sac, with erythema and swelling of the overlying skin. There is usually a history of nasolacrimal duct obstruction.

Diagnosis

The priority is to rule-out excessive tear *production* as the cause of excessive tearing before diagnosing nasolacrimal duct obstruction. Photophobia, eyelid closure (blepharospasm), ciliary flush, pain, and nasal discharge suggest excessive production. See Table 16.1 for the differential diagnosis of excessive tearing.

Table 16.1 Differential diagnosis of excessive tearing

Diagnosis	Differentiating features
Congenital glaucoma	Buphthalmos, corneal clouding, photophobia
	Nasal discharge
Corneal foreign body or abrasion	Sudden onset of tearing
	Blepharospasm, pain
Iritis	Ciliary flush, miosis, photophobia
	May have a history of trauma
Nasolacrimal duct obstruction	Onset in second or third month of life
	Discharge, recurrent conjunctivitis
	Dermatitis of lids

Consider a foreign body or corneal abrasion if the tearing started suddenly, especially if it is accompanied by pain and blepharospasm. The diagnosis of glaucoma is confirmed by evaluation of the intraocular pressure. Consider iritis after trauma which should result in pain in the affected eye when light is shone in the contralateral unaffected eye (due to consensual pupillary reflex).

The diagnosis of nasolacrimal duct obstruction is suggested by constant tearing beginning in the second or third month of life, associated with concurrent eye discharge. There may be swelling of the lacrimal sac with reflux of material from the punctum when digital pressure is applied to the side of the nose overlying the lacrimal sac. Dacryocystitis is likely if there is erythematous swelling of the lacrimal sac accompanied by tenderness.

ED Management

The management of excessive tearing secondary to a foreign body (p. 552) or conjunctivitis (pp. 555–557) is detailed elsewhere. Glaucoma and iritis require immediate ophthalmologic consultation.

Dacryostenosis

In most cases, dacryostenosis clears spontaneously by 6–12 months of age. Prescribe a topical ophthalmic antibiotic (erythromycin ointment, bacitracin ointment, or poly-myxin-trimethoprim drops) tid to suppress infection. Refer the patient to an ophthalmologist for evaluation if the condition does not clear by the sixth month, especially if there have been frequent infections or significant dermatitis.

Hydrops

Refer immediately to an ophthalmologist

Dacryocystitis

Culture any material in the palpebral fissure and treat with oral and topical antibiotics. Use amoxicillin-clavulanate (875/125 formulation; 45 mg/kg/day div bid) or cephalexin (25–50 mg/kg/day div tid). If there is a significant prevalence of MRSA in the community, treat with clindamycin (20 mg/kg/day divided q 6–8h). Topical ophthalmic antibiotics (bacitracin, erythromycin, or moxifloxacin) qid and warm compresses qid are useful adjunctive therapies. Urgent referral to an ophthalmologist is indicated, as probing of the nasolacrimal duct may be necessary in order to avoid recurrence.

Follow-up

- Dacryocystitis: return in 2–3 days if there is no improvement.

Indications for Admission

- Congenital glaucoma
- Dacryocystitis, if close outpatient follow-up is not ensured

Bibliography

Adil E, Huntley C, Choudhary A, Carr M. Congenital nasal obstruction: clinical and radiologic review. *Eur J Pediatr.* 2012;**171**(4):641–650.

Ali MJ. Pediatric acute dacryocystitis. *Ophthal Plast Reconstr Surg.* 2015;**31**(5):341–347.

Giangiacomo A, Beck A. Pediatric glaucoma: review of recent literature. *Curr Opin Ophthalmol.* 2017;**28**(2):199–203.

Schnall BM. Pediatric nasolacrimal duct obstruction. *Curr Opin Ophthalmol.* 2013;**24**(5):421–424.

Eyelid Inflammation

The eyelids can be affected by dermatologic conditions that also involve other areas of the skin, although the unique structures of the eyelids make them prone to particular and characteristic diseases. The protective function of the eyelids, their constant movement, and their prominent location make abnormalities particularly noticeable and troubling.

Clinical Presentation and Diagnosis

Hordeolum

A hordeolum, or stye, is an infection (*Staphylococcus* most commonly) of a sebaceous or sweat gland of the lid (gland of Zeis or Moll). It usually presents as a localized erythematous swelling of the lid margin, although the entire lid may be affected. The area is tender, and the abscess may point at the base of a lash. Several styes may be present simultaneously.

Chalazion

A chalazion is a granulomatous swelling of the other sebaceous gland of the lid (Meibomian gland). It begins as a firm, painless, circular swelling within the lid itself. There may be multiple chalazia. Secondary infection leads to increased swelling and pain, with the abscess pointing onto the skin surface or the conjunctival side of the lid.

Blepharitis

Blepharitis is inflammation of the margin of the lid, usually secondary to *Staphylococcus aureus* infection. Blepharitis is often chronic and may contribute to the development of hordeola and chalazia. Typically, the lid margins are erythematous, crusted, and swollen. There may be an associated conjunctivitis. Pruritus, burning, foreign body sensation, tearing, blurry vision, and loss of lashes are common complaints.

Seborrheic Dermatitis

Seborrheic dermatitis is an erythematous, scaly, or crusting eruption with overlying yellowish greasy scale. The eyelids can be affected, in addition to the scalp, postauricular areas, ears, and neck. Conjunctivitis is uncommon.

Herpes Simplex

Herpes simplex (pp. 124–126) presents with grouped vesicles on an erythematous base. Eyelid involvement may be the sole finding or may be part of a more generalized herpetic infection. The surrounding skin and lips may also be affected. There may be associated conjunctivitis, keratitis, iritis, and preauricular lymphadenopathy. Recurrences are common.

Varicella

The characteristic maculopapular, vesicular, and crusting rash of varicella may affect the eyelids and surrounding skin. Conjunctivitis can be present, particularly if the lid margin is affected. Photophobia, iritis, pupillary abnormalities (irregular or sluggishly reacting), and loss of vision occur rarely. Zoster causes pain in the affected area, followed by swelling of the eyelids. Several days later, the characteristic vesicles develop.

Molluscum Contagiosum

Molluscum appear as 1–5 mm flesh-colored umbilicated papules, sometimes associated with similar lesions on the periorbital skin. Patients are usually asymptomatic, although involvement of the lid margins can produce a concomitant, chronic conjunctivitis.

Parasitic Infestation

The crab louse (*Pthirus pubis*) can infest the eyelids. The infestation is pruritic, and lice and ova or "nits" (tiny white dots) can be seen attached to the lashes and eyebrows. Severe conjunctivitis can result.

ED Management

Hordeolum and Chalazion

Treat hordeola and infected chalazia with warm (not hot) compresses for 3–5 minutes three times a day. Apply 2–3 mm of an ophthalmic antibiotic ointment (erythromycin, bacitracin) tid after the compress. Treat any associated blepharitis (see below) to prevent recurrence. Usually a hordeolum disappears within a week. Refer the patient to an ophthalmologist if improvement does not occur within 2–3 days. A chronic chalazion may remain for weeks to months and may require excision.

Blepharitis

Blepharitis is a chronic disorder, and treatment is directed at controlling the condition. Use warm-water compresses to loosen the scales at the base of the lashes. The scales can then be removed with an applicator stick or clean finger moistened with diluted baby shampoo. Apply erythromycin or bacitracin ophthalmic ointment TID to reduce bacterial overgrowth.

Seborrhea

Treat seborrhea with gentle cleansing with diluted baby shampoo to remove the crusts. Shampoo the scalp every other day with a keratolytic shampoo (Sebulex, Selsun). Ophthalmologic referral is needed before treatment with topical corticosteroids.

Herpes Simplex

If conjunctivitis is present or keratitis is suspected, immediately consult with an ophthalmologist for antiviral therapy.

Varicella and Zoster

Varicella and zoster eyelid infections do not require treatment unless intraocular or corneal involvement is suspected. If the patient demonstrates ciliary flush, photophobia, pupillary abnormalities or visual loss, immediately consult with an ophthalmologist.

Molluscum Contagiosum

Molluscum is usually a self-limited disease, so no treatment is necessary unless the lesions are cosmetically unacceptable, increase in number, or occur at the lid margin and are associated with conjunctivitis. Refer to an ophthalmologist for incision and curettage.

Lice

Treat pediculosis with ophthalmic ointment bid (Lacri-Lube or erythromycin) for ten days, to the base and length of the lashes. Repeat at weekly intervals to kill the emerging lice. Defer forceps removal of lice and nits to an ophthalmologist. Check for and treat pubic lice, and thoroughly wash clothing and bedding. Investigate the child's sleeping arrangements and the possibility of infestation in other household members.

Follow-up

- Chalazion, blepharitis, seborrhea, and lice: primary care follow-up in 1–2 weeks.

Bibliography

Duss DN, Grigorian AP, Medow NB. Management of recurrent chalazia. *J Pediatr Ophthalmol Strabismus*. 2012;**49**(6):327–328.

Hammersmith KM. Blepharokeratoconjunctivitis in children. *Curr Opin Ophthalmol*. 2015;**26**(4):301–305.

Wagner RS. When is a chalazion not a chalazion? *J Pediatr Ophthalmol Strabismus*. 2016;**53**(4):205.

Ocular Trauma

Consider ocular trauma in cases of sudden reduction of vision, sudden onset of eye pain, blepharospasm (uncontrollable closure of one or both eyes), facial trauma, and high-velocity projectile injury. In the setting of multiple trauma, delay the search for and treatment of ocular injuries only until more serious injuries have been addressed. If trauma to the eye is suspected, apply a protective shield until it can be adequately evaluated. Eye trauma may also be the presentation of abuse.

Clinical Presentation

Lid Lacerations

Lid lacerations, particularly if vertical, are easily seen. However, a search for lid lacerations is required in all cases of facial trauma. There may be associated injury to the underlying globe. Vertical lacerations through the lid margin result in wide gaping of the wound because of the circular nature of the orbicularis oculi muscle. Lacerations through the medial one-sixth of the lid margin may be associated with a severed canaliculus.

Ruptured Globe

Always suspect a ruptured or lacerated globe in cases of blunt facial trauma or when there is an eyelid laceration. The findings may be subtle and can include reduction of vision, subconjunctival hemorrhage, swelling of the conjunctiva, deformity or obvious laceration of the cornea or sclera, shallowing or absence of the anterior chamber, deformity of the iris, cataract, softness of the globe, and extrusion of intraorbital contents. Choroid tissue, which is contiguous with the iris, may plug the perforation, so the only finding may be a distorted pupil (teardrop, peaked, pointed, pulled to one side, or flattened on one side). Staining the tears with fluorescein can help diagnose a subtle perforation of the cornea. Clear aqueous stream leaking from the perforation becomes more obvious with fluorescein (Seidel test). Do not use an open solution of fluorescein because of possible bacterial contamination, particularly with *Pseudomonas aeruginosa*.

Hyphema

A hyphema is caused by rupture of blood vessels of the iris with leakage of blood into the anterior chamber. It is usually associated with blunt trauma, but a spontaneous hyphema can occur with iris neovascularization or intraocular tumors (malignant and benign). The findings can be subtle, particularly in the supine patient, if small amounts of blood are mixed with the aqueous. Look for obscuration of the iris markings. Larger quantities of blood are more obvious and cast a reddish glow on the iris. In the upright patient, gravity causes blood to settle, and a blood–aqueous level can usually be seen. The vision can be reduced, conjunctival hyperemia is common, and the pupil is often irregular and pointed. Pain is almost always present. Look for associated injuries (ruptured globe).

A dangerous rise in intraocular pressure may result, especially in patients with sickle cell disease or trait. Persistent hyphemas may cause blood staining (opacification) of the cornea with vision loss. Rebleeding can occur, usually within the first five days after the injury, and is associated with the sudden onset of pain and increased intraocular pressure.

Corneal and Conjunctival Abrasions

Superficial abrasions of the conjunctiva and cornea present with pain that can be severe, photophobia, conjunctival hyperemia, and tearing. The vision is variably affected. An abrasion can often be seen as an irregularity of the normally smooth surface of the globe or as a shadow cast on the iris when a light is directed into the eye.

Fluorescein dye instilled into the cul-de-sac will stain areas of epithelial cell loss and glow bright yellow-green under cobalt blue or Wood's lamp. A subtle perforation of the cornea can be diagnosed when fluorescein is used to stain the tears and reveals clear aqueous leaking from the perforation site (Seidel test).

Foreign Bodies

Superficial foreign bodies present with poorly localized discomfort. Vision is variably affected, but tearing, photophobia, and blepharospasm are common. Lid eversion may be required for the object to be seen, and magnification may be needed if the object is small or transparent. A foreign body can adhere to the conjunctiva of the upper lid at the edge of the tarsal ridge and cause vertical linear abrasions of the superior cornea. There may be one or more foreign bodies.

Intraocular foreign bodies may present with variable signs of ocular irritation. The expected findings of visual reduction, irritation, pain, and signs of penetration may be absent. A high index of suspicion is required, particularly if the patient experienced pain or a foreign body sensation while hammering nails or other metal objects. The history is very important in establishing the diagnosis.

Orbital Fracture

An orbital fracture is caused by blunt trauma to the bony walls of the orbit. A ruptured globe may occur as well. Edema and ecchymosis of the lids and surrounding tissues are usually present; swelling and tenderness of periorbital tissues can limit the examination.

Fracture of the floor or walls of the orbit can injure the extraocular muscles or surrounding tissues and result in decreased ocular mobility and diplopia (double vision). Enophthalmos can result from orbital contents prolapsing into a sinus. Fracture of the floor of the orbit can result in injury to the infraorbital nerve, with resultant hypesthesia in the lower lid and cheek. Air may be introduced subcutaneously from the affected sinus, causing crepitus (orbital emphysema). Injury to the ciliary ganglion causes dilation of the pupil and loss of accommodation (ability to focus) so that near vision is more affected than distance vision.

Burns

Thermal and chemical burns can cause both immediate and delayed damage. Burns due to acids coagulate and denature surface proteins but generally do not penetrate the eye, whereas alkali burns penetrate and damage internal ocular structures. In addition to the globe, the skin of the face and lids may be affected. Presentation depends on the extent of the injury but may include blepharospasm, tearing, photophobia, decreased vision, conjunctival swelling, hyperemia or ischemia, loss of corneal clarity, and variable pain.

Iris Tear

A tear of the iris can occur after blunt or penetrating injuries to the eye. Since the muscles of the iris are circular and radial, a tear causes deformity in the size, shape, and motility of the iris. Always look for an associated hyphema.

Retrobulbar Hemorrhage

A retrobulbar hemorrhage causes acute proptosis, chemosis, variable subconjunctival hemorrhage, reduction of vision, pain, reduced corneal clarity, glaucoma, and limitation of ocular motion. It can occur after blunt or penetrating injury and may lead to loss of vision due to central retinal vessel occlusion.

Traumatic Iritis

Traumatic iritis is due to exudation of protein and inflammatory cells into the aqueous humor and can occur after any injury to the eye. It is characterized by reduction of vision, photophobia, conjunctival hyperemia, ciliary flush, and miosis (papillary constriction). Symptoms may be delayed by several days.

Child Abuse

Non-accidental trauma (pp. 604–608) may present with any of the following: injury to the face and eyelids, subconjunctival hemorrhage, hyphema, pupillary abnormalities, traumatic cataract, eye movement abnormalities, papilledema, and retinal hemorrhages.

Diagnosis

A thorough history and determination of visual acuity in each eye with and without glasses are the first steps in the evaluation of all cases of possible ocular injury. *The exception is chemical (especially alkali) burns to the eye, which require immediate lavage.* For all other injuries, ascertain the precipitating event, whether there were witnesses, the time of the injury, visual loss or disturbance in one or both eyes, onset of pain and injection, presence of light intolerance, and any previous trauma or other ocular abnormality.

Check vision with a standard Snellen chart (see also pp. 540–543). Test the uninjured eye first in order to reduce anxiety. Unless a ruptured globe is suspected, place one drop of an anesthetic in the eye (e.g., proparacaine 0.5%) to reduce pain and aid in the evaluation. Note the eye tested, the vision test used, the distance from the object of regard to the examined eye, and the result.

Examine the face, lids, lashes, and brows. Look for ptosis and deformity of the lid and the surrounding orbit. Observe the extraocular movements, look for strabismus, and note any complaint of diplopia, limitation of movement, or pain caused by movement. Examine the palpebral and bulbar conjunctiva, and look for evidence of laceration, localized injection, or foreign body.

To evert the upper lid, hold an applicator stick horizontally at the midportion of the lid. Grasp the lid lashes with the thumb and forefinger of the other hand and evert, using the applicator stick to help form a hinge. Inspect for foreign bodies at the ridge formed by the top of the tarsal plate or lodged deep in the upper or lower fornix (junction of bulbar and palpebral conjunctivae).

Check the clarity of the cornea, and look for lacerations, particularly at the corneoscleral junction. Suspect a ruptured globe if the anterior chamber is shallower or deeper than that of the other eye or if the pupil is distorted.

A hyphema can be as obvious as a definite aqueous-blood level in the anterior chamber or as subtle as a faint red tinge to the iris or the loss of distinct iris markings. It may be visible only on magnification with a biomicroscope (slit lamp). Pupillary distortion and pain often accompany a hyphema.

An abrasion can be delineated with fluorescein dye instilled in the cul-de-sac, which will adhere to areas of epithelial cell loss and fluoresce bright yellow-green under cobalt blue or Wood's lamp.

The red reflex of light from the direct ophthalmoscope illuminating the pupil can be used to estimate and compare the clarity of the ocular media. In a darkened room, set the dial of the ophthalmoscope to zero, stand one foot away from the patient's eyes, and direct the light beam so that the two pupils are equally illuminated and can be viewed through the aperture of the instrument (you may have to change the dial setting of the ophthalmoscope to focus on the iris). A shadow of a corneal abrasion or cataract may be illuminated in the red pupillary reflex, and there can be a difference in the color and brightness of the reflex. Use the ophthalmoscope to examine the optic nerve head for papilledema and the retina for hemorrhage, tears, or detachment.

The diagnosis of a foreign body may require ultrasound, radiography, or computed tomography (CT) scanning. Avoid magnetic resonance imaging (MRI) if a magnetic foreign body is suspected.

To evaluate a possible orbital fracture, compare the position of the eyes by standing above and behind the patient and sight down the forehead. With the patient's eyes open, evaluate the position of the most forward point of each cornea. With the patient's eyes closed, compare the most anterior point of the upper lid. Palpate the orbital rim for any irregularity.

ED Management

Topical cycloplegics are not necessary in the initial evaluation of the patient, but topical anesthesia can be very helpful with chemical burns, abrasions, and foreign bodies. If a ruptured globe is suspected, avoid increasing intraocular pressure and do not manipulate the eyes (see below).

Lid Lacerations

Consult an ophthalmologist if the laceration is vertical through the lid margin, extends through the full thickness of the lid, or affects the nasal one-sixth of the lid and may therefore damage the tear excretory apparatus. Always check for injuries to the underlying globe.

Ruptured Globe

Consult an ophthalmologist immediately. Delay radiographs to search for foreign bodies until after the evaluation. *Avoid topical agents* and do not remove pigmented material from the surface of the globe, as it may be intraocular contents. Tape a protective shield from forehead to cheekbone over the injured eye until a definitive diagnosis can be made, but do not use a bulky pad under the shield to prevent exerting pressure on the globe. Place the patient supine, with the head of the bed elevated 30°, and avoid excessive movement. Assume surgical intervention will be required and keep the patient NPO. Keep the patient calm so as not to raise intraocular pressure and avoid invasive procedures (IV placement) if it will upset the child.

Hyphema

Immediately consult with an ophthalmologist. Put the patient at rest in a quiet area with the head of the bed elevated to 30°, place a protective shield, and avoid excessive manipulation. Do not give aspirin or NSAIDs, which may prolong bleeding time. Test for sickle hemo-globinopathy when appropriate.

Corneal Abrasion

Prescribe a topical ophthalmic antibiotic (e.g., polysporin-trimethoprim, erythromycin, bacitracin) tid. Do not use occlusive dressings, as they have not been shown to shorten healing time or decrease pain and may facilitate developing an infection. Avoid repeated instillation of topical anesthetics because they interfere with healing and can cause keratitis. Next-day referral to an ophthalmologist is indicated if the abrasion is large, pain or photophobia are still present, vision is affected, or the eye remains red. Small corneal abrasions often heal within a day. If pain seems out of proportion to the size of the abrasion or if there is corneal haze around the abrasion, consider a corneal ulcer and immediately refer the patient to an ophthalmologist.

A contact lens wearer potentially has more virulent bacteria on the ocular surface so prescribe a more potent, fluoroquinolone topical antibiotic (moxifloxacin, besifloxacin) qid. There is a greater potential for corneal ulcer, so refer the patient to an ophthalmologist to be seen the next day.

Foreign Bodies

Superficial corneal and conjunctival foreign bodies may be irrigated off the anesthetized eye with a forceful stream of sterile saline or other ocular irrigating solution (Dacriose). A cotton swab can be used to remove or loosen a foreign body and the remainder irrigated off the eye. Check for multiple foreign bodies. Treat any remaining corneal or conjunctival abrasion as above. Immediately consult with an ophthalmologist if the foreign body cannot be easily removed or there is a retained rust deposit.

Intraocular and intraorbital foreign bodies require an immediate ophthalmologic consultation. Apply a protective shield.

Orbital Fracture

Immediately consult with an ophthalmologist for any patient with an orbital fracture, particularly if there is enophthalmos, limitation of extraocular motion, diplopia, pupillary inequality, or hypesthesia in the region of the infraorbital nerve. Treat with amoxicillin-clavulanic acid (20 mg/kg/day div tid) if a sinus is involved and advise the patient to use a nasal decongestant and avoid blowing the nose. Refer the patient to an ophthalmologist within five days so that surgical repair, if necessary, can be performed in a timely fashion.

Burns

Chemical burns require *immediate* lavage with 1–2 liters of sterile saline. Tap water may be used if sterile saline is not available. Use a topical anesthetic. A Morgan lens (a clear plastic scleral shell with cannula attached) will deliver irrigation to the eye more thoroughly, but a lid speculum can also be used. Sweep the fornices with applicator sticks to remove foreign bodies, and check the pH of the tears with litmus paper 30 minutes after irrigation is complete to ensure that neutralization has occurred. Normally, tears are approximately neutral (pH 7). Do not use an irrigant of opposite pH, as more damage will occur. Consult an ophthalmologist immediately.

Thermal burns are rarely isolated to the lids or globe except in cases of cigarette burns, which are treated as a simple abrasion with antibiotic ointment. Extensive facial burns require ophthalmologic evaluation of the eye and lid function.

Traumatic Iritis

Refer immediately to an ophthalmologist for evaluation of the globe and treatment with topical cycloplegics and possibly topical steroids.

Retrobulbar Hemorrhage

Immediate ophthalmologic evaluation is necessary for treatment with pressure-lowering drugs (intravenous mannitol), surgery (lateral canthotomy), and intravenous steroids.

Follow-up

- Corneal abrasion: return the next day.
- Hyphema: daily ophthalmology visits.

Indications for Admission

- Ruptured globe
- Hyphema, if compliance with follow-up visits and bedrest cannot be assured
- Lid laceration requiring surgical repair in operating room
- Intraocular foreign body
- Orbital fracture, if there is muscle entrapment or compliance with follow-up care cannot be assured
- Retrobulbar hemorrhage

Bibliography

Abbott J, Shah P. The epidemiology and etiology of pediatric ocular trauma. *Surv Ophthalmol.* 2013;**58** (5):476–485.

Binenbaum G, Forbes BJ. The eye in child abuse: key points on retinal hemorrhages and abusive head trauma. *Pediatr Radiol.* 2014;**44**(Suppl. 4):S571–S577.

Haring RS, Sheffield ID, Frattaroli S. Detergent pod-related eye injuries among preschool-aged children. *JAMA Ophthalmol.* 2017;**135**(3):283–284.

Micieli JA, Easterbrook M. Eye and orbital injuries in sports. *Clin Sports Med.* 2017;**36**(2):299–314. doi: 10.1016/j.csm.2016.11.006.

Shetawi AH, Lim CA, Singh YK, Portnof JE, Blumberg SM. Pediatric maxillofacial trauma: a review of 156 patients. *J Oral Maxillofac Surg.* 2016. pii: S0291-2391(16)00265-2.

The Red Eye

The conjunctiva is normally transparent. When inflamed, the numerous fine blood vessels become engorged, causing a "pink eye." Inflammation is most often secondary to infection. Organisms include bacteria (*Staphylococcus aureus, Streptococcus viridans, Streptococcus pneumoniae, Haemophilus influenzae, Enterococci, Neisseria gonorrhoeae*), viruses (herpes simplex, adenovirus, enterovirus, molluscum contagiosum), and *Chlamydia trachomatis* (trachoma).

Conjunctival hyperemia can be secondary to keratitis (superficial corneal inflammation) or uveitis. Keratitis is most often caused by ocular trauma or infection (adenovirus, herpes, *Chlamydia, Staphylococcus, Streptococcus, Haemophilus influenzae*). The anterior uvea (iris and ciliary body) can be inflamed by trauma, infection (herpes simplex, Lyme disease, varicella), or a corneal foreign body.

Other causes of a red eye include allergy and reaction to dust, smoke, foreign bodies, chemicals, and other irritants. Finally, conjunctival hyperemia can accompany serious acute conditions such as preseptal and orbital cellulitis, erythema multiforme, Kawasaki disease, or intraorbital tumor.

Clinical Presentation and Diagnosis

Preseptal and Orbital Cellulitis

The orbital septum connects to both the periosteum of the orbital bones and the tarsal plates of the lid and separates the lid structures from the orbital contents. Infections can spread from contiguous structures or be blood-borne from distant sites. The organisms most frequently implicated are *S. aureus, S. pyogenes*, and *S. pneumoniae*.

Both preseptal (periorbital) and orbital cellulitis present with lid swelling, erythema, and pain. Preseptal cellulitis can arise from a break in the skin (insect bite, laceration), trauma, dacryocystitis, chalazia, hordeola, or sinusitis. Vision is usually normal.

Orbital cellulitis is characterized by proptosis, limitation of extraocular movement, diplopia, and pain with extraocular movement. Vision may be decreased, an afferent pupillary defect (APD) may be present, and there may be ethmoid, frontal, or pansinusitis.

A patient with orbital cellulitis can appear toxic, with fever and lethargy. Most often, there is a history of recent upper respiratory symptoms, and the sinuses are involved. In addition, there is a risk of intracranial spread with subsequent dural sinus thrombosis and brain abscess. Obtain a CT scan with contrast to determine the extent of sinus and/or bony involvement, or if intracranial involvement is suspected.

Conjunctivitis

Inflammation of the bulbar and palpebral conjunctival mucous membranes produces vascular engorgement. Although itching or a "sandy" sensation is frequently noted, there is no ocular pain, and photophobia, if present, is mild. Visual acuity is normal. On examination, there may be a discharge ranging from mucous and crusting to frank pus, along with lid edema and erythema.

A viral cause is suggested by a watery or mucoid discharge during a URI, especially if there is preauricular adenopathy or an associated pharyngitis (typical of adenovirus, which may be called pharyngoconjunctival fever). With enteroviral infection, there may be associated subconjunctival hemorrhage. *Herpes simplex* can be diagnosed from viral culture or immunofluorescence. A bacterial cause is more likely if the child is younger than six years, presents in winter, if they complain of a glued eye in the morning, or if there is a purulent eye discharge on exam. Allergy is suggested by a seasonal pattern (spring or autumn), watery or mucoid discharge, edema, pruritus, and multiple creases and discoloration of the lower lid. In general, the quality of the eye discharge is not diagnostic of the etiology of the conjunctivitis, and there is some overlap in the clinical picture among causes.

Neonatal conjunctivitis was more frequent in the past when silver nitrate prophylaxis was used routinely in the delivery room. Currently, a purulent discharge in the first week of life suggests a gonococcal or chlamydial infection, but a definite diagnosis cannot be made without confirmatory tests. Gram-negative intracellular diplococci and PMNs are found on Gram-stained smears of eye discharge caused by *N. gonorrhea*. Confirm *Chlamydia trachomatis* by cell culture or direct fluorescent antibody staining of conjunctival scrapings.

Obtain the specimen by rolling a saline-moistened sterile swab along the lower palpebral conjunctiva. A sample of the exudate is not adequate, as it often yields a false-negative result. Do not use a topical anesthetic when obtaining the culture of the discharge, as preservatives in the anesthetic can interfere with growth.

Allergic conjunctivitis can be caused by environmental or contact exposure. Signs and symptoms include itching, watery eyes, and swelling. It can involve the lids or bulbar and/or palpebral conjunctiva of one or both eyes. It may occur in isolation or with other allergic symptoms.

Vernal keratoconjunctivitis (VKC) is an atopic condition affecting the bulbar and palpebral conjunctivae. It typically occurs in spring with annual recurrences but can be perennial. It is characterized by severe itching, ropy white discharge, and blepharospasm. Vision can be affected. Gray or white limbal nodules (Horner–Trantas dots) are characteristic and are typically found at the superior limbus, though they can be circumferential. Giant papillae may be seen on the palpebral conjunctiva of the upper lid on lid eversion.

Corneal Disease (Keratitis)

Corneal involvement is generally accompanied by conjunctival hyperemia. Pain, photophobia, and reduction in vision are common. Confirm the diagnosis of a disruption of the corneal epithelium by fluorescein staining of the cornea, followed by illumination with a cobalt blue or Wood's light. Areas of epithelial disturbance or loss will fluoresce a bright green in the midst of the yellow fluorescein.

Uveitis

Inflammation of the pigmented vascular structures of the eye can be associated with conjunctival hyperemia. The presentation is variable and may include photophobia, reduced vision, conjunctival hyperemia, ciliary flush (a halo of dilated episcleral vessels that surround the cornea), and pupillary miosis.

Erythema Multiforme

Stevens–Johnson syndrome (pp. 120–121; formerly erythema multiforme major), is a bullous eruption with skin and mucous membrane involvement. Bullae form on the conjunctiva, which can result in symblepharon (adhesions between the bulbar and palpebral conjunctiva) with shrinkage of the fornices, loss of tear production, and resultant dry eye. There may be purulent conjunctival discharge, conjunctivitis, keratitis with corneal ulceration, or uveitis. Long-term sequelae include entropion and trichiasis.

Kawasaki Disease

Kawasaki disease (pp. 414–417) is characterized by a constellation of symptoms including prolonged fever, cervical lymphadenopathy, stomatitis, erythematous polymorphous rash, edema of the peripheral extremities, and transient conjunctivitis without discharge. Ocular signs can be a presenting feature of the disease. These include bilateral, painless, nonexudative bulbar conjunctival injection with limbic sparing, bilateral anterior uveitis (usually mild), and, less commonly, superficial punctate keratitis, vitreous opacities, and papilledema.

ED Management

The determination of visual acuity is of paramount importance; any acute reduction is an indication for immediate ophthalmologic consult. Evidence of intraocular involvement includes severe photophobia or ocular pain, limbal flush, and pupillary abnormalities. Always inquire about a history of ocular trauma.

Preseptal and Orbital Cellulitis

Treat mild preseptal cellulitis on an outpatient basis with oral amoxicillin-clavulanate (875/125 formulation, 90 mg/kg/day of amoxicillin div bid or cephalexin (40 mg/kg/day div qid). If MRSA is a concern, either use clindamycin (20 mg/kg/day div q 6–8h) or add trimethoprim-sulfamethoxazole (8 mg/kg/day of TMP div bid) to one of the above regimens.

   If orbital cellulitis cannot be ruled out, obtain a CT scan with contrast of the orbits. If orbital involvement is confirmed, admit the patient, obtain a blood culture prior to giving IV antibiotics, perform a lumbar puncture if meningeal or cerebral signs are present, and consult an otolaryngologist if sinus involvement is suspected. Treat with IV antibiotics (amoxicillin-sulbactam 25–50 mg/kg div q 6h above one month of age). In communities with MRSA prevalence, depending on local antibiograms, add either vancomycin 40–60 mg/kg/day div q 6h or clindamycin 30–40 mg/kg/day div q 8h. Vancomycin must be given if there is any possibility of intracranial involvement. Consult an ophthalmologist, particularly if there is an ocular abscess and drainage is needed.

Conjunctivitis

In general, bacterial cultures are not needed. If bacterial conjunctivitis is suspected, treat with a topical ophthalmic antibiotic, either tid–qid application of either a solution (ciprofloxacin, ofloxacin, polymyxin B/trimethoprim, tobramycin) or an ointment (bacitracin, erythromycin, tobramycin). The antibiotics will rapidly treat most uncomplicated bacterial cases and retard secondary bacterial infection if the origin is viral. *Do not prescribe steroid preparations without ophthalmologic consultation.* Continue treatment for 5–7 days or for two days after clinical resolution. Instruct the patient or parent of a younger child to gently wipe away any crust with a warm, damp gauze pad or cottonball before instilling the drops. Meticulous hygiene (no shared towels or washcloths) and frequent handwashing are also necessary. Advise the patient to discard any eye makeup or contact lens cases. Contact lenses should not be worn. Refer the patient to an ophthalmologist if there is persistent infection, severe photophobia or pain, visual complaints, or if the patient developed conjunctivitis while wearing contacts.

Neonatal Conjunctivitis

The presence of Gram-negative diplococci in PMNs is diagnostic of gonococcal conjunctivitis until cultures are available. Admit the infant and treat with one dose of ceftriaxone (25–50 mg/kg, 125 mg maximum) IM or IV. Isolate the infant for 24 hours and remove any discharge with frequent sterile saline irrigations, taking care to avoid splashing the pus into the caregiver's eyes.

If the Gram stain in an infant 1–12 weeks of age with a purulent discharge reveals PMNs but few organisms, and antigen detection or culture for *Chlamydia* are not available, treat for presumed *Chlamydia* conjunctivitis with either erythromycin (50 mg/kg/day PO div q 6h) for two weeks or azithromycin (20 mg/kg PO as one daily dose, for three days) to avoid systemic complications such as pneumonitis. Use topical erythromycin ointment QID for three days as well.

Allergic Conjunctivitis

Treat with a topical antihistamine and mast cell stabilizer (olopatadine, ketotifen) beginning two weeks before the start of the allergy season. Alternatively, use a topical nonsteroidal anti-inflammatory (ketorolac) alone. Topical combination drugs (naphazoline/pheniramine, naphazoline/antazoline) are convenient. *Do not prescribe steroid preparations without ophthalmologic consultation.* If there is no improvement in seven days or the symptoms worsen, refer the patient to an ophthalmologist. Cold compresses are useful. If VKC is suspected, begin treatment with a topical antihistamine–mast cell stabilizer and refer to an ophthalmologist.

Immediately refer all cases of keratitis and uveitis to an ophthalmologist.

The treatment of erythema multiforme major (pp. 120–121) requires an ophthalmologist and includes topical antibiotics, steroids, and lubricants. Surgery, including lysis of synechiae, is sometimes necessary.

Follow-up

- Preseptal cellulitis: 1–2 days
- Conjunctivitis: five days, if no improvement

Indications for Admission

- Orbital cellulitis
- Preseptal cellulitis if compliance not assured

- Stevens–Johnson syndrome
- Gonococcal conjunctivitis

Bibliography

Beal C, Giordano B. Clinical evaluation of red eyes in pediatric patients. *J Pediatr Health Care.* 2016. pii: S0891-5245(16)00063-8.

Divya S, Khan FI. Causes and management of red eye in pediatric ophthalmology. *Curr Allergy and Asthma.* 2011;**11**:212–219.

Palejwala NV, Yeh S, Angeles-Han ST. Current perspectives on ophthalmic manifestations of childhood rheumatic diseases. *Curr Rheumatol Rep.* 2013;**15**(7):341.

Seth D, Khan FI. Causes and management of red eye in pediatric ophthalmology. *Curr Allergy Asthma Rep.* 2011;**11**(3):212–219.

Wong MM, Anninger W. The pediatric red eye. *Pediatric Clin N Am.* 2014;**61**:591–606.

The White Pupil (Leukocoria)

Light entering the eye is absorbed by the pigmented interior and does not leave in sufficient quantity to illuminate the pupil. If an opacity exists in the normally clear optical media, light will reflect off the opacity and be seen in the pupil as a white reflection (leukocoria).

The most common causes of leukocoria are cataracts, infections (syphilis, *Toxocara*, toxoplasmosis, tuberculosis), intraocular hemorrhage, retinopathy of prematurity, detached retina, retinoblastoma, coloboma, and persistent hyperplastic primary vitreous. Therefore, opacities can represent static conditions that interfere with vision (cataracts), active diseases that can lead to visual difficulties (early retinal detachment), or life-threatening illnesses (retinoblastoma).

Clinical Presentation and Diagnosis

Examine both pupils, using a direct ophthalmoscope set at zero at a distance of 12–18 inches from the eye. Normally, the red reflex is symmetrical and the pupil size equal. If there is an opacity in the media, all or part of the pupil will appear dark or off-white instead of red. Depending on the extent of the abnormality, the eyes and/or pupils may be asymmetric in size. There may be no pupillary light response, or it may be slower than in the opposite eye.

Leukocoria can be unilateral or bilateral. If a unilateral problem is suspected, covering the "good" eye will upset a small child, while covering the affected eye will not change the child's behavior.

ED Management

Consult an ophthalmologist immediately whenever leukocoria is suspected

Indications for Admission

- Any case of leukocoria if adequate outpatient follow-up cannot be assured

Bibliography

Damasco VC, Dire DJ. A child with leukocoria. *Pediatr Emerg Care.* 2011;**27**(12):1170–1174.

Olitsky SE, Huse D, Plummer LS, et al. Disorders of the retina and vitreous. in Kliegman RM, Stanton BF, St Geme JW, Schor NF (eds.) *Nelson Textbook of Pediatrics* (20th edn.). Philadelphia, PA: Elsevier; 3049–3056.

Patel N, Salchow DJ, Materin M. Differentials and approach to leukocoria. *Conn Med.* 2013;**77** (3):133–140.

Varughese R, Frith P. Fifteen minutes consultation: a structured approach to the child with a white red reflex. *Arch Dis Child Educ Pract Ed.* 2014;**99**(5):162–165.

Orthopedic Emergencies

Sergey Kunkov, James A. Meltzer, and Katherine J. Chou

Back Pain

In contrast to adults, back pain is a relatively uncommon complaint in children. Back pain in a prepubertal child is particularly concerning and may indicate significant underlying pathology.

Etiologies of pediatric back pain can be classified as musculoskeletal, infectious, inflammatory, neoplastic, and miscellaneous. Of note, idiopathic scoliosis is not a cause of pediatric back pain.

Clinical Presentation

Musculoskeletal Conditions

Spondylolysis and Spondylolisthesis

Spondylolysis and spondylolisthesis are the most common causes of back pain in children older than ten years of age. Spondylolysis is a defect in the pars interarticularis, a bony process on the posterior spine, usually caused by repetitive stress. This is most common at L5 and may present as a fracture, stress fracture, or sclerotic change. The incidence is higher in children who participate in activities involving hyperextension of the spine (dancing, figure skating, gymnastics, football, tennis, and weight training).

A patient with spondylolysis may complain of low back pain worsened by activity, often associated with tight hamstrings and buttock pain. Spondylolysis may become complicated by spondylolisthesis, which is a forward slippage of one vertebra upon another (usually L5 on S1). The physical examination may be normal or there may be a palpable step-off in the lower lumbar region, along with tight hamstrings and limited forward flexion.

Scheuermann's Kyphosis

Excessive kyphosis in the thoracic or lumbar regions is a frequent cause of back pain in adolescents. The patient complains of dull pain over the deformity, which is worsened by activity. On examination, the kyphosis is obvious, accentuated by bending forward, and persists despite the patient's conscious efforts to stand erect. Lateral spine radiographs will show anterior wedging of at least 5° in three or more adjacent vertebral bodies.

Intervertebral Disk Injury

A disk may be injured (bulging) or herniated, most often at L4–L5 and L5–S1. Patients are usually older than ten years and complain of back pain with or without sciatica (pain down the back of the thigh). Physical examination findings include decreased lumbar lordosis, limited forward flexion, paraspinal muscle spasm, and a positive straight leg-raising test (see below).

Lumbar Sacral Sprain

This is an injury or tearing of the ligaments and/or muscle fibers (interspinous or paraspinal) that connect one vertebra to another or support a vertebra. The most common mechanism of injury is a sudden twisting motion in an inflexible and overweight patient. This injury can also occur in children who carry heavy backpacks.

Trauma

Fractures of the spine are uncommon and usually are associated with a significant amount of force. Occasionally, trauma to the back can lead to an epidural hematoma that can compress the spinal cord as it expands, especially in patients with hemophilia or other clotting disorders.

Infectious Etiologies

Orthopedic infections including diskitis, osteomyelitis (pp. 585–586), and spinal epidural abscess can cause back pain.

Diskitis

Diskitis is a rare condition that occurs most often in younger children (average three years old). The patient may present with fever, malaise, low back pain, refusal to walk or crawl, and associated hip or abdominal pain. On physical examination, there may be tenderness over the involved disk, decreased back motion, and pain with hip flexion. The WBC is often normal, but the ESR and CRP are usually elevated. The blood culture is usually negative but sometimes yields an organism, most often *S. aureus*.

Vertebral Osteomyelitis

Vertebral osteomyelitis presents similarly to diskitis, but is more common in the older child (average seven years old). Unlike diskitis, the blood culture is positive in about 50% of cases (usually *S. aureus*). Uncommon entities, such as *B. Henselae*, Salmonella, and tuberculosis (TB), can also cause vertebral osteomyelitis but generally are associated with recognized risk factors (cat scratch, sickle cell anemia, risks for TB).

Epidural Abscess

An epidural abscess most often results from hematogenous spread of bacteria into the epidural space, but it can also occur secondary to direct extension from an underlying osteomyelitis or superinfection of a traumatic hematoma. In some cases, there will be no fever or back pain, so the patient may present later, with neurologic symptoms. The microbiology of epidural abscesses is similar to that of vertebral osteomyelitis. Children with infections (i.e., abscess or pyomyositis) involving the paraspinal or pelvic muscles often complain of back pain. In addition, various non-orthopedic infections, such as pyelonephritis, pneumonia, and pancreatitis, can occasionally present with back pain.

Nonspinal Infections

Pneumonia, endocarditis, pyelonephritis, pelvic inflammatory disease, retrocecal appendicitis, pancreatitis, and myositis of spinal muscles may also cause back pain.

Inflammatory Rheumatologic Diseases

Ankylosing Spondylitis

Ankylosing spondylitis is a spondyloarthropathy involving the sacroiliac joints and lumbar spine. It is most common in adolescent boys, and the majority of affected patients are HLA-B27 positive. The patient may experience transient arthritis of large joints, followed by back involvement later in the disease course. Pain in the lower back, hips, and thighs is associated with morning stiffness that is relieved by movement. There may also be an acute iridocyclitis and/or aortitis. The spinal involvement begins in the sacroiliac joints and ascends progressively to involve the rest of the spine, including the cervical vertebrae. In contrast, juvenile idiopathic arthritis (JIA) affects the cervical spine, but spares the lumbar spine.

A patient with inflammatory bowel disease may have associated spondylitis similar to ankylosing spondylitis. The patient may present with low back pain prior to the onset of gastrointestinal symptoms.

Neoplasm

Spinal Tumor

A spinal tumor is a rare but concerning cause of back pain in children. The majority are benign, including osteoid osteomas, eosinophilic granulomas, and unicameral bone cysts. Malignancies include Ewing sarcoma, osteosarcoma, and metastatic lesions (neuroblastoma, etc.). A history of nighttime pain, pain not associated with activity, or a painful scoliosis raises the concern of a tumor. Leukemia may present as persistent back pain secondary to infiltration of the bone marrow.

Sickle Cell Crisis

Back pain is a common complaint in children with sickle cell disease. Most patients will be identified early in life on the newborn screen, unless they come from a country where there is no routine newborn screening for sickle hemoglobinopathies.

Miscellaneous Conditions

Reflex Sympathetic Dystrophy (RSD)

The hallmark of this syndrome is severe pain associated with autonomic dysfunction (swelling, edema, skin color changes, mottling). RSD may occur in the back after trauma, although the initial injury may be a sprain or a disk injury, with ongoing pain out of proportion to what is expected for the original injury (allodynia, dysthesias).

Diagnosis

A thorough history is essential in determining whether the patient's back pain requires urgent or immediate intervention. Determine the onset of the pain, its timing, severity, and radiation, as well as factors that alleviate or trigger it. Inquire about sports participation, including the intensity of the involvement and the initiation of any new sports. Ask specifically about trauma. Evaluate the child's activity level since the onset of symptoms; back pain that forces the child to refrain from usual activities requires a thorough evaluation.

Determine whether the pain is related to sleep or resting in bed. Specific difficulty in moving from side to side in bed may suggest a disk problem or lumbar sprain. A patient awakened and kept awake by back pain must be thoroughly evaluated for a tumor, infection, or inflammatory condition. In contrast, back pain from overuse syndromes, muscle pain, Scheuermann's disease, or spondylolysis (with or without spondylolisthesis) usually improves with rest.

Always check for the presence of systemic symptoms, such as fever, malaise, irritability, or weight loss. In these children, ask about pets (i.e., kittens) and risk factors for TB such as travel to or from endemic areas. A positive history for ankle or foot weakness, changes in bowel or bladder function, and/or an altered gait, is suggestive of neurologic impairment. Ask about medications or therapies already tried, including chiropractic manipulation and acupuncture. Note any chronic medications that cause osteoporosis (i.e., steroids), because these increase the risk for fracture.

Physical Examination

Have the patient undress down to his or her underwear and observe the gait and posture. Note any muscle asymmetry and signs of splinting. Assess the back for a midline defect or lesion such as a tuft of hair or hemangioma. Carefully check for tenderness by palpating over the vertebrae, spinous processes, vertebral spaces, and interspinal ligaments, as well as the shoulders and paraspinal muscles.

For the lumbar spine, evaluate forward flexion, lateral rotation, lateral bending, and extension. The forward bend test helps reveal any deformities of the spine; low back pain increased by hyperextension suggests spondylolysis and/or spondylolisthesis.

Perform a complete neurological examination, paying particular attention to symmetry and deep tendon reflexes (knee jerk and ankle jerk). Look for quadriceps and hamstring asymmetry, which can result from a low back problem. Check the strength of each lower extremity, isolating each joint and comparing it to the other: hip (flexion, extension, abduction, and adduction), knee (flexion and extension), and ankle/foot (plantar flexion/dorsiflexion, inversion, eversion). Lower limb weakness may be a sign of spinal cord compression and is a particularly ominous finding requiring immediate attention. Also check for signs of meningeal irritation (Kernig's and Brudzinski's signs).

A straight leg-raising test will frequently be positive in a patient with disk herniation: with the patient supine, grasp the ankle, and with the knee held in extension, bring the leg upward to assess range of flexion of the hip joint. Note the angle and location of any elicited pain. Then repeat the maneuver and dorsiflex the foot as the painful angle is approached, which will aggravate the pain. Back pain radiating down the back of the leg indicates sciatic nerve irritation and a herniated disk.

Radiological Studies

A patient with abnormal physical findings, pain that has lasted three months or more despite conservative treatment, nighttime or constant pain, or pain due to significant trauma requires radiological evaluation. Obtain anteroposterior and lateral radiographs of the spine and add oblique lumbar spine views if spondylolysis is suspected. Obtain a technetium-99 bone scan if a febrile patient has an examination that is consistent with diskitis or osteomyelitis, if the plain films are normal. A CT scan can further define spinal pathology located by bone scan and a fine-cut CT scan (1–3 mm cuts) is useful in diagnosing and evaluating spondylolysis. Obtain an MRI for any abnormal neurologic findings. The MRI is a valuable tool in evaluating spinal cord tumors, tethered cords, disk herniations, diskitis, and other spinal pathology, but clinically insignificant disk herniations or

Table 17.1 Clinical features of back pain requiring immediate evaluation

Symptom	Significance
Age <4 years	Benign back pain very uncommon in this age
Duration >1 month	Concern for neoplasm/infection
History of malignancy	Concern for spinal metastases
Neurological abnormalities: foot or ankle weakness, altered gait, abnormal DTRs or Babinski, asymmetric strength, meningeal signs, bladder or bowel dysfunction	Concern for root compression/epidural abscess
Nocturnal or constant pain	Concern for spinal tumor or infection
Pain radiating below buttocks	Concern for nerve root compression
Point tenderness over spine or intervertebral space	Concern for spinal infection or fracture

degenerative disk disease may be over-read. A concern about spinal cord compression is one of the few indications for an emergent MRI.

Laboratory Studies

If a medical cause is suspected, order a CBC, serum electrolytes, CRP, ESR, urinalysis, and a blood culture. If a rheumatologic cause is suspected, also obtain an ANA, rheumatoid factor, and HLA-B27 screening.

ED Management

The priority is to identify conditions requiring immediate treatment, including mass lesions, diskitis, or osteomyelitis. If the patient has any of the clinical features outlined in Table 17.1, arrange for immediate radiological evaluation (see above) and consultation with a neurologist and/or orthopedist. Immediately consult a neurosurgeon if the patient has any signs of spinal cord compression.

If an older child with back pain for less than one month appears well, has a normal neurological examination, and does not have point tenderness, nighttime pain, or restriction of daily activities, refer him or her to a primary care provider, orthopedist, or sports medicine specialist for follow-up within one week. In general, management will include referral to a physical therapist, avoidance of the offending activity (usually hyperextension), and occasionally, a back brace. However, bed rest has virtually no role in the management of back pain. Encourage the patient to walk and go to school as soon as possible. Reserve ibuprofen (10 mg/kg q 6h) for acute pain (sprains, fractures, disk injuries).

Follow-up

- Within one week; patient to return immediately for worsening pain, especially at night, neurologic symptoms, or systemic symptoms

Indications for Admission
- Diskitis, osteomyelitis, or spinal epidural abscess
- Suspected neoplasm

Bibliography

Dizdarevic I, Bishop M, Sgromolo N, Hammoud S, Atanda A Jr. Approach to the pediatric athlete with back pain: more than just the pars. *Phys Sportsmed*. 2015;**43**(4):421–431.

Houghton KM. Review for the generalist: evaluation of low back pain in children and adolescents. *Pediatr Rheumatol Online J*. 2010;**8**:28.

MacDonald J, Stuart E, Rodenberg R. Musculoskeletal low back pain in school-aged children: a review. *JAMA Pediatr*. 2017;**171**(3):280–287.

Moreno MA. Low back pain in children and adolescents. *JAMA Pediatr*. 2017;**171**(3):312.

Shah SA, Saller J. Evaluation and diagnosis of back pain in children and adolescents. *J Am Acad Orthop Surg*. 2016;**24**(1):37–45.

Common Orthopedic Injuries
Upper Extremity

Clavicle

Clavicular fractures are particularly common in newborns (5 per 1000 births). They are associated with a breech or difficult delivery but may not be noticed until about one week of age, when a grossly obvious callus is found in the area of the fracture. In older children, they are caused by a fall on an outstretched hand (FOOSH) or by a direct blow, and present with swelling and tenderness. It is important to tell parents to expect a large, possibly tender, swelling (callus) 7–10 days after the injury. Most clavicle fractures heal with minimal supportive treatment. Either immobilize the arm with a sling or apply a figure-of-eight clavicle splint. A full return of function requires 3–4 weeks.

True sternoclavicular and acromioclavicular (AC) joint dislocations are relatively uncommon in children and more often are, in fact, physeal fractures. However, the treatment is usually the same (outpatient management with a sling). Rarely, the clavicle may be severely displaced and require reduction. Medial clavicular injuries require particular attention when displaced posteriorly because they may compress the trachea, great vessels, and brachial plexus. An emergent CT scan and orthopedic consultation are required if this injury is suspected.

Shoulder

Shoulder dislocations are rare in childhood, as the proximal humeral epiphysis is weaker than the shoulder joint capsule. As the growth plate closes, shoulder dislocations can occur with a FOOSH, forced abduction of an externally rotated arm, or a posterior blow to an elevated, abducted arm. Anterior dislocation is the most common, presenting with the arm held slightly abducted and in external rotation, with a squared-off appearance to the shoulder. There may be numbness and tingling of the arm. The recurrence rate approaches 90% after an initial dislocation in a teenager.

Except for a patient with a history of a shoulder dislocation, obtain radiographs prior to reduction as a superior humeral fracture can resemble a dislocation. Test for neurovascular compromise before and after any attempt at shoulder reduction by comparing bilateral brachial pulses and examining sensation over the deltoid muscle. Reduce an anterior shoulder dislocation with the Stimson method. After providing adequate sedation (pp. 715–722), have the patient lie prone on a stretcher, with the affected arm hanging down. Application of a 5–10 lb weight to the arm will cause gradual reduction over 15–30 minutes. During the reduction rotate the inferior edge of the scapula medially with gentle pressure. Place the arm in a sling and obtain post-reduction radiographs to evaluate for an associated fracture.

Proximal Humerus

Injuries to the proximal humerus usually involve the growth plate or metaphysis, occurring after a FOOSH. Neurovascular compromise is rare. This area has tremendous remodeling potential, so growth disturbances are uncommon. Angulations up to 30° and displacement of up to 50% may not require reduction. Treat with a sling and immobilization. More significantly displaced fractures require reduction.

Overhand sports (baseball pitching, swimming, etc.) can place stress and injure the proximal humeral physis by the same mechanism that causes a rotator cuff injury in older athletes. Typically, the pain has a gradual onset over months and is most severe when performing the overhand activity. Patients often present with tenderness over the proximal humerus, but many are asymptomatic at rest. Radiographs of the humerus may be normal or show widening of the physis, fragmentation, demineralization, or sclerosis. Treat with rest, ice, analgesia, and a slow return to sports.

Humeral Shaft

These fractures are less common than proximal and distal humeral fractures. They can be associated with a unicameral bone cyst of the humerus. Carefully assess the radial nerve (wrist dorsiflexion), which may be injured as it passes close to the bone in the distal half of the shaft. Treat with a sling, as few of these injuries require reduction.

Elbow Injuries

If a fracture is suspected, splint the extremity and obtain true AP and lateral radiographs. If there is an obvious deformity, do not test passive range of motion, because of the risk of displacing a fracture. Apply ice and elevate the extremity above the level of the heart to reduce swelling.

Since a child's elbow is a maze of growth centers, surrogate markers for fracture are often helpful when a fracture line is not obvious. On the lateral radiograph, the anterior humeral line normally intersects the middle third of the capitellum on a true lateral; if it does not, suspect a fracture. Similarly, the radius typically aligns with the capitellum; if it does not, suspect a dislocation. Also on the lateral radiograph, a normal elbow will have a visible thin anterior fat pad that is flush up against the humerus. The posterior fat pad normally lies deep in the olecranon fossa and is not visible when the elbow is flexed. When the joint capsule is distended by blood or an effusion, however, the anterior fat pad is lifted away from the humerus (sail sign) and the posterior fat pad becomes visible as it is pushed posteriorly out of the olecranon fossa.

Supracondylar Fractures

These account for about two-thirds of elbow fractures and typically occur in children <10 years of age who FOOSH with a hyperextended elbow. Fractures of the distal end of the humerus pose a high risk (12%) of neurovascular compromise, most often involving the median and radial nerves. Supracondylar fractures may present with ischemic pain in the forearm from a compartment syndrome or injury to the brachial artery. An attempt to extend the fingers may cause considerable pain. This is a more reliable sign of ischemia than the absence of the radial pulse. Prompt orthopedic intervention is required to prevent a Volkmann's contracture. If compartment syndrome is suspected, arrange for immediate measurement of compartment pressure.

Treat nondisplaced fractures with *in situ* immobilization; these heal well. Displaced fractures require accurate anatomic reduction and immobilization, often necessitating pin fixation. Admit a patient with a displaced supracondylar fracture and/or marked swelling for repeated neurovascular checks.

Fractures of the Lateral and Medial Condyles and Epicondyles

These represent Salter IV fractures involving both the growth plate and the elbow joint. Lateral epicondyle fractures are one of the few types of pediatric fractures that may proceed to nonunion. Radiographs may not reveal the true extent of the displacement; an arthrogram may be required. Suspect a fracture if there is instability on valgus and varus stress. Treat nondisplaced fractures with immobilization, but displaced fractures require surgery for precise anatomic reduction.

Little League elbow is a common overuse injury that results in an apophysitis about the medial epicondyle. The act of throwing places excessive valgus stress on the medial epicondyle. Typically, the pain worsens during throwing and improves with rest. Examination may be normal or demonstrate point tenderness over the medial epicondyle. Radiographs may be normal or show a widened physis, fragmentation, or hypertrophy about the medial epicondyle. Treatment consists of rest, ice, and analgesia similar to other overuse injuries.

Fractures of the Proximal Radius

These can also occur from a FOOSH. Characteristic findings are pain over the radial head and decreased forearm pronation and supination. Neurovascular compromise is unusual. Other parts of the elbow are frequently injured (50%), so obtain a dedicated ipsilateral elbow radiograph if only a forearm x-ray was taken. Normally, a line drawn through the shaft of the radius always intersects the capitellum, no matter how the arm is positioned. In the absence of any angulation or displacement, treat symptomatically with a sling and range of motion exercises beginning the next day. Otherwise, consult an orthopedist for evaluation and possible reduction because of the increased risk of avascular necrosis and subsequent loss of function.

Nursemaid's Elbow (Radial Head Subluxation)

This is a common problem that typically occurs when a young child's (1–3 years) arm is suddenly pulled while the elbow is extended and the arm pronated, or after a minor fall. It may be recurrent, but can be managed without radiographs or orthopedic consultation. The patient will often be comfortable but refuse to actively flex the elbow, preferring an extended, internally rotated position. Examine the affected arm in the extended position to ensure there is no swelling or tenderness around the elbow or wrist prior to any attempt at reduction. If the patient has any tenderness with palpation, obtain radiographs to evaluate for fracture.

To reduce a nursemaid's elbow, cup the elbow in one hand and the wrist in the other. Rapidly supinate the forearm while simultaneously flexing the elbow. Usually a click is felt, and within 10–15 minutes (sometimes longer) the child actively flexes the elbow. If the success of the reduction is in question, obtain radiographs of the elbow to evaluate for an occult fracture before attempting to reduce again. Note some patients with nursemaid's elbow, however, will demonstrate a joint effusion on elbow radiographs. Hyperpronation of the forearm is another technique useful for reduction.

Elbow Dislocations

Posterior dislocations of the elbow are the most common type, although neurovascular compromise is unusual, but critical to identify. Contact orthopedics for reduction. Afterward, obtain post-reduction radiographs to look for associated fractures, which occur frequently, and admit the patient for observation for compartment syndrome.

Forearm Fractures

These are the most common fractures of childhood and are usually caused by falls. About 75% occur in the distal third of the forearm and most others in the middle third. Over half are greenstick fractures presenting with pain and swelling without significant deformity. If only one forearm bone is fractured, image the elbow and wrist to evaluate for concurrent dislocation of the other bone.

Treat a nondisplaced fracture with splinting or casting. A displaced or angulated fracture requires closed reduction and casting under sedation. Use a long arm cast for a midshaft fracture, but a short arm cast will suffice for a distal fracture. In a patient under ten years of age, the forearm and wrist will remodel with no lasting deformity, if proper reduction is achieved. Treat a buckle fracture of the distal radius with a removable volar splint to allow for increased comfort and early return of function.

Wrist and Hand Fractures

Carpal fractures are uncommon in children, although the scaphoid (navicular) is the most frequently fractured, usually by a FOOSH (see Hand Injuries, pp. 744–749). Carpal fractures present with pain in the wrist, with deformity or swelling, and sometimes without definite radiologic abnormalities. Point tenderness in the anatomic snuff box suggests a scaphoid fracture, as does pain in the snuffbox with axial loading of the thumb. Obtain a wrist radiograph with dedicated scaphoid views. Treat nondisplaced scaphoid fractures with a thumb spica cast. Displacement is a sign of wrist instability and requires open reduction and internal fixation. Radiographs may not detect subtle scaphoid fractures so place all patients with snuffbox tenderness and negative x-rays in a thumb spica splint.

Metacarpal fractures are usually the result of fighting. The neck of the fifth metacarpal is most often affected (boxer's fracture). The patient may present 1–2 days after the injury with swelling of the dorsum of the hand and decreased range of motion. In the absence of significant angulation or displacement, treat with a radial and/or ulnar gutter splint depending on the affected bone. Consult orthopedics for multiple metacarpal fractures or when there is an associated rotational deformity causing finger overlap.

Finger Fractures and Injuries

Most finger fractures are simple, nondisplaced distal phalangeal shaft injuries. A subungual hematoma is often associated with the fracture due to crush injury.

Reduction is indicated if there is a displaced phalangeal fracture with >20° of volar angulation. Use a dorsal splint to immobilize a fractured digit, maintaining the MCP joints at 35–40° of flexion, ensuring that the rotational alignment of the digits is preserved. Injuries to the base of the thumb may require a thumb spica cast, and significantly unstable fractures may require pin fixation.

Finger dislocations are easily recognized from the deformity of the digit. The most frequently dislocated metacarpophalangeal joint is the second. Anesthetize the finger using a digital nerve block and reduce the finger dislocation with simple traction. Afterward, splint for 7–10 days.

Lower Extremity

Pelvic Fractures

Fractures of the pelvis are rarely isolated, occurring most often in a multiple-trauma victim who has pain with movement or palpation of the pelvis. There may be associated injuries to the viscera and bladder or a vaginal or rectal laceration. If there is any suspicion of a pelvic injury, obtain pelvic radiographs as part of a multiple trauma work-up. Most pelvic fractures are stable, so treatment is directed toward fluid resuscitation and hemodynamic stabilization. Pelvic fractures that cause widening of the sacroiliac joints can result in a substantial amount of blood loss. For a patient whose pelvic ring is substantially disrupted or who remains hemodynamically unstable, apply lateral pressure with a pelvic binder, or bedsheets, wrapped around the femoral heads.

Do not insert a urinary catheter in any patient with blood at the urethral meatus, a high-riding prostate or scrotal hematoma, or a vaginal laceration because of the risk of converting a partial urethral tear into a complete one. Consult urology for an emergent urethrogram. For a female, because the urethra is so short, urethroscopy may be more helpful.

Pelvic apophyseal injuries are common and usually isolated injuries in children. These occur after an acute strong contraction of the attached muscle, most often in an athlete who presents with localized pain. Overuse injuries (apophysitis) are more chronic and improve with rest. The anterior superior and inferior iliac spines, the iliac crest, and the ischial tuberosity are the sites most often involved. Pelvic radiograph findings vary from a widening of the physis to complete avulsion. Treat simple apophyseal injuries symptomatically with analgesia, ice, and rest. Consult an orthopedist for complete avulsion fractures.

Hip Injuries

Hip fractures are rare, occurring with significant high-energy trauma. In 30% of cases, there are associated injuries. Observe how the patient holds the leg while lying supine. The affected leg is shortened and externally rotated, while the hip may be flexed. Obtain AP and lateral (frog-leg) radiographs. Prompt surgical reduction is required to prevent avascular necrosis, especially with femoral neck fractures and hip dislocation. A delay in treatment can cause permanent deformity.

A traumatic hip dislocation is rare, and most are posterior. It occurs when the hip is flexed and forced posteriorly (kneeling football player, sitting in motor vehicle). It is associated with significant morbidity if not relocated within six hours.

Femoral Shaft Fractures

Typically, femur fractures are easily identified, presenting with swelling, deformity, and tenderness in the thigh. Occasionally, they may be detected while evaluating a crying child who refuses to bear weight on the affected leg. Look for other injuries, such as ipsilateral hip dislocation, femoral neck fracture, epiphyseal injury, tibial fracture, and fracture of the contralateral femur. While a femoral shaft fracture can occur with falls and play, suspect child abuse in non-ambulatory children or those with other signs of inflicted trauma (pp. 604–608). When caused by high-energy trauma, a substantial amount of blood can extravasate into the surrounding tissue and result in shock. Consult orthopedics for definitive management.

Knee Injuries

The knee is a common site of sports injuries, especially in football players and skiers. The history of the mechanism of injury, including the position of the knee and foot at the time of injury, and whether there was any contact, help suggest the most likely diagnosis. The patient may complain of pain or swelling or may be limping or unable to bear weight. A sensation of "tightness" behind the knee suggests a small effusion.

Obtain AP and lateral radiographs of the knee to rule-out fracture in patients that have any bony tenderness, are unable to bear weight, or cannot flex their knee to 90°. Order an additional patellar skyline view if the patient has tenderness over the patella. Obtain a CT scan of the knee when the clinical suspicion for a fracture is high but the radiographs are not definitive. It is quite common for an acutely injured knee to be so swollen and painful that an examination is impossible. Use the RICE protocol with a knee immobilizer, and refer the patient to an orthopedist for definitive diagnosis and treatment. If a fracture is present, immediate consultation is required.

Knee Sprains

Knee sprains are rare in young children; they occur more frequently in adolescents with closed or closing growth plates. The medial collateral ligament (MCL) is the most common site of sprain, caused by a lateral blow to the knee. Injuries to the anterior cruciate ligament (ACL) can occur without contact by abrupt deceleration maneuvers, jumping, missed landing, or "cutting" maneuvers such as those seen in basketball, football, or tennis. Lateral collateral ligament (LCL) and posterior cruciate injuries are less common.

After the initial evaluation of the injured extremity, the integrity of the knee ligaments must be checked. For each ligament, assess the range of motion and whether there is a definite endpoint, using the other side as a reference. With the patient supine, the hip extended, and the knee at 0° (fully extended), place one hand above the ankle and the other on the lateral aspect of the distal femur. Abducting the lower leg then causes valgus knee stress, testing the MCL. Place the upper hand on the medial aspect of the distal femur, and adduct the lower leg (varus stress, LCL). If there is instability (no definite endpoint), stop the examination; if the knee is not unstable, repeat the exam at 30° flexion. MCL sprains cause medial pain; LCL injuries result in pain on the lateral side of the knee.

Next, test the cruciate ligaments by performing a Lachman test. With the knee flexed 20°, stabilize the femur with one hand and draw the tibia downward with the other. A sharp endpoint indicates ACL integrity. Then flex the hip to 45° and the knee to 90° with the foot flat on the table. Sit on the patient's toes, place four fingers of both hands on either side of the patient's calf and your thumbs on the femoral condyles, and pull the tibia forward (anterior draw, ACL), feeling for a definite endpoint. Then push it backward (posterior draw, posterior cruciate).

With ACL tears the patient or bystanders may report having heard a "pop" or "snap," the patient refuses to bear weight, and swelling begins almost immediately. Treat knee sprains with a knee immobilizer and crutches. Radiographs may demonstrate an avulsion fracture of the superior lateral tibia (Segond fracture).

Meniscal Injuries

Meniscal injuries occur on weight-bearing with the foot externally rotated, pushing off, often during squatting and twisting (baseball catchers); lateral meniscus injuries are uncommon. Meniscal injuries present with painful ambulation and inability to fully extend the knee. To evaluate the menisci, perform McMurray's test. While the knee is hyperflexed, rotate it internally and externally by applying torque at the ankle. Palpitate over the medial and lateral joint lines; clicking or grinding reflects a positive test. Treat with a knee immobilizer.

Patellar Dislocation

A lateral patellar dislocation is most common in adolescent girls. It can be caused without contact by an acute strong contraction of the quadriceps muscles or by a direct blow to the knee. A ripping sound is often reported by the patient, and the knee is held semi-flexed, appears deformed, and cannot be straightened. Patellar dislocation is obvious when the patella is lateral to the joint, and the anterior aspect of the knee appears concave and empty. Reduction can usually be achieved by manipulating the patella medially while the quadriceps muscle is at its shortest – that is with the knee fully extended and the hip flexed. Many patients often present after self-relocation, complaining of knee pain with no obvious deformity. The patellar apprehension test is useful if relocation has occurred. Slightly flex the knee and prepare to push the patella laterally. The patient will become anxious and stop the procedure. Apply a knee immobilizer and give the patient crutches. Consult an orthopedist if reduction is unsuccessful or if there is an associated fracture on x-ray.

Knee Fractures

Intra-articular fractures of the knee are uncommon, although pain, deformity, decreased range of motion, and fluid in the knee joint suggest the possibility. The distal femoral growth plate (which can be displaced and lead to growth disturbance), tibial tubercle, and proximal tibial metaphysis are the most common areas fractured. Movements that would normally cause an ACL tear in an adult will cause a fracture of the tibial spine in a child. Fractures of the patella are uncommon, resulting from a forceful blow directly to the knee.

Perform a careful neurovascular examination to ensure that the popliteal vessels are intact. If there is neurovascular compromise, apply gentle longitudinal traction in line with the extremity. Comparison x-rays are helpful in assessing the degree of displacement of the tibial tubercle and tibial spine. Treatment of tibial fractures usually consists of closed reduction, but fractures of the distal femoral epiphysis usually require surgical reduction and fixation. Admit the patient for neurovascular checks if there is severe swelling; otherwise discharge home with crutches, analgesia, and instructions to keep leg elevated whenever possible.

Osgood–Schlatter Disease

Osgood–Schlatter disease is an apophysitis of the tibial tuberosity. It typically presents in athletes who complain of anterior knee pain and swelling worsened by exercise. The patient will have point tenderness over the tibial tubercle. Radiographs are not needed to confirm the diagnosis but demonstrate thickening of the patellar tendon and, often, fragmentation of the tibial tubercle. The disease is self-limited and improves with rest, ice, and nonsteroidal anti-inflammatories (NSAIDS), such as ibuprofen (10 mg/kg q 6h, 800 mg/dose maximum).

Tibia and Fibula Fractures

These are most frequently caused by motor vehicle accidents and falls from height. Many are greenstick-type fractures. Spiral fractures of the tibia, caused by rotational force on a foot that is fixed, are a common sports injury. Pain and swelling may not be seen in isolated fibula fractures. Beware of any signs of compartment syndrome (see p. 574). Treat tibial fractures with long leg casting.

A toddler's fracture is a nondisplaced fracture of the distal diaphysis of the tibia. It most commonly occurs between nine months and three years of age, sometimes without a history of significant trauma. The child presents with a limp, and the initial radiograph may show a faint line in the tibial shaft. A callus can be seen on repeat films one week later. If a toddler's fracture is missed, however, it will heal without sequelae.

Isolated fibula fractures are rare, and pain and swelling may be absent. Careful examination and radiographs are necessary to rule-out any displacement and joint disruption. An isolated nondisplaced fibula fracture requires supportive care only.

Ankle Injuries

Patients with these common injuries often present after twisting or "rolling" their ankle, with localized pain, swelling, and decreased range of motion. While older teenagers are more likely to sprain their ankle, younger children are more likely to have a fracture. Carefully examine the ankle for tenderness over the medial and lateral malleoli. Always examine the ipsilateral foot and knee for associated injuries.

If the radiograph does not demonstrate a fracture and the patient has closed physes, treat with RICE therapy. Crutches may be used until the patient is able to bear weight on the affected ankle.

Skeletally immature patients (i.e., with open physes) may have a Salter 1 fracture although the radiograph appears normal. Immobilize the ankle and repeat the radiograph in 10–14 days. This may demonstrate callous formation as evidence of the fracture. Immobilize a patient with medial malleolar (tibial) tenderness in a short leg cast or a posterior splint; give crutches and instructions for non-weight-bearing. Place a patient with lateral malleolar tenderness into an air-cast or splint, and permit walking because the fibula is a non-weight-bearing bone.

Consult orthopedics for radiographically evident physeal fractures. Some ankle fractures may need additional "stress view" radiographs to evaluate for ankle joint instability. Tillaux and triplane fractures can occur during adolescence when the tibial physes are beginning to close. Operative treatment may be required and subsequent growth arrest can be significant. Displacement of ankle fractures usually requires operative management.

Tarsal and Metatarsal Injuries

These most commonly occur secondary to a direct blow to the foot. Ninety percent of foot fractures occur in the metatarsals, presenting with pain and swelling. Treat with a padded support dressing and protected weight-bearing with crutches. A common error is confusing the growth center of the first metatarsal (located proximally) as a fracture; the growth centers of the other metatarsals are located distally.

Avulsion fractures of the base of the fifth metatarsal are common injuries, but they can be confused with secondary ossification centers. These fractures most commonly occur with an inversion injury and present with point tenderness and mild swelling. Treat them like most other metatarsal fractures with a short-leg walking cast.

A true "Jones fracture" occurs at the proximal diaphysis of the fifth metatarsal, is perpendicular to the long axis of the bone, and extends into the joint between the fourth and fifth metatarsals. Because of the risk of nonunion, treat with a short-leg cast or posterior splint, crutches, and non-weight-bearing.

Tarsometatarsal Dislocation

A dislocation of the tarsometatarsal joint can occur when violent plantar flexion of the forefoot occurs if the foot is in the "tiptoe" position (foot used to break a fall from a bicycle or motorcycle). These dislocations are generally accompanied by metatarsal shaft or neck fractures. The patient presents with swelling of the dorsum of the foot overlying the tarsometatarsal joints, with marked pain and tenderness and inability to bear weight. Often, a deformity is not present because of the high rate of spontaneous reduction. Reduction, with immobilization or pinning, is required.

Fractures of the Phalanges of the Foot

These are rare in young children but more common in adolescents. They are caused by direct trauma secondary to a falling object or kicking a hard object. The patient presents with pain, swelling, and, occasionally, deformity. Treat with alignment, buddy taping, and hard-soled shoe to prevent movement.

Indications to Consult an Orthopedist

- Compound, complete, open, or pathologic fracture
- Displaced fracture requiring reduction
- Growth plate injury other than Salter I
- Suspected neurovascular compromise
- Specific fractures: supracondylar, pelvis, hip, femur
- Specific dislocations: elbow, hip, knee, tarsometatarsal

Follow-up

- Fracture treated with casting: immediately for pain out of proportion to the injury, color change of the distal extremity, and numbness or tingling; otherwise as per orthopedist
- Injury treated with sling, splint, or immobilizer: immediately for unremitting pain; otherwise 1–2 weeks
- Nursemaid's elbow: 24 hours, if the child is not moving the arm in a normal fashion

Bibliography

Desai N, Caperell KS. Joint dislocations in the pediatric emergency department. *Clin Pediatr Emerg Med.* 2016;**17**(1):53–66.

Hosseinzadeh P, Hayes CB. Compartment syndrome in children. *Orthop Clin North Am.* 2016;**47**(3):579–587.

Laine JC, Kaiser SP, Diab M. High-risk pediatric orthopedic pitfalls. *Emerg Med Clin North Am.* 2010;**28**(1):85–102.

Royal Children's Hospital Melbourne. Paediatric fractures guidelines. www.rch.org.au/clinicalguide/fractures (accessed May 30, 2017).

Su AW, Larson AN. Pediatric ankle fractures: concepts and treatment principles. *Foot Ankle Clin.* 2015;**20**(4):705–719.

Thornton MD, Della-Giustina K, Aronson PL. Emergency department evaluation and treatment of pediatric orthopedic injuries. *Emerg Clin North Am.* 2015;**33**(2):423–449.

Fractures, Dislocations, and Sprains

Skeletal injuries account for 10–15% of all injuries in children; 15% of these involve the physis or growth plate. Always consider the possibility of child abuse in young children.

Clinical Presentation and Diagnosis

Obtain a complete history, including the mechanism of the injury; location of maximal pain; previous orthopedic or rheumatologic problems (fractures, dislocations, joint pain or swelling); chronic medical problems (rickets, renal failure, liver disease, malignancy); and drug use (phenytoin can produce a rickets-like picture). For open fractures, ascertain the patient's tetanus status and whether the trauma occurred in a dirty environment (farm and field injuries are at risk for clostridial infections).

On physical examination, focus on the area(s) of pain and tenderness, as well as the joints above and below the suspected injury. Perform a complete examination, looking for associated and/or additional traumatic injuries.

Begin the examination with assessment of the neurovascular status of the affected extremity. Palpate the pulses; check the warmth, capillary filling, and active motion of the fingers or toes; and evaluate sensation, using the uninjured limb for comparison. The presence of any of the "six Ps" distal to the fracture site suggests compartment syndrome and neurovascular compromise: pain, pulselessness, pallor, paralysis, paresthesias, and painful passive motion. Painful passive motion is the most sensitive sign. While the presence of a pulse does not assure adequate circulation, assume that absence of a pulse means compromise. For upper-extremity injuries, check for nerve injury by ensuring the child can form, with the hand of the affected extremity, a "rock" (median nerve), "paper" (radial nerve), "scissors" (ulnar nerve), and an "ok" sign (anterior interosseous nerve).

Inspect the extremity and compare it to the uninjured side, looking for asymmetry, swelling, abrasions, ecchymoses, and deformity. Check for point tenderness, which is often, but not always, associated with a fracture. In some cases, the pain may not be well localized, but usually is near the fracture site. Next, evaluate the joints. Have the patient attempt an active range of motion of the injured joint, using the other side for comparison. If the child is unable to complete a full range of motion, gently perform a passive examination of joint mobility.

Toddlers and young children may take an unwitnessed fall and present with crying or unwillingness to bear weight on the affected leg. Paradoxical irritability (more crying when picked up by a caregiver) can be a sign of rib or clavicle fracture. Consider child abuse if the injury either was not witnessed or inconsistent with the observer's history.

Fracture

A fracture is a break in the continuity or architecture of a bone. It is described by the skin integrity (open or closed) overlying the site of the injury; the name of the bone; the location within the bone (intra-articular, distal, proximal, or midshaft); the character of the fracture (comminuted, spiral, greenstick, transverse, oblique); and the direction of displacement of the distal fragment (displaced, nondisplaced 10°, dorsally angulated, etc.).

A fracture usually presents with point tenderness, ecchymosis, and swelling after an episode of trauma. An infant or toddler, however, may merely refuse to use the affected limb, which is neither swollen nor markedly tender. Significant blood loss, leading to shock, can occur with a fracture of the femur or pelvis.

Open Fracture

An open or compound fracture communicates with the outside environment by means of a puncture or laceration through the skin.

Pathologic Fracture

A pathologic fracture can occur in areas of bone weakness. Causes include rickets, bone cysts, osteogenesis imperfecta, and malignancies.

Buckle Fracture

A buckle or torus fracture is caused by compression of the metaphysis in a young child's bone. There is disruption of at least one side of the cortex, without a visible fracture line.

Greenstick Fracture

A greenstick fracture, which usually involves the diaphysis, occurs when a force breaks one, but not both, sides of the cortex.

Complete Fracture

A complete fracture is a cortical break through both sides of the bone.

Plastic Deformation (Traumatic Bowing)

This is bowing of a bone without obvious radiographic fracture.

Epiphyseal Injury

Determining if a growth plate is injured is critical. Although many growth plate injuries do not result in growth arrest, serious deformity and disability can result despite optimal medical care. The Salter classification scheme of epiphyseal injury (Figure 17.1) is useful for describing the fracture. This system correlates well with the degree of injury and is useful in treatment and prognosis.

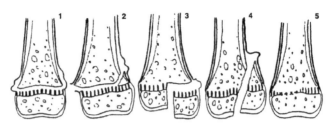

Figure 17.1 Salter–Harris classification of growth plate injuries.
Adapted from Salter RB, Harris WR. Injuries involving the epiphyseal plate. *J Bone Joint Surg* 1963;45A:587.

Dislocation

A dislocation is a complete disruption of the normal articular relationships of a joint. The most common sites are the shoulder (anterior), metacarpophalangeal and interphalangeal finger joints (pp. 744–745), and patella. Posterior elbow, knee, and hip dislocations are uncommon, but can cause significant vascular compromise.

Subluxation

A subluxation is an incomplete dislocation and occurs most commonly in the radial head of a toddler (nursemaid's elbow).

Sprain

A sprain is disruption of a ligament. Young children are more likely to have fractures than sprains because of the relative weakness of their bones (more porous, presence of physis) compared to the surrounding ligaments. Joint injuries and dislocations are therefore less common in the young child. Sprains occur more frequently in the adolescent whose bones are more ossified and have closed or closing growth plates.

Sprains present as joint swelling, with ecchymosis and tenderness over the affected ligament. Usually there is a clear history of trauma. There may be pain on palpation over the ligament without any instability (grade I), increased joint laxity upon stress (grade II), or total joint instability (grade III).

Strain

In contrast to a sprain, a strain is an injury to the musculotendinous unit.

Dislocation

A dislocated joint appears deformed, with limited, painful range of motion.

Radiographs

Anteroposterior (AP) and lateral radiographs are indicated if there is an obvious deformity, point tenderness, or marked swelling or ecchymosis. Although CT, MRI, and bone scan are helpful in making a detailed assessment of a fracture or dislocation, these are not the primary means of diagnosis. Splint the extremity first, and obtain views that include the joints above and below the site of injury. Comparison views of the uninjured extremity are not routinely indicated. Obtain oblique views if a "toddler's fracture" is suspected but not confirmed on the standard views.

For patients with an ankle injury, use the Ottawa ankle rules and obtain ankle films for patients with any of the following: tenderness over the distal 6 cm of the fibula or tibia, medial or lateral malleolus tenderness, navicular or fifth metatarsal tenderness, or inability to bear weight both immediately and in the emergency department (four steps). In the case of a knee injury, obtain knee films if there is isolated tenderness to the patella, tenderness at the fibular head, and/or inability to bear weight both immediately and in the emergency department (four steps).

When viewing the radiographs, carefully follow the cortex, looking for any discontinuity, which is diagnostic of a fracture. Evaluate the growth plates and joints for displacement, disruption, or widening. Pay particular attention to the metaphysis, which is often the site of buckle fractures.

The differentiation between sprains and Salter I epiphyseal injuries can be difficult, as both can present with minimal swelling over the growth plate and normal radiographs. Growth plate injuries, however, are more common in young children, while sprains are more likely in adolescents. With a sprain, the ligament is tender and the joint may be lax, while Salter I injuries cause tenderness over the growth plate.

A number of fractures are suspicious for child abuse: metaphyseal (bucket-handle), rib (especially posterior), scapular, spinous process, and sternal fractures and long-bone fractures in young non-ambulating children. Other injuries that are associated with inflicted trauma include epiphyseal separations, vertebral body fractures and subluxations, digital fractures, complex skull fractures, and multiple fractures, especially if bilateral or in various stages of healing.

ED Management

Time is critical with neurovascular compromise, open fractures, and joint sepsis. These orthopedic emergencies demand prompt intervention to avoid complications and possible loss of limb. Obtain radiographs only after the initial assessment is conducted.

After stabilization of vital signs and assessment of non-orthopedic injuries, the priority is assessment of the neurovascular status of the injured extremity. As discussed above, the presence of any of the "six Ps" suggests neurovascular compromise and is an indication for immediate reduction. If orthopedic consultation is not immediately available, place the extremity in longitudinal traction and align any gross deformities.

Pain relief is the next priority. Splint the extremity (pp. 587–594) in a comfortable position, elevate, and apply ice to minimize swelling. Splints can be made from any firm material and tape. Give acetaminophen (15 mg/kg PO) or ibuprofen (10 mg/kg PO). Treat severe pain with morphine, 0.1 mg/kg IV or IM.

If there is an open fracture, priorities before obtaining radiographs are to cover the wound with sterile dressings, start an IV, give the first dose of antibiotics (cefazolin 25 mg/kg; clindamycin 10 mg/kg if penicillin-allergic), and give a tetanus vaccine unless there is documentation of adequate immunization.

Fractures

Definitive treatment ranges from a simple sling to complex surgical reconstruction. In general, most nondisplaced extremity fractures can be treated with *in situ* immobilization with a cast or splint. Refer all displaced fractures and growth plate fractures to an orthopedist. These usually require reduction to an anatomic position, followed by immobilization.

If the patient must travel to see an orthopedist, splint the extremity in a physiologic position to avoid further displacement.

Dislocations

Reduce a finger dislocation promptly, with axial traction, after finger block anesthesia. See below for the reduction of a glenohumeral dislocation. Elbow, hip, and knee dislocations are at risk of neurovascular compromise and therefore require orthopedic consultation.

Contusions and First-Degree Sprains

Treat with RICE therapy: Rest, Ice (for 24–48 hours), Compression (with an elastic bandage), and Elevation (to reduce swelling). Advise the patient that activities can be resumed as tolerated. Most minor injuries will resolve over 5–7 days. Instruct the patient to follow-up with an orthopedist if there is no improvement.

Severe Sprains

A second- or third-degree sprain requires splinting for several weeks. In the ED, apply any of the commercially available splints or a Jones dressing. Give crutches if the patient has a severe sprain of a lower extremity.

Cast Care

After casting, follow-up must be arranged with the orthopedist. Instruct the patient to keep the extremity elevated, move the fingers or toes, keep the cast dry, and avoid putting any objects into the cast. Advise the family to check for pain out of proportion to the injury, color change of the distal extremity, and numbness or tingling. These signs suggest excessive cast tightness or neurovascular compromise and require an immediate return to the ED.

Bibliography

Beckenkamp PR, Lin CC, Macaskill P, et al. Diagnostic accuracy of the Ottawa Ankle and Midfoot Rules: a systematic review with meta-analysis. *Br J Sports Med*. 2017;51(6):504–510.

Chasm RM, Swencki SA. Pediatric orthopedic emergencies. *Emerg Med Clin North Am*. 2010;28(4):907–926.

Flaherty EG, Perez-Rossello JM, Levine MA, Hennrikus WL. Evaluating children with fractures for child physical abuse. *Pediatrics*. 2014;133(2):e477–e489.

Graff DM, Brey J, Herr S. Traumatic pediatric orthopedic emergencies: an approach to evaluation and management. *Clin Pediatr Emerg Med*. 2016;17(1):3–12.

Meyer CL, Kozin SH, Herman MJ, Safier S, Abzug JM. Complications of pediatric supracondylar humeral fractures. *Instr Course Lect*. 2015;64:483–491.

Pannu GS, Herman M. Distal radius-ulna fractures in children. *Orthop Clin North Am*. 2015;46(2):235–248.

Trionfo A, Cavanaugh PK, Herman MJ. Pediatric open fractures. *Orthop Clin North Am*. 2016;47(3):565–578.

Limp

Limp in children is most often secondary to trauma. Other causes are infections, connective tissue disorders, malignancies, and sickle cell disease (Table 17.2). In addition, if the pain can be localized to either the hip or knee joint, there are specific age-related disorders to consider.

Table 17.2 Etiologies of limp

Arthritis

Acute rheumatic fever

Henoch–Schönlein purpura

Inflammatory bowel disease

Juvenile rheumatoid arthritis

Serum sickness

Systemic lupus erythematosus

Hip diseases

Developmental dysplasia (DDH)

Legg–Calvé–Perthes disease

Slipped capital femoral epiphysis

Transient synovitis

Knee diseases

Chondromalacia patellae

Osgood–Schlatter disease

Osteochondritis dissecans

Infections

Intervertebral diskitis

Lyme disease

Osteomyelitis

Septic arthritis

Viral infections

Other

Abdominal or pelvic pathology

Neoplasm

Sickle cell disease

Trauma

Dislocation

Foreign body

Fracture

Soft tissue injury (bruise)

Sprain

Clinical Presentation

Trauma

The etiology may be a minor trauma (e.g., ill-fitting shoe or a foreign body in the sole of the foot) or a more serious injury, such as fracture, sprain, or dislocation, with ecchymosis, swelling, localized tenderness, decreased range of motion, ligamentous laxity, or obvious deformity. A history that is inconsistent with the traumatic injury raises the concern for possible child abuse.

Infections

Osteomyelitis

Osteomyelitis (pp. 585–586) causes fever and limp or unwillingness to use the extremity. Point tenderness is typical, with or without overlying cellulitis.

Septic Arthritis

Septic arthritis presents with the sudden onset of fever and limp or complete unwillingness to move the leg. There is erythema, increased warmth, and tenderness over the affected joint, and the patient resists passive range of movement. When the hip is affected, it is maintained in flexion, external rotation, and abduction. Classically, a patient with septic arthritis will be unable to bear weight on the affected limb, and will have fever (>38.9 °C; 102°F) and elevations of the ESR (>60 mm/h), CRP (>2.0 mg/dL), and WBC (>15,000/mm^3).

Lyme Disease

During the early localized and early disseminated stages of Lyme disease (pp. 417–420), there may be arthralgias and the patient may favor an extremity. Fever, lethargy, and headache may occur along with the pathognomonic rash, erythema migrans. Frank arthritis (especially of the knee) is a manifestation of the late or chronic stages. Typically, the joint is swollen and tender but not warm or erythematous.

Intervertebral Diskitis

Intervertebral diskitis is an infectious or inflammatory disease occurring primarily in 2–7-year-olds. The patient may present with limp, back pain, refusal to sit or walk, irritability, and low-grade fever. Physical examination findings include localized tenderness directly over the spine, paravertebral muscle spasm, and limited straight leg raising.

Viral Infections

Many viral infections can present with, or be followed by, arthritis or arthralgias, which is usually symmetric and polyarticular. Possible etiologies include herpesviruses (HSV, varicella, EBV, CMV), parvovirus, hepatitis, rubella, HIV, mumps, adenovirus, Coxsackie, and echovirus. Children may also experience arthralgia or arthritis after receiving the MMR or rubella vaccine.

Hip Diseases

With hip diseases, the pain may be in the groin or anterior thigh, or it may be referred to the anteromedial aspect of the knee.

Transient Synovitis

Transient synovitis is a benign, self-limited, inflammatory hip disease that occurs predominantly in 3–8-year-olds. There is an acute or gradual onset of limp and either hip or referred knee pain. Fever is variable and the child does not appear toxic, but there may be a URI. The hip is held in mild flexion, external rotation, and abduction, but there is no erythema or increased warmth. Abduction and internal rotation are limited by pain only at the extremes of motion. WBC, ESR, and CRP are generally normal or slightly elevated. Radiographs and sonography may show a hip effusion. Transient synovitis is a diagnosis of exclusion and must be distinguished from an early septic arthritis of the hip.

Legg–Calvé–Perthes Disease

Legg–Calvé–Perthes disease, or osteochondrosis of the femoral head, usually occurs in 4–9-year-old boys. There is a gradual onset of limp and pain in the hip, groin, or medial knee. Abduction and internal rotation of the hip are limited. The radiographic findings may be confused with avascular necrosis associated with corticosteroid use, sickle cell disease, or Gaucher's disease.

Slipped Capital Femoral Epiphysis

A slipped capital femoral epiphysis (SCFE) is a displacement of the normal relationship between the femoral head and neck. Between 10% and 20% of cases are bilateral and some patients with short stature may have associated hypothyroidism. The typical patient is an obese adolescent who presents with a limp and subacute or chronic groin pain, which may be referred to the anterior thigh or knee. The hip is held in flexion and external rotation. Passive hip flexion may accentuate the external rotation deformity, while internal rotation and abduction may be limited. Long-term morbidity (i.e., arthritis) is directly linked to the degree of displacement on presentation.

Developmental Dysplasia of the Hip (DDH)

DDH occurs most often in girls who underwent a breech delivery. A patient who is not diagnosed in the newborn period will develop a limp once walking begins. Unlike many other causes of limp, these children are often pain-free.

Knee Diseases

Although there are a number of specific disorders that affect the knee, hip diseases can present with knee pain. Therefore, examine the hips carefully in any patient with knee pain.

Osgood–Schlatter Disease

Osgood–Schlatter disease, or apophysitis of the tibial tuberosity, is a self-limited "overuse" disorder that usually occurs in physically active adolescents. The patient typically presents with a gradual onset of limp, especially after exercise. On examination, there is unilateral or bilateral tenderness and swelling over the tibial tuberosity, but the knee joint is otherwise normal.

Chondromalacia Patellae

Also known as "runner's knee" or "painful patella syndrome," this overuse injury is thought to be due to misalignment of the patella in the femoral groove, which leads to erosion of the cartilage. Typical findings of chondromalacia patellae include patellar pain after activity (especially stair climbing), episodes of buckling (but not locking), and crepitance and tenderness on palpation of the patellar articular surface. The "patella grind test" will be painful in a patient with this condition; while the patient is supine with the knee extended, gently push the patella inferiorly while the patient contracts the quadriceps muscle. A joint effusion is uncommon and suggests other diagnoses.

Osteochondritis Dissecans

With osteochondritis dissecans, an area of bone, usually on the lateral aspect of the medial femoral condyle, develops ischemic necrosis and subsequent fracture. A piece of bone and cartilage may then break loose into the joint. This causes intermittently painful limp after exercise, buckling, locking, and a tender medial femoral condyle. The cause is unknown but is most common in adolescent boys involved in organized sports.

Lower Leg Diseases

Sever Disease (Calcaneal Apophysitis)

Sever disease is an apophysitis that affects the calcaneus at the site of insertion of the Achilles tendon. It presents with uni- or bilateral chronic heel pain, exacerbated by wearing footwear lacking support (flip-flops) or heel cleats (particularly soccer cleats). Physical examination reveals tenderness upon palpation of the Achilles insertion site into calcaneus.

Other Causes

Arthritis

Arthritis (nonseptic) presents with swelling, erythema, tenderness, decreased range of motion, and increased warmth of single or multiple joints (pp. 700–704). Associated findings may include fever, rash, heart murmur, generalized adenopathy, and hepatosplenomegaly.

Sickle Cell Disease

Sickle cell bone infarcts (pp. 370–372) can cause diffuse bone pain with tenderness and limp. Associated findings may include fever, jaundice, abdominal pain, and, in younger children, swelling of the dorsum of the hands and feet (dactylitis).

Neoplasms

Rare causes of limp include both benign (osteoid osteoma, osteochondroma) and malignant (osteosarcoma, Ewing's sarcoma) bone tumors. Metastatic bone cancer (i.e., neuroblastoma) and leukemia and can also present as bone pain and limp.

Abdominal or Pelvic Pathology

Diseases that irritate the psoas or obturator muscles, such as pelvic inflammatory disease or appendicitis, can cause hip or thigh pain which then manifests as limping.

Diagnosis

The priority is the prompt diagnosis of a septic arthritis, osteomyelitis, or SCFE. Inquire about trauma, rate of onset (acute versus chronic), similar previous episodes, past medical history, fever, weight loss, malaise, easy bruising, and location and radiation of the pain. Perform a full physical examination, looking for a source for the limp, paying particular attention to the abdomen, back, and genitals. Observe the patient's gait, if able, while barefoot, attempting to locate the area of concern. Next, thoroughly evaluate the affected extremity(ies), looking for erythema, warmth, and tenderness. Put all joints through complete active and passive ranges of motion, then evaluate the neurovascular status of the extremity.

Thoroughly examine the hip of any child with a complaint of knee pain. Flex and extend the hip from 0° to maximal flexion. While the hip is flexed, check internal and external rotation. Pain on rotation may be the first sign of hip disorders.

Unless it is clear that the cause of the limp is minor trauma, obtain standard AP and lateral radiographs of the suspicious areas. If the limp is associated with decreased hip range of motion, obtain AP pelvis and frog-leg lateral radiographs of both hips. Possible findings include fractures, SCFE (on the frog-leg view), joint space widening (septic arthritis, transient synovitis, Legg–Calvé–Perthes disease), increased density of the femoral epiphysis (Legg–Calvé–Perthes disease), or subchondral bone fragmentation (osteochondritis dissecans). An MRI is needed to diagnose early Legg–Calvé–Perthes disease. X-rays of the knee are not necessary when Osgood–Schlatter disease is suspected, and radiographs are normal in chondromalacia patellae. Similarly, radiographs are not needed to diagnose Sever disease and are only indicated for atypical presentations (acute onset, inability to bear weight, systemic symptoms).

If the limp is associated with back pain, consider diskitis or osteomyelitis, particularly if the patient is febrile. Obtain plain radiographs and arrange for an MRI scan.

Obtain a CBC, ESR, CRP, and Lyme titer (in endemic areas) when there are fever and/or constitutional symptoms and no definite history of trauma. Leukocytosis, a shift to the left, and an increased ESR (>60 mm/h) and CRP (>2.0 mg/dL) may occur in inflammatory conditions such as septic arthritis, osteomyelitis, and diskitis. With transient synovitis, the ESR is elevated, but usually <60 mm/h and the CRP is <2.0 mg/dL.

ED Management

It may be impossible to make a specific diagnosis of the cause of a limp. If the fever is not high, the WBC, ESR, and CRP are normal, and the radiographs are unremarkable, the patient may be discharged with close follow-up. Many such children have a soft tissue injury without fracture or transient synovitis. Instruct the patient to return at once if there is high fever or an inability to ambulate or bear weight.

Infection

If septic arthritis or osteomyelitis is suspected, refer the patient immediately to an orthopedist for aspiration of joint fluid or subperiosteal pus. Intravenous antibiotics are then indicated. The treatment of septic arthritis, osteomyelitis (pp. 585–586), and Lyme disease (pp. 417–420) are detailed elsewhere. Since diskitis is difficult to distinguish from osteomyelitis, admit the patient for bed rest and IV antibiotics (p. 586).

Hip Diseases

Transient Synovitis

Patients who are well-appearing, with a normal WBC and an ESR <60 mm/h, CRP (<2.0 mg/dL) may be treated at home with bed rest and acetaminophen (15 mg/kg q 4h) or ibuprofen

(10 mg/kg q 6h) until the symptoms have resolved. For a patient with more severe symptoms, consult an orthopedist and admit for bed rest and skin traction, until the range of motion is normal.

SCFE

Immediately obtain orthopedic consultation, as minor trauma can cause complete displacement of the femoral epiphysis. Weight bearing must be discontinued and the patient placed at rest. Long-term morbidity (i.e., arthritis) is directly linked to the degree of displacement on presentation. If the patient has short stature, obtain thyroid function tests in addition to any labs needed prior to surgery.

Legg–Calvé–Perthes

Although no emergency treatment is required, refer the patient to an orthopedist so that a comprehensive plan of treatment can be arranged.

Knee Diseases

Osgood–Schlatter Disease

Treat with ibuprofen (as above) and limitation of activity until the acute symptoms resolve (2–6 weeks). Then, increase the activity level slowly.

Chondromalacia Patellae

The treatment is the same as for Osgood–Schlatter disease. In addition, recommend quadriceps-strengthening exercises (straight leg lifting).

Osteochondritis Dissecans

Refer a patient with suspected osteochondritis dissecans to an orthopedist, since treatment usually requires immobilization or possible surgery.

Lower Leg Diseases

Sever Disease (Calcaneal Apophysitis)

Treatment is the same as for Osgood–Schlatter disease. In addition, recommend wearing bilateral heel cups or lifts and performing calf-strengthening exercises.

Follow-up

- Transient synovitis: 2–3 days, if symptoms have not resolved
- Legg–Calvé–Perthes, osteochondritis dissecans: orthopedist in 1–2 weeks
- Osgood–Schlatter, chondromalacia patellae, Sever disease: primary care follow-up in 2–4 weeks

Indications for Admission

- Slipped capital femoral epiphysis
- Possible septic arthritis, osteomyelitis, diskitis, rheumatic fever, or neoplasm
- Transient synovitis with fever, leukocytosis, ESR >60 mm/h, CRP (>2.0 mg/dL), or markedly decreased range of motion

Bibliography

Cook, CP. Transient synovitis, septic hip, and Legg–Calvé–Perthes disease: an approach to the correct diagnosis. *Pediatr Clin North Am.* 2014;**61**(6): 1109–1118.

Gill KG. Pediatric hip: pearls and pitfalls. *Semin Musculoskelet Radiol.* 2013;**17**(3):328–338.

Herman MJ, Martinek M. The limping child. *Pediatr Rev.* 2015;**36**(5):184–197.

Jain N, Sah M, Chakraverty J, Evans A, Kamath S. Radiological approach to a child with hip pain. *Clin Radiol.* 2013;**68**(11):1167–1178.

Smith E, Anderson M, Foster H. The child with a limp: a symptom and not a diagnosis. *Arch Dis Child Educ Pract Ed.* 2012;**97**(5):185–193.

Osteomyelitis

Osteomyelitis is a bacterial bone infection, caused by organisms introduced either hematogenously or by direct spread from a contiguous local focus. The usual site is the metaphysis, and the distal femur and proximal and distal tibia are the most commonly involved bones. In the newborn, the proximal humerus is a frequent location.

Staphylococcus aureus causes approximately two-thirds of the cases. Other etiologies include group A *Streptococcus, S. pneumoniae* and *Kingella* in young children and toddlers, and group B Streptococcus and enteric bacteria in neonates. Children with hemoglobinopathies (sickle cell disease) are at risk for infection with *Salmonella. Pseudomonas* can infect the bones of the foot after a puncture wound through the sole of a shoe.

Clinical Presentation

The usual presentation in a child or adolescent is pain and point tenderness at a long-bone site, with decreased range of motion in the adjacent joints. Swelling, erythema, and warmth are generally not seen unless purulent material ruptures through the cortex and spreads to the subcutaneous tissues. The patient may be febrile and often refuses to use or bear weight on the limb, holding it as motionless as possible. With vertebral osteomyelitis, there is chronic back pain or torticollis with spasms of the paraspinal muscles.

An infant may occasionally have nonspecific signs, such as fever, irritability, vomiting, and decreased mobility of an extremity, but more often there is swelling and tenderness of the affected area. As a result of the relatively thin cortex and loose periosteum in an infant, osteomyelitis spreads to contiguous structures in muscle and joints more often than in an older patient. Seventy percent of neonates have an associated septic arthritis.

Diagnosis

The diagnosis of osteomyelitis is clinical. The typical combination of fever, point tenderness, and unwillingness to use an extremity is not invariably seen, but when present is highly suggestive of osteomyelitis. The CRP and ESR are almost always elevated, whereas elevation of the WBC count is not as consistent. Aspiration of the pus from the bone and positive blood cultures confirm the diagnosis.

Plain films may show soft tissue changes and swelling as early as three days after onset of symptoms. However, routine radiographs do not show bone changes until 10–20 days after the onset of the infection. In contrast, a 99mTc phosphate bone scan can detect bone changes earlier than plain films, and prior aspiration of the bone does not affect results.

MRI has emerged as the most sensitive tool for detecting osteomyelitis and gauging the extent of the disease. However, bone scan is less expensive, usually does not require sedation in young children, and can detect multiple foci of infection.

Osteomyelitis is an unusual entity and can mimic many common diagnoses. Trauma can cause pain, swelling, and limitation of movement. Usually there is a history of an injury or radiographic evidence of a fracture, and the ESR and CBC are normal. Cellulitis of a distal extremity can be mistaken for a manifestation of osteomyelitis, although there is no point tenderness over the bone.

Sickle cell disease can cause pain secondary to infection or vaso-occlusive crisis. Distinguishing between the two may be difficult, although the pain of a crisis tends to recur in the same sites, can be in several locations at once, and often resolves with IV hydration. Pain in a single bone that has not been affected in the past is suspicious for osteomyelitis.

Other considerations include bone tumor, Caffey's disease (infantile cortical hyperostosis), and Langerhans' cell histiocytosis. All of these can be excluded by radiographs.

ED Management

When osteomyelitis is suspected, obtain a blood culture, CBC with differential, ESR, CRP, and radiographs of the extremity. If the diagnosis is in doubt, order an MRI or scintigraphy. Consult with an orthopedist to perform needle aspiration to drain the pus and provide specimens for culture and Gram's stain. If no pus is obtained, send bone marrow for culture and Gram's stain. Needle aspiration can also exclude a sickle cell vaso-occlusive crisis when the clinical picture is unclear.

Admit a patient with osteomyelitis and, once a specimen is obtained from the aspiration, choose empiric IV treatment based on local bacterial resistance. When MRSA prevalence is >10%, start with IV clindamycin (40 mg/kg/day div q 8h, 2.7 g/day maximum). Monotherapy with a first-generation cephalosporin or an anti-staphylococcal penicillin is not adequate in such communities.

The increased prevalence of clindamycin-resistant, methicillin-susceptible *S. aureus* (MSSA) makes first-generation cephalosporin or an anti-staphylococcal penicillin the preferred initial option in some areas. Use oxacillin (150–200 mg/kg/day div q 6h, 6 g/day maximum) *or* cefazolin (100–150 mg/kg/day div q 8h, 6 g/day maximum) *or* vancomycin (40–60 mg/kg/day div q 6h, 4 g/day maximum). Give dual IV treatment with one of these agents *plus* clindamycin in severe cases.

Add *Salmonella* coverage (ceftriaxone 100 mg/kg/day div q 12h) for a patient with a hemoglobinopathy such as sickle cell disease and *Pseudomonas* coverage (piperacillin/tazobactam 250 mg/kg/day IV div q 6h or ceftazidime 100 mg/kg/day div q 8h) for osteomyelitis of the foot secondary to a puncture through a shoe. Treat a neonate with cefotaxime (150 mg/kg/day div q 8h) and either nafcillin or vancomycin.

Indication for Admission

- Osteomyelitis

Bibliography

Arnold JC, Bradley JC Osteoarticular infections in children. *Infect Dis Clin North Am.* 2015;**29** (3):557–574.

Dodwell ER. Osteomyelitis and septic arthritis in children: current concepts. *Curr Opin Pediatr.* 2013;**25**(1):58–63.

Peltola H, Pääkkönen M. Acute osteomyelitis in children. *N Engl J Med.* 2014;**370**(4):352–360.

Yagupsky P. *Kingella kingae*: carriage, transmission, and disease. *Clin Microbiol Rev.* 2015;**28**(1):54–79.

Splinting

Many simple, nondisplaced fractures can be managed with splinting alone. Splinting is also useful in the treatment of ligamentous injuries, soft tissue injuries and infections, and joint infections.

Equipment

1. Cotton padding (Webril) between the fingers or toes to prevent maceration, and against the skin to be covered by plaster or fiberglass
2. Plaster of Paris, fiberglass rolls, or Ortho-Glass
3. Elastic bandages.

Splint Application

Wrap cotton padding around the affected limb; be sure to separate the fingers or toes. Measure the appropriate length of the splint needed and cut the plaster or fiberglass to that size. For elbows and ankles, cut a notch where the splint bends to allow for a smooth corner about the joint. Dip the plaster or fiberglass into a basin of room-temperature water until no bubbles are seen. Roll or "squeegie" the slab until excess water is removed. Smooth the plaster to avoid wrinkles, and apply it to the affected limb in the position desired. Roll a layer of Webril, followed by an elastic bandage, over the splint. Smooth and mold the splint with the palms of both hands, taking care to avoid using fingertips or excessive force (Figure 17.2).

In many institutions, the traditional plaster or fiberglass rolls have been replaced by Ortho-Glass, which consists of a roll of fiberglass with a cotton covering. Measure the appropriate length of material and then cut that amount from the larger roll. Wet the Ortho-Glass under the faucet and then pat it dry using a towel. Make certain that the edges of the fiberglass are covered because when dry they will become sharp and may hurt the patient. Apply the splint and cover it with an elastic bandage. Smooth and mold the splint into the desired position.

As a splint hardens, heat will be generated and the splint will shrink slightly. After the splint hardens, perform a careful neurovascular examination of the fingers or toes. Instruct the patient and family about rest, ice, and elevation in the first 24 hours, and arrange follow-up to reassess the injury and remove the splint at the appropriate time.

Suggested Lengths of Immobilization

Contusions or abrasions: 1–3 days

Mild sprains: 5–7 days

Soft tissue lacerations: 5–7 days

Fractures: As per orthopedist

Tendon lacerations: As per orthopedist or plastic surgeon

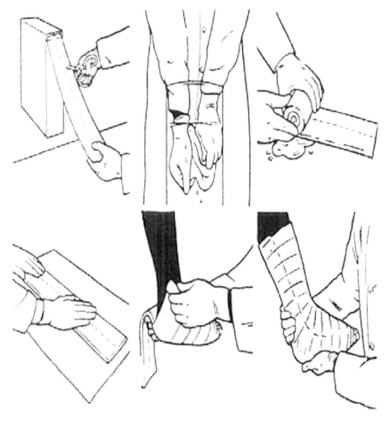

Figure 17.2 Splint application.
Adapted from Roberts JR, Hedges JR. *Clinical Procedures in Emergency Medicine* (3rd edn.). Philadelphia, PA: Saunders, 1997, with permission.

Commonly Used Splints

See Table 17.3 for the indications for various splints.

Volar Splint

This splint (Figure 17.3) extends from the distal aspect of the metacarpals to the proximal aspect of the forearm, leaving the phalanges and elbow free. Apply the splint along the volar surface of the arm with the wrist in a neutral or slightly extended (10–20°) position.

Sugar Tong Forearm Splint

This type of splint (Figure 17.4) will immobilize the elbow, preventing pronation and supination. Apply Webril from above the elbow to the distal edge of the palm. With the elbow in 90° of flexion, apply the plaster or fiberglass in a U-shape, starting at the distal edge of the palm, wrapping around the elbow, and ending just proximal to the knuckles. Place the wrist in a neutral to slightly extended (10–20°) position and allow the thumb to move freely.

Table 17.3 Common splinting indications

Splint	Indications
Buddy tape/dorsal finger	Simple phalangeal fracture
	Reduced interphalangeal dislocation
Long posterior arm	Reduced elbow dislocation
	Supracondylar fractures
	Nondisplaced radial head or midshaft forearm fracture
Long posterior leg	Knee injuries
Radial gutter	Second or third metacarpal or proximal phalange fracture
Short posterior leg	Ankle sprain
	Fracture of the foot, ankle, or distal fibula
Sugar tong forearm	Simple and buckle distal forearm fractures
Thumb spica	Scaphoid fracture
	Ulnar collateral ligament injury (gamekeeper's thumb)
	Nonangulated, nonrotated, thumb or first metacarpal fracture
Ulnar gutter	Fourth or fifth metacarpal or proximal phalange fracture
Volar wrist	Wrist sprain, contusion, soft tissue injury

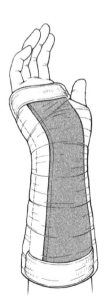

Figure 17.3 Volar forearm splint.
Adapted from Roberts JR, Hedges JR. *Clinical Procedures in Emergency Medicine* (3rd edn.). Philadelphia, PA: Saunders, 1997, with permission.

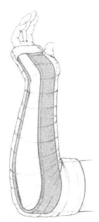

Figure 17.4 Sugar tong splint.
Adapted from Roberts JR, Hedges JR. *Clinical Procedures in Emergency Medicine* (3rd edn.). Philadelphia, PA: Saunders, 1997, with permission.

(a)   (b)

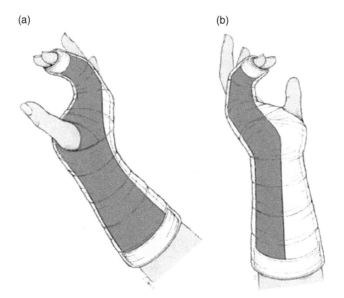

Figure 17.5 Gutter splint.
Adapted from Roberts JR, Hedges JR. *Clinical Procedures in Emergency Medicine* (3rd edn.). Philadelphia, PA: Saunders, 1997, with permission.

Gutter Splint

Separate the fingers with gauze or Webril, apply the plaster along either the radial or ulnar aspect of the forearm, and wrap it around the two fingers to be immobilized (Figure 17.5). Flex the metacarpophalangeal joints to 90° and the interphalangeal joints to 10–20°. Place the wrist in the neutral position or hyperextend it slightly (10–20°). Note that for the radial gutter, a hole must be cut to allow the thumb to move freely.

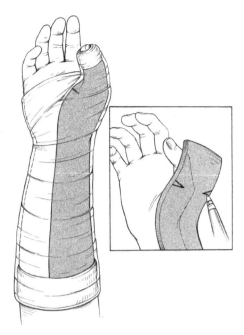

Figure 17.6 Thumb spica splint.
Adapted from Roberts JR, Hedges JR. *Clinical Procedures in Emergency Medicine* (3rd edn.). Philadelphia, PA: Saunders, 1997, with permission.

Thumb Spica

Apply the splint (Figure 17.6) along the radial aspect of the forearm and wrap it around the thumb, extending to the thumbnail. Keep the wrist in a neutral or slightly extended position (10–20°) and the thumb abducted and slightly flexed (10–20°).

Posterior Arm Splint

Apply the plaster to the posterior aspect of the upper arm and forearm, extending to the midpalmar area (Figure 17.7). Flex the elbow to 90°, and place the wrist in a neutral or slightly extended (10–20°) position. Put the arm in a sling after the splint is applied. While these splints are useful in managing many types of fractures, consult an orthopedist for more complicated fractures (i.e., supracondylar).

Posterior Leg Splint

Apply a short leg splint from the head of the metatarsals to the midcalf, with the ankle in as close to a neutral position (90°) as possible. For a long leg posterior splint, extend the plaster to the mid-thigh and keep the knee in slight flexion (Figure 17.8).

Finger Splints

Perform a careful examination of the injured finger and review the radiographs to determine the presence of a rotational or unacceptably angulated deformity, growth plate injury, or collateral ligament injury, all of which require orthopedic consultation.

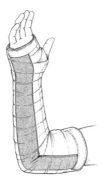

Figure 17.7 Posterior arm splint.
Adapted from Roberts JR, Hedges JR. *Clinical Procedures in Emergency Medicine* (3rd edn.). Philadelphia, PA: Saunders, 1997, with permission.

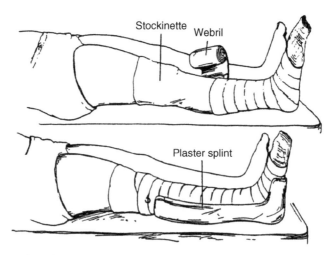

Figure 17.8 Posterior leg splint.
Adapted from Roberts JR, Hedges JR. *Clinical Procedures in Emergency Medicine* (3rd edn.). Philadelphia, PA: Saunders, 1997, with permission.

A simple phalangeal fracture or a reduced interphalangeal dislocation may be managed with splinting alone. A soft tissue injury or laceration will also benefit from finger splinting. Dynamic splinting, or "buddy taping" (Figure 17.9), permits movement at the MCP joint and slight movement at the IP joints. Splint the injured finger to the adjacent finger, or "buddy," to provide support.

An alternative splint is the foam-backed aluminum splint (Figure. 17.10), which may be cut and bent to fit. It is preferably applied to the dorsal surface of the finger, which preserves dexterity more effectively than splints applied to the volar surface. The splint should immobilize as few joints as possible; measure it to include only one joint above and one joint below the injury. Place the finger in the position of function or slightly flexed (10–20°) at the IP joints. Two-finger injuries require specific splinting techniques other than buddy taping or dorsal splinting.

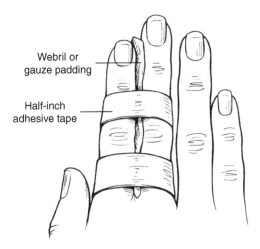

Webril or
gauze padding

Half-inch
adhesive tape

Figure 17.9 Dynamic splinting.
Adapted from Roberts JR, Hedges JR. *Clinical Procedures in Emergency Medicine* (3rd edn.). Philadelphia, PA: Saunders, 1997, with permission.

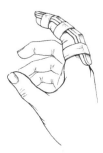

Figure 17.10 Foam splint.
Adapted from Roberts JR, Hedges JR. *Clinical Procedures in Emergency Medicine* (3rd edn.). Philadelphia, PA: Saunders, 1997, with permission.

Mallet Finger

The mallet finger is caused by a rupture of the extensor tendon at the DIP joint. Splint the finger over the dorsal aspect of the DIP only, in full extension or slight hyperextension. The splint must remain for at least eight weeks, and the finger must not be flexed at any time during that period.

Boutonnière Deformity

The boutonnière deformity is a rupture of the central slip of the extensor digitorum communis tendon, resulting in the PIP "buttonholing" through the torn extensor hood. Splint the finger over the dorsal aspect of the PIP only, in full extension or slight hyper-extension. Keep the splint in place for at least four weeks, during which time the finger must not be permitted to flex.

Bibliography

Cheung JP, Fung B, Ip WY. Review on mallet finger treatment. *Hand Surg.* 2012;**17**(3):439–447.

Gaston RG, Chadderdon C. Phalangeal fractures: displaced/nondisplaced. *Hand Clin.* 2012;**28**(3):395–401.

Hill CE, Masters JP, Perry DC. A systematic review of alternative splinting versus complete plaster casts for the management of childhood buckle fractures of the wrist. *J Pediatr Orthop B.* 2016;**25**(2):183–190.

Williams KG, Smith G, Luhmann SJ, et al. A randomized controlled trial of cast versus splint for distal radial buckle fracture: an evaluation of satisfaction, convenience, and preference. *Pediatr Emerg Care.* 2013;**29**(5):555–559.

Yeung DE, Jia X, Miller CA, Barker SL. Interventions for treating ankle fractures in children. *Cochrane Database Syst Rev.* 2016;**4**:CD010836.

Chapter 18

Physical Abuse

Kristine Fortin and Olga Jimenez

Abandonment and Neglect

Neglect is broadly defined as failure to meet a child's basic needs. Neglect is the most common form of child maltreatment, and its effects on health can be as injurious as those of physical or sexual abuse. There are different types of neglect, including:

- physical neglect: failure to provide basic needs such as housing or food;
- supervisory neglect: failure to provide adequate supervision for the child's developmental level;
- medical neglect: failure to provide prescribed medical care or to seek care in a timely manner;
- psychological/emotional neglect: failure to provide adequate support, affection, nurturance.

Abandonment is an extreme form of neglect. It occurs when a child has been left by parents whose whereabouts are unknown, or when the parents fail to maintain contact for a significant period of time.

Clinical Presentation

Concern for neglect may arise during the emergency department visit, although abandoned and neglected children may be brought to the emergency department by Child Protective Services (CPS) for medical evaluation. Other possible presentations include complications of a chronic disease due to medical neglect, significant delays in seeking medical care, failure to thrive, and injuries or intoxications occurring in the setting of lack of supervision.

Diagnosis

Perform a thorough physical examination, with particular attention to a general assessment of the state of hydration, nutrition, vital signs, growth parameters, and hygiene. Undress and examine the child thoroughly for physical stigmata of abuse or neglect. Other physical findings could include dental caries or dermatological problems (infections, infestations). Abandoned and neglected children can also have significant behavioral and emotional health issues that require immediate attention.

In some cases the need for a CPS report will be clear, such as a toddler intoxicated by an illegal substance, while other cases are more nuanced. There are no clear guidelines for deciding when to report medical or supervisory neglect. In a complex case, utilize an interdisciplinary approach, possibly including social work, primary care, pharmacy, and inpatient teams. Assess the patient's risk of imminent harm. Evaluate whether there is an immediate health risk to the child, and characterize the nature and severity of potential or actual health consequences. Also note any risk factors, family strengths, availability of resources to assist with identified concrete needs, patterns of neglect, prior CPS involvement, and the results of prior interventions.

ED Management

If the patient is at imminent risk of harm in the current living environment, await a safe discharge plan from CPS, or admit to the hospital if indicated for medical or safety reasons. In a case where decision-making about the need to report to CPS extends beyond the emergency department visit and there is not imminent risk of harm, meticulously document the evaluation to date, and communicate clearly with the inpatient team and/or primary care provider.

In cases of abandonment, report to CPS and/or the police, per local child abuse reporting laws and protocols. If possible locate the parent or another family member known to the child. Disposition options in the management of an abandoned child include CPS transferring custody to an approved relative, or alternatively placement in a temporary shelter or foster care. If medical care is necessary, or if community-based resources do not exist, admit the patient to the hospital.

Indications for Admission

- Abandoned or neglected child who requires medical care
- Abandoned or neglected child at imminent risk of harm, when community placement resources do not exist

Bibliography

Fong HF, Christian CW. Child neglect: a review for the primary care pediatrician. *Pediatr Ann.* 2012;**41**:e254–e258.

Potter D, Nasserie T, Tonmyr L. A review of recent analyses of the Canadian Incidence Study of Reported Child Abuse and Neglect (CIS). *Health Promot Chronic Dis Prev Can.* 2015;**35**(8–9):119–129.

Schilling S, Christian CW. Child physical abuse and neglect. *Child Adolesc Psychiatr Clin N Am.* 2014;**23**(2):309–319.

Stoltenborgh M, Bakermans-Kranenburg MJ, van Ijzendoorn MH. The neglect of child neglect: a meta-analytic review of the prevalence of neglect. *Soc Psychiatry Psychiatr Epidemiol.* 2013;**48**(3):345–355.

Teeuw AH, Derkx BH, Koster WA, van Rijn RR. Educational paper: detection of child abuse and neglect at the emergency room. *Eur J Pediatr.* 2012;**171**(6):877–885.

Welch GL, Bonner BL. Fatal child neglect: characteristics, causation, and strategies for prevention. *Child Abuse Negl.* 2013;**37**(10):745–752.

Chart Documentation in Cases of Suspected Child Abuse

Medical professionals evaluating children in whom child abuse diagnosis is a consideration must ensure that the medical record is complete, comprehensive, objective, and fact-oriented. A well-documented medical record is essential in these circumstances and is a critical tool in child abuse investigations. The data entered in the record provides information about the statements provided, diagnoses considered, and ancillary tests performed, as well as the medical provider's assessment, treatment, and recommendations made.

Chart documentation that occurs soon after the evaluation of the child takes place is more reliable than notes written after a significant amount of time has passed. It is important to document the date, time, and place of the interviews, who was present, the language spoken, and if translator services were utilized. Also include any additional information obtained from other sources, such as police reports, child protective workers, etc.

History of the Presenting Problem

The principal diagnostic component of the child abuse assessment lies in the history obtained from the parent(s), and the child suspected of being abused. Interview the parents first, and separately, and if the child is verbal, interview him/her alone. In suspected physical abuse cases, gather information in a non-accusatory, but meticulous manner in order to determine if the injuries found could be explained by the history provided. It is crucial to interview the person(s) who was with the child at the time of the injury and it is especially important to ask if they actually witnessed the child when he/she sustained the injury. Document a detailed history of what happened and where and when it occurred. Note how the child was before and after the injury and the order in which symptoms developed. It is essential to clearly document the child's account of how he/she sustained the injury. In those cases in which a child is suspected of being sexually abused, document the circumstances surrounding the disclosure and what the parents know about the suspected sexual abuse.

Most children being evaluated for sexual abuse do not have specific medical findings. Therefore, the history provided *by the child* is the most important part of the evaluation. This will enable the clinician to make appropriate medical and protective decisions. When interviewing a child, allocate time to establish rapport before introducing the topic of concern. Rapport building allows the child to feel comfortable and it provides the clinician an opportunity to assess the child's developmental level to guide the choice of appropriate language during the interview.

Use open-ended questions during the interview. These questions usually begin with "who," "how", "what," "when," "where," or "why." These types of questions allow the child the freedom to describe details of what happened without jeopardizing the integrity of the interview. For example, you can ask: "Tell me, why you are here today?" Or, "Tell me, what happened that brought you to the hospital?" If the child discloses that her stepfather touched her inappropriately, avoid using leading or suggestive questions such as: "Did he touch you on your vagina?" In contrast, a non-leading question might be phrased "Where did your stepfather touch you?" Record the child's statements without correcting grammatical errors or paraphrasing the child. Use quotations as often as possible. Describe the child's demeanor and emotional state during the medical evaluation.

Statements made by a child are often considered "hearsay," a statement made out of court offered into evidence in order to establish the truth of the matter asserted in the statement. In other words, the child's words are offered in court to prove that what the child said is actually the truth. Generally, hearsay statements are not admissible in court, although two pertinent exceptions are the *excited utterance* exception and the *medical diagnosis or treatment* exception. Documentation of the features that allow a statement to qualify as a hearsay exception increases the chances the child's words will be admissible in court.

Excited Utterance

The excited utterance exception is a hearsay statement that relates to a stressful event. Three requirements are necessary for a statement to fall under this exception: the child must have experienced a stressful event; the child's statement must be associated with the event; and the child must still be experiencing the emotions caused by the event. Document the type of stressful event, the amount of time that passed between the event and when the child first made the statement, the child's speech (including spontaneity and emotions), what questions led to the disclosure, and when was the first secure opportunity the child had to disclose.

Medical Diagnosis or Treatment Exception

This relates to the belief that people are honest with medical professionals and therefore the information provided is trustworthy. Under this exception the information obtained in the medical history including chief complaint, review of systems, past medical history, and the child's description of the cause of injury are admissible in court. It is important to document the characteristics of the patient's statements that enhance their reliability, including the child's advanced knowledge of anatomy, description of distinctive sensory/visual details of sexual acts, and emotions displayed when the statement was made.

Past Medical History

Birth History

Document if the pregnancy was planned, as well as any complications during pregnancy or delivery, traumatic birth, prematurity, etc. Certain injuries are related to birth trauma and may go unnoticed by medical providers. Request the child's birth medical record and pictures or videos of the baby taken at birth to correlate with the medical findings.

Developmental History

Documenting the patient's developmental capabilities is crucial when trying to correlate the mechanism of injury with the story provided. Ask the parents to provide a video of the child performing a certain activity (rolling over, climbing, etc.) if they report a milestone has been met but not observed by the clinician. Note whether the examiner or another objective observer was able to substantiate the information provided.

Medical Conditions

Certain medical conditions can mimic abuse or may play a role in the injury noted. List the child's medical problems provided by the parent and inquire about those pertinent to the case (e.g., rickets and inherited bone disorders when evaluating a fracture). Documenting pertinent negatives informs the person reviewing the medical record that a certain diagnosis was considered in the differential.

Medications

Note any medications, alternative medicine, or vitamins given to the child, as the parents may give the patient medications that can cause serious medical problems without their knowledge. Also consider the effects of mislabeling and dispensing and dosage errors in the differential diagnosis.

Hospitalizations/Injuries

Note any hospitalizations, motor vehicle accidents, fractures, burns, or other serious injuries for which the child was treated in the past. If possible, obtain the patient's medical records. These may reveal injuries or medical conditions not recalled by parents or the child. Document this information in the medical record, including the source used.

Primary Care Provider

Note the name and contact information of the child's primary care medical provider. Also obtain the patient's immunization record. Some children who are neglected/abused may not be up to date with their vaccinations or have a regular health care provider.

Surgeries

It is important to include anogenital surgeries or procedures that may have left residual findings.

Review of Systems

When evaluating a child for sexual abuse, pay particular attention to the genitourinary and gastrointestinal systems. Note the presence of specific symptoms and the time of presentation in relationship to the sexual contact reported. Ask about a history of vaginal pain, bleeding, discharge, vaginal foreign bodies, self-stimulation, genital trauma, and the use of tampons. Inquire about dysuria, frequency, urgency, or enuresis. Dysuria, pain, and bleeding are highly associated with genital-to-genital contact.

Document any history of constipation, anal pain, bleeding, itching, hemorrhoids, encopresis, or infections. In cases of possible physical abuse, document the time line of changes in mental status, irritability, seizures, vomiting, breathing difficulties, and loss of consciousness. If a fracture is suspected, note the presence of any decreased range of motion, swelling, or deformity.

Behavior

Children that are abused or neglected may exhibit changes in their behavior. Inquire and document whether the child has been exhibiting any behavioral changes, sexualized behavior, or advanced sexual knowledge. Depression, suicidal ideation or attempts, self-injurious behavior, running away, and substance abuse could be indicators of abuse.

With the recent advances in technology and easy access to internet and cameras in multiple electronic devices, there are increased reports of exposure to pornographic images and inappropriate photographs or videos. It is important to inquire and document if the child has been found with or watching pornographic materials. In addition, ask the child/parent if inappropriate pictures or videos of the child have been taken/found. These pictures/videos corroborate the child's account and can assist in the prosecution of child sexual abuse cases.

Family History

Include any condition that may predispose the patient to injuries, such as osteogenesis imperfecta, bleeding disorders, etc., although these conditions could coexist with abuse. Also note a parental history of abuse or psychiatric illness.

Social History

Document the names of all of the child's caretakers, including daycare providers and whether any of these people reside in the patient's home. A history of substance or alcohol abuse and intimate partner violence can put a child at risk for abuse/neglect. Knowledge of these risk factors will help determine if it is safe for the child to go home.

Documentation of the Physical Examination

A thorough and complete physical examination is indicated for all children and adolescents suspected of being abused or neglected. Include the following in the medical record.

Growth Parameters

These are especially important when evaluating a child for failure to thrive and possible neglect. Chart current values on a growth curve and compare them with previous measurements if available.

Injuries

Describe the pattern, shape, location, size, and color of any marks, bruises, burns, bites, scars, and/or other lesions concerning for abuse. Look for sentinel injuries, which are poorly explained minor injuries in infants, such as subconjunctival hemorrhages or a torn frenulum. These injuries have been noted in children in whom serious physical abuse was later diagnosed. Include a careful inspection of the skin and oral mucosa, particularly of areas where injuries are easily missed, such as the labial and sublingual frena, ears, scalp, anogenital area, hands, and feet. Include all positive and pertinent negative findings (e.g., no retinal hemorrhages noted in a child with suspected inflicted head trauma).

Emergency medical providers may need to perform examinations on children suspected of being sexually abused when a child abuse expert is not immediately available. In order to properly document genital findings, refer to American Professional Society on the Abuse of Children (APSAC) published guidelines for standardized language to describe normal, variants of normal, and abnormal genital findings. Use the clock face to describe the location of the injury. The 12 o'clock position is anterior (urethra being at 12 o'clock). The anal examination can be performed in the lateral decubitus, supine, or knee–chest position. Document the following about the anogenital examination:

1. Position in which the patient was examined (e.g., supine, knee–chest).
2. Sexual maturation stage.
3. Use of magnification (colposcope or other magnifying instrument).
4. Whether the exam was photographed or video-recorded (see Photographic Documentation below).
5. The presence or absence of lesions, bruises, petechiae, etc. of each anatomical structure (labia, clitoris, vestibule, hymen, fossa navicularis, posterior fourchette, vagina).
6. The shape of the hymen (crescentic, annular, redundant, etc.). Make note of the presence of warts, bruises, tears, petechiae, and/or ecchymosis (e.g., "hymen crescentic-shaped with an acute complete transection at 6 o'clock, few petechiae noted at 3 and 5 o'clock"). Avoid terms like "virginal" or "intact."
7. Utilize body and/or genital diagrams demonstrating the site and type of injury.

8. Anal tags, fissures, bruises, lacerations, scars, rashes, discharge, bleeding, and/or other lesions. Note the normal variants of the anal examination so that these are not confused with abnormal findings.
9. For the male genitalia, write a description of the penis and scrotum, noting the presence of circumcision and any lacerations, scars, ecchymoses, rashes, discharge, erythema, and/or other lesions.

Photographic Documentation

Documentation of medical findings with photographs is an essential element of the child abuse evaluation. Photographs give clinicians an opportunity for later review of the medical findings; in some cases additional information initially overlooked may be found. If a second opinion is sought, the photos can be reviewed instead of having the child endure repeated examinations. In court, photographs provide a visual impact that may surpass the best-written description. In addition, photographs can be used to compare examinations over time, although they are not a substitute for a detailed description of the injury.

It is the role of the medical personnel caring for the child to photograph the injuries found. Before taking a picture, explain to the child in simple language what is going to happen, who will see the pictures, and why pictures are being taken. Label the photographs, including the date, patient's name, and medical record number, as well as the name of the photographer. Take an identifying picture of the child's face and as many pictures as needed of each injury, including an anatomic landmark. For example, include a knee, elbow, or other body part in order to identify the location of the injury. When the child presents with burns, it is particularly important to take pictures before debridement is done or a dressing is applied. For bite marks, take the photograph such that the angle of the camera lens is directly over and perpendicular to the plane of the bite to avoid distortion. Include in the picture a measuring device. The ABFO No. 2 reference scale was developed specifically for this purpose as well as for documenting patterned injuries. Consult with an odontologist or forensic odontologist as necessary. Photo or video-colposcopy is helpful for documenting the genital exam.

Although digital photography is now widely utilized for legal reasons, one must not alter the images in any way. Each institution must have a policy for photographing, storing, releasing, and handling pictures.

Laboratory and Radiological Tests

Document the results of all laboratory tests performed. If cultures for sexually transmitted infections (STIs) are taken, document the type of culture and the site from which it was obtained (e.g., vagina, rectal). At the present time, cultures are still the gold standard for evaluating STIs in children suspected of being sexually abused. Follow the Centers for Disease Control and American Academy of Pediatrics recommendations for testing children and adolescents in the context of sexual abuse. Include in the medical record the interpretations of radiographs, MRIs, and CT scans performed. Order a skeletal survey, looking for occult fractures (acute and chronic) for any child under the age of two years in whom physical abuse is strongly suspected.

Impression and Recommendations

1. Clearly document the result and interpretation of the medical findings.
2. Avoid using terms such as "alleged sexual assault" or "rule-out abuse." It is important to note that a normal genital or anal examination does not exclude sexual abuse and that most sexually abused children do not have medical findings. Therefore, a normal examination does not rule-out sexual abuse and "normal" does not mean that nothing happened.
3. If there are concerns for physical abuse, document the type of injury and clearly state if the story provided could be consistent with the medical findings. In certain cases, consultation with a child abuse pediatrician and other specialists is indicated to determine if the mechanism described is plausible.
4. List any medications prescribed, including dosages and length of treatment.
5. Document recommendations made by subspecialists.
6. In acute sexual abuse/assault cases, in which forensic evidence was collected, document the name and badge number of the police officer receiving the forensic evidence. It is of utmost importance to maintain the "chain of custody" at all times.
7. Increasing rates of adolescent sexual assault have been associated with the availability of drugs used to incapacitate the victim. If "rape drugs" are suspected, collect a drug-facilitated sexual assault kit with the adolescent's signed consent. Maintaining the chain of custody is vital.
8. In cases in which collected evidence is not immediately handed to the police, follow hospital policy for storing, discarding, and releasing the evidence.
9. If a report to CPS was made, note the name of the child protective worker and any detectives or police officers involved.
10. Document if a referral was made to a specialized program for a sexual and/or physical abuse evaluation. In most cases of sexual abuse, a comprehensive evaluation including a detailed genital examination can be deferred until a later date in a more appropriate setting. Consult the hospital's child abuse pediatrician or affiliated child advocacy center.
11. Referral to a mental health professional with expertise in caring for abused children and their families.
12. Ensure and document medical follow-up of the patient.
13. Collaborate with child protective and law enforcement agencies to establish the safest environment for the child. A representative for CPS will decide between the child staying at home and being placed in foster care. At times, however, the treating medical staff may disagree with CPS and feel that the disposition decision is not in the child's best interests. In such cases, ask to speak with the representative's supervisor.

Bibliography

Adams JA, Kellogg ND, Farst KJ, et al. Updated guidelines for the medical assessment and care of children who may have been sexually abused. *J Pediatr Adolesc Gynecol*. 2016;**29**(2):81–87.

Christian CW. Committee on Child Abuse and Neglect: the evaluation of suspected child physical abuse. *Pediatrics*. 2015;**135**(5):e1337–e1354.

Jenny C. *Child Abuse and Neglect: Diagnosis, Treatment and Evidence*. St. Louis, MO: Elsevier Saunders, 2011.

Jenny C, Crawford-Jakubiak JE, American Academy of Pediatrics Committee on Child Abuse and Neglect. The evaluation of children in the primary care setting when sexual abuse is suspected. *Pediatrics*. 2013;**132**:e558–e567.

Leetch AN, Woolridge D. Emergency department evaluation of child abuse. *Emerg Med Clin North Am*. 2013;**31**(3):853–873.

Myers JEB. *The APSAC Handbook on Child Maltreatment* (3rd edn.). Thousand Oaks, CA: Sage Publishing, 2011.

Sheets LK, Leach ME, Koszewski IJ, et al. Sentinel injuries in infants evaluated for child physical abuse. *Pediatrics*. 2013;**131**(4):701–707.

Commercial Sexual Exploitation of Children

Commercial sexual exploitation of children (CSEC) refers to sex crimes (examples: sex trafficking, pornography, prostitution, performance in strip clubs/sexual venues) against children for economic gain.

Clinical Presentation

CSEC is associated with many physical and mental health problems that could lead to emergency department visits. Victims could present for treatment of injuries, sexual assault, sexual health concerns (pregnancy, infections), uncontrolled chronic medical conditions, infections, or substance abuse issues, as well as mental health concerns including depression, suicidality, and posttraumatic stress disorder.

Diagnosis

Identifying victims of CSEC can be challenging, as they usually do not spontaneously disclose their abuse to healthcare providers. Examples of history or physical examination findings that could prompt provider concern include changing information about home address or other demographics, the child being accompanied by an adult who is unrelated and/or who dominates the conversation, history of multiple sexually transmitted infections, history of running away repeatedly, tattoos suggestive of branding, or presence of inflicted injuries.

When there is a concern for CSEC, ask the patient about a history of having sex in exchange for money or other needs (housing, food), having sexual pictures posted online, or being asked to have sex with a third party. Ask questions in a non-judgmental or threatening way, after establishing rapport.

ED Management

Address any identified medical issues including injuries, infections, acute sexual assault, suicidal ideation, or other mental health concerns. Consider prophylactic treatment for sexually transmitted infections in the context of risk factors for infection and difficulty in ensuring medical follow-up. Offer post-coital contraception if applicable. Make a report to authorities according to local mandatory reporting laws; local administrators can assist in determining if reports should be made to child protective services and/or law enforcement. Some jurisdictions clearly recognize CSEC as a form of child maltreatment, and have specialized response teams. Local resources for CSEC victims may include child advocacy centers offering forensic interviews, specialized shelters, and trauma-informed mental health services. In addition to local resources the National Human Trafficking Resource Center Hotline (1-888-373-7888) can provide assistance with reporting questions and locating services for victims.

Follow-up

- Child abuse specialist: within 1–2 days if there is concern for injury on examination. Otherwise, with a physician within two weeks, to repeat testing for pregnancy and sexually transmitted infections, as indicated
- If HIV post-exposure prophylaxis is initiated, with a physician in two weeks to monitor medication tolerance. Also, follow-up HIV and RPR serology at six weeks and twelve weeks post-exposure as indicated. If not using fourth-generation HIV testing, also follow-up six months post-exposure.
- Mental health professional: as soon as possible

Indications for Admission

- Patient at risk for ongoing contact with the alleged perpetrator if discharged, and CPS is unable to establish a safety plan.
- Medical need that requires inpatient care (vaginal or rectal bleeding, suicidal ideation, etc.)

Bibliography

Chaffee T, English A. Sex trafficking of adolescents and young adults in the United States: healthcare provider's role. *Curr Opin Obstet Gynecol.* 2015;**27**(5):339–344.

Chung RJ, English A. Commercial sexual exploitation and sex trafficking of adolescents. *Curr Opin Pediatr.* 2015;**27**(4):427–433.

Greenbaum J, Crawford-Jakubiak JE, Committee on Child Abuse and Neglect. Child sex trafficking and commercial sexual exploitation: health care needs of victims. *Pediatrics.* 2015;**135**(3):566–574.

Moore JL, Kaplan DM, Barron CE. Sex trafficking of minors. *Pediatr Clin North Am.* 2017;**64** (2):413–421.

Rafferty Y. Challenges to the rapid identification of children who have been trafficked for commercial sexual exploitation. *Child Abuse Negl.* 2016;**52**:158–168.

Physical Abuse

Physical abuse is defined as non-accidental physical injury inflicted on a child. In all states, health professionals are legally mandated to report their suspicions of abuse to their state CPS.

Clinical Presentation

The recognition of abusive injuries can be challenging. Young children and infants may present with obvious signs/symptoms of trauma, such as extremity swelling or deformity, or they may have nonspecific symptoms, such as fussiness or vomiting. Abusive injuries may also be detected incidentally in a child who presents for unrelated medical issues (e.g., rib fractures identified on a chest radiograph performed for evaluation of respiratory distress). Older children and teenagers may present after making a disclosure of physical abuse.

Diagnosis

The primary concerns in the differential diagnosis of physical abuse are accidental injuries and underlying medical conditions mimicking or predisposing to injury. Birth trauma is also a consideration in a young infant.

Recognize injury patterns that suggest physical abuse. These include bruising with a distinctive pattern, such as slap marks and ligature marks, as well as curvilinear, parallel linear, or loop-shaped marks from a wire, cord, or belt. Bruising in non-mobile infants is unusual, as "those who don't cruise rarely bruise." Locations of bruises that raise a concern for inflicted injury include the ears, neck, genitals, and torso/abdomen. Burns in a glove or stocking distribution with uniform depth and clearly demarcated margins can result from abusive immersion burns. Fractures with a high specificity for abuse are scapular, sternal, classic metaphyseal, and rib, especially if posterior.

Gather detailed information about the reported accidental mechanisms of injury and document any changes in the history provided, or differences among the interviewees. Ask about timing of incidents, as well as onset of symptoms, noting delays in seeking care. Take a detailed developmental history. On review of systems and past medical history, ask about symptoms associated with injuries to other organ systems (musculoskeletal, abdominal, neurological), prior injuries, as well as signs and symptoms of underlying medical conditions (e.g., hemophilia, neuromuscular diseases, rickets). Ask about a family history of hereditary diseases that can mimic abuse, such as bleeding disorders and osteogenesis imperfecta. Take a detailed social history, and determine if there are other siblings in the home who could also be potentially at risk for harm.

Remove all of the child's clothing and examine the skin carefully for injuries. Bruising to the ears and neck could be missed without careful attention to these areas. Assess for frenulum tears, which are especially concerning in non-mobile infants, and check the scalp for traumatic alopecia. Photograph injuries if possible.

Evaluate the patient for dysmorphic features associated with genetic conditions, such as osteogenesis imperfecta (blue sclera, triangular facies). Note whether the growth parameters suggest failure to thrive, or a disproportionally large head size worrisome for an intracranial process. Also, check the fontanelles and perform a thorough neurological examination. On musculoskeletal examination check for deformities, palpable calluses, or any abnormal range of motion. Assess for signs of abdominal injury. Maintain a high level of suspicion, as a young child can have head, abdominal, or musculoskeletal injuries that can be undetected on physical examination.

Continue the evaluation based on the patient's age and clinical findings. If there is concern for physical abuse in a child under two years of age, obtain a complete skeletal survey for trauma. For an older patient, if the physical examination suggests a fracture, obtain specific radiographs. Since infants with intracranial injury can be asymptomatic, neuroimaging (head CT or MRI) is indicated in cases of infants with physical abuse.

An ophthalmological examination alone is not an adequate screening tool for head trauma, although a funduscopic examination by an ophthalmologist is indicated if there are intracranial findings detected on neuroimaging. Abdominal injuries can be occult in a young child, so check for elevated liver enzymes, which suggests that further work-up is needed. If abdominal injury is suspected, obtain a CT scan with IV, but not oral, contrast.

Additional studies may be indicated to evaluate for medical conditions that mimic or predispose to injuries based on clinical findings. A CBC and coagulation studies are basic screening tests for bleeding disorders in a patient with significant bruising or intracranial hemorrhage. In the setting of multiple fractures of different ages, obtain an alkaline phosphatase, calcium, phosphorous, and 25-hydroxyvitamin D. Table 18.1 lists some other medical conditions that can be mistaken for abuse with distinguishing clinical, laboratory, and radiologic features.

In some cases, an accidental or medical cause will be obvious after the emergency department assessment. Diagnose accidental trauma when the reported mechanism explains the patient's injury, and is consistent with the child's developmental level. Also, some injuries are more typical of accidental injuries, such as a toddler's fracture (spiral fracture of the distal tibia in an ambulatory toddler). Some accidental injuries may raise concern for neglect – for example, injuries occurring when a young child is left home alone. In other cases, a medical

Table 18.1 Distinguishing features and laboratory studies for some medical diagnoses that can mimic or predispose to injury

Findings	Differential diagnosis	Distinguishing features and tests
Abusive head trauma		
	Benign external hydrocephalus	No history of trauma MRI helps differentiate blood from CSF
	Glutaric aciduria type 1	Urine organic acids: ↑ glutaric acid or 3-hydroxyglutaric acid
		MRI: brain atrophy with widening of Sylvian fissures and basal ganglia lesions
	Menkes' disease	Hair: pili torti ↓ Copper, ceruloplasmin
Bruising and/or bleeding		
	Hemangioma	History of long-standing lesion, changes slowly over time
	Hemophilia	↑ PTT, ↓ factor VIII or IX
	Henoch–Schönlein purpura	Palpable purpura particularly on the lower extremities
		May have hematuria
	ITP	Generalized petechiae and purpura ↓ Platelets
	Purpura fulminans	Clinical appearance (findings of sepsis) ↓ Platelet count
	Vitamin K deficiency	History of inadequate vitamin K supplementation at birth ↑ PT, aPTT
	Von Willebrand disease	History of abnormal bleeding Abnormal Von Willebrand panel

Table 18.1 (cont.)

Findings	Differential diagnosis	Distinguishing features and tests
Burns		
	Ecthyma, impetigo	Crusting lesions of varying sizes
	Phytophotodermatitis	History of contact with psoralen (lime. lemon) and UV exposure
Fractures and bony abnormalities		
	Caffey disease	Hyperostosis in first six months of life No metaphyseal changes
	Hypophosphatasia	Demineralization and rachitic changes ↓ Alkaline phosphatase
	Osteogenesis imperfecta	May have blue sclerae and/or dysmorphic features May have a positive family history X-rays with ↓ bone density
	Osteopenia of prematurity	Very low birth weight ↑ Alkaline phosphatase X-ray: enlarged epiphysis
	Rickets	↑ Alkaline phosphatase X-ray: cupping at ends of long bones and widened metaphysis
Oncologic		
	Leukemia	Abnormal peripheral smear, bone marrow, biopsy
	Osteogenic malignancy	Positive x-ray

explanation for the findings will be evident because of a previously known underlying medical condition or a clear new diagnosis that accounts for the findings. Examples include a child with a known diagnosis of osteogenesis imperfecta presenting with fracture, or a new diagnosis of idiopathic thrombocytopenic purpura in a patient presenting with petechiae.

ED Management

Once the patient is medically stabilized, *report any suspicion* of abuse to CPS. Also notify the parents about your intention to report. The CPS worker must evaluate the case and decide whether the child can safely return home or must go to a different living environment for safety, such as with a relative under a CPS safety plan, a temporary shelter, or foster care setting. Hospitalize the child if medical care is needed or if the inpatient setting is the only option to ensure safety. CPS investigators also address safety of siblings and other household contacts. Physical examination of the siblings, as well as a skeletal survey for those aged under two years, is indicated.

Working with the families of abused children can be a difficult experience. Avoid an accusatory attitude and take a supportive approach, keeping the parents informed and involved. Emphasize that the goal of all concerned is to keep the child safe and, when possible, the family together. Explain the role of the social worker and supportive services, and assure confidentially. Careful documentation is critical (see pp. 596–602), as the record will be needed for legal reference.

Follow-up

- Patient discharged home or to a shelter: primary care follow-up within one week
- Patient under two years with abnormal or equivocal findings on initial skeletal survey, or strong clinical suspicion for abuse: repeat skeletal survey in two weeks (can omit skull, pelvis, and spine)

Indications for Admission

- Medical care required, including treatment of injuries and/or additional medical work-up
- Extent of injury uncertain
- Need for protection unavailable through community resources

Bibliography

Anderst JD, Carpenter SL, Abshire TC, et al. Evaluation for bleeding disorders in suspected child abuse. Pediatrics. 2013;**131**(4):e1314–e1322

Campbell KA Olsen LM, Keenan HT. Critical elements in the medical evaluation of suspected child physical abuse. *Pediatrics*. 2015;**136**(1):35–43.

Christian CW, American Academy of Pediatrics Committee on Child Abuse and Neglect: the evaluation of suspected child physical abuse. *Pediatrics*. 2015;**135**(5):e1337–e1354.

Flaherty EG, Perez-Rossello JM, Levine MA, Hennrikus WL, American Academy of Pediatrics Committee on Child Abuse and Neglect. Evaluating children with fractures for child physical abuse. *Pediatrics*. 2014;**133**(2):e477–e489.

Jenny C, Crawford-Jakubiak JE, American Academy of Pediatrics Committee on Child Abuse and Neglect. The evaluation of children in the primary care setting when sexual abuse is suspected. *Pediatrics*. 2013;**132**(2):e558–e567.

Sexual Abuse

Using force or threats to engage a person of any age in sexual activity constitutes abuse. Child sexual abuse occurs when a child is engaged in sexual activity, regardless of whether or not force is used. Children are legally unable to consent to sexual activity, the age of which is set by each individual state. Perpetrators of sexual abuse are often adults known to children who use coercion or manipulation as opposed to physical force.

Clinical Presentation

Seeking medical care after a child tells a trusted adult about sexual abuse is a common clinical presentation. Less frequently, victims of sexual abuse present to care with physical findings such as trauma to the hymen, sexually transmitted infections, or pregnancy. Sexual abuse victims may also have nonspecific symptoms such as school difficulties, behavior changes, suicide gestures, sleep disturbances, enuresis, and encopresis. These symptoms, however, can also result from medical conditions and other psychosocial stressors and are therefore not diagnostic of sexual abuse. Sexualized behavior that deviates from developmental norms is more specific, although this too can result from other psychosocial stressors and is not diagnostic of sexual abuse in and of itself. Parental concern that their child may have been sexually abused may also prompt consultation.

Diagnosis

Evaluation of sexual abuse requires a multidisciplinary team that can include professionals from social work, CPS, law enforcement, child advocacy centers, and clinicians. Diagnostic certainty is not needed to report abuse, as healthcare workers are mandated to report when there is a *reasonable suspicion* of abuse.

A careful and thorough history is a key component of sexual abuse evaluations. Obtain information from adult caregivers accompanying the child. In some cases, investigators can also provide information if their involvement precedes the emergency department visit. Physicians may also obtain information from children, but avoid repetitive interviews about the abuse. Many communities have children's advocacy centers that can conduct forensic interviews. In cases where caregivers or investigators can provide information necessary for medical decision-making, and an investigative interview has already been completed or is anticipated, an additional interview about the abuse is not necessary. In cases where the child does need to be interviewed by emergency department providers, keep in mind that young children are more suggestible than adults. Avoid leading questions, and instead use open-ended questions that allow the child to provide a narrative, such as "Tell me why you came to the hospital today" or "tell me everything that happened". Children should be interviewed individually, without the alleged perpetrator present during the evaluation process. Document the questions asked and the child's answers, using quotes when possible.

It is important to document when the most recent sexual abuse occurred, because there is a window of time, in many circumstances 72 hours, for both forensic evidence collection and the initiation of prophylactic medications. In cases where children have not yet developed the concept of telling time, ask caregivers about the last possible contact with the alleged perpetrator.

Knowledge of the nature of abuse will also inform clinical decisions. For example, receptive anal penetration is associated with the highest risk of HIV transmission from sexual contact, while voyeurism without physical contact would not place a child at risk for sexually transmitted infections. If available, information about the alleged perpetrator, such as known history of HIV or other sexually transmitted infections, as well as IV drug use or other risk factors for HIV, can be useful in assessing the child's risk for infection. Noting whether the perpetrator lives in the home, or could otherwise have ongoing access to the child, is important in assessing safety and child protection needs. In the review of systems, assess for physical symptoms of trauma and infection such as genital discharge or bleeding. Also assess for psychological symptoms of trauma, with careful attention to suicidal ideation requiring urgent psychiatric treatment.

Perform a complete and careful physical examination, including of the genitals, looking for marks, bruises, or other signs of physical injury or illness. However, the vast majority of sexual abuse victims have normal physical examinations, and a normal genital–anal

Table 18.2 Possible laboratory studies in sexual abuse

Chlamydia trachomatis: vagina/urethra, rectum culture or NAAT per local protocol

Neisseria gonorrhea: oropharynx, vagina/urethra, rectum culture or NAAT per local protocols

Hepatitis B: surface antibody unless patient has received three doses of hepatitis B vaccine

HIV serology

Pregnancy test (if appropriate)

Syphilis serology

Trichomonas vaginalis: NAAT, rapid antigen detection test, wet mount, and/or culture of vaginal discharge per local protocols

If HIV post-exposure prophylaxis is initiated: complete blood count, basic metabolic panel, liver function panel

appearance does not rule-out sexual abuse. Do not force a patient if the examination is refused. In prepubertal girls use the frog-leg, supine, or knee–chest prone position; the supine lithotomy position can be used for teenagers and taller children. Separation and traction of the labia majora are needed to visualize internal vestibular structures including the hymen, but a speculum is not needed to visualize these structures and would not be tolerated by prepubertal girls. For rare cases presenting with ongoing genital–anal bleeding or significant lacerations, consult with a pediatric gynecologist or pediatric surgeon on the need for examination under anesthesia.

In boys, examine the penis and scrotum for bruises, swelling, teeth marks, erythema, or other signs of trauma. In both boys and girls, spread the buttocks with both hands to examine the anus and perineal area. If possible, photo-document injuries.

Use the information gathered to determine the need for laboratory testing for pregnancy and sexually transmitted infections (Table 18.2). Nucleic acid amplification testing (NAAT) has replaced culture for chlamydia and gonorrhea testing in many centers, and local laboratory experts can inform protocols for confirmation of positive NAATs. Depending on the time since the most recent incident of abuse, follow-up testing may also be needed. Follow-up HIV testing is indicated at 6 and 12 weeks post-exposure, if using fourth-generation tests.

ED Management

Consider medical, child protection, and forensic aspects of care. Medical management includes treatment of any identified injuries or infections, as well as prophylactic treatment for HIV and other sexually transmitted infections. The time window to initiate HIV post-exposure prophylaxis (PEP) is 72 hours, so give the first dose as soon as possible. Consider perpetrator characteristics, nature of the sexual contact, and patient-level factors when assessing risk for HIV. Examples of risk factors include anal or genital penetration or trauma, perpetrator with known infection or unknown to patient, and reports of exposure to blood or semen. PEP requires a 28-day, three-drug regimen. Provide the family with a starter pack of medications, as it can be difficult to obtain these medications from community pharmacies. In addition to local resources, there is a National Clinician's Post-Exposure Prophylaxis Hotline (PEPLine; 1-888-448-4911) to assist with decision-making.

The approach to prophylactic treatment for *Chlamydia, gonorrhea,* and *Trichomonas* differs between prepubertal and postpubertal patients. The latter are at risk for pelvic inflammatory disease, asymptomatic infection, and poor compliance with follow-up visits, so give prophylactic treatment with ceftriaxone 250 mg IM in a single dose, *plus* azithromycin 1 g orally in a single dose, *plus* if ≥ 45 kg metronidazole 2 g orally in a single dose. Treat prepubertal children only if they have a positive test, and reserve prophylactic treatment for special circumstances such as perpetrator with known infection, or evidence of trauma from penetration. Offer a post-coital contraceptive to postmenarchal females with negative pregnancy tests seen within 72–120 hours. Plan B is an FDA-approved emergency contraceptive, and other options can be found on the Emergency Contraception website (http://ec.princeton.edu/questions/dose.html). Also address mental health needs through community referrals or, when indicated, emergency psychiatric care.

Healthcare providers are mandated to report suspected abuse. An immediate response from the child protection agency is needed when the alleged perpetrator lives in the child's home or could have ongoing access to the child.

Law enforcement agencies also investigate allegations of sexual abuse, and forensic evidence can be collected in some cases depending on the timing and nature of the abuse. In many jurisdictions, the time window for forensic collection is 72 hours, but this can vary according to local guidelines. Most emergency departments have sexual assault evidence-collecting kits for this purpose, with instructions on how to proceed with collection. Kits contain collection bags for clothes, swabs for the anus, genitals, and body, patient DNA sample for comparison, as well as forms for consent and documentation. Many kits also allow for collection of specimens for drug testing in cases where drug-facilitated sexual assault is suspected. Label all specimens taken for evidence, and place them in the envelopes provided in the kit. Once completed and sealed, hand the kit to police or hospital security, or per local procedures for chain of custody.

Follow-up

- Child abuse specialist: within 1–2 days if there is concern for injury on examination. Otherwise, with a physician within two weeks to repeat testing for pregnancy and sexually transmitted infections, as indicated
- If HIV post-exposure prophylaxis is initiated, with a physician in two weeks to monitor medication tolerance. Also, follow-up HIV and RPR serology at 6 and 12 weeks post-exposure as indicated. If not using fourth-generation HIV testing, also follow-up six months post-exposure
- Mental health professional: as soon as possible

Indications for Admission

- Patient at risk for ongoing contact with the alleged perpetrator if discharged, and child protective services is unable to establish a safety plan
- Injury such as active vaginal or rectal bleeding

Bibliography

Adams JA, Kellogg N, Farst KJ, et al. Updated guidelines for the medical assessment and care of children who may have been sexually abused. *J Pediatr Adolesc Gynecol.* 2016;29(2):81–87.

Clinician consultation center, University of California, San Francisco. PEP: post-exposure prophylaxis. http://nccc.ucsf.edu/clinician-consultation/pep-post-exposure-prophylaxis (accessed December 12, 2016).

Jenny C, Crawford-Jakubiak JE, American Academy of Pediatrics Committee on Child Abuse and Neglect. The evaluation of children in the primary care setting when sexual abuse is suspected. *Pediatrics.* 2013;**132**(2):e558–e567.

Office of Population Research at Princeton University. The emergency contraception website. Table 1. Oral contraceptives that can be used for emergency contraception in the United States. http://ec .princeton.edu/questions/dose.html (accessed December 10, 2016).

Workowski KA, Bolan GA, Centers for Disease Control and Prevention. Sexually transmitted disease treatment guidelines, 2015. *MMWR Recomm Rep.* 2015;**64**:104–110.

Chapter 19

Psychological and Social Emergencies

Scott Miller and Loretta Sonnier

Death in the Emergency Department

The loss of a child has a devastating effect on a family, particularly when it is unexpected or without any readily identifiable cause. These families do not have the opportunity for "preparatory grief." Proper ED management is critical to the family's long-term adjustment.

Clinical Presentation and Diagnosis

When the ED is notified of the transport of a child in extremis, assign a resuscitation team member to work with the parents. Take the parents to a quiet area not far from the resuscitation scene, and have that team member act as a liaison to keep the family informed. In some centers, parents will be present in the resuscitation room, but a staff member who can interpret the events must accompany them.

At the time of the child's death, notify the parents privately, clearly, and directly. Specify the word "dead" to avoid any confusion. Avoid using euphemisms like "He has passed." Once the death has been communicated, the management phase begins.

ED Management

Family members may display many emotional reactions, from hysterical screaming, to anger, to silence. All responses are normal. Once the immediate reaction has had time to occur, be available to answer any questions. There is no need for excuses, although parents may appreciate expressions of personal emotion and concern. Respond to parental expressions of guilt with a realistic appraisal of the circumstances. Also try to obtain additional history that may be helpful in establishing a diagnosis. If abuse (pp. 604–608) is suspected, it will be confirmed at autopsy, so there is no need to confront the grieving family.

Provide the family with assistance: phone, water, tissues. Do not assume that they want a particular relative or clergyman unless they so request.

Encourage parents to see the child's body once it has been prepared for their viewing (removal of medical equipment, soiled linen, etc.). Allow parents to hold the child's body and say their farewells. A prayer or closing ritual said over the body is a good way to bring closure after a brief period of contact with the child.

Inform the family of any requirements concerning an autopsy. In most states an autopsy is not mandated if the child had a chronic condition in which death was expected. If there are no requirements, encourage an autopsy in order to answer any questions pertaining to the cause of death. Also discuss the possibility of organ/tissue donation with the family.

Instruct a trusted family member or friend about hospital policy on claiming the body and other necessary arrangements.

Give the parents your contact information in written form for follow-up questions and concerns, and document the chart and death certificate appropriately. Contact the child's primary care provider, along with any relevant subspecialists, to notify them of the child's death. Afterward, a brief staff meeting may pull staff members together and allow them to express their feelings.

Bibliography

American Academy of Pediatrics Committee on Pediatric Emergency Medicine, American College of Emergency Physicians Pediatric Emergency Medicine Committee, Emergency Nurses Association Pediatric Committee. Death of a child in the emergency department. *Pediatrics*. 2014;**134**(1):198–201.

Dudley N, Ackerman A, Brown KM, et al. Patient- and family-centered care of children in the emergency department. *Pediatrics*. 2015;**135**(1):e255–e272.

Garstang J, Griffiths F, Sidebotham P. What do bereaved parents want from professionals after the sudden death of their child: a systematic review of the literature. *BMC Pediatr*. 2014;**14**:269.

Harrison ME, Walling A. What do we know about giving bad news? A review. *Clin Pediatr (Phila)*. 2010;**49**(7):619–626

McAlvin SS, Carew-Lyons A. Family presence during resuscitation and invasive procedures in pediatric critical care: a systematic review. *Am J Crit Care*. 2014;**23**(6):477–484.

O'Meara M, Trethewie S. Managing paediatric death in the emergency department. *J Paediatr Child Health*. 2016;**52**(2):164–167.

Interpersonal Violence

Interpersonal violence is an altercation between two or more non-caretaker individuals in which at least one of the participants intended to harm the other. These altercations frequently occur in the school, schoolyard, or street. In general, it is not useful to apply the terms "victim" and "perpetrator," as the "victim" that presents to the ED may have instigated the fight that he or she subsequently "lost." It has recently been reported that as many as 25% of all adolescents seen in a pediatric ED were treated for injuries resulting from interpersonal violence.

In contrast, family violence, such as child abuse and domestic violence, is characterized by one individual having significant power over another within the relationship. While most healthcare systems have protocols for the management of family violence, there is no mandated reporting system for interpersonal violence.

Clinical Presentation and Diagnosis

Violently injured patients present with a wide range of injuries and injury severity. Prior to the interview, assure the patient that all responses are confidential, with the exceptions of suicidal or homicidal statements and the disclosure of child abuse. Let the patient tell the story in his or her own words, in private, and listen non-judgmentally. After the interview,

Table 19.1 Priorities in the evaluation of the violently injured patient

Circumstances

Police involvement

Relationship to the other participants

Use or appearance of weapons at the scene

What caused the event

Safety issues

Access to weapons

Depression: long-term plans, presence of family and close friends

Retaliation plans by patient, family, or friend[a]

Suicidal ideation[b]

[a] Requires immediate referral to police.
[b] Requires immediate referral to psychiatry and social work.

ask the youth's permission to involve the family in the discussion. Enlisting the help of the family can often facilitate follow-up and ongoing support for the patient.

The responses to a few suitable questions can determine the need for immediate referral to social work, mental health, or law enforcement (Table 19.1). Clearly document these responses in the medical record. The legality of access to the medical record by law enforcement agencies varies among communities, so contact the hospital's legal counsel regarding local statutes and recommendations pertaining to documentation.

A thorough evaluation of the violently injured patient includes an understanding of what caused the event, the location and time of the episode, the relationship of the patient to others involved in the incident, and the use or appearance of weapons at the scene. Explore issues related to the patient's safety. Ask specific questions regarding any intention to hurt themselves or others. Also inquire if a family member or friend plans to retaliate. Although open-ended questions such as "Once you leave here, what are you going to do?" can clue a physician into potentially dangerous plans, ask directly about retaliation and suicidal thoughts. Similarly, ask the patient about drug selling, access to weapons, and possible gang affiliation. When present, these risk factors may predict the lethality of future actions. When asking about substance use and abuse, also inquire about the patient's friends and acquaintances, to determine potential exposure to that lifestyle. If the patient admits to using marijuana or other drugs, ask "why." The responses to these questions may help confirm that the adolescent is self-medicating.

Assess the patient's present emotional state and reaction to the trauma. Since there is a strong correlation between depression and the risk of violent injury, ask about the patient's long-term plans for the future and the presence or absence of close friends or family members as confidants and allies.

ED Management

The primary psychological goals of ED care of a violently injured youth are to stabilize the patient, ensure the immediate safety of the patient and other participants, and to assess the patient's risk for further injury. If the patient reveals suicidal or homicidal intent, contact a psychiatrist immediately. Also, the medical staff is obligated to contact the police if there are legitimate concerns about retaliation.

It is also important to assess and address the psychosocial comorbidities, including depression, substance abuse, school failure, and family violence. Refer a depressed or hopeless patient to a psychiatrist urgently. Provide psychosocial support to all violently injured patients, regardless of the situation that caused the injury. Consult a social worker, who can help provide access to available community resources. Give contact information for appropriate crisis hotlines, community support groups, and available local shelters. Information about these resources is often also available from municipal social service agencies.

If the patient is being admitted, communicate any safety concerns to the inpatient medical and nursing staff, security officers, and social workers. One-to-one observation is necessary for suicidal or homicidal patients. If there is any concern for gang retaliation, it may be necessary to admit the patient under an alias to ensure his or her safety.

Follow-up

- Primary care, mental health, or social work follow-up in one week

Indication for Admission

- Active suicidal or homicidal ideation

Bibliography

Anixt JS, Copeland-Linder N, Haynie D, Cheng TL. Burden of unmet mental health needs in assault-injured youths presenting to the emergency department. *Acad Pediatr.* 2012; **12**:125.

Cunningham RM, Carter PM, Ranney M, et al. Violent reinjury and mortality among youth seeking emergency department care for assault-related injury: a 2-year prospective cohort study. *JAMA Pediatr.* 2015;**169**:63.

Cunningham RM, Ranney M, Newton M, et al. Characteristics of youth seeking emergency care for assault injuries. *Pediatrics.* 2014;**133**:e96.

Ramirez M, Wu Y, Kataoka S, et al. Youth violence across multiple dimensions: a study of violence, absenteeism, and suspensions among middle school children. *J Pediatr.* 2012;**161**:542.

Munchausen Syndrome by Proxy

Munchausen syndrome (MS) was first described in adults who subject themselves to diagnostic tests and therapeutic procedures in order to gain the safety and security of being hospitalized. Munchausen syndrome by proxy (MSBP) is a subset of the child abuse syndrome in which signs or symptoms of medical illnesses are either feigned by the parent or produced in the child, so that the parent and child can be hospitalized. It is therefore an extension of MS in adults with similar psychopathology. The difference is that in MSBP, the child is used by the parent as the focus of medical attention.

Clinical Presentation

MSBP has many varied presenting signs and symptoms, including apnea, brief resolved unexplained events (BRUE) or near-miss SIDS episodes, hematuria, hematochezia, hematemesis, fever, seizures, frequent infections, failure to thrive, hypoglycemia, and poisonings. Virtually any complaint can be feigned or artificially produced in MSBP. In some series, MSBP has a 10% mortality rate.

Diagnosis

A high index of suspicion is required to diagnose MSBP. Suspect it in any clinical situation that has baffled physicians at other centers or has a "one of a kind" dimension. The identified parental characteristics include a parent (the mother in 90% of cases) who has some medical background, is often by the bedside, appears very devoted, and is invested in the illness. MSBP parents are usually very intelligent, verbal, and appealing to the medical staff. Generally, the parent who is implicated is the same one that notes the episodic nature of the signs and symptoms. In addition, the parent is usually distant from her spouse, and she may have a history of being a patient herself.

ED Management

MSBP is rarely diagnosed in the ED, as careful observation over time is required. The ED staff should be alert to parents who seem to be frequent, inappropriate ED users or who seem to exaggerate their children's symptoms. If the diagnosis is suspected in the ED, admit the child and notify the child abuse team. Depending on the nature of the MSBP, there are many strategies for proving the diagnosis, including laboratory tests (blood type, insulin level, etc.), blood cultures, covert videotaping of the parent, monitoring devices, and limitation of parental visitation. If the ED staff can make the diagnosis of MSBP by direct observation, report the case to the Child Protection Services (CPS) and place the child in a protected environment.

Indication for Admission
- Suspected victim of MSBP

Bibliography

Bass C, Glaser D. Early recognition and management of fabricated or induced illness in children. *Lancet.* 2014;**383**(9926):1412–1421.

Brown P, Tierney C. Munchausen syndrome by proxy. *Pediatr Rev.* 2009;**30**(10):414–415

Flaherty EG, Macmillan HL, Committee on Child Abuse and Neglect. Caregiver-fabricated illness in a child: a manifestation of child maltreatment. *Pediatrics.* 2013;**132**(3):590–597.

Isaacs D. Induced illness in children. *J Paediatr Child Health.* 2015;**51**(11):1049–1050.

Squires JE, Squires RH. A review of Munchausen syndrome by proxy. *Pediatr Ann.* 2013;**42**(4):67–71.

Psychiatric Emergencies

As a consequence of the scarcity of mental health services for children, the ED often serves as a portal of entry into the mental health system. In the ED, the priorities in the psychiatric assessment are to determine if the patient is suicidal or homicidal, and whether the child can be cared for safely in an environment less restrictive than a psychiatric hospital.

Clinical Presentation

Depression

The depressed patient may present with recurrent somatic complaints for which no organic cause can be found, or the patient may exhibit acting-out behavior, running away, stealing, fire-setting, or being accident-prone. The caretaker may express concern about social withdrawal, a loss of appetite, declining school performance, poor grooming and self-care, or a change in sleep pattern.

Psychosis

The psychotic patient may have delusional beliefs, hallucinations, and bizarre or disorganized behavior. A prodrome of psychotic symptoms may develop gradually and precede the acute presentation to the ED. Psychotic adolescents may have catatonia or negative psychotic symptoms, including blunting or flattening of emotional expression, psychomotor retardation, and poverty of thought.

Violent or Aggressive Behavior

Many different kinds of mental pathology underlie aggression, including problems with impulse control, mood, communication, cognition, or perception. Comorbid disorders are often present in children with disruptive behavior disorder and heighten the likelihood of aggressive acts. Determining the underlying cause of the aggression will help to establish whether the behavior is impulsive and reactive or planned and purposeful.

Diagnosis and ED Management

Depression

Children with depression often lack awareness of their affliction, but caretakers can describe changes in a child's functioning and mood. Consider whether a chronic organic disorder (hypothyroidism, diabetes, HIV, Lyme disease, etc.) may be making the patient depressed. A patient who has considered suicide must be evaluated in the ED by a trained mental health professional and cannot be discharged without the evaluation.

Psychosis

The first step is to rule-out an organic etiology for the psychosis, the most common of which is drug ingestion (LSD, PCP, Ecstasy, amphetamines, cocaine, anticholinergics, over-the-counter cough remedies). Teenagers who are "thrill seeking" will often experiment with multiple substances, confusing their presentation and complicating their medical management. Other causes of psychosis are delirium, pain, infection, sepsis, encephalitis, seizures, increased intracranial pressure, and medication or substance withdrawal syndrome.

Ask about possible drug ingestion, and have the family bring in all medications from the child's home and from the homes of friends or relatives the patient has visited recently. Stimulants commonly used to treat attention-deficit disorder can induce psychotic symptoms, even at pharmacologic doses. Therefore, determine if the patient has recently started

Table 19.2 Medications for restraint of uncontrolled patients

Drug	Dose	Route
Lorazepam[1]	0.5–2 mg	PO/IM
Olanzapine[2]	2.5–10 mg	SL/PO/IM
Risperidone	0.25–2 mg	SL/PO

[1] Beware of paradoxical disinhibition with lorazepam.
[2] Do not give IM olanzapine within one hour of any IM benzodiazepine due to risk for respiratory depression.

taking a new medication. Inquire about a family history of schizophrenia or mood disorders. With an organic psychosis, the onset is acute and hallucinations are often visual, olfactory, tactile, or gustatory, rather than auditory. With schizophrenia and other functional psychoses, the hallucinations are typically auditory, the onset is more insidious, and hallucinations fit into the patient's delusional belief system.

On physical examination, there may be fever (anticholinergic or amphetamine ingestion, brain abscess, encephalitis), tachycardia (sepsis, hallucinogen, anticholinergic or amphetamine ingestion), and hypertension (anticholinergic, amphetamines, cocaine, LSD, or PCP ingestion). Note the pupillary size and reactivity; there may be inequality (mass lesion, brain abscess), mydriasis (hypoglycemia or LSD, amphetamine, cocaine, or anticholinergic ingestion), or miosis (cholinergics, opiate, or PCP ingestion).

Immediately order a CT scan for patients with any focal neurologic abnormalities, signs of increased intracranial pressure, or central nervous system infection. If the CT is normal, febrile patients require a lumbar puncture. Also obtain a CBC, electrolytes, serum glucose, liver function tests, and a urinalysis.

Unless an organic cause for the psychosis can be definitely ruled out in the ED, admit the patient to a pediatric service to continue the evaluation after consultation with a psychiatrist. Consult psychiatry before initiating antipsychotic medications. If sedation is required for agitation or uncontrolled acting out, use an agent listed in Table 19.2, but attempt de-escalation techniques before medication is used. When prescribing medication for agitation, start at a low dose, avoid medication combinations, and use a medication that treats the underlying primary psychiatric diagnosis when possible.

Violent Behavior and Aggression

In managing children with aggression, the goals are to (1) ensure the safety of the child, family, and staff; (2) rule-out medical conditions; and (3) gather information for appropriate disposition.

If a medical condition or an intoxicant is inducing the aggression, acute medical hospitalization is indicated. If an underlying psychiatric disorder is the cause of aggression, psychiatric hospitalization may be indicated for further evaluation and management to prevent worsening.

Follow-up

• Medically stable patient: as per the mental health consult

Indications for Admission

- Suicidality (see Suicide, pp. 621–623)
- Depression with inability to function
- Psychosis
- Behavior that may harm self or others
- Acute medical complications of substance abuse

Bibliography

Carubia B, Becker A, Levine B. Child psychiatric emergencies: updates on trends, clinical care, and practice challenges. *Curr Psychiatry Rep.* 2016;**18**:41.

Chun TH, Mace SE, Katz ER, et al. Evaluation and management of children and adolescents with acute mental health or behavioral problems. Part I: common clinical challenges of patients with mental health and/or behavioral emergencies. *Pediatrics.* 2016;**138**:e1–e22

Giles MM, Martini DR. Psychiatric emergencies. In Dulcan MK (ed.) *Dulcan's Textbook of Child and Adolescent Psychiatry* (2nd edn.). Arlington, VA: American Psychiatric Publishing, 2016; 621–636.

Guiner A, Chandnani H, Chao D. Approach to the adolescent psychiatric and behavioral health emergency. *Adolesc Med State Art Rev.* 2015;**26**(3):552–569.

Marzullo, L. Pharmacologic management of the agitated child. *Pediatr Emerg Care.* 2014;**30**(4):269–275.

Sudden Infant Death Syndrome

Sudden infant death syndrome (SIDS) is defined as "the sudden death of an infant or young child, unexpected by history, in which a thorough postmortem examination and death scene investigation fail to demonstrate an adequate cause for death." SIDS is the leading cause of death among infants one month to one year old.

Clinical Presentation

The peak incidence is at 2–4 months, although there have been autopsy-proven occurrences up to 12 months of age. The incidence is higher in males, premature infants, and if the mother is a smoker, drug addict, or of lower socioeconomic status. Most cases occur between midnight and 9 a.m. during the cold-weather months. Typically, a previously healthy baby either does not awaken for a morning feed or is found cold and lifeless in the crib.

On occasion, the infant is found pale or cyanotic, apneic, or limp, and resuscitation is initiated at home or enroute to the ED. It is not clear if these episodes are part of the SIDS spectrum.

While no single explanation accounts for all cases of SIDS, prone positioning during sleep has been most strongly implicated, and the incidence of SIDS has dramatically decreased since the advent of the "Back to Sleep" campaign. In addition, the American Academy of Pediatrics (AAP) recommends a firm sleep surface, removal of soft objects and loose bedding from the crib, room sharing but no co-sleeping, cessation of maternal smoking during and after pregnancy, offering a pacifier at sleep time, and avoidance of overheating, swaddling of infants who attempt or are able to roll, and car seats for sleeping. The AAP also discourages sleep positioning devices and home monitors.

Diagnosis

SIDS is a diagnosis of exclusion and cannot be confirmed until an autopsy and other postmortem studies have ruled out other possible causes of sudden death in infancy, including adrenal insufficiency, overwhelming pneumonitis, bacterial sepsis (especially in sickle cell disease), child abuse, and poisoning. Near-miss episodes and BRUE may also result from prolonged sleep apnea, gastroesophageal reflux-induced apnea, cardiac dysrhythmias, metabolic disorders, and seizures (see The Critically Ill Infant, pp. 799–806).

ED Management

The management of the SIDS victim requires a detailed history of the circumstances surrounding the infant's death. An autopsy must be performed by the medical examiner. The management of a bereaved family is discussed on pp. 613–614.

If the resuscitation of a near-miss victim is successful, admit the infant to an ICU for continuous cardiopulmonary monitoring and further evaluation. Obtain an ECG with rhythm strip, chest x-ray, and blood for a CBC with differential, electrolytes, glucose, and culture. Perform a lumbar puncture for cytology, chemistries, a viral encephalitis panel, and culture, and obtain a urinalysis and urine culture.

Indications for Admission

- Near-miss episode requiring resuscitation

Bibliography

Bechtel K. Sudden unexpected infant death: differentiating natural from abusive causes in the emergency department. *Pediatr Emerg Care.* 2012;**28**(10):1085–1089.

Centers for Disease Control and Prevention. Sudden unexpected infant death and sudden infant death syndrome. www.cdc.gov/sids/aboutsuidandsids.htm (accessed May 24, 2017).

Moon RY, Task Force on Sudden Infant Death Syndrome. SIDS and other sleep-related infant deaths: evidence base for 2016 updated recommendations for a safe infant sleeping environment. *Pediatrics.* 2016;**138**. pii: e20162940.

Tieder JS, Bonkowsky JL, Etzel RA, et al. Brief resolved unexplained events (formerly apparent life-threatening events) and evaluation of lower-risk infants. *Pediatrics.* 2016;**137**(5). pii: e20160590.

Suicide

Suicide is the third leading cause of death in the United States among individuals 10–14 years of age, and the second leading cause of death among those 15–24 years of age. Death by suicide occurs four times more often in males than females, although females are three times more likely to attempt suicide. Firearms are the most common mechanism of suicide by males, whereas suffocation is the most common in females. The ratio of suicide attempts to suicide death in youth is estimated to be about 25:1, although this is likely an underestimate.

Clinical Presentation and Diagnosis

Suicide most often occurs in the setting of depression. The attempt is usually triggered by a "crisis" situation, such as the death or departure of a loved one, a fight with a boyfriend or

Table 19.3 Risk and protective factors for suicide

Risk factors	Protective factors
Family history of suicide	Effective care for mental and substance abuse disorders
Family history of child abuse	Easy access to clinical interventions and support
Previous suicide attempt(s)	Family and community support
History of substance abuse	Cultural and religious beliefs that discourage suicide
Feelings of hopelessness	Ongoing medical and mental healthcare relationships
History of mental disorders, particularly clinical depression	Skills in problem-solving, conflict resolution, and nonviolent ways of handling disputes
Impulsive or aggressive tendencies	
Local epidemics of suicide	
Sense of isolation from other people	
Inability to access mental health treatment	
Loss (relational, social, work, financial)	
Physical illness	
Easy access to lethal methods	
Stigma of mental health and substance abuse disorders	
Cultural and religious beliefs that suicide is a noble resolution of a personal dilemma	

Adapted from Centers for Disease Control and Prevention. Suicide: risk and protective factors. www.cdc.gov/violenceprevention/suicide/riskprotectivefactors.htm

girlfriend, or an argument with a parent. There are a number of risk and protective factors that affect the likelihood of someone attempting suicide (Table 19.3).

In the ED, these patients may present as victims of trauma or in an altered mental status due to overdose or an unknown cause. Every child older than ten years who takes a medication overdose or ingests a household product (caustics, hydrocarbons, insecticides) is making a suicide attempt until proven otherwise.

ED Management

The patient's clinical condition and severity of suicidal intent determine the priorities of ED management. Greater lethality of intent is supported by the presence of planning or precautions against discovery. Examples of planning include writing a suicide note, obtaining items for the attempt, and researching methods of suicide on the internet. Lethal intent is also suggested by absence of communication of intent to others, failure to call for help after the attempt, taking action that is clearly lethal, and expression of regret that death was not the outcome of the attempt. The degree of lethal intent helps differentiate between a suicide "attempt" and a "gesture." The former is a sincere effort to die while a gesture inflicts physical pain, relieves emotional distress, and/or communicates to others. Individuals who self-harm may not require hospitalization if they can be discharged into a safe environment with appropriate psychiatric follow-up.

A trained mental health professional must evaluate any patient making a suicidal gesture or attempt. Hospitalize those with medical complications in a pediatric unit. Transfer patients who are medically stable to an acute inpatient psychiatric unit unless, after evaluation, mental health professionals (1) believe the patient can be treated safely in a less restrictive environment and (2) a follow-up treatment plan has been established and agreed to by caretakers. In the case of discharge, ED providers must discuss removing firearms, sharp objects, and medications from the patient's home.

Follow-up
- Primary care follow-up in one week
- Psychiatric follow-up as soon as possible (within three days)

Indications for Admission
- Suicide attempt that requires medical care
- High lethality intent
- Lack of immediate, outpatient mental health follow-up
- Failure of established outpatient care

Bibliography

Babeva K, Hughes JL, Asarnow J. Emergency department screening for suicide and mental health risk. *Curr Psychiatry Rep*. 2016;**18**(11):100.

Centers for Disease Control and Prevention. Suicide: risk and protective factors. www.cdc.gov/violenceprevention/suicide/riskprotectivefactors.html (accessed May 24, 2017).

Dilillo D, Mauri S, Mantegazza C, et al. Suicide in pediatrics: epidemiology, risk factors, warning signs and the role of the pediatrician in detecting them. *Ital J Pediatr*. 2015;**41**:49.

Shain B, Committee on Adolescence. Suicide and suicide attempts in adolescents. *Pediatrics*. 2016;**138** (1). pii: e20161420.

Wilcox HC, Wyman PA. Suicide prevention strategies for improving population health. *Child Adolesc Psychiatr Clin N Am*. 2016;**25**(2):219–233.

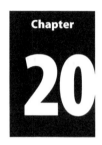

Pulmonary Emergencies

Sergey Kunkov and Sandra J. Cunningham

Asthma

Asthma is characterized by reversible hyperresponsiveness, obstruction, and inflammation of the lower airways. About 13% of children are affected and, despite recent therapeutic advances, morbidity continues to be substantial, especially among inner-city residents.

Common triggers include irritants (cigarette smoke), viral infections, weather changes, allergens (dust, animals), exercise, cold air, and emotional stress. Children with a history of bronchopulmonary dysplasia (BPD) or other acute lung injury (smoke inhalation, hydrocarbon ingestion, near-drowning) are at increased risk for hyperactive airways or asthma. The greatest risk of mortality is in children who have a history of respiratory failure or hypoxic seizures, are under-treated (at home or after a medical visit), or delay seeking medical attention.

Clinical Presentation

Acute asthma presents with dyspnea, cough, and expiratory and, to a lesser extent, inspiratory, wheezing. Cough-variant asthma presents with episodes of dry or productive cough and little or no wheezing. Airway obstruction can lead to retractions and decreased air entry, with little or no audible wheezing. Tachycardia, tachypnea, and, in severe attacks, cyanosis may be present; altered mental status (agitation, lethargy) occurs with impending ventilatory failure. URI is also often present.

Complications

Atelectasis is common. Pneumomediastinum, which requires no specific treatment, and, rarely, pneumothorax, which may be under tension and requires immediate evacuation, can also occur. Respiratory failure may occur suddenly from large-airway collapse or exhaustion.

Diagnosis

Immediately evaluate a patient with a reported asthma exacerbation or wheezing. After the initial brief assessment, institute treatment promptly. While the first bronchodilator treatment is given, perform a focused history and physical examination related to the acute exacerbation. A more detailed history and physical examination can be delayed until after the initial therapy is given.

A trial of an inhaled β_2 agonist (albuterol) may simultaneously confirm the diagnosis and provide clinical improvement. Relief of airway obstruction occurs in <15 minutes (often

RR >60 Infant, >40 older child, Tachy HR >160.

<5 minutes), and peak flow (PEFR) typically improves by >20% from baseline. Less improvement may occur with severe or prolonged episodes associated with more inflammation, leaving the diagnosis uncertain unless the patient has a history of previous wheezing episodes. Laboratory studies do not help in establishing the diagnosis of asthma, and chest x-rays are not necessary for most first episodes of wheezing. A chest x-ray may be indicated in the setting of localized posttreatment findings in association with significant tachypnea (rate >60/min in infants, >40/min in older children) or persistent tachycardia (rate >160/min) 20–30 minutes after the completion of a β_2 agonist treatment in an afebrile child.

Inquire about a history of prematurity, mechanical ventilation, BPD, previous wheezing episodes, or heart disease. Check for a family history of asthma, recurrent bronchitis, eczema, allergic rhinitis, or other allergies.

Consider the possibility of complicating factors or a diagnosis other than asthma if a child or infant has protracted (more than three days), recurrent, or persistent localized wheezing in the face of adequate therapy for asthma. See Table 20.1 for the differential diagnosis and Table 20.2 for selected risk factors for death in asthma.

ED Management

Acute Treatment

>5yrs – measure Peak Flow.

Rapidly assess the airway and breathing, measure the peak flow in all children older than 5–6 years of age, and determine whether the patient has a mild, moderate, or severe asthma exacerbation (Table 20.3). To facilitate evaluation of the PEFR and changes following therapy, always record the PEFR as a percentage of the child's predicted normal PEFR from a table of standards by height or best value (if known), rather than an absolute number. Provide supplemental oxygen (40% by mask) to a patient with mild or moderate wheezing; use 100% oxygen if the attack is severe. In addition, some patients may have an initial drop in pO_2 during β_2 agonist therapy due to ventilation–perfusion (V/Q) mismatch, particularly if the aerosol is administered with room air rather than oxygen. Monitor a severely ill patient with pulse oximetry, and consider obtaining an ABG if the breath sounds are barely audible and do not improve within 5–10 minutes following the initial therapy.

Inhaled β_2 Agonists

Give 0.15 mg/kg (2.5 mg minimum; 10 mg maximum) of albuterol every 20 minutes for three doses, then 0.15–0.3 mg/kg every 1–4 hours as needed for mild to moderate exacerbations. As an alternative, give 0.25 mg for a patient weighing <20 kg and 5 mg if ≥20 kg. Substitute 4–8 puffs of an albuterol MDI (90 mcg/puff) with a spacer every 20 minutes for nebulized albuterol if the patient is cooperative. The onset of action is within five minutes and the duration is 4–6 hours. Give repeat doses every 20–30 minutes until no further improvement is noted in peak flow, oxygen saturation, or respiratory rate. For severe exacerbations, give 0.5 mg/kg/hour by continuous administration. Levalbuterol does not appear to provide superior therapeutic effect or diminish adverse effects. Reserve it for patients with a history of extreme tachycardia following albuterol administration.

Subcutaneous Epinephrine and Terbutaline

A dose of subcutaneous epinephrine or terbutaline may be given for severe attacks (peak flow <15% predicted or nearly absent breath sounds) when aerosolized medication may not

Xopenex – not better than Albuterol
nor less side effects
only indication is to avoid Tachy after Albuterol

Table 20.1 Differential diagnosis of asthma

Diagnosis	History	Physical examination	Radiography/laboratory
Upper airway obstruction			
Anaphylaxis	Exposure to allergen May have vomiting	May have urticaria Stridor and/or wheezing	None
Bacterial tracheitis	Indolent onset Worsening croup	Respiratory distress	Anteroposterior and lateral neck radiographs with "ragged" trachea
Croup	Cough Fever	Barking cough Inspiratory stridor	"Steeple" sign Radiographs usually unnecessary
Epiglottitis	Acute onset High fever	Muffled stridor Sniffing dog position, toxic appearance	Do not obtain if patient is in distress "Thumbprint sign" on lateral neck radiograph
Foreign body aspiration	Choking episode	Upper: inspiratory stridor Lower: localized wheezing	Radiopaque object Expiration: contralateral mediastinal shift
Laryngotracheomalacia		Degree of stridor depends on body positioning	Laryngo- or bronchoscopy usually diagnostic
Retropharyngeal abscess	Fever	Drooling Inspiratory stridor	Lateral neck: wide retropharyngeal space
Vascular rings/laryngeal webs		Localized wheeze	Bronchoscopy usually diagnostic
Vocal cord dysfunction	Adolescents May have psych history	Monophasic wheeze loudest over glottis Can mimic severe asthma attack	None

Lower airway obstruction

Atypical pneumonia (Mycoplasma, Chlamydia)	Cough Fever	Bilateral wheezing 40–50% with (+) cold agglutinins	Patchy bilateral infiltrates
Cardiac asthma		Tachycardia, heart murmur Hepatomegaly Pedal edema	Cardiomegaly Pulmonary overperfusion
Cystic fibrosis	Malabsorption Failure to thrive Excessive salt loss		
Gastroesophageal reflux	Nighttime cough	Bilateral wheezing, poorly responsive to bronchodilators	

Table 20.2 Selected risk factors for death from asthma

≥2 hospitalization in the past year

Difficulty in perceiving asthma symptoms

Hospitalization or ED visit for asthma during past month

Low socioeconomic status or inner-city residence

Previous severe asthma exacerbation necessitating ICU care or intubation

Psychological/psychiatric problems

Table 20.3 Clinical severity classification of acute asthma exacerbation

	Symptoms	Peak expiratory flow rate
Mild	Dyspnea only during activity	≥70% predicted or personal best
Moderate	Dyspnea interferes with usual activity	40–69% predicted or personal best
Severe	Dyspnea at rest Interferes with speech	<40% predicted or personal best
Life-threatening	Too dyspneic to speak	<25% predicted or personal best

Adapted from National Heart, Lung, and Blood Institute, *Guidelines for the Diagnosis and Management of Asthma*, Bethesda, MD: National Heart, Lung, and Blood Institute, 2007.

[handwritten: Epinephrine 1:1000, 0.01 mL/kg SC max dose 0.3 mL]

reach the target small airways. The epinephrine dose is 0.01 mL/kg to 0.3 mL maximum of the 1:1000 preparation. For terbutaline, use 0.01 mL/kg up to 0.25 mL maximum. Common epinephrine side effects include nausea, palpitations, tachycardia, agitation, tremor, and, less frequently, hypertension and ventricular dysrhythmias. Terbutaline may cause less nausea and vomiting. Simultaneously begin nebulized β_2 agonist treatments.

Corticosteroids

Promptly give an oral dose of a corticosteroid if the patient meets any of the following criteria:

- requires ≥2 β_2 agonist aerosol treatments;
- oxygen saturation is <93% on any assessment;
- >2 days of coughing or awakening from sleep due to asthma in the past week;
- chronically uses (every day or every other day) oral corticosteroids;
- ED visit within the past two weeks, has had a past ICU admission;
- hospitalized (for asthma) within the past two weeks;
- ≥3 hospitalizations during the past year;
- has maximized β_2 agonist treatment at home.

Use prednisone or prednisolone, 1 mg/kg (40 mg maximum) or dexamethasone 0.6 mg/kg (10 mg maximum). If the patient cannot tolerate oral medication, give IM dexamethasone (same dose as above). For a patient with impending respiratory failure,

[handwritten: Prednisone Prednisolone 1 mg/kg max 40 mg PO Dexamethasone Or 0.6 mg/kg max 10 mg PO or IM.]

Impending RF – CH3 prednisone – Bolus IV 2mg/kg, max 125mg followed by 1 mg/kg IV q 6h.

give a bolus of IV methylprednisolone (2 mg/kg, 125 mg maximum, followed by 1 mg/kg q 6h).

Mix Albuterol 0.25mg 20kg > 5mg

Ipratropium Bromide
Ipratropium – 250 µg < 12 yrs > 500 µg

Ipratropium bromide is an <u>anticholinergic</u> that produces bronchodilation by antagonizing the activity of acetylcholine at the level of airway smooth muscle. Compared to inhaled β-agonists, the effect on airway obstruction is modest and generally results in approximately a 10% improvement in FEV_1. Dilute albuterol (<20 kg: 0.25 mg; ≥20 kg: 5 mg) in a vial of ipratropium (250 mcg <12 years of age or 500 mcg ≥12 years of age). <u>Give three consecutive</u> ipratropium–albuterol inhalations to a patient with a severe exacerbation. The onset of action of ipratropium is relatively slow (20 minutes), and the peak effect occurs in about 60 minutes.

Ipratropium, unlike atropine, is poorly absorbed across mucous membranes, has little toxicity at the stated dose, and does not inhibit mucociliary clearance. There are, however, infrequent reports of <u>paradoxical bronchoconstriction</u> with the administration of anticholinergic agents. Monitor the patient carefully, and stop the nebulization if there are any signs or symptoms of worsening asthma.

Magnesium Sulfate

The IV administration of magnesium sulfate may be useful for a patient whose condition worsens or fails to improve significantly (peak flow increases <50% from presentation and is <60% of predicted; intercostal retractions persist; or oxygen saturation <93%) after administration of β-agonists and systemic corticosteroids. The dose is 50–75 mg/kg (2 g maximum) in 50 mL of normal saline administered IV over 30 minutes. Side effects include hypotension, mild sedation, and cutaneous flushing; do not use the drug in patients with significant hypotension or renal failure. Monitor the blood pressure every ten minutes during the infusion and every 30 minutes thereafter for four hours, but do not stop the infusion for mild reductions in blood pressure in the absence of hypotensive symptoms.

Hydration

Encourage oral fluids and provide IV hydration if the patient is seriously ill, but limit IV hydration to maintenance plus replacement of ongoing losses. If a patient with absent or minimal breath sounds or a PEFR <15% of expected has been vomiting or drinking poorly, assess the hydration status and obtain blood for electrolytes when placing the IV line. In general, most hospitalized asthma patients do not need an IV placed.

Heliox

Heliox (a mixture of helium and oxygen) can be used as a nebulizing agent for albuterol when there has been a poor response to conventional therapy. Heliox provides a low-density gas mixture which can decrease turbulence in air flow though constricted airways and improve gas exchange and albuterol delivery. Request Heliox <u>(70% helium/30% oxygen)</u> in a premixed tank from the respiratory therapy department, then administer a continuous nebulization of albuterol via a nonrebreathing mask at 10 L/min. Discontinue Heliox if the oxygen saturation is <93% and initiate treatment with 100% oxygen via a nonrebreather mask. *70% He, 30% O2.*

Trial Bipap - 10/5cm H2O

Mechanical Ventilation

If the above-described therapy fails to achieve adequate oxygenation, attempt a trial of BPAP (bilevel positive airway pressure), if available, with an initial expiratory positive airway pressure (EPAP) of 4–5 cmH$_2$O and inspiratory positive airway pressure (IPAP) of 8–10 cmH$_2$O.

If the patient's respiratory mechanics fail to improve, endotracheal intubation and mechanical ventilation are necessary. Use ketamine (1–2 mg/kg) to provide sedation and bronchodilation. Use smaller tidal volumes than average (6–8 mL/kg) on a volume-preset ventilator, with normal-to-somewhat-lower respiratory rates for age, and long expiratory times. The required inspiratory pressures can exceed 50–60 cm H$_2$O. Assess breath sounds and obtain an ABG. Permissive hypercapnia may lessen the risk of barotrauma, so the goal is incomplete correction of the respiratory acidosis (permit a pCO$_2$ up to 50–60 mg Hg). An intubated patient will usually require a sedative (midazolam 0.1–0.3 mg/kg IV q 1–2h, 5 mg maximum) and a neuromuscular relaxant (vecuronium 0.05–0.1 mg/kg IV q 1–2h, 10 mg maximum) to minimize barotrauma.

Discharge Management

A patient with acute asthma can be discharged home when the peak flow is >60–70% predicted for height, the oxygen saturation is >92% in room air, wheezing is minimal, there are no signs of significant obstruction (retractions, tachypnea, decreased air entry), and the patient denies having trouble breathing. Ensure that the parent can give the medications confidently, knows how to use a spacer device with an MDI, can monitor the child frequently, and is able to return to the ED if necessary. Ongoing bronchodilator therapy is usually necessary for two weeks. Prepare a written asthma action plan for worsening symptoms and a follow-up appointment within a week or two of the ED visit.

β$_2$ Agonist

Inhaled β$_2$ agonists are preferred for all patients with documented asthma and are first-line therapy, sometimes as single-drug therapy, but more commonly in combination with steroids. Infants and young children can use an MDI attached to a spacer with the proper-sized facemask, while older children do not need a face mask. The albuterol MDI dose is two puffs every 4–6 hours. For a nebulizer, use albuterol 0.5% (<20 kg: 0.5 mL; ≥20 kg: 1.0 mL) or levalbuterol (<10 kg: 0.63 mg; ≥10 kg: 1.25 mg) in 3 mL of normal saline given over 5–10 minutes.

Corticosteroids

Give an outpatient course of oral steroids if the patient required two or more acute albuterol treatments or has required acute therapy twice (or more) within 24 hours or three times in the past week. Avoid steroids in a child who has been exposed to viruses in the herpes family (*especially varicella*). Give oral prednisone or prednisolone (1 mg/kg/day q day or div bid, 40 mg/day maximum) for 3–4 more days. A single dose of oral dexamethasone (0.6 mg/kg q day, 10 mg maximum) is an alternative.

Prescribe inhaled steroids to patients whose risk (likelihood of exacerbations) and impairment (frequency and intensity of symptoms and functional limitations) character-istics classify them as having persistent asthma (see Table 20.4). Use fluticasone (44 mcg/puff 4–11 years; 110 mcg/puff ≥12 years) one puff bid. Prescribe budesonide inhalation

Table 20.4 Assessing asthma severity using risk and impairment

Risk	Impairment		Severity
Exacerbations requiring oral steroids	Symptoms	Nighttime awakenings	
0–1/year	≤2 days/week	0	Intermittent
≥2 in six months	>2 days/week	1–2/month	Mild persistent
≥2/year	>2 days/week	3–4/month	Moderate persistent
≥2/year	Throughout day	Often 7/week	Severe persistent

Adapted from Expert Panel Report 3: *Guidelines for the Diagnosis and Management of Asthma*. US Department of Health and Human Services National Institutes for Health. National Heart, Lung and Blood Institute, 2007

suspension for nebulization (0.25–0.5 mg) for children 0–4 years of age whose other asthma medications are given via nebulizer.

Follow-up
- Mild to moderate first wheezing episode >1 year of age, new or altered medications or steroids prescribed: primary care follow-up in 1–2 weeks

Indications for Admission
- Status asthmaticus: continued moderate or severe wheezing or other evidence of significant airway obstruction after therapy with nebulized β_2 agonists, ipratropium, corticosteroids, or subcutaneous epinephrine, or any wheezing after IV magnesium sulfate
- Repeated emergency visits over several days when therapy is maximal or compliance uncertain
- Persistent tachypnea, inability to tolerate fluids or medications, altered mental status
- Hypercapnia: pCO_2 >40 mg Hg
- Hypoxemia: pO_2 <60 mg Hg or oxygen saturation < 93% in room air despite aggressive therapy
- Pneumothorax, pneumomediastinum, or significant atelectasis

Bibliography
Bozzetto S, Carraro S, Zanconato S, Baraldi E. Severe asthma in childhood: diagnostic and management challenges. *Curr Opin Pulm Med*. 2015;21(1):16–21.

Carroll CL, Sala KA. Pediatric status asthmaticus. *Crit Care Clin*. 2013;29(2):153–166.

Konradsen JR, Caffrey Osvald E, Hedlin G. Update on the current methods for the diagnosis and treatment of severe childhood asthma. *Expert Rev Respir Med*. 2015;9(6):769–777.

Powell CV. Acute severe asthma. *J Paediatr Child Health*. 2016;52(2):187–191.

Watnick CS, Fabbri D, Donald H, Arnold DH. Single-dose oral dexamethasone is effective in preventing relapse after acute asthma exacerbations. *Ann Allergy Asthma Immunol*. 2016;116 (2):171–172

MC - Life-threatening Bacterial infection...

Bacterial Tracheitis

age = 4 yrs .

Bacterial tracheitis (BT) is the most common life-threatening bacterial infection of the airway, including the larynx, trachea, and bronchi. The pathology involves copious purulent secretions and pseudomembranes within the trachea. *Staphylococcus aureus* is most frequently implicated, followed by *Streptococcus pyogenes, Moraxella catarrhalis,* and *Streptococcus pneumoniae. Influenza* type A is often detected as well, suggesting a primary viral process followed by bacterial superinfection.

Clinical Presentation

like

Any age patient can be affected, although the mean is about four years of age. Following a brief prodrome of cough, rhinorrhea, and low-grade fever, the initial presentation resembles moderate to severe viral croup, with hoarseness, sore throat, barking cough, and stridor. Then, instead of the expected improvement after several days, the patient develops high fever with significant respiratory distress. Drooling is uncommon.

Diagnosis

Suspect BT in a febrile child with stridor that does not respond to racemic epinephrine administration or that gets worse after a number of days (when croup is usually resolving), particularly if the cough seems productive. In a stable patient, a portable lateral neck radiograph obtained in the ED may reveal an irregular tracheal margin characteristic of BT. Viral croup (pp. 638–641), epiglottitis (pp. 641–643), retropharyngeal abscess (pp. 166–167) and foreign body aspiration (pp. 643–645) are major differential diagnostic considerations.

ED Management

If BT is suspected, allow the patient to assume a position of comfort on the parent's lap. Provide supplemental oxygen in an unobtrusive manner, but defer completing a physical examination or inserting an IV. Immediately notify an anesthesiologist and otolaryngologist to prepare for laryngoscopy and possible orotracheal intubation in the operating suite. If the patient's respiratory status suddenly deteriorates (usually due to movement of a pseudomembrane within the airway) perform bag-mask ventilation.

Definitive treatment includes airway stabilization, most frequently with tracheal intubation in the operating suite and meticulous pulmonary toilet and suctioning of secretions. Treat with broad-spectrum antibiotics, cefotaxime (150 mg/kg/d IV divided q 6h, 8 g/day maximum) *plus* MRSA coverage with vancomycin (40 mg/kg/day div q 6h, 4 g/day maximum) *or* clindamycin 40 mg/kg/day IV div q 8h, 4.8 g/day maximum).

Indications for Admission

- Suspected bacterial tracheitis

Bibliography

Kuo CY, Parikh SR. Bacterial tracheitis. *Pediatr Rev.* 2014;35(11):497–499.

Mandal A, Kabra SK, Lodha R. Upper airway obstruction in children. *Indian J Pediatr.* 2015;82 (8):737–744.

Miranda AD, Valdez TA, Pereira KD. Bacterial tracheitis: a varied entity. *Pediatr Emerg Care*. 2011;**27**(10):950–953.

Shargorodsky J, Whittemore KR, Lee GS. Bacterial tracheitis: a therapeutic approach. *Laryngoscope*. 2010;**120**(12):2498–2501.

Bronchiolitis   < 2 yrs ,

Bronchiolitis is the most common wheezing-associated respiratory illness in children under two years of age. Epidemics in the winter (December through early February) are most frequently caused by respiratory syncitial virus (RSV). Human metapneumovirus (hMPV) causes bronchiolitis in somewhat older children (median age 11 months), typically in the spring (March through April). Less common causes of bronchiolitis include parainfluenza, influenza, and adenovirus, *Mycoplasma, pertussis, Chlamydia*, and *Ureaplasma*.

Clinical Presentation

A prodrome of URI with rhinorrhea and coryza is followed by cough, audible wheezing, and varying degrees of respiratory distress. An infant with severe disease has tachypnea (>50/min), subcostal and intercostal retractions, poor feeding, nasal flaring, and grunting. In all cases, symptoms are likely to be most prominent at night. Fever is variable and usually low-grade. Although wheezing is the typical auscultatory finding, rhonchi and coarse rales may also be heard. In most patients, the condition worsens for 3–4 days and then rapidly resolves, although some patients may have a persistent cough for weeks afterward. Neonates and young infants may present with apnea and a sepsis-like picture.

Diagnosis

Acute wheezing, cough, and respiratory distress in a young infant are most often secondary to bronchiolitis. Other diagnoses include the following.

Asthma

Asthma (reactive airway disease) can cause a clinical picture with wheezing that is indistinguishable from bronchiolitis. Some infants with a first RSV exposure may already manifest hyperreactive airways. Consider asthma if the patient has had previous episodes of wheezing that were responsive to bronchodilators, a history of bronchopulmonary dysplasia, eczema, or a family history of asthma or atopic disease.

Foreign Body Aspiration

An aspirated foreign body may present with wheezing after a coughing or choking episode in an infant typically more than six months of age. There is no URI prodrome. Unless there is acute infection distal to the foreign body, there is usually no fever. Auscultatory findings are often localized. An esophageal foreign body can impinge on the trachea and also cause respiratory distress.

Congenital Malformations

These conditions can cause airway obstruction and wheezing, which are exacerbated by a URI. Consider congenital lobar emphysema and intrapulmonary cysts (bronchogenic or cystadenomatoid malformation) when the wheezing is unilateral or localized. The chest x-ray is often diagnostic. With tracheomalacia, stridor from inspiratory collapse of a floppy trachea predominates over expiratory wheezing. Wheezing from a vascular ring is typically loudest over the trachea and midlung fields.

Congestive Heart Failure

Congestive heart failure can occasionally present with pulmonary edema, which can mimic bronchiolitis. Other possible findings are significant tachycardia and a gallop, hepatomegaly, jugular venous distension, and cardiomegaly noted on chest x-ray.

ED Management

Inquire about a history of apnea, wheezing, prematurity, or mechanical ventilation (BPD), and check for a family history of asthma or allergies. Perform the examination with the infant undressed from the waist up and sitting on the parent's lap. Obtain an accurate respiratory rate, note any signs of respiratory distress (flaring, grunting, retractions, cyanosis) or heart disease (murmur, hepatosplenomegaly), and assess the activity level and ability to drink.

Respiratory Rate >60/min or Signs of Respiratory Distress

Check the oxygen saturation in room air by pulse oximetry and suction the nares, if necessary. Provide supplemental oxygen (usually 30–40% by oxyhood or nasal prongs) to hypoxic patients to maintain an oxygen saturation >90% or a pO_2 >65 mm Hg. Do *not* use albuterol, racemic epinephrine, hypertonic saline, or oral steroids. Start an IV and give maintenance fluids with D_5 ½ NS unless the patient is dehydrated (see pp. 245–249). If there is no substantial improvement, admit the patient as clinical deterioration, with persistent hypoxemia, elevation of pCO_2, or the development of acidosis may portend exhaustion and respiratory failure requiring mechanical ventilation.

Respiratory Rate 40–60/min

Supportive therapy (fluids, acetaminophen as necessary) is all that is needed if the infant is alert, tolerating fluids well, and has no signs of distress. Close follow-up is warranted.

Chest radiographs are not routinely indicated in patients with bronchiolitis. Obtain a chest x-ray if the infant has known underlying pulmonary or heart disease or does not respond to aggressive inpatient management.

Follow-up

- Persistent tachypnea (>60/min), difficulty feeding: return at once
- All infants in 24 hours for reevaluation of feeding, respiratory effort, weight

Indications for Admission

- Respiratory rate >70/min, regardless of clinical appearance
- Respiratory rate 60–70/min with lethargy or poor oral intake
- Infant <3 months of age with a respiratory rate 60–70/min after maximal ED therapy
- Respiratory distress, oxygen saturation <90% or pO_2 <65 mm Hg in room air, or normal-to-elevated pCO_2 (>40 mm Hg)

- Infants with congenital heart disease, chronic lung disease, or immunodeficiency (at risk for complications of RSV infection) in the progressive stage (first day or two) of the illness
- Parents uncomfortable with the severity of illness or with limited resources at home (especially if the infant is <3 months of age)

Bibliography

Castro-Rodriguez JA, Rodriguez-Martinez CE, Sossa-Briceño MP. Principal findings of systematic reviews for the management of acute bronchiolitis in children. *Paediatr Respir Rev.* 2015;**16** (4):267–275.

Cunningham S, Rodriguez A, Adams T, et al. Oxygen saturation targets in infants with bronchiolitis (BIDS): a double-blind, randomised, equivalence trial. *Lancet.* 2015;**386**(9998):1041–1048.

Florin TA, Plint AC, Zorc JJ. Viral bronchiolitis. *Lancet.* 2017;**389** (10065):211–224.

Meissner, HC. Viral bronchiolitis in children *N Engl J Med.* 2016;**374**(1):62–72.

Ralston SL, Lieberthal AS, Meissner HC, et al. Clinical practice guideline: the diagnosis, management, and prevention of bronchiolitis. *Pediatrics.* 2014;**134**(5):e1474–e1502.

Cough

Cough is a very common symptom that is most often caused by a minor URI. However, a cough may also signal a more serious problem, such as pneumonia, asthma, or congestive heart failure. A thorough clinical evaluation is necessary before assuming that the patient just has a "cold."

Clinical Presentation and Diagnosis

The clinical presentation varies, depending on the etiology (Table 20.5). Usually these can be differentiated with a careful history and physical exam, with only the occasional need for laboratory tests. Three features of a cough that help determine the cause are its quality, timing, and whether it is productive of sputum.

Barking – Croup. Honking, Loud Psychogenic
Pertusis – Paroxymal, No breath F/U Apnea, Cyanosis, Whoop

Quality
Quality refers to both the sound and pattern of the coughing episodes; it is best ascertained from hearing the cough, rather than relying on the history. Coughs are often described as "wet" or "dry"; however, these descriptions may not be useful. A <u>barking cough</u> suggests <u>croup</u>, and a loud, honking cough is often associated with a psychogenic cough. <u>Paroxysmal episodes</u> (a series of coughs with no breathing between them), especially when followed by <u>apnea, cyanosis, or a whoop</u>, are consistent with a <u>pertussis syndrome.</u> A staccato cough (a series of coughs with short breaths between them) suggests an "afebrile pneumonia" (<u>*Chlamydia, Mycoplasma*</u>). *Staccato – Chlaydia, Mycoplasma.*

Timing
Cough that is related to feeds and includes either choking or emesis suggests aspiration. The possible causes include gastroesophageal reflux (cough may be the only symptom), mechanical abnormalities (tracheoesophageal fistula), and neurologic abnormalities. Night cough is consistent with asthma, sinusitis, postnasal drip, gastroesophageal reflux (GERD) and croup. An early-morning cough suggests a suppurative process. Seasonal cough, exercise-

Table 20.5 Differential diagnosis of cough

Anatomic site	Emergent/potentially emergent	Common/other
Upper airway	Aspiration	Gastroesophageal reflux
	Congenital anomalies	Noxious fumes
	Croup (severe)	Pharyngitis
	Foreign body aspiration	Sinusitis
	Laryngeal edema	Tracheal compression
	Pertussis	Upper respiratory infection
Lower airway	Anaphylaxis	Cystic fibrosis
	Asthma	Foreign body aspiration
	Bronchiolitis	Pulmonary hemosiderosis
	Congestive heart failure	
	Pneumonia	
	Congestive heart failure	
Nonrespiratory	Impaired gag reflex	Aural foreign body
		Diaphragmatic irritation
		Phrenic or vagus nerve irritation
		Psychogenic cough

related cough, and cold-air-related cough occur with reactive airway disease. Finally, "school day-only cough" suggests a psychogenic origin.

The patient's age suggests different causes. During infancy, consider congenital anomalies, pertussis, bronchiolitis, *Chlamydia*, and pulmonary edema (usually cardiogenic). Cough during the first two months of life is more probably related to serious pathology than at any other age. Consider foreign body aspiration in toddlers and young children. Among adolescents, consider smoking and mediastinal masses.

Sputum Production

Sputum production is difficult to judge, as children tend to swallow sputum. Green sputum reflects leukocyte breakdown and not necessarily a bacterial process. Blood-streaked sputum suggests pneumococcal pneumonia. Hemoptysis may reflect foreign body aspiration, a chronic suppurative process (cystic fibrosis), tuberculosis, and, more rarely, pulmonary hemosiderosis.

Physical findings help localize the origin to a specific part of the respiratory tract. Pharyngitis, otitis media, rhinorrhea, swollen turbinates, sinus tenderness, snoring, and stridor are consistent with upper airway disease. Wheezing, rales, rhonchi, and decreased breath sounds occur with lower respiratory tract pathology. Also look for signs of congestive heart failure (gallop, hepatomegaly, jugular vein distention) and diaphragmatic irritation (right or left upper quadrant tenderness).

ED Management

The priority is prompt recognition and treatment of respiratory distress and emergent conditions. Assess oxygenation and perfusion, and initiate appropriate resuscitation, if necessary. Look for signs of upper airway obstruction, assess the patient's preferred position of breathing, and listen carefully for stridor (place the stethoscope on the side of the neck). If there are any signs of obstruction, maintain the patient in the position of maximal airway opening (see p. 5). If oxygenation and perfusion are compromised, consider the potentially emergent and most common causes for each age group (Table 20.5). If the history and physical examination are not conclusive, obtain a chest x-ray and room air pulse oximetry to screen for serious pathology.

Infants Under Two Months

Rule-out serious pathology (pneumonia, bronchiolitis, pulmonary edema), as this age group is at relatively high risk for apnea. Potential emergencies include pertussis, *Chlamydia* and other afebrile pneumonias (*Ureaplasma* and *Mycoplasma*), bronchiolitis, aspiration, and congenital mechanical obstruction. Measure the oxygen saturation, and obtain a chest x-ray and CBC looking for lymphocytosis (pertussis) or eosinophilia (*Chlamydia*).

URIs and GERD are common non-emergent causes. Treat a URI with normal saline nose drops and suctioning, but avoid neosynephrine nose drops, which may cause dysrhythmias (SVT) and severe rebound congestion. For reflux, if there is associated apnea, consult with a gastroenterologist or pulmonologist to determine whether an immediate upper GI series is needed. Otherwise, further work-up can be deferred to the outpatient setting.

Older Infants and Children

Emergent etiologies include pneumonia, reactive airway disease (bronchiolitis/asthma), and pulmonary edema. Upper airway obstruction in this age group is usually related to foreign body aspiration or laryngeal edema (croup).

Common causes of cough in this age group include asthma, sinusitis, postnasal drip, and GERD. Asthma may have no corroborating physical findings, and the peak flow may be normal. If the history is suggestive (night cough, family history of atopy, other atopic symptoms, exercise-induced cough), a diagnostic/therapeutic trial of bronchodilators is warranted (pp. 624–625). If the history and physical examination suggest sinusitis (worsening rhinorrhea for more than seven consecutive days, periorbital swelling, halitosis, swollen turbinates), treat with a 14-day course of antibiotics (pp. 168–169).

GERD can cause persistent cough, despite the absence of GI symptoms, and should be suspected when systematic investigation for other common causes of cough are negative. Although a 24-hour esophageal pH monitoring study can confirm the diagnosis, first assess the response to an empiric trial of anti-reflux medication (ranitidine, 4–5 mg/kg/day div bid).

Older Children and Adolescents

ED management is similar to the approach outlined above. Emergency resuscitation and upper airway clearance are the priorities. Common causes are similar to those in younger children. If a patient presents with persistent symptoms, obtain a chest x-ray (mediastinal mass) and check for a history of exposure to TB.

Finally, treat the cause of the cough and not the cough itself. Consider cough suppression only when the cause is known and the cough severely impairs the patient's daily life (sleep deprivation, not permitted in school). In such cases, try a cough suppressant with 100% dextromethorphan, but do not use codeine. ✓

Follow-up
- Refer a patient with chronic cough (more than two weeks) to a primary care provider

Indications for Admission
- Respiratory distress or patient requires oxygen
- Pertussis (infant under six months old)
- Bronchiolitis or *Chlamydia* pneumonia (infant under two months, because of risk of apnea)
- Interstitial pneumonia (infant under two months)
- Lobar pneumonia (infant under six months)
- Pulmonary edema
- Foreign body aspiration
- Persistent upper airway obstruction from any cause
- Laryngeal edema
- Croup with significant upper airway obstruction and stridor at rest

Bibliography
Chang AB, Oppenheimer JJ, Weinberger M, et al. Children with chronic wet or productive cough: treatment and investigations – a systematic review. *Chest.* 2016;**149**(1):120–142.

Chang AB, Oppenheimer JJ, Weinberger M, et al. Use of management pathways or algorithms in children with chronic cough: systematic reviews. *Chest.* 2016;**149**(1):106–119.

Gardiner SJ, Chang AB, Marchant JM, Petsky HL. Codeine versus placebo for chronic cough in children. *Cochrane Database Syst Rev.* 2016;7:CD011914.

Kantar A Update on pediatric cough. *Lung.* 2016;**194**(1):9–14.

Smith SM, Schroeder K, Fahey T. Over-the-counter (OTC) medications for acute cough in children and adults in community settings. *Cochrane Database Syst Rev.* 2014;**11**:CD001831.

Croup   6 mths - 3 yrs , MC - 1st year.
Laryngotracheobronchitis, or croup, is an acute subglottic inflammatory process generally caused by parainfluenza virus, types 1 and 3, during the late fall and early winter months. Other causes are *Influenza* viruses A and B, measles, *Mycoplasma pneumoniae*, human metapneumovirus, and respiratory syncitial virus. Croup primarily occurs between six months and three years of age, but morbidity is greatest in the first year of life, when the subglottic airway is relatively narrow. Although exhaustion may lead to obstruction of the airway by mucus, death is infrequent.

Spasmodic croup is likely an allergic disease that occurs mainly in patients with personal or family histories of asthma and allergies.

Clinical Presentation

Patients with croup present with inspiratory stridor, suprasternal retractions, tachypnea, and tachycardia. Croup usually begins with low-grade fever and rhinorrhea, followed by hoarseness and a barking, "seal-like" cough. The degree of stridor is highly variable, but with increasing obstruction there are suprasternal and intercostal retractions, decreased air entry, increased work of breathing, and stridor at rest. The illness lasts 3–5 days, with the second or third day being the peak of clinical symptoms. High fever, dysphagia, and drooling are usually absent. Patients with preexisting upper airway problems (congenital or acquired subglottic stenosis, webs, tracheomalacia, choanal narrowing, micrognathia, macroglossia) are at particular risk.

Spasmodic croup presents in the middle of the night with the sudden onset of loud stridor and croupy cough which resolves quickly and often improves with cool mist. There is little or no viral prodrome, and dysphagia, drooling, high fever, and toxicity are notably absent. The croup may recur on successive nights, and recurrent episodes are common. Some children have recurrent croup-like illnesses induced by infection or allergens that may have associated reversible lower airway obstruction suggestive of asthma.

Diagnosis

Croup is a clinical diagnosis based on history and physical findings. When epiglottitis cannot be ruled out clinically, or when other entities are being considered, soft tissue neck (high kilovoltage [kV]) radiographs are helpful. A lateral neck film can exclude entities such as epiglottitis, bacterial tracheitis, or a retropharyngeal abscess. With croup, the upper airway is narrowed to appear like a "steeple," and the infraglottic region is hazy.

Epiglottitis

The onset of epiglottitis (pp. 641–643) is sudden, sometimes suggestive of spasmodic croup, although a patient with epiglottitis is toxic, with high fever, dysphagia, and drooling. The barking cough is absent, and there is a tendency to adopt a characteristic "sniffing" position, sitting up with the neck extended. On lateral neck x-ray there is classic "thumb"-shaped epiglottis and swelling of the aryepiglottic folds, the normal cervical lordosis is lost, and the hypopharynx is distended with air.

Foreign Body

An upper airway foreign body (pp. 643–645) can present with the sudden onset of stridor. The object may be seen only on radiograph or by direct visualization. Hoarseness and the "barking" cough are not usually present.

Bacterial Tracheitis

Bacterial tracheitis (p. 632) is a form of acute subglottic obstruction usually caused by *S. aureus*. It generally occurs in patients who have had croup for several days, and resembles epiglottitis, with the sudden onset of high fever, toxicity, and severe respiratory distress. Anteroposterior and lateral soft tissue neck radiographs will demonstrate a "ragged" trachea indicative of the presence of pseudomembrane formation.

Laryngomalacia and Subglottic Stenosis

These are common causes of stridor in infants. The stridor is accentuated during respiratory infections and is not associated with hoarseness, and the child's activity is usually normal.

Retropharyngeal Abscess

Fever is accompanied by drooling and dysphagia. Respiratory distress is variable but may be pronounced, and meningismus or torticollis may also be present (pp. 166–167). Examination of the oropharynx may reveal bulging tissue in the rear of the mouth. Lateral neck radiograph demonstrates widening of the retropharyngeal space anterior to the vertebral bodies.

ED Management

Mild to Moderate Croup

Make a rapid assessment of color, perfusion, work of breathing, retractions, and air entry. If the patient is in mild-to-moderate distress, administer humidified oxygen, 4 L/min by facemask. Some infectious croup episodes and almost all spasmodic croup attacks will respond to mist with diminished stridor and lessened respiratory distress. Give a dose of oral or IM dexamethasone (0.3–0.6 mg/kg, 10 mg maximum) to a patient with a barking cough or cough with hoarseness or rhonchi.

Most often, the condition of a patient with spasmodic croup is markedly improved by the time of ED arrival; however, caution the parents that the illness may recur the following night.

Severe Croup

Administer humidified oxygen, 4 L/min by facemask. Use 100% O_2 delivered by a non-rebreather mask for a patient with severe distress, and continuously monitor with a pulse oximeter. Treat a patient with stridor at rest, or respiratory distress, with either nebulized racemic epinephrine (0.05 mL/kg [max. 0.5 mL] in 3 mL NS) or L-epinephrine (1:1000, 0.5 mL/kg in 3 mL NS; <4 years 2.5 mL maximum, ≥4 years 5 mL maximum) over 5–10 minutes. Epinephrine acts as a local vasoconstrictor that shrinks airway swelling. The effects last approximately two hours unless steroids are given. Therefore, to prevent a rebound in the airway swelling, give dexamethasone afterwards to any patient who receives nebulized epinephrine treatment and observe for at least two hours prior to discharge from the ED. Maintain the humidified oxygen after the treatment.

Discharge a patient who clearly has croup, if there is no significant stridor at rest during at least two hours of observation following treatment with epinephrine and dexamethasone. Arrange for follow-up in the next 24–48 hours.

A patient whose severe respiratory distress persists despite racemic epinephrine or L-epinephrine and dexamethasone may require intubation. *Use a tube at least 0.5 mm smaller than usual* to prevent pressure necrosis of the airway lumen. Start an IV if the patient is not drinking adequately and administer a 20 mL/kg bolus of isotonic crystalloid if the patient appears dehydrated. Obtain an ABG after epinephrine treatment if the child is agitated or has increased work of breathing, as carbon dioxide retention can occur in a young infant with moderate-to-severe croup. In addition, obtain radiographs of the chest and lateral neck if the patient is in moderate-to-severe distress or the diagnosis is unclear.

Follow-up

- Immediately if stridor at rest develops at home, otherwise daily for the first 2–3 days

Indications for Admission

- Stridor at rest that fails to resolve with epinephrine and dexamethasone
- Rebound during a two-hour observation period following epinephrine and dexamethasone treatment for stridor at rest
- Inadequate fluid intake
- Impending respiratory failure (pCO_2 >40 mm Hg; O_2 saturation <93% in room air)

Bibliography

Bjornson CL, Johnson DW. Croup in children. *CMAJ.* 2013;**185**(15):1317–1323.

Bjornson C, Russell K, Vandermeer B, Klassen TP, Johnson DW. Nebulized epinephrine for croup in children. *Cochrane Database Syst Rev.* 2013;**10**:CD006619.

Joshi V, Malik V, Mirza O, Kumar BN. Fifteen-minute consultation: structured approach to management of a child with recurrent croup. *Arch Dis Child Educ Pract Ed.* 2014; **99**(3):90–93.

Moraa I, Sturman N, McGuire T, van Driel ML. Heliox for croup in children. *Cochrane Database Syst Rev.* 2013;**12**:CD006822.

Petrocheilou A, Tanou K, Kalampouka E, et al. Viral croup: diagnosis and a treatment algorithm. *Pediatr Pulmonol.* 2014;**49**(5):421–429.

Epiglottitis

Epiglottitis (supraglottitis) is a life-threatening bacterial infection of the upper airway almost always caused by *Haemophilus influenza* type b (HIB). The incidence has declined dramatically as a result of the HIB vaccine. Other causes of supraglottic inflammation are *S. aureus*, herpesvirus, and *Candida albicans* infections and thermal injury from hot liquid aspiration. Immediate, aggressive management of the airway in a child with suspected epiglottitis is the first priority to ensure survival without morbidity from the complications of sudden upper airway obstruction.

Clinical Presentation

Most patients with epiglottitis are 3–8 years of age, although it occurs in young infants as well as adults. Typically there is a sudden onset of fever, lethargy, and respiratory distress with stridor. Drooling occurs in about 50% of patients, and the barking cough of croup is notably absent. Occasionally a patient (usually older child or teenager) presents in a more indolent fashion with mild stridor and a severe sore throat.

Most patients with epiglottitis will place themselves in the position of comfort, the "sniffing" position, sitting up with the neck extended. Physical findings include respiratory distress, tachypnea, stridor, and, often, retractions (suprasternal). If the obstruction is more severe, the child may have signs of respiratory failure, including obtundation, cyanosis, absent breath sounds, or apnea.

Diagnosis

The clinical picture is usually so characteristic that the diagnosis is suspected immediately. Epiglottitis is most safely and efficiently confirmed by direct visualization of the inflamed upper airway in an operating room. If a cooperative older child can open his or her mouth wide, direct visualization of the cherry-red epiglottis may be possible in the ED. Do not use a tongue depressor as there is the potential danger of causing acute airway obstruction. When epiglottitis is *not* the primary suspected diagnosis, using a tongue depressor to visualize the oropharynx is generally safe. Be careful when evaluating a patient with an upper airway problem, especially when there may be secretions or a foreign body in the posterior pharynx.

If epiglottitis is *unlikely* (prolonged course, low-grade fever) but has not been ruled out clinically, order a lateral neck radiograph of the soft tissues. Obtain a portable film in the ED, with the emergency staff and airway equipment at the child's bedside. Allow the patient to remain in the sitting position for the x-ray, with the parent at the bedside. Radiographic findings reveal a distended hypopharynx, an obliterated vallecula, a large and indistinct epiglottis (thumbprint), thickened aryepiglottic folds, and loss of the normal cervical lordosis. The subglottic region appears normal.

Croup (pp. 638–641) is most common in infants from six months to three years of age, although it does occur in older children. The onset is more indolent, with low-grade fever, hoarseness, a "barking" cough, and varying degrees of stridor. Often a normal supraglottic region can be seen during a careful examination of the oropharynx. If obtained, the lateral neck radiograph is normal in the supraglottic region, and there may be some subglottic haziness.

A retropharyngeal or parapharyngeal abscess most commonly occurs in a young child <3–4 years of age. Fever is usually accompanied by excessive drooling and dysphagia. Respiratory distress is variable but may be pronounced, and meningismus or torticollis may also be present. Examination of the oropharynx may reveal bulging tissue in the rear of the mouth. The lateral neck radiograph shows a swollen prevertebral soft tissue space (much more than half the width of the vertebral bodies).

Foreign body aspiration (pp. 643–645) with upper airway obstruction is generally of very acute onset, with cough and varying degrees of stridor. Aspiration is most common in children six months to five years of age. Fever is unusual, and the chest radiographs may be normal or a radiopaque density may be seen in the upper airway.

Bacterial tracheitis (p. 632) is an acute bacterial infection of the trachea associated with a membranous obstruction. It is usually caused by *S. aureus*, and it most often affects children 2–10 years of age. Most characteristic is the severe stridor. A lateral neck radiograph will reveal a ragged trachea secondary to pseudomembranes. Diagnosis is usually made by direct visualization of the normal supraglottic region and intubation of the airway with suctioning of thick inspissated secretions.

ED Management

The management varies according to the clinical presentation.

Epiglottitis Likely, Airway Stable

Place the patient in a position of comfort, with the parents, in a room with immediate access to airway equipment. Give supplemental oxygen if possible, but *do not agitate the child*. Pulse oximetry is advisable if it does not upset the patient. Immediately notify the operating room staff, and assemble the physician team best able to handle airway intubation (usually an attending anesthesiologist and otolaryngologist). Delay IV placement and laboratory studies until after the child is taken to the operating suite. The airway can be secured best under light general anesthesia without neuromuscular relaxation.

Epiglottitis Likely, Patient in Extremis With an Unstable Airway

Place the child supine, and open the airway with a chin lift. Perform bag-valve-mask ventilation with a tight seal and 4–5 cmH_2O pressure to maximize air entry past the obstructing epiglottis. Occasionally this will not be sufficient, and intubation will be necessary. Rarely, needle cricothyrotomy (children under ten years old) is required to provide a temporary airway until a team can assemble in the ED to manage the airway.

Mild Suspicion of Epiglottitis, Airway Stable

Obtain a lateral neck radiograph to differentiate among the other potential problems. If there is significant stridor or respiratory distress, perform the radiograph in the ED with the physician at the bedside. If epiglottitis is confirmed, proceed with operating room management.

Indications for Admission
- Suspected or confirmed epiglottitis
- Undiagnosed upper airway obstruction with stridor at rest

Bibliography

Mandal A, Kabra SK, Lodha R. Upper airway obstruction in children. *Indian J Pediatr*. 2015;**82** (8):737–744.

Richards AM. Pediatric respiratory emergencies. *Emerg Med Clin North Am*. 2016;**34**(1):77–96.

Foreign Body in the Airway

Aspirated foreign bodies cause more deaths in the United States than croup and epiglottitis combined. Diagnosing a foreign body requires an accurate history, a high degree of clinical suspicion, and often a direct visualization of the airway. The peak incidence is 1–2 years of age, with nuts causing 42% of aspirations.

Clinical Presentation

Aspiration of a foreign body classically presents with an immediate episode of coughing, gagging, choking, or cyanosis. In infants and small children, a foreign body lodged in the esophagus can impinge on the trachea, causing respiratory distress.

Extrathoracic (Laryngeal or Tracheal)

The patient presents with stridor, a croupy cough, varying degrees of dyspnea, or acute hypoxemia and cyanosis. The symptoms may vary with the degree of obstruction of the airway. The sound elicited by air moving over the object varies with the size of the airway and degree of inflammation induced.

Intrathoracic (Lower Trachea and Bronchial)

A lower airway foreign body presents with an initial choking episode and varying periods of quiescence, followed by persistent and often progressive symptoms. Commonly, there is cough, wheezing, and dyspnea. With inflammation or secondary atelectasis, fever and signs of pneumonia may predominate, leading to a misdiagnosis of asthma or recurrent pneumonia. A focal foreign body may produce unilateral hyperinflation with widening of intercostal spaces. On auscultation, localized or diffuse wheezing, rales, or decreased air entry may be appreciated.

Diagnosis

The clinical symptoms of a foreign body aspiration may be subtle. Suspect an aspiration if an afebrile patient presents with the sudden onset of significant respiratory distress, an "asthmatic" has localized wheezing or decreased breath sounds, or a patient has recurrent pneumonias on the same side. The only certain method for verifying the diagnosis is with bronchoscopy. However, if foreign body aspiration is suspected and the patient is not in extreme respiratory distress, obtain radiographs, which can assist in the diagnosis.

Extrathoracic

Radiographs of the lateral neck and chest are generally normal, as only a small number of aspirated foreign bodies are radiopaque. There may be signs of upper airway obstruction, such as ballooning of the hypopharynx, gastric distention, or diminished lung volumes. Esophageal foreign bodies can occasionally compress the trachea from behind; these tend to be larger objects that are more likely to be radiopaque. Orientation of a radiopaque foreign body in the sagittal plane on the PA film of the chest (slit-like image) confirms its presence in the trachea or larynx.

The differential diagnosis of an extrathoracic foreign body includes epiglottitis, croup, bacterial tracheitis, tracheomalacia, retropharyngeal abscess, and congenital anomalies of the airway. The abrupt onset suggests aspiration, but in cases with moderate symptoms bronchoscopy is required to confirm the diagnosis.

Intrathoracic

Most are radiolucent, but there is a high incidence of abnormal chest radiographs (80%). Hyperinflation, atelectasis, and pneumonia are the most common abnormalities. In rare instances, a pneumothorax may be present. In an older child, inspiratory and expiratory chest films may reveal persistent hyperinflation of the ipsilateral side during expiration. Unilateral hyperinflation on the inspiratory film may be seen, but it is less common. For a toddler, when cooperation for an inspiratory film is unlikely, obtain bilateral decubitus films, which may reveal increased lucency and hyperinflation on the affected side, when that side is dependent. Fluoroscopy may sometimes be useful to distinguish small areas of air trapping or mediastinal shifting.

An intrathoracic foreign body is often confused with asthma, pneumonia, congenital lobar emphysema, or other syndromes associated with hyperinflation or atelectasis. History, clinical response to therapy (i.e., bronchodilators in asthma), and chronicity may help distinguish these entities.

ED Management

Assess the patency of the airway and breathing. Complete obstruction demands immediate BLS maneuvers: five back blows followed by five chest compressions in a patient <12 months of age and 6–10 subdiaphragmatic abdominal thrusts (Heimlich maneuver, see p. 9) for an older child. If there is an incomplete obstruction, place the child in the sniffing position (maximal airway opening), provide supplemental oxygen, and permit the patient's own ventilation through a partly occluded airway to be maintained. Maneuvers that dislodge the foreign body may move the object to the central airways, causing complete obstruction. Keep the patient calm and avoid performing procedures that would upset the child (e.g., IV insertion). Continuously monitor the patient with pulse oximetry while awaiting an anesthesiologist and bronchoscopist (pediatric surgeon or otolaryngologist) to perform rigid bronchoscopy, preferably in the operating room.

Lower airway foreign bodies generally present with less severe signs of obstruction. Chest physiotherapy may cause occlusion of a major airway and hypoxemia, and is therefore contraindicated. Provide supplemental oxygen, and arrange for semi-elective removal by rigid bronchoscopy under general anesthesia.

Indications for Admission

- Clinical suspicion of an airway foreign body
- Respiratory symptoms after expulsion of an airway foreign body

Bibliography

Berdan EA, Sato TT. Pediatric airway and esophageal foreign bodies. *Surg Clin North Am.* 2017;**97** (1):85–91.

Green SS. Ingested and aspirated foreign bodies. *Pediatr Rev.* 2015;**36**(10):430–436.

Oncel M, Sunam GS, Ceran S. Tracheobronchial aspiration of foreign bodies and rigid bronchoscopy in children. *Pediatr Int.* 2012;**54**(4):532–535.

Pugmire BS, Lim R, Avery LL. Review of ingested and aspirated foreign bodies in children and their clinical significance for radiologists. *Radiographics.* 2015;**35**(5):1528–1538.

Sink JR, Kitsko DJ, Mehta DK, et al. Diagnosis of pediatric foreign body ingestion: clinical presentation, physical examination, and radiologic findings. *Ann Otol Rhinol Laryngol.* 2016;**125** (4):342–350.

Hemoptysis

Hemoptysis is the expectoration of blood from the lower respiratory tract. Hemoptysis is uncommon in childhood; most suspected cases are the result of vomiting blood swallowed from the esophagus, nasopharynx, or oropharynx. The cause of true hemoptysis is usually a pulmonary infection or other pulmonary disease (Table 20.6).

Clinical Presentation

Hemoptysis usually presents with signs and symptoms of the underlying disease, an acute exacerbation of that process, or a pulmonary infection. For example, pneumonia presents with fever, cough, tachypnea, and rales or decreased breath sounds. A patient with cystic fibrosis may have chronic diarrhea and failure to thrive.

Bronchiectasis

Bronchiectasis can occur with cystic fibrosis, tuberculosis, fungal infections (e.g., coccidi-oidomycosis). Airway erosion leads to acute hemorrhage that is frightening but usually self-

Table 20.6 Etiologies of hemoptysis

Infectious causes (bronchiectasis, airway erosion)

Bacterial infections

Bronchopulmonary dysplasia

Coccidioidomycosis

Cystic fibrosis

Measles

Tuberculosis

Noninfectious causes

Foreign body aspiration

Airway compression: carcinoid, bronchogenic cyst, cystadenomatoid malformation, mediastinal tumor

Arteriovenous malformation

Bleeding diathesis

Pulmonary embolus

Pulmonary hemosiderosis

Pulmonary sequestration

Rib fracture with pulmonary contusion

Wegener's granulomatosis

limiting, although the bleeding may be life-threatening if a major vessel is affected. The usual presentation is fever, cough, and expectoration of blood.

Foreign Body

An airway foreign body generally presents with cough, localized wheezing, and varying degrees of respiratory distress. A chronic foreign body may cause erosion of a bronchus or distal bronchiectasis.

Trauma

Trauma to the chest and airways is often associated with rib fractures and pulmonary contusion. In most instances, there is point tenderness over the rib, pleuritic chest pain, and dyspnea in addition to the hemoptysis.

Mass

A patient with an intrinsic pulmonary or endobronchial mass may be relatively asymptomatic, or they may have cough or wheezing. Weight loss or fatigue can also occur.

Bleeding Diathesis

The patient will have other manifestations of bleeding (petechiae, ecchymoses, hematemesis, epistaxis, hematochezia).

Diagnosis

Initially, confirm that the blood is truly pulmonary in origin and exclude the oral cavity, nasopharynx, or GI tract as the site of the bleeding. If necessary, pass a nasogastric tube to exclude an upper GI bleed.

Inquire about a history of possible aspiration of a foreign body, trauma, acute infection, or exposure to fungus or TB. Check for an underlying history of bronchopulmonary dysplasia, cystic fibrosis, or bleeding dyscrasia.

Perform a careful physical examination of the chest, including observation of abnormality in chest excursion, palpation for external tenderness, and auscultation for air entry and adventitious sounds (rales or wheezes). The area of pulmonary hemorrhage may not alter the breath sounds heard over the chest wall.

Radiographs of the chest may demonstrate an infiltrate, evidence of a foreign body (hyperinflation of the affected side, radiopaque foreign body, or infiltrate distal to the foreign body), or a mass or density. With pulmonary hemosiderosis, there may be fluffy infiltrates that change location with each episode.

ED Management

Admit a patient with true hemoptysis (estimated volume >60 mL) and consult with a pulmonologist or thoracic surgeon. Obtain a chest radiograph, CBC, platelet count, PT, PTT, and type and cross-match. If the patient has tachypnea or respiratory distress, measure the oxygen saturation with either pulse oximetry or an ABG. Insert a large-bore IV and transfuse packed RBCs (pp. 377–378) for volume depletion or evidence of significant ongoing blood loss. Place a 5 TU PPD (0.1 mL) if the patient is not known to have a positive skin test.

Hemoptysis with blood-streaked mucus can be treated on an outpatient basis if the patient is not in respiratory distress. The ED management of pneumonia (pp. 648–652), foreign body aspiration (pp. 643–645), and a bleeding diathesis (pp. 353–357) is discussed elsewhere.

Follow-up

• Pulmonology or primary care follow-up within one week

Indications for Admission

• Hemoptysis >60 mL
• Hematocrit <30% or signs of acute severe blood loss
• Underlying chronic disease requiring parenteral antibiotics or inpatient therapy
• Mediastinal mass or peripheral lung density
• Suspected foreign body aspiration, pulmonary embolus, TB

Bibliography

Bannister M. Paediatric haemoptysis and the otorhinolaryngologist: systematic review. *Int J Pediatr Otorhinolaryngol.* 2017;**92**:99–102.

Simon DR, Aronoff SC, Del Vecchio MT. Etiologies of hemoptysis in children: a systematic review of 171 patients. *Pediatr Pulmonol.* 2017;**52**(2):255–259.

Singh D, Bhalla AS, Veedu PT, Arora A. Imaging evaluation of hemoptysis in children. *World J Clin Pediatr.* 2013;**2**(4):54–64.

Pneumonia

Pneumonia is a common disease with an incidence of 1–4.5 cases per 100 children per year. Pathogens can reach the lung parenchyma via either microaspiration or hematogenous spread. While just 20–30% of pneumonias are bacterial in origin, these are responsible for the majority of severe complications.

Streptococcus pneumoniae remains the most common bacterial pathogen. Universal immunization has decreased the frequency of pneumococcal infections, but severe disease continues to occur, and some organisms have become relatively penicillin-resistant.

RSV is the most frequent viral cause and *Pneumocystis jiroveci* (previously *Pneumocystis carinii*) is the most likely opportunistic infection in HIV-positive infants. Methicillin-resistant *Staphylococcus aureus* (MRSA) has emerged as an important pathogen, especially in very ill-appearing children with pleural effusions. Table 20.7 lists the most likely etiologies in each age group.

Table 20.7 Etiologies of pneumonia

Age	Agent
<2 weeks	Coliform bacteria
	Group B *Streptococcus*
	Respiratory syncitial virus (RSV)
	Staphylococcus aureus
≥2 weeks–3 months	*Chlamydia trachomatis*
	Haemophilus influenzae type b (extremely rare)
	Parainfluenza virus
	Respiratory syncitial virus
	Staphylococcus aureus
	Streptococcus pneumoniae
≥3 months–5 years	*Haemophilus influenzae* type b (extremely rare)
	Streptococcus pneumoniae
	Viral (especially respiratory syncitial virus, influenza)
≥5 years	*Chlamydia pneumoniae*
	Mycoplasma pneumoniae
	Streptococcus pneumoniae
	Chlamydia pneumoniae
Other agents to consider	*Legionella* sp.
	Mycobacterium tuberculosis
	Pertussis (<1 year old)
	Pneumocystis carinii (HIV-positive)

Clinical Presentation

Cough, tachypnea, and fever are the common symptoms of childhood pneumonia, while pallor, fatigue, decreased oral intake, and other constitutional symptoms are variable. A neonate or young infant may present with tachypnea, decreased activity, and poor feeding. With progression of the pneumonia, there may be signs of respiratory distress, including nasal flaring, intercostal or substernal retractions, dyspnea, cyanosis, or apnea. On auscultation, inspiratory rales may be heard or the breath sounds may be locally decreased or tubular, although adventitious sounds are harder to appreciate in a young child. Dullness and diminished breath sounds may indicate an effusion. Abdominal pain can occur with lower lobe pneumonia and meningismus with upper-lobe infection.

Chlamydia trachomatis is the most common non-viral cause of pneumonia in infants between two weeks and three months of age. The classic presentation is a staccato cough in an afebrile, tachypneic infant with nasal congestion and fine rales. There may be a history of or concurrent conjunctivitis in approximately 50% of cases, as well as wheezing, bilateral patchy infiltrates on chest x-ray, and eosinophilia (>300/mm^3).

Mycoplasma pneumoniae and *Chlamydia pneumoniae* present with the gradual onset of a nonproductive hacking cough in a school-age child. The patient does not appear very sick, wheezing is more common than rales, headache and myalgias may also occur, and other family members may have had a similar illness.

Infection with *Bordetella pertussis* (pp. 429–430) may also lead to a secondary lobar or diffuse pneumonia. Typically there is a URI with rhinorrhea (catarrhal stage), which progresses to a harsh, episodic cough (paroxysmal stage), followed by the resolution of the cough over weeks to months (convalescent stage).

Staphylococcus aureus infection can be present in a very ill child with clinical signs of pneumonia. Pneumatoceles may be noted on the chest x-ray. Consider MRSA in a patient with concurrent soft tissue or bone/joint infection and in any patient with suspected empyema.

Diagnosis

Pneumonia can be diagnosed clinically when fever, cough, and localized rales are present; a radiograph does not often alter the patient's management. Obtain a chest x-ray (PA and lateral) when the patient is in respiratory distress, the diagnosis is uncertain, there is concern about a pleural effusion, or when an infant under two months of age has respiratory signs (including cough). Also obtain a chest radiograph if a patient is being hospitalized or is not responding to appropriate therapy. Various patterns on the radiograph may help with the differential diagnosis (Table 20.8). Generally, pyogenic bacterial infections appear as bronchopneumonia or lobar infiltrates, sometimes with pleural effusion. Viral infections often present with diffuse airway involvement and hyperinflation. Point-of-care ultrasound is an emerging tool for the diagnosis of pneumonia. It is highly sensitive and specific diagnostic, and in centers with trained clinicians it can be used in place of radiographs.

The abdominal pain sometimes associated with pneumonia can suggest gastroenteritis or early appendicitis, although a history of cough as an early symptom and a higher temperature suggest a primary respiratory disease.

Table 20.8 Chest x-ray pattern as a guide to etiology

Diffuse pattern

Viral (90%) of cases

Chlamydia trachomatis (afebrile infants, eosinophilia common)

Fungi (uncommon)

Haemophilus influenzae type b (extremely rare)

Mycobacteria (uncommon)

Mycoplasma pneumoniae and Chlamydia pneumoniae (school-age children)

Pneumocystis carinii (usually central pattern, elevated LDH, hypoxia)

Rickettsia (uncommon)

Lobar pattern

Streptococcus pneumoniae (90%)

Haemophilus influenzae type b (extremely rare)

Staphylococcus aureus

Other bacteria (uncommon)

Pneumonia with effusion

Streptococcus pneumoniae (most common cause of effusion)

Adenovirus (small effusion)

Group A *Streptococcus*

H. influenzae type b (extremely rare)

Mycobacteria (unilateral effusion can occur without pneumonia)

Mycoplasma pneumoniae (effusions uncommon)

Staphylococcus aureus (often cavitation and/or empyema)

Asthma

Asthma, which may be difficult to distinguish from pneumonia, can predispose to pneumonia, and accompanying atelectasis can lead to localized decreased breath sounds. Asthma is suggested by the presence of diffuse wheezing and a response to bronchodilators.

Congestive Heart Failure

Congestive heart failure can present with tachycardia, tachypnea, rales, a gallop, and evidence of the primary cause (muffled heart sounds in myocardial disease, a murmur in volume overload shunts, poor perfusion or diminished pulses with left ventricular obstruction). Hepatosplenomegaly may be noted, and cardiomegaly and pulmonary congestion can be seen on the chest radiograph.

Foreign Body Aspiration

A foreign body can cause decreased breath sounds or predispose to pneumonia. The history and radiographs may be suggestive, but bronchoscopy is often required for a definitive diagnosis.

Inhalation Injury

Inhalation injury or any pulmonary toxic agent may induce findings consistent with intrapulmonary inflammation, mimicking pneumonia.

Recurrent Pneumonia

Recurrent pneumonia is usually associated with asthma but may be caused by immunologic dysfunction, cystic fibrosis, foreign body aspiration, or external airway compression (tumor, node).

ED Management

Most children have infections with viral agents and require only supportive care (fever control, fluids). Nonetheless, it is critical to immediately assess the adequacy of breathing. If the patient is dyspneic or in respiratory distress, assess the oxygen saturation with pulse oximetry. Consider an ABG if the patient has poor breath sounds and is lethargic, and administer supplemental oxygen if the patient is in distress or has decreased oxygenation (oxygen saturation <90%; pO_2 <60–65 mm Hg). The goal is an oxygen saturation >92% or pO_2 >65 mm Hg. Obtain a chest radiograph, if indicated (see above). Perform a lumbar puncture to exclude meningitis if there is fever and irritability, obtundation, lethargy, or meningismus. If the patient is febrile, give antipyretics to decrease the temperature and its effects on work of breathing (acetaminophen 15 mg/kg; ibuprofen 10 mg/kg).

Under Six Months Old

Admit all patients under six months of age with lobar pneumonia and all infants with interstitial pneumonia under two months of age. Obtain a CBC, blood culture, and chest radiograph, and if the patient appears toxic or is under two months of age, perform a lumbar puncture and obtain serum electrolytes. Secure an IV if the patient appears toxic or is not taking oral fluids adequately. See pp. 391–393 for the treatment of an infant under eight weeks of age. Treat a patient under eight weeks of age with either cefuroxime (150 mg/kg/day div q 8h, IM or IV) or ceftriaxone (75 mg/kg/day div q 12h IV). If *C. trachomatis* pneumonitis seems likely, obtain a nasopharyngeal culture and treat with oral erythromycin (40 mg/kg/day div q 6h) for 14 days or, as an alternative, oral azithromycin (20 mg/kg q day) for three days. Treat wheezing with a β_2 agonist (pp. 624–631).

Six Months Old and Older

Obtain an oxygen saturation (pulse oximetry) if the patient is tachypneic (respiratory rate >60/min <2 years of age; 40–60/min >2 years of age) or has moderate retractions. An ABG is indicated if the patient has poor color and poor breath sounds. Indications for admission include a pO_2 <60–65 mm Hg, oxygen saturation <90%, or pCO_2 > 40 mm Hg.

  If the pneumonia is lobar, treat with amoxicillin (90 mg/kg/day div bid for ten days). Give an initial dose of parenteral ceftriaxone (50 mg/kg IM or IV, 500 mg maximum) before oral therapy if the patient is vomiting, although this does not hasten recovery. If the patient is being admitted to the hospital, treat with IV ampicillin (200 mg/kg/day div q 6h) or penicillin (200,000–250,000 units/kg/day, div q 4–6h) or IV cefuroxime (150 mg/kg/day div q 8h) or ceftriaxone (50–75 mg/kg/day div q 12h). Add IV vancomycin (40 mg/kg/day div q 6h) *or* clindamycin (40 mg/kg/day div q 6h) if MRSA pneumonia is suspected.

Treat a child older than five years with oral azithromycin (10 mg/kg, once on day 1, followed by 5 mg/kg q day on days 2–5), or clarithromycin (15 mg/kg div bid, 1 g maximum) for lobar or presumed *Mycoplasma* pneumonia.

If *P. jiroveci* pneumonia (PJP) is suspected (pp. 397–398), obtain a chest radiograph and LDH. Admit and treat with TMP-SMX (20 mg/kg/day TMP div q 6h) if the LDH is elevated or the x-ray is consistent with PCP.

Significant pleural effusion is an indication for admission for diagnostic thoracocentesis and parenteral antibiotics.

Follow-up

- Respiratory distress at home: at once
- Lobar pneumonia: 24 hours
- Patient <2 years of age with suspected viral pneumonia: 24–48 hours
- All patients: at the end of treatment or about two weeks after presentation to assess for improvement. Because chest x-ray abnormalities can persist for 8–12 weeks after the acute illness, and symptoms (especially cough) can persist for weeks, wait at least 8–12 weeks after presentation to consider the need for a follow-up chest x-ray, unless the patient is worsening

Indications for Admission

- Patient <2 months of age with pneumonia
- Patient <6 months of age with lobar pneumonia
- Patient with pO_2 <65 mm Hg, oxygen saturation <90%, pCO_2 >40 mm Hg
- Patient not taking fluids, dehydrated, or with parents unable to comply with instructions
- Presence of significant pleural effusion
- Suspicion of PCP

Bibliography

Bradley JS, Byington CL, Shah SS, et al. The management of community-acquired pneumonia in infants and children older than 3 months of age: clinical practice guidelines by the Pediatric Infectious Diseases Society and the Infectious Diseases Society of America. *Clin Infect Dis.* 2011;53(7):e25–e76.

Gardiner SJ, Gavranich JB, Chang AB. Antibiotics for community-acquired lower respiratory tract infections secondary to *Mycoplasma pneumoniae* in children. *Cochrane Database Syst Rev.* 2015;1: CD004875.

Gereige RS, Laufer PM. Pneumonia. *Pediatr Rev.* 2013;34(10):438–456.

Pereda MA, Chavez MA, Hooper-Miele CC, et al. Lung ultrasound for the diagnosis of pneumonia in children: a meta-analysis. *Pediatrics.* 2015;135(4):714–722.

Tam PY. Approach to common bacterial infections: community-acquired pneumonia. *Pediatr Clin North Am.* 2013;60(2):437–453.

Pulse Oximetry

Pulse oximetry is a simple and noninvasive means of measuring the oxygen saturation of hemoglobin. It is based on the principle that deoxygenated blood absorbs more light in the red spectrum, while oxygenated blood absorbs more infrared light. The oximeter measures the two different light absorbencies, and then calculates the oxygen saturation. The light

Table 20.9 Factors affecting accuracy of pulse oximetry

Condition	Effect on oxygen saturation estimate
Anemia (severe)	False sense of adequate oxygenation
Bilirubin	May underestimate
Carboxyhemoglobin	Overestimates
Dark nail polish	Underestimates
Methemoglobin	Over- and underestimates
Neonate	Accuracy varies with hemoglobin level
Profound hypoxia (O_2 saturation <80%)	Not reliable
Sickle cell anemia	May overestimate (not significantly)

source and sensor of the oximetry probe must be placed opposite one another in an accessible area, such as a finger, toe, or earlobe. Verify the oximeter pulse rate reading by correlation with a manually obtained pulse rate. Several factors affect the accuracy of pulse oximetry and may limit its use (see Table 20.9).

Bibliography

Langley R, Cunningham S. How should oxygen supplementation be guided by pulse oximetry in children: do we know the level? *Front Pediatr.* 2017;27;4:138.

Sinha IP, Mayell SJ, Halfhide C. Pulse oximetry in children. *Arch Dis Child Educ Pract Ed.* 2014;99 (3):117–118.

Respiratory Distress and Failure

Respiratory distress or respiratory failure may be the endpoint of a multitude of clinical disorders in children, both pulmonary and nonpulmonary in origin. Airway obstruction is the leading cause of life-threatening acute respiratory distress and can be caused by bacterial tracheitis, croup, foreign body aspiration and, rarely, epiglottitis. Asthma or bronchiolitis produce lower airway obstruction. Other disorders that can lead to respiratory distress or failure are abnormalities of the neuromuscular control of breathing (seizures, central apnea, meningitis, encephalitis, head trauma), problems with the mechanics of breathing (congenital, acquired, or traumatic chest wall deformities), and alveolar disorders (pneumonia). Nonpulmonary disorders include cardiac disease and heart failure, sepsis, and disorders of oxygen delivery (CO poisoning, methemoglobinemia, severe anemia).

Clinical Presentation and Diagnosis

Respiratory distress is manifested by difficulty breathing, fatigue, diminished activity and/or feeding, varying degrees of exhaustion, and symptoms associated with the cause. Signs include pallor or cyanosis, tachypnea, grunting, retractions, diminished air entry, tachycardia (bradycardia with severe respiratory failure with hypoxemia), and/or signs of the specific origin of the distress.

Upper airway obstruction usually presents with stridor. Radiographs may delineate supraglottic disorders such as epiglottitis or a foreign body, although direct visualization of the airway in a controlled setting is the diagnostic and therapeutic procedure of choice.

Lower airway obstruction presents with hyperinflation, expiratory prolongation, and wheezing. Localized signs are noted more with foreign body aspiration.

Neurologic diseases lead to depressed level of consciousness, poor respiratory effort or apnea, depressed airway reflexes, and less effective cough.

Mechanical problems present with ineffective chest wall excursion or distorted lung inflation.

Alveolar causes present with general signs of respiratory distress, hypoxemia, and tachypnea. The findings on examination include rales or decreased breath sounds.

Congestive heart failure can present with tachycardia, a gallop, a murmur, diminished heart sounds, venous distention, and sometimes hepatomegaly. Severe anemia presents with pallor and a low hemoglobin.

Nonpulmonary disorders (CO poisoning [pp. 466–467]; methemoglobinemia [p. 449]) require laboratory studies to confirm the diagnosis.

Criteria for Respiratory Failure

- pO_2 <50 mm Hg (oxygen saturation <84%) on 60% FIO_2 (except in cyanotic congenital heart disease)
- pCO_2 >50 mm Hg and rising (with pH <7.30) or >40 mm Hg with exhaustion
- In neuromuscular and central disorders, central apnea, or decreased vital capacity (<12–15 mL/kg) with exhaustion

ED Management

Provide 100% oxygen and perform a rapid cardiopulmonary assessment: assess airway patency, count the respiratory rate, check the stability of the airway (maintainable or unmaintainable), and evaluate color, breath sounds (air entry), heart rate, pulses, capillary refill, and blood pressure. Monitor the oxygen saturation. Ascertain the cause of respiratory failure, and begin immediate therapy.

If the airway is not patent, elevate the patient's shoulders in the supine patient to prevent neck flexion, and use the jaw thrust and suction. If respiratory failure is present, continue with 100% O_2 and institute bag-valve-mask ventilation. Intubate patients who are unable to maintain a stable airway for an extended period (pp. 11–15). Establish IV access and give broad-spectrum antibiotics if infection is likely (cefuroxime 150 mg/kg/day div q 8h or ceftriaxone 100 mg/kg/day div q 12h).

Noninvasive Positive Pressure Ventilation (NPPV)

NPPV is the delivery of positive pressure ventilation (PPV) through a nasal or oronasal mask. NPPV may reduce the work of breathing and improve gas exchange, without resorting to intubation. It is useful for patients who are alert and able to maintain their own airway, but have evidence of respiratory distress such as retractions, decreased breath sounds, and hypoxia despite 100% oxygen via a nonrebreather mask. Do not use NPPV if the mask does not fit well or the patient is hemodynamically unstable, agitated, unconscious, has facial or neck trauma, or is unable to maintain the airway or handle oral secretions/ongoing emesis.

Compared to traditional PPV through a tracheal tube, NPPV use reduces the risk of upper airway trauma, avoids postextubation laryngeal edema and vocal cord dysfunction, decreases the risk of nosocomial respiratory infections, eliminates the need for muscle relaxants, and reduces the need for sedation, and potentially reduces the length of hospitalization.

Continuous Positive Airway Pressure (CPAP)

CPAP delivers uninterrupted pressure support, regardless of the stage of the respiratory cycle. Provide CPAP for infants via nasal prongs. Set the initial positive airway pressure at 4 cmH$_2$O and titrate up to 10 cmH$_2$O, as needed, to reduce the work of breathing.

Bilevel Positive Airway Pressure (BiPAP)

BiPAP provides inspiratory pressure support during inhalation (IPAP) while providing baseline pressure support during exhalation (EPAP). Use BiPAP for older children and adolescents with a well-fitted nasooral mask. Consult with a pediatric pulmonologist to determine whether BiPAP is indicated and the initial settings to be used. Monitor the patient closely for one hour following the initiation of BiPAP. Signs of improvement include decreased respiratory rate and work of breathing and improved oxygenation. Lack of improvement suggests the need for intubation.

Mechanical Ventilation

<10 kg

Use a pressure-limited ventilator. Adjust inspiratory pressure (IP) to obtain adequate chest movement and audible breath sounds. In disorders with minimal alteration of lung compliance, start with an IP of 20 cm and a rate of 20–25 breaths per minute. Higher pressures are required in more restrictive (less compliant) disorders.

≥10 kg

Use a volume-preset ventilator set to deliver 8–10 mL/kg of tidal volume (lower in disorders with hyperinflation), a rate of 15–20 breaths per minute, and an I:E 1:2.

With either ventilator, consider positive end expiratory pressure (PEEP; 4–5 cmH$_2$O) to maintain end-expiratory lung volume and thereby minimize atelectasis and intrapulmonary shunting (except in a patient with hyperinflation). Assess the adequacy of ventilation by chest excursions and breath sounds. Start with an FIO$_2$ of 1.0 and slowly wean as tolerated to maintain an oxygen saturation >90%. Ensure that the patient is adequately sedated to decrease pain and work of breathing, and to prevent dislodgement of the endotracheal tube.

Check an ABG after 15 minutes, and obtain other laboratory studies as indicated to ascertain a diagnosis (chest radiograph, lateral neck radiograph, serum electrolytes, respiratory cultures, ECG, lumbar puncture, EEG, CT scan). Subsequent laboratory tests and changes in the ventilator settings are guided by the clinical status, pulse oximetry, and ABG results.

Indications for Admission

- Respiratory failure requiring mechanical ventilation or intensive monitoring
- Respiratory distress not reversible with definitive therapy

- New oxygen requirements
- Pulmonary infection requiring parenteral antibiotics

Bibliography

Conti G, Piastra M. Mechanical ventilation for children. *Curr Opin Crit Care*. 2016;**22**(1):60–66.

Mayfield S, Jauncey-Cooke J, Hough JL, et al. High-flow nasal cannula therapy for respiratory support in children. *Cochrane Database Syst Rev*. 2014;**3**:CD009850.

Pediatric Acute Lung Injury Consensus Conference Group. Pediatric acute respiratory distress syndrome: consensus recommendations from the Pediatric Acute Lung Injury Consensus Conference. *Pediatr Crit Care Med*. 2015;**16**(5):428–439.

Schibler A, Franklin D. Respiratory support for children in the emergency department. *J Paediatr Child Health*. 2016;**52**(2):192–196.

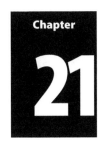

Radiology

James A. Meltzer, Robert Acosta, Dan Barlev, and
C. Anthoney Lim

Pediatric Emergency Bedside Ultrasound

Over the past 20 years, bedside ultrasound (BUS) has emerged as an essential tool in the
pediatric emergency department. Its applications are designed to answer specific questions,
similar to other point-of-care tests. BUS supplements the overall clinical evaluation and does
not replace more complete diagnostic imaging *performed by radiologists*. BUS applications
require a minimal amount of training for proficiency and they can significantly expedite time
to diagnosis and definitive management. See Table 21.1 for BUS indications and findings.

Table 21.1 Bedside ultrasound indications and findings.

Indications	Findings
E-FAST	
Blunt or penetrating trauma: identify hemothorax, pneumothorax, pericardial tamponade, hemoperitoneum	Significant intrathoracic or intraperitoneal hemorrhage appear as anechoic or hypoechoic stripes seen in potential spaces Negative E-FAST alone does not rule-out a significant injury
Abdominal ultrasound	
Rule-out appendicitis	Normal appendix: blind-ended, compressible, tubular structure with a diameter <7 mm, extending from the cecum Appendicitis: non-compressible structure with a diameter >7 mm, hypoechoic edematous layers with loss of anatomic differentiation
Rule-out intussusception	Transverse view: concentric rings ("target or donut sign") Longitudinal view: "pseudokidney" or "trident" sign
Transabdominal and/ or transvaginal ultrasound	
Rule-out ectopic pregnancy	IUP: presence of a yolk sac (five weeks) or a fetal pole (six weeks) Ectopic: may appear as tubal ring, complex adnexal mass, or an extra-uterine gestation sac

Table 21.1 (cont.)

Indications	Findings
Cardiac ultrasound	
Pericardial effusion	Subxiphoid view: anechoic pericardial fluid between the liver and the heart Parasternal views: anechoic pericardial fluid posterior to heart but anterior to descending aorta
Pericardial tamponade	Right ventricular compression during diastole
Cardiac function	Calculate the ejection fraction: EF = (EDD – ESD)/EDD; Poor EF = <30%
Shock	Volume overload (cardiogenic, obstructive shock): full IVC with minimal collapse with respiration Volume depletion (hypovolemic, distributive shock): narrow IVC that completely collapses with respiration
Pulmonary embolus	Apical four-chamber view: bowing of the septum and right ventricle > left ventricle Parasternal short view: flattened intraventricular septum, left ventricle produces a "D" sign
Orthopedic ultrasound	
Hip joint effusion	Width of the anterior synovial recess >5 mm or the difference in width from the contralateral hip is >2 mm
Elbow joint effusion	Normal: posterior humeral fat pad within the protuberances of the olecranon fossa Effusion: elevated fat pad beyond olecranon fossa protuberances or hypoechoic fluid within the fat pad
Fracture	Discontinuity in the normally continuous hyperechoic periosteum May have an overlying hypoechoic hematoma
Skin ultrasound	
Abscess/cellulitis	Abscess: hypoechoic fluid collection with hyperechoic walls and increased surrounding vascular flow on color Doppler Cellulitis: thickened hyperechoic dermal layers with a "cobblestoned" appearance due to interstitial edema and inflammation
Foreign body	Hyperechoic anterior surfaces and posterior shadowing
Vein identification	Vein: thin-walled, compressible structure with internal color flow Artery: thick-walled, non-compressible, with pulsatile internal color flow
Regional nerve block	Nerve: reticular "honeycombed" structure that exhibits "anisotropy" or variable echogenicity and resolution, depending on the angle of visualization Tendons: more hyperechoic, will move with muscle activity, but also exhibit anisotropy Vascular structures: exhibit color flow.

EDD: end diastolic diameter; EF: ejection fraction; ESD: end systolic diameter; IUP: intrauterine pregnancy; IVC: inferior vena cava

Extended Focused Assessment With Sonography for Trauma (E-FAST)

For patients who have sustained blunt or penetrating trauma, a bedside E-FAST is indicated to rapidly identify potentially life-threatening hemoperitoneum, hemothorax, pneumothorax, and pericardial tamponade. The Advanced Trauma Life Support guidelines include the E-FAST as an adjunct to the primary survey and it can be performed simultaneously with resuscitation efforts. The investigation for free fluid can also be useful when evaluating other non-traumatic etiologies (e.g., appendicitis, para-pneumonic effusion, ruptured ectopic, ovarian cyst).

A complete E-FAST consists of four torso views (right upper quadrant, left upper quadrant, subxiphoid, bladder) and bilateral lung views. If possible, place the patient in the Trendelenburg position to allow for free fluid to collect in the upper quadrants, and ask the patient to inhale during the exam to improve visualization.

The normal absence of free fluid in potential spaces is reassuring, demonstrated as a hyperechoic interface between the visceral and parietal peritoneum. Free fluid will appear as an anechoic (i.e., black) collection that settles in dependent areas. Note that a small amount of normal physiologic free fluid may be seen in the retrovesical space in females.

In the setting of trauma, anechoic or hypoechoic stripes seen in potential spaces are indicative of clinically significant intrathoracic or intraperitoneal hemorrhage. These findings may obviate the need for time-consuming computed tomography (CT). Obtain emergent surgical intervention if there is a positive E-FAST in a hemodynamically unstable patient who has not responded to the initial volume resuscitation. In a hemodynamically stable trauma patient, a positive E-FAST indicates the need for further diagnostic testing and surgical consultation. However, a negative E-FAST alone does *not* rule-out a significant injury.

Abdominal Ultrasound

A point-of-care bedside ultrasound examination can be useful in the evaluation of patients with right lower quadrant pain or unopposed vomiting, in whom there is a suspicion for appendicitis (pp. 241–244). A point-of-care ultrasound can also aid in the diagnosis of intussusception (pp. 273–274) in infants and toddlers. Obtain prompt surgical and radiologic consultations *for official imaging* following an abdominal BUS.

Appendicitis

A normal appendix, which can be more difficult to find than an inflamed one, appears as a blind-ended, compressible, tubular structure extending from the cecum, measuring <7 mm in diameter. It often appears as three parallel lines representing a hyperechoic collapsed mucosal lumen surrounded by alternating layers of muscularis and serosa with varying echogenicity. Conversely, appendicitis appears as a non-compressible structure with a diameter >7 mm, with hypoechoic edematous layers with loss of anatomic differentiation. Secondary signs of appendicitis include surrounding free fluid or complex fluid collections, presence of an appendicolith, signs of peritonitis, and localized ileus.

Intussusception

In a negative examination, there will normally be thin multilayered intestinal walls with hypoechoic contents exhibiting peristalsis. Identify intussusception in transverse view as concentric rings ("target or donut sign") and in longitudinal section as "pseudokidney" or "trident" sign, formed by the edematous bowel walls of the intussusceptum within the intussuscipiens. Color flow often reveals increased vascular flow within the intestinal layers.

Early Pregnancy

A BUS is indicated for any pregnant female with vaginal bleeding and/or abdominal pain, as these symptoms place the patient at risk for an ectopic pregnancy. In a young female who is not receiving fertility treatments, the presence of an intrauterine pregnancy (IUP) on bedside ultrasound effectively rules-out ectopic pregnancy.

If a transabdominal ultrasound is performed, ensure the patient has a full bladder, which will provide optimal images by acting as a "sonographic window" and displacing air-filled bowel. A transvaginal ultrasound is best performed, however, with an empty bladder to allow for a more comfortable examination. Transvaginal ultrasound is more sensitive than transabdominal ultrasound and can identify gestational structures earlier.

Although a gestational sac is usually visualized at four weeks' gestation on a transvaginal ultrasound, its presence is *not sufficient* to rule-out ectopic pregnancy. A patient with an ectopic pregnancy may have a pseudo-gestational sac or a decidual cyst that can mimic the anechoic appearance of a gestational sac. Only the presence of a yolk sac (five weeks) or a fetal pole (six weeks) confirms that the patient has an IUP and not an ectopic pregnancy. Obtain obstetrical consultation if the ultrasound does not yield the expected findings by the appropriate post-gestation time. A small amount of intraperitoneal free fluid may be physiologic; however, moderate to large amounts of free fluid in this setting, particularly in Morrison's pouch, are an ominous finding that is concerning for ectopic rupture.

Ectopic pregnancy, occurring most commonly in the fallopian tube, can occasionally be visualized as a tubal ring, complex adnexal mass, and rarely as an extra-uterine gestation sac complete with a yolk sac, fetal pole, and fetal heart.

Cardiac/Inferior Vena Cava (IVC)

Cardiac ultrasound can help determine the presence of a heartbeat, a pericardial effusion, volume overload (i.e., obstructive or cardiogenic shock) or volume depletion (i.e., distributive or hypovolemic shock), and a pulmonary embolus. It will also assess the overall function of the heart. There are five primary cardiac views: parasternal long view, parasternal short view, subxiphoid view, apical four-chamber view, and inferior vena cava view.

Pericardial Effusion

Anechoic pericardial fluid is often first seen in the most dependent regions. On subxiphoid view, this is the region between the liver and the heart; on the parasternal views, this region is posterior to the heart. To distinguish a pericardial effusion from a pleural effusion in the parasternal long view, note whether the fluid crosses anterior (pericardial) or posterior (pleural) to the descending aorta. Pericardial tamponade is present when the right ventricle becomes compressed during diastole by the pericardial effusion, resulting in obstructive shock.

Cardiac Function

This is best evaluated on the parasternal long view. Often visual inspection of the size of the left ventricle at end systole and end diastole will suffice to evaluate function. Calculate the ejection fraction using the following formula:

$$\text{Ejection fraction} = (\text{end diastolic diameter} - \text{end systolic diameter}/ \\ \text{end diastolic diameter}).$$

An ejection fraction <30% represents poor function.

Shock

Volume overload (i.e., cardiogenic, obstructive shock) has a full IVC that has minimal collapse with respiration versus volume depletion (i.e., hypovolemic, distributive shock) that demonstrates a narrow IVC that completely collapses with respiration.

Pulmonary Embolus

Substantial right heart strain consistent with a pulmonary embolus presents with bowing of the septum and a right ventricle that is larger than the left ventricle on the apical four-chamber view. Similarly, on the parasternal short view, the intraventricular septum will be flattened and the left ventricle produces a "D" sign.

Orthopedic Ultrasound

Use BUS to identify the presence of joint effusion in the setting of trauma, infection, or inflammation, and to identify fractures and help guide their reduction. Use a high-frequency linear probe to obtain images of the affected extremity and the contralateral side for comparison.

Hip Joint Effusion

The anechoic anterior synovial recess is the concave space defined by the anterior border of the femoral neck and the posterior border of the ileopsoas muscle. An effusion is present if the width of the anechoic anterior synovial recess is >5 mm, or the difference in width from the contralateral hip is >2 mm. BUS cannot differentiate between a septic hip and transient synovitis.

Elbow Joint Effusion

A normal posterior humeral fat pad lies within the protuberances of the olecranon fossa. The presence of a lipohemarthrosis (i.e., hypoechoic fluid within the fat pad) or an elevated posterior fat pad beyond these protuberances is suggestive of a joint effusion which, in the setting of trauma, is concerning for a fracture. In the absence of trauma, evaluate the patient for infectious and rheumatologic etiologies.

Fracture

A fracture appears as a discontinuity in the normally continuous hyperechoic periosteum, sometimes associated with a hypoechoic overlying hematoma. Once a fracture is located, measure the amount of displacement between the distal and proximal parts of the fracture. If reduction is needed, repeat the measurement after every reduction attempt until satisfactory alignment is obtained. Compared to bedside C-arm, BUS is preferred for fracture reduction because it eliminates the radiation risk associated with multiple pre- and post-reduction images.

Skin Infections/Foreign Body

In a patient with a possible skin infection, BUS can help differentiate among an abscess, cellulitis, and angioedema. BUS can also identify phlegmons and lymphadenitis, and facilitate drainage while preventing damage to nearby structures. Also use BUS to identify and help remove foreign bodies embedded in soft tissues. It is especially useful in identifying small and radiolucent foreign bodies that are not visible on plain films.

Technique

Cellulitis is demonstrated by thickened hyperechoic dermal layers and a "cobblestoned" appearance on ultrasound due to interstitial edema and inflammation. An abscess is a hypoechoic fluid collection with hyperechoic walls and increased surrounding vascular flow on color Doppler. With foreign bodies, there are hyperechoic anterior surfaces and posterior shadowing. Once visualized, obtain orthogonal views to determine the extent of the abscess, the orientation of the foreign body, and any anatomical structures that should be avoided during drainage or removal.

To improve the visualization of shallow foreign bodies or abscesses, use a step-off pad (commercially available or made with a glove filled with water) placed between the skin and probe, or immerse the extremity in a basin of water and hold the probe above the suspected area. Use BUS prior to the procedure for diagnosis or "real-time" to provide continuous visualization of internal structures (e.g., abscess or foreign body) throughout the procedure.

Vascular Access

Use BUS statically to identify the location of veins prior to attempting cannulation or dynamically by maintaining visualization of the target vessel and the needle throughout the procedure. Use of BUS decreases unsuccessful attempts at peripheral access, and reduces complications from central line access.

Technique

For the static technique, with a tourniquet in place as needed, place a high-frequency probe transversely over the desired area for cannulation. Visualize the vein as a thin-walled, compressible structure with internal color flow, as opposed to arteries, which are thick-walled, non-compressible, and exhibit pulsatile internal color flow. Slide the probe slightly proximal or distal to approximate the course of the vein, and use a skin marker to denote its position. The probe may then be placed aside and intravenous access performed using standard methods.

For the dynamic technique, prepare overlying skin and/or the ultrasound probe in sterile fashion as needed; begin as above to identify the target vein. Keeping the vein in the middle of the visual field, enter the skin with the needle at a 45° angle, at the same distance distal to the probe head as the vein depth, and advance in the direction the vein courses. The needle tip will enter the screen and appear as a hyperechoic point with posterior shadowing. Make small rocking movements of the probe to follow the needle tip to the vein wall, which will be seen to indent then rebound as the needle tip enters the vessel. Complete cannulation of the vein using standard methods.

Proper restriction of movement and use of anxiolysis and pain control are necessary, as vessel position will change with movement, especially at joints. In dynamic placement, light downward pressure allows for accurate measurement of vein depth and more accurate needle entry. Confirm successful cannulation by displaying the "wire in vessel," or by flushing the catheter and visualizing turbulence within the vein using color flow.

Regional Nerve Block

In patients undergoing a potentially painful procedure, ultrasound-guided regional nerve blocks can provide adequate analgesia, eliminating the need for procedural sedation. This is particularly useful when caring for children in whom sedation is contraindicated, such as those with a difficult airway, concomitant head injuries requiring monitoring, or allergy to sedative medications.

Sonographically, nerves appear as reticular "honeycombed" structures that exhibit "anisotropy" or variable echogenicity and resolution depending on the angle of visualization. Keeping the nerve in the middle of the screen, enter the skin with the needle at a 45° angle at the same distance distal to the probe as the nerve depth and advance until the tip of the needle enters the ultrasound screen, appearing as a hyperechoic point with posterior shadowing. Slowly pan the probe to follow the needle tip to the nerve periphery, and infiltrate enough local anesthetic to completely surround the nerve; check distally for anesthesia.

Nerves must be identified and distinguished from nearby anatomic structures for regional nerve blocks to be successful. Tendons, which also exhibit anisotropy, tend to be more hyperechoic and will move with muscle activity. Avoid puncturing nearby vascular structures which exhibit color flow. As the needle tip approaches the nerve, if paresthesias are elicited, withdraw the needle slightly prior to instilling anesthetic to avoid intraneural infiltration and potential nerve injury. Since extremities often have overlapping areas of innervation, multiple nerve distributions may require regional anesthesia to ensure proper analgesia.

Bibliography

Guttman J, Nelson BP. Diagnostic emergency ultrasound: assessment techniques in the pediatric patient. *Pediatr Emerg Med Pract*. 2016;**12**(12):1–28.

O'Brien AJ, Brady RM. Point-of-care ultrasound in paediatric emergency medicine. *J Paediatr Child Health*. 2016;**52**(2):174–180.

Rowlands R, Rippey J, Tie S, Flynn J. Bedside ultrasound vs x-ray for the diagnosis of forearm fractures in children. *J Emerg Med*. 2017;**52**(2):208–215.

Sivitz AB, Cohen SG, Tejani C. Evaluation of acute appendicitis by pediatric emergency physician sonography. *Ann Emerg Med*. 2014;**64**(4):358–364.

Zhan C, Grundtvig N, Klug BH. Performance of bedside lung ultrasound by a pediatric resident: a useful diagnostic tool in children with suspected pneumonia. *Pediatr Emerg Care*. 2016. Epub ahead of print.

Ordering Radiologic Examinations

To maximize the value of ED radiographic imaging, adhere to the following guidelines:

- Order a study if the results will alter the care and management of the patient. For example, the clinical diagnosis of sinusitis is evident in a child who has fever, several days of cough, purulent nasal discharge, and tenderness over the maxilla, so sinus x-rays will

Table 21.2 Suggested radiologic procedures

	Procedure	Findings	Notes
Abdomen			
Appendicitis	Abdomen film Abdominal ultrasound (AUS) CT of abdomen	Plain film may be normal Presence of appendicolith associated with perforation AUS: blind-ending noncompressable structure >7 mm in diameter CT: nonfilling of appendix (with oral contrast), >7 mm in diameter, with thickened wall, and usually with surrounding edema	No imaging necessary if clinically positive CT performed with rectal and IV contrast
Cholecystitis	Abdominal ultrasound (AUS) HIDA scan	AUS: stones or thickened GB wall HIDA scan: cystic duct obstruction	
Foreign body ingestion	Abdominal films Chest x-ray	Note shape, size and location; thoracic inlet, aortic arch, and lower esophageal sphincter are usual areas of concern	Younger children may allow for both chest and abdomen in one view. Button batteries will appear to have a "double ring" appearance.
Intussusception	Abdominal films Abdominal ultrasound (AUS) Contrast/air enema for therapy	Plain films: crescent or target sign and lack of gas in transverse colon AUS: target or pseudokidney sign Enema for reduction	Hydrate patient prior to reduction attempt Hydrostatic reduction contraindicated if peritoneal signs are present
Malrotation/volvulus	Abdominal films Abdominal ultrasound (AUS) Upper GI series (UGI)	AUS: may show reversal of SMA and SMV or whirlpool sign UGI: may show corkscrew sign with dilatation of duodenum	Plain films may be normal UGI always done through a nasogastric tube

Condition	Imaging study	Findings	Comments
Pyloric stenosis	Abdominal ultrasound (AUS)	Pyloric muscle thickness >3 mm Pyloric channel length >16 mm	Not an emergency study, can wait until the next morning if middle of the night presentation
Meckel's diverticulum	Meckel's scan	Gastric mucosa takes up radiotracer	Findings can be easily obscured by previous barium studies
Cardiology			
Congestive failure	Chest x-ray	Large heart and increased central pulmonary blood volume with indistinct vessels	
Endocarditis	Chest x-ray	May be normal	
Pericarditis	Chest x-ray	May be normal	
ENT			
Cervical adenitis	Imaging usually not indicated		Consider ultrasound if node is enlarging or resistant to antibiotic therapy
Croup	Airway films (usually not necessary)	Steeple sign on frontal view Infraglottic edema on lateral view	
Epiglottitis	Clinical diagnosis Soft tissue neck film only if diagnosis is *unlikely*	Edematous epiglottis and aryepiglottic folds Pharyngeal distension	Do not leave patient unattended Emergent intubation/tracheostomy may be needed
Mastoiditis	CT of temporal bones and mastoids	Opacification of mastoid air cells may be seen Coalescence of air cells represents bony septal destruction	IV contrast not usually necessary, but may be administered if epidural abscess suspected
Orbital cellulitis	CT of orbits	CT Distinguish preseptal from postseptal disease CT Orbital abscess easily seen	IV contrast allows easier abscess identification.
Peritonsillar abscess	Imaging not indicated		

Table 21.2 (cont.)

	Procedure	Findings	Notes
Retropharyngeal abscess	Soft tissue neck film CT of neck	Abnormal retropharyngeal soft tissue swelling with/without gas bubbles CT: low-density center may be seen (IV contrast: ring enhancement)	Obtain CT if there is no clinical improvement on IV antibiotics.
Sinusitis	Sinus films usually not necessary Sinus CT	Plain films: opacification of sinus or air-fluid level CT: more sensitive in select cases	Limited CT is sufficient (coronal images only, one slice through each sinus) IV contrast not needed
Genitourinary			
Epididymitis	Scrotal ultrasound (US)	Enlarged epididymis with increased color Doppler flow	
Testicular torsion	Scrotal US Testicular (nuclear) scan	US: absent or decreased flow (especially diastolic flow) on Doppler evaluation Nuclear scan: absent uptake, but a missed torsion may appear as a doughnut sign.	If diagnosis is clear, do not delay surgery to obtain imaging studies
Gynecology			
Ectopic pregnancy	Transvaginal ultrasound	Extra-uterine gestation Fluid in cul-de-sac	Study can confirm an intrauterine pregnancy Twin ectopic pregnancy is very unlikely
Ovarian torsion	Pelvic ultrasound	Enlarged ovary with peripheral follicles	Blood flow may be seen, since ovaries have a dual blood supply

Neurology

Condition	Imaging	Notes
Acute ataxia Acute hemiparesis Headache Non-febrile seizure	CT of brain MRI of brain	CT: quickly assesses for hydrocephalus, cerebral lesions or acute bleeding MRI: more sensitive for posterior fossa (cerebellar) lesions	CT and MRI can be done pre-/post-IV contrast No imaging needed for febrile seizure
Head trauma	Noncontrast CT of brain Skull films	Epidural bleed: convex (lens shaped) density. Subdural bleed: crescentic density which could cross suture lines Subarachnoid bleed: blood within sulci Brain contusion: focal bleed or edema (hypodense)	Do not give IV contrast Acute blood is dense (white) on CT Calvarial fractures may be easier to see on plain films Basilar fractures easier to see on CT
VP shunt evaluation	Shunt series Noncontrast CT of brain Abdominal ultrasound (AUS)	Plain films: identify breaks or kinks in shunt CT: evaluate ventricular size AUS: identify CSF pseudocyst	IV contrast not needed for CT Compare CT to prior studies to assess change in ventricular size

Orthopedics

Condition	Imaging	Notes
Osteomyelitis	Plain films Bone scan MRI (test of choice)	Plain film: periosteal elevation, bone destruction Bone scan: hot focus	Plain films not positive for 10+ days Bone scan positive in 24–48 hours
SCFE	AP and frog lateral hip x-rays	Widening of the proximal femoral growth plate with irregularity of the metaphysis may be the earliest sign (pre-slip slip)	Always image the contralateral side for comparison, but SCFE can also be bilateral

Pulmonary

Condition	Imaging	Notes
Asthma Bronchiolitis	Imaging usually not indicated		

Table 21.2 (cont.)

	Procedure	Findings	Notes
Foreign body aspiration	Chest x-rays in inspiration and expiration	Airway obstruction could cause atelectasis, hyperinflation, or hyperlucency	Expiration films in young children may be obtained with decubitus views or by timing the exposure during a cry Ask an older child to "blow out" an imaginary birthday candle for the expiration exposure
Pneumonia	Chest x-ray	Bacterial (pneumococcal) pneumonia usually presents as a focal pleural-based opacity	Decubitus views or ultrasound are useful for evaluating for a pleural effusion
Tuberculosis	Chest x-ray	Lung opacities Hilar and mediastinal adenopathy	
Trauma			
Abdomen	Abdominal film Abdominal CT	May see free air or loss of normal fat stripes on plain film CT with IV contrast (no PO contrast) is very sensitive for visceral organ injury	Do not obtain a CT if the patient is unstable
Cervical spine	Plain films (lateral, AP, open mouth) Cervical spine CT Cervical spine MRI	CT is usually more readily available than MRI in the ED setting	Plain x-ray does not exclude injury CT is limited for soft tissue injury MRI can evaluate soft tissues and bony structures
Chest	Chest x-ray Chest CT	Pneumothorax, pulmonary contusion, rib fractures, pleural effusion, pneumomediastinum CT can better delineate injury seen on plain films	CT is contraindicated if the patient is unstable

Pericardial tamponade	Chest x-ray Echocardiogram	Enlarged heart may be seen on plain film Echocardiogram can better evaluate size of fluid collection
Renal	CT with contrast	Renal laceration, fracture or pedicle avulsion Consider delayed scans or delayed abdominal film (after IV contrast injection) to assess bladder (Foley must be clamped beforehand)
Soft tissue foreign body	Plain films Ultrasound	Most glass is radiopaque and will be seen on x-ray

not affect the ED management. However, radiographs might confirm (or help eliminate) the diagnosis of acute sinusitis in a patient with frontal headache and infraorbital swelling, but without purulent rhinorrhea or facial tenderness.

• Consult with a member of the radiology department prior to ordering a test, particularly when the patient's presentation is not straightforward. Discuss the child's signs and symptoms to determine, with the radiologist, the best test or sequence of tests to perform. This may vary by institution or time of day, based on the availability of equipment and expertise of the personnel.

• Inform the radiologist, either in person or when ordering the test, of the location of the patient's findings as well as the tentative diagnosis. Never simply write, for example, "rule-out pneumonia" when ordering a chest radiograph. Instead, specify the pertinent history and the nature of the physical findings.

• When ordering radiographic studies for children, limiting the amount of radiation exposure is a critical consideration. Younger patients are at greater risk for radiation damage and have a longer life span during which time sequelae such as cancer can develop. Always use a non-ionizing study if it will yield the answer to your question (i.e., think ultrasound before CT).The natural background radiation exposure in one year is approximately 3 mSv (millisieverts). Among the more common radiographic studies, the exposure is: chest x-ray (PA and lateral), 0.16 mSv; abdominal x-ray, 0.25 mSv; adult abdominal CT, 10 mSv; and neonatal abdominal CT, 20 mSv. Note that, compared with an adult, a neonate's organs will receive twice the amount of radiation with an abdominal CT.

Table 21.2 contains suggested radiologic examinations when a patient presents with a particular finding or when a particular diagnosis is being considered.

Bibliography

Baker N, Woolridge D. Emerging concepts in pediatric emergency radiology. *Pediatr Clin North Am.* 2013;60(5):1139–1151.

Frush K. Why and when to use CT in children: perspective of a pediatric emergency medicine physician. *Pediatr Radiol.* 2014;44(Suppl. 3):409–413.

Miglioretti DL, Johnson E, Williams A, et al. The use of computed tomography in pediatrics and the associated radiation exposure and estimated cancer risk. *JAMA Pediatr.* 2013;167(8):700–707.

Mills AM, Raja AS, Marin JR. Optimizing diagnostic imaging in the emergency department. *Acad Emerg Med.* 2015;22(5):625–631.

Tomà P, Cannatà V, Genovese E, Magistrelli A, Granata C. Radiation exposure in diagnostic imaging: wisdom and prudence, but still a lot to understand. *Radiol Med.* 2017;122(3):215–220.

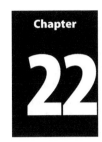
Renal Emergencies

Sandra J. Cunningham and Beatrice Goilav

Acute Glomerulonephritis

Acute glomerulonephritis (AGN) is a clinical syndrome caused by an immune-mediated injury to the glomerulus. Clinical features are reduction in glomerular filtration rate (GFR), oliguria or anuria, azotemia, proteinuria (possibly nephrotic range), microscopic or gross hematuria with RBC casts, pyuria, and evidence of volume overload (hypertension, peripheral edema, vascular congestion). The degree of renal dysfunction and azotemia can range from very mild (subclinical) to severe.

Most cases of AGN result from deposition of preformed immune complexes in glomerular structures (systemic lupus erythematosus [SLE]) or *in situ* fixation of complement and specific antibody with antigen trapped within glomeruli (post-infectious glomerulonephritis [PIGN]). Other forms of AGN are caused by activation of the classical or alternative complement pathway (membranoproliferative glomerulonephritis [MPGN]), direct antibody-mediated injury (Goodpasture's syndrome), or damage from infiltrated inflammatory cells (Wegener's granulomatosis).

Although hereditary nephritis (Alport syndrome) is considered a form of nephritis, it is caused by a genetic mutation resulting in a structural abnormality of the glomerular basement membrane with subsequent glomerular dysfunction. In IgA nephropathy (Berger's disease), deposition of IgA in the glomerular tuft leads to secondary inflammation. Systemic etiologies that can cause secondary renal injury, but are not a form of glomerulonephritis by definition, include vasculitis (Henoch–Schönlein purpura [HSP]), thrombotic microangiopathy (hemolytic-uremic syndrome [HUS]), subacute bacterial endocarditis (SBE), and shunt (ventriculoatrial) nephritis.

Clinical Presentation

As the GFR falls, oliguria/anuria ensues, leading to the clinical symptoms that are the hallmark of AGN: edema (gravity-dependent: periorbital in the morning and lower extremities in the evening), weight gain, hypertension (both systolic and diastolic), decreased urine output, and tea- or cola-colored urine due to gross hematuria (80% of patients). There may be constitutional symptoms, such as back or abdominal pain, and nausea and vomiting, in addition to the clinical features of the underlying disease. CNS symptoms such as lethargy, irritability, headache, mental status changes, and seizures may occur due to a rapid rise in blood pressure and/or azotemia. Water and salt retention can lead to congestive heart failure and pulmonary edema.

Post-Infectious Glomerulonephritis

The most common etiology of PIGN is Group A beta-hemolytic *Streptococcus* (GAS). The disease is most common in school-aged males and typically starts 1–3 weeks after a sore throat during winter months. Impetigo can precede nephritis by up to six weeks and this presentation is most frequently seen in preschool-aged children during the summer months. Onset of PIGN that is synchronous with pharyngitis is suggestive of IgA nephropathy, but may still be caused by GAS (synpharyngitic PIGN). The onset of the AGN is abrupt, with microscopic/macroscopic hematuria, periorbital edema, and mild–moderate hypertension. More than 90% of children with PIGN will have a full recovery.

Systemic Lupus Erythematosus

AGN with or without nephrotic syndrome can be the initial presentation of SLE. Other manifestations of the disease are also usually present, including weight loss, fatigue, rashes, polyserositis, or arthritis.

Henoch–Schönlein Purpura

HSP may present with a purpuric rash, abdominal pain, hematochezia, and arthritis (see pp. 683–684). Renal involvement is common, but usually is clinically silent.

Membranoproliferative Glomerulonephritis

MPGN causes an illness that may be indistinguishable from PIGN. However, it is more common in older children, particularly adolescent girls, and is characterized by persistent (more than six weeks) hypocomplementemia.

Alport's Syndrome

Alport's syndrome, which is associated with sensorineural and ocular disorders in males, can present with gross hematuria and can cause an acute decline in renal function during an intercurrent infection.

Diagnosis

Obtain a careful history, including whether there is a family history of persistent microscopic hematuria, hearing loss, autoimmune diseases, or kidney failure. On physical examination, check the blood pressure manually with an appropriate-sized cuff, note the presence of edema, examine the fundi, skin, heart, lungs, and joints, and assess hearing, mental status, and neurologic function.

If AGN is suspected, order a urinalysis. In glomerular disease, regardless of the etiology, dysmorphic RBCs and RBC casts are almost always present and are diagnostic of this disorder. In renal diseases associated with non-glomerular hematuria, such as nephrolithiasis, trauma, or a bleeding diathesis, the RBCs are eumorphic and RBC casts are not seen. If there is gross hematuria, examine an unspun urine specimen. WBCs may predominate over RBCs early in the course of the disease, suggesting the diagnosis of a urinary tract infection, but the urine culture remains negative. Proteinuria >2+ on a dipstick is virtually always present. Also obtain a CBC, platelet count, ESR, CRP, serum electrolytes, calcium, BUN, creatinine, total protein, albumin, cholesterol, triglycerides, and complement (C3, C4, C50). Hypocomplementemic forms of AGN include PIGN, MPGN, shunt nephritis, and embolic renal disease (SBE).

If the clinical picture is compatible with PIGN, obtain a throat culture, or a skin culture if the patient has impetigo. Antistreptolysin (ASLO) or streptozyme titers will be positive in PIGN caused by GAS, but will be negative with other infections. If SLE is a consideration, obtain an ANA and anti-dsDNA antibody titer.

ED Management

Consult a nephrologist for all patients with AGN. Immediate priorities include management of hypertension and hyperkalemia. Because hypertensive encephalopathy can occur at a minimally increased blood pressure, especially in PIGN, treat hypertension promptly and aggressively. For an asymptomatic patient, use oral nifedipine (0.25 mg/kg, 10 mg maximum). The onset of action of nifedipine is immediate after the patient bites the capsule and swallows its contents. For a slower reduction in BP in an asymptomatic patient, give amlodipine (0.1 mg/kg/dose), or if the child does not have a history of asthma, oral labetalol (2 mg/kg/dose).

For a patient with *acute* symptoms (headache, seizures, altered mental status, chest pain, blurred vision), treat with IV nicardipine or labetalol (contraindicated in asthma and pulmonary edema) (see Hypertension, pp. 684–688). The goal of the initial antihypertensive therapy is a 20% reduction in the mean blood pressure (diastolic BP + 1/3 [systolic BP – diastolic BP]).

The cornerstone of medical management is fluid and sodium restriction (see Acute Kidney Injury, pp. 674–679). Restrict fluids to insensible losses plus urine output, regardless of whether the patient is oliguric. Withhold potassium until the patient voids and eukalemia is documented (see Hyperkalemia, pp. 186–188). When the child can eat, limit the sodium to 2 g/day.

Conservative medical therapy is the rule, with renal replacement therapy reserved for severe volume overload with pulmonary edema, life-threatening hyperkalemia ($\geq$7 mEq/L), intractable acidosis, intractable hypocalcemia with seizures, or symptomatic uremia (pleuritis, pericarditis, GI bleeding, encephalopathy).

Follow-up

- Normotensive patient with mild edema, and normal urine output: the next day for a BP check. Ongoing follow-up is needed until the blood pressure and complements normalize and proteinuria resolves.

Indications for Admission

- AGN with pulmonary edema, hypertension, or oliguria.

Bibliography

Davin JC, Coppo R. Henoch–Schönlein purpura nephritis in children. *Nat Rev Nephrol.* 2014;**10** (10):563–573.

Eison TM, Ault BH, Jones DP, Chesney RW, Wyatt RJ. Post-streptococcal acute glomerulonephritis in children: clinical features and pathogenesis. *Pediatr Nephrol.* 2011;**26**(2):165–180

Kambham N. Postinfectious glomerulonephritis. *Adv Anat Pathol.* 2012;**19**(5):338–347.

VanDeVoorde RG 3rd. Acute poststreptococcal glomerulonephritis: the most common acute glomerulonephritis. *Pediatr Rev.* 2015;**36**(1):3–12.

Table 22.1 Classification of acute kidney injury

Prerenal	Postrenal	Renal
Mechanism		
Hypotension	Obstruction – mechanical	Ischemia
Hypovolemia	Obstruction – functional	Glomerulonephritis
Hypoxia		Nephrotoxin
Etiologies		
Anaphylaxis	Neurogenic (HSV, MS, spina bifida)	Antibiotics (amphotericin, gentamicin, vancomycin)
Antihypertensives	Intra-abdominal tumor	Acute interstitial nephritis
Burn	Posterior urethral valves	ATN not treated expeditiously
Cardiopulmonary arrest	Renal vein thrombosis	Heavy metals
Congestive heart failure		Myo- or hemoglobinuria
Dehydration		
Hemorrhage		
Hyperthermia		
Sepsis		

ATN: acute tubular necrosis; HSV: herpes simplex virus; MS: multiple sclerosis

Acute Kidney Injury

Acute kidney injury (AKI; formerly acute renal failure) is characterized by an acute decrease in the glomerular filtration rate (GFR), associated with increases in blood urea nitrogen and serum creatinine concentrations (azotemia). Oliguria (≤ 0.5 mL/kg/h) is a frequent, but not invariable, finding.

The causes of AKI can be divided into three pathophysiologic categories: prerenal, postrenal, and renal parenchymal disease (Table 22.1). Prerenal AKI reflects a decline in renal function in the absence of primary structural injury. It is a consequence of inadequate kidney perfusion secondary to hypovolemia (dehydration or blood loss), hypotension, or ischemia/hypoxia. The GFR is rapidly restored to normal when renal blood flow is increased; however, severe renal hypoperfusion may lead to acute tubular necrosis (ATN). Postrenal AKI is secondary to urinary tract obstruction affecting both kidneys (i.e., at the level of the bladder or the urethra). Intrarenal AKI can result from glomerular diseases (AGN, HUS), or tubular injury secondary to nephrotoxins, rhabdomyolysis, or tubular ischemia, as well as acute interstitial nephritis.

Clinical Presentation

The clinical presentation of AKI depends on the etiology, but signs of significant renal dysfunction such as fluid overload, hypertension, nausea and vomiting, hypocalcemic tetany, as well as neurologic symptoms (coma, seizures) can occur in all forms. Prerenal

AKI is suggested by loss of peripheral pulses, prolonged capillary refill time or hypotension (hypovolemic shock), lethargy and fever (sepsis), cutaneous burns, or bleeding. Difficulty voiding and an abnormal urinary stream (obstruction) suggest postrenal AKI. Illnesses associated with jaundice (hemoglobinuria), rhabdomyolysis (myoglobinuria), pallor and bloody diarrhea (HUS), rash, abdominal pain, arthralgias (HSP), or gross hematuria in the context of an antecedent sore throat or URI (PIGN) are associated with intrarenal AKI.

Diagnosis

Make a rapid assessment of the patient's volume status, looking for clinical signs of dehydration (orthostatic vital sign changes, poor capillary refill, weak peripheral pulses, cool extremities, hypotension) or volume overload (edema, rales, palpable liver, cardiac gallop). It is essential to identify the cause of oliguria as quickly as possible and to institute immediate treatment. Prerenal azotemia is a reversible condition early in its course, but failure to recognize a prerenal etiology (hypovolemia) can lead to ATN.

Estimate the GFR by using the modified Schwartz formula:

$$GFR = [\text{the patient's height(in cm)} \times k]/\text{serum Cr(in mg/dL)}.$$

The constant k depends on age and sex of the patient; LBW infants: $k = 0.33$; AGA and term infants: $k = 0.45$; children; and adolescent females: $k = 0.55$, adolescent males: $k = 0.7$.

An increase in creatinine of 0.3 mg/dL from baseline is suspicious for kidney injury, despite a serum creatinine level that is still within the range of normal

If the patient is unable or unwilling to void spontaneously, insert a Foley catheter to obtain urine and monitor the urine output. To differentiate among the causes of oliguria, obtain urine for specific gravity, sodium and creatinine, and microscopy. Look for blood, protein, and RBC casts (AGN) or pyuria >5 WBC/hpf). Concentrated urine with a high specific gravity is a feature of prerenal AKI, while isosthenuria with a specific gravity ≤1.010 and few or no cells or proteinuria is seen in interstitial nephritis. Hematuria on dipstick examination, but without RBCs seen on microscopy, is consistent with myoglobinuria or hemoglobinuria. Hematuria with macroscopic clots or microscopic crystals suggests kidney stones.

Obtain blood for electrolytes, BUN, and creatinine. Calculate the fractional excretion of sodium (FE_{Na}, Table 22.2):

$$[(\text{Urine Na/Plasma Na})]/[(\text{Urine Cr/Plasma Cr})]$$

When urine is unavailable or the urinary findings are pending, but there is *no evidence of volume overload* and *obstruction has been ruled out* (sonogram), attempt to discriminate intrarenal AKI from prerenal azotemia by rapidly infusing 20 mL/kg of an isotonic solution (normal saline). If oliguria persists and there are no signs of volume overload, repeat the bolus until it is clear that the patient is not volume-depleted (based on vital signs and capillary refill). If there is no diuresis, place a Foley catheter and give one dose of IV furosemide (1–2 mg/kg; higher doses increase the risk of ototoxicity). If oliguria continues, the diagnosis of *intrinsic renal disease* (frequently ATN) is probable. If urine output increases with these measures, the patient has *prerenal insufficiency*, which will return to normal provided adequate maintenance fluid therapy is given. If a sonogram cannot be obtained immediately, a distended bladder suggests a *postrenal* problem.

Table 22.2 Laboratory findings in acute kidney injury

Diagnosis	U_{SG}[1]	U_{NA}[2] (mEq/L)	BUN/Cr[3]	FENA[4] (%)	U/A[5]
Acute glomerulonephritis (early)	>1.020	<20	>20	<1	RBC casts, dysmorphic RBCs
Acute tubular necrosis	1.008–1.012	>40	<20	>1	Tubular epithelial cells
Prerenal azotemia	>1.020	<20	>20	<1	Nonspecific
Postrenal	1.008–1.012	>40	<20	>1	Nonspecific

[1] U_{SG} = urine specific gravity.
[2] U_{Na} = urine sodium concentration.
[3] BUN/Cr = ratio of BUN to creatinine.
[4] FENA = fractional excretion of sodium; $(U_{Na} \times P_{Cr})/(P_{Na} \times U_{Cr})$.
[5] U/A = typical urinalysis finding.

ED Management

Prerenal AKI

See above.

Intrarenal AKI

Fluid

If a hemodynamically stable patient remains oliguric, fluid restriction is required: Limit fluids to insensible losses plus urine output. Estimate insensible losses to be 400 mL/m^2/day; losses are higher with fever and burns and lower with mechanical ventilation.

Sodium

If the patient is dehydrated and hyponatremic, the goal is to correct the sodium to at least 135 mEq/L. In a patient with sodium >120 mEq/L, restore the deficit slowly, (2–4 mEq/L q 4h) using the following calculation for the sodium deficit:

$$(135 \text{–patient's sodium}) \times (\text{body weight in kg}) \times 0.6 = \text{mEqNa}.$$

Obtain repeat electrolytes every 3–4 hours and adjust the correction rate as needed.

Initiate a rapid correction for patients who are seizing, or are symptomatic and have a sodium <120 mEq/L. Administer hypertonic (3%) saline, which contains 513 mEq/L of Na (every 2 mL contains 1 mEq Na). Calculate the amount of 3% NaCl as follows:

$$3\% \text{ NaCl(mEq/L)} = (125 \text{–measured Na}) \times \text{body weight(kg)} \times 0.6$$

Multiply this result by 2 to determine the volume in mL.

Potassium

Hyperkalemia often occurs in AKI as a result of renal dysfunction and an acidosis-induced shift of potassium to the extracellular space. Dietary restriction (1 g/day) is sufficient if the potassium is <6 mEq/L. If the potassium is ≥6 mEq/L, immediately obtain an ECG to identify cardiac conduction abnormalities such as peaked T-waves (T-wave ≥ one-half the R- or S-wave) and a shortened QT interval. Later changes include lengthening of the PR interval and QRS duration.

The treatment of hyperkalemia primarily entails enhancing potassium excretion or increasing the movement of potassium into cells as a temporary measure, as well as minimizing cardiac effects. Aggressive IV therapy is necessary for patients who are symptomatic (muscle weakness or cramps/tetany) or have ECG changes. Give 0.5–1 g/kg of glucose (2–4 mL/kg of a 25% dextrose solution) over 30 minutes *concurrently with* regular insulin (1 unit per 5 g of glucose given). The potassium-lowering effect occurs in 10–20 minutes, but carefully monitor the serum glucose for both hyper- and hypoglycemia. In an infant, IV dextrose alone may be sufficient. Nebulized β-agonists, such as albuterol, are also effective at shifting potassium into the cells, but are less predictable than other therapies. The peak effect is 40–80 minutes after administration. The dose is 10–20 mg in 4 mL normal saline (4–8 times the dose used for the treatment of asthma).

In the absence of peaked T-waves, treat with polystyrene sulfonate (Kayexalate), 1 g/kg dissolved in 4 mL of water, with sorbitol (PO or PR). This dose lowers the serum potassium by 0.5–1 mEq/L by enhancing GI excretion, but the onset is slow and duration is variable. In a patient who is not anuric, give furosemide (1–2 mg/kg). The onset of action is within one hour, and the dose may be repeated every six hours.

Calcium

In a patient with hyperkalemia, calcium will stabilize the myocardium without affecting the serum potassium level. If there are EKG changes or a cardiac arrhythmia is noted, give IV 10% calcium gluconate solution (100 mg/kg), which will be effective in 1–3 minutes. Do not exceed a rate of 100 mg/min. Complications include hypercalcemia and bradycardia; continuously monitor the EKG, and stop the calcium if the patient becomes bradycardic. Use the same regimen to treat hypocalcemia causing tetany, laryngospasm, arrhythmias, or seizures. When the symptoms have resolved, add maintenance calcium to the IV solution (100 mg elemental calcium/kg/day).

Bicarbonate

Sodium bicarbonate may be helpful for severe acidosis, but do not use it just to lower the serum potassium. To correct acidosis, use the following equation:

$$\text{mEq bicarbonate} = (\text{desired} - \text{observed bicarbonate}) \times \text{patient weight(kg)} \times 0.5$$

Dialysis

Absolute indications for dialysis include life-threatening hyperkalemia (serum potassium ≥7 mEq/L) not responsive to pharmacological treatment, anuria, intractable acidosis, symptomatic volume overload (CHF, pulmonary edema), and symptomatic uremia (pleuritis, pericarditis, encephalopathy, GI bleeding).

Hypertension

Hypertension is frequent in AKI and may be mild and asymptomatic or life-threatening. Treat mild hypertension with salt restriction and oral antihypertensives, but more severe hypertension requires IV medication (pp. 686–687) and dialysis when secondary to fluid overload.

Postrenal AKI

Immediately consult with a urologist to determine the appropriate therapy.

Indications for Admission

- Acute kidney injury, except for patients with prerenal etiologies who have responded to fluid therapy and can maintain hydration status

Bibliography

Alobaidi R, Basu RK, Goldstein SL, Bagshaw SM. Sepsis-associated acute kidney injury. *Semin Nephrol.* 2015;35(1):2–11.

Fortenberry JD, Paden ML, Goldstein SL. Acute kidney injury in children: an update on diagnosis and treatment. *Pediatr Clin North Am.* 2013;60(3):669–688.

Kumar G, Vasudevan A. Management of acute kidney injury. *Indian J Pediatr.* 2012;79(8):1069–1075.

Merouani A, Flechelles O, Jouvet P. Acute kidney injury in children. *Minerva Pediatr.* 2012;**64** (2):121–133.

Shah SR, Tunio SA, Arshad MH, et al. Acute kidney injury recognition and management: a review of the literature and current evidence. *Glob J Health Sci.* 2015;**8**(5):120–124.

Hematuria

Hematuria is defined as ≥2–5 RBCs/hpf in fresh unspun urine or ≥5–10 RBCs/hpf in centrifuged fresh urine. Up to 5% of school-age children have microscopic hematuria on a single specimen, and 1–2% have this finding subsequently confirmed. The incidence increases with age and is greater in girls. Gross hematuria reflects RBCs in the urine that are visible upon inspection.

Hematuria can be classified as either traumatic or non-traumatic in origin. Non-traumatic hematuria can be divided into upper and lower genitourinary tract. Upper tract bleeding usually refers to glomerular causes, but can be of non-glomerular origin (e.g., papillary necrosis in a patient with sickle cell disease).

Clinical Presentation

Traumatic Bleeding

See Renal and Genitourinary Trauma, pp. 299–302.

Non-Traumatic Bleeding

Lower Genitourinary Tract

Lower urinary tract bleeding is most often caused by a urinary tract infection (UTI) and is usually accompanied by suprapubic pain and dysuria. A bacterial UTI presents with urgency, frequency, pyuria, and bacteriuria, although these signs and symptoms are often absent in the infant or young child. Viral cystitis (adenovirus) can occur in association with URI symptoms and is accompanied by fever, suprapubic tenderness, and gross hematuria. Urine cultures will be negative, and the hematuria resolves within 5–7 days without any specific treatment. Schistosomiasis is a parasitic cause of terminal microscopic and gross hematuria in recent immigrants from or travelers to endemic areas (sub-Saharan Africa, the Middle East). A stool sample is needed to detect characteristic eggs.

A urethral foreign body typically presents with dysuria in an afebrile toddler. Urolithiasis can present with microscopic or gross hematuria and intense renal colic. Often the patient has a history of urinary tract abnormalities or infections. Some drugs (cyclophosphamide, ifosfamide) are toxic to the bladder and can cause hemorrhagic cystitis.

Upper Genitourinary Tract – Glomerular

Hallmarks of glomerular bleeding, which may be microscopic or gross, include RBC casts and dysmorphic RBCs, with or without proteinuria. In addition, edema, hypertension, and oliguria can occur (see Glomerulonephritis, pp. 671–673). There may be a history of a sore throat or impetigo in the previous two weeks or 1–2 days (IgA nephropathy). A family history of early deafness and renal disease predominantly in males defines X-linked Alport's syndrome (hereditary nephritis). Palpable purpura of the lower extremities, abdominal pain, hematochezia, and arthralgias occur with HSP (pp. 683–684). Hematuria can be the presenting sign of SLE (pp. 709–711), although generally there are associated findings (malar rash, polyserositis, arthritis, hematologic abnormalities).

Upper Genitourinary Tract – Non-Glomerular

Urinary RBCs are eumorphic and RBC casts are absent. Sickle cell trait is associated with gross or microscopic hematuria without other obvious manifestations of renal disease. Wilms' tumor can cause gross hematuria in children under six years of age, although the most common presentation complaint is an abdominal mass.

Congenital and anatomic abnormalities such as polycystic kidney disease, renal hemangioma, and hydronephrosis can also present with hematuria after minor blunt abdominal trauma. Compression of the left renal vein between the aorta and the proximal superior mesenteric artery (nutcracker syndrome), can cause asymptomatic hematuria or left flank pain. Idiopathic hypercalciuria, in the absence of urolithiasis, is a common cause of non-glomerular painless hematuria, which can be microscopic or gross. There is often a positive family history of urolithiasis.

Diagnosis

Hematuria must be confirmed by microscopic examination of the urine, since not all red urine and not all dipstick-positive urine contains RBCs. Foodstuffs such as beets, red dyes, and drugs such as rifampin and phenazopyridine can give the urine a red tint. In infants, urate crystals may stain the diaper pink. A false-positive urine dipstick can occur if there is free hemoglobin or myoglobin in the specimen. In addition, hematuria may be incorrectly diagnosed when a menstruating female provides a voided urine specimen.

Gross hematuria can be bright red, brown, or cola-colored. The urine sample from a patient with gross hematuria is always turbid due to the presence of RBCs. This is in contrast to pigmenturia due to myoglobin or hemoglobin, which can be differentiated by centrifugation of a sample of serum. A pink tinge is found with hemoglobin, whereas the serum is clear with myoglobin.

A careful urinalysis is critical for locating the source of the bleeding. With non-glomerular hematuria, the RBCs appear eumorphic. Gross non-glomerular hematuria may be associated with clots. With glomerular hematuria there usually are RBC casts, and the RBCs are dysmorphic. In gross hematuria of glomerular origin, the urine is cloudy and dark brown (cola- or tea-colored) and not associated with clots.

Idiopathic hypercalciuria is suggested by a spot urine Ca:Cr ratio >0.2 in children over two years of age, with slightly higher normal ratios in younger infants. Confirmation requires a 24-hour urine collection with a calcium excretion >4 mg/kg/day.

ED Management

Obtain a thorough history, including current symptoms (fever, dysuria, suprapubic pain, URI, pharyngitis, gastroenteritis, joint pain), recent genitourinary trauma, medication use, previous episodes of hematuria or sickle cell trait/disease, recent weight gain suggestive of edema, and family history of renal disease (hereditary nephritides such as Alport's syndrome). Priorities on the physical examination include measuring the blood pressure and evaluating the patient for rash or purpura, abdominal mass, signs of a bleeding disorder, edema, and arthritis.

Traumatic Hematuria

See Genitourinary Trauma, pp. 299–302.

Non-Traumatic Hematuria

In the absence of edema, hypertension, an abdominal mass, proteinuria, or oliguria, the work-up of non-traumatic hematuria can be performed on an outpatient basis. If the bleeding is non-glomerular, obtain a urine culture, sickle prep, and measurement of urinary calcium and creatinine. Order an ultrasound if there is gross hematuria. When there is isolated hematuria (no proteinuria) of glomerular origin, minimal testing is warranted. Obtain a BUN, creatinine, and C3 and C4 levels if there is a history of hematuria for more than six months or associated hypertension.

Admit patients with acute glomerulonephritis and fluid overload, hypertension, elevated BUN/creatinine, or oliguria. In addition to the initial work-up outlined above, further evaluation includes urine protein-to-creatinine ratio, serum albumin, serology (ANA, HIV, HBV, HCV), and consultation with a nephrologist. The management of acute kidney injury is detailed elsewhere (pp. 671–673).

Follow-up

- Non-traumatic hematuria (<50 RBC/hpf) with a normal physical examination and without signs of glomerulonephritis or renal dysfunction: primary care or nephrology follow-up in 2–4 weeks

Indications for Admission

- Acute glomerulonephritis with edema, hypertension, or oliguria
- Acute kidney injury
- Hematuria associated with an abdominal mass

Bibliography

Leung JC. Inherited renal diseases. *Curr Pediatr Rev.* 2014;**10**(2):95–100.

VanDeVoorde RG 3rd. Acute poststreptococcal glomerulonephritis: the most common acute glomerulonephritis. *Pediatr Rev.* 2015;**36**(1):3–12.

Vogt B. Nephrology update: glomerular disease in children. *FP Essent.* 2016;**444**:30–40.

Hemolytic-Uremic Syndrome

Hemolytic-uremic syndrome (HUS) is characterized by the triad of microangiopathic hemolytic anemia, thrombocytopenia, and AKI. Although the mortality from renal failure has decreased, renal sequelae occur in approximately 40% of patients. Late renal deterioration, with hypertension, proteinuria, and reduced renal function, can occur after apparent resolution of the disease. HUS is divided into two major subtypes: infection-associated (typical) and genetic (atypical).

The diarrheal form of HUS accounts for the majority of cases (>90%) and generally affects previously healthy children who have ingested foods contaminated with *E. coli* O157: H7 that produce a Shiga toxin. *Shigella, Salmonella, Yersinia,* and *Campylobacter* also have been implicated. Most patients are 1–10 years of age, with a peak incidence at 1–4 years of age. There is a seasonal pattern, with most cases occurring in the summer. Commonly associated foods include hamburger meat and unpasteurized dairy products or cider. Less frequently, typical HUS is associated with pneumonia due to *Streptococcus pneumoniae.*

Atypical HUS accounts for fewer than 10% of cases and tends to occur in younger patients (infants), with no seasonal predilection. There is no diarrheal prodrome, although an antecedent URI is often reported.

Clinical Presentation

In typical HUS, a generalized, toxin-mediated, thrombotic microangiopathy occurs, presenting as a diffuse colitis with abdominal pain and hematochezia or bloody diarrhea. The diarrhea prodrome lasts from 1–15 days, followed by a short period of recovery, and then the abrupt onset of pallor and/or jaundice. Fever is generally absent. Renal impairment presents with hypertension, hematuria, proteinuria, and oligo-anuria. Electrolyte disturbances are common and include metabolic acidosis and hyperkalemia. There may also be neurologic symptoms secondary to the microangio-pathy, uremia, and hypertension (headaches, coma, seizures), as well as manifestations of fluid overload (edema, hypertension, congestive heart failure). Petechiae may be present due to thrombocytopenia.

Diagnosis

Obtain a CBC with peripheral smear, PT/PTT, Coombs test, LDH, haptoglobin, electrolytes, bilirubin, BUN/Cr, urinalysis, and stool for antigen studies specific for *E. coli* O157:H7 (routine stool cultures will not detect *E. coli* O157:H7). Consistent laboratory features include a peripheral blood smear that shows intravascular hemolysis (schistocytes) and thrombocytopenia. Anemia can be severe with hemoglobin as low as 5 g/dL. Thrombocytopenia (generally <60,000/mm^3) is a consistent finding. The Coombs test is negative, and the PT, PTT, and coagulation factors are normal. LDH and bilirubin are elevated and haptoglobin is decreased, indicating intravascular hemolysis. BUN/Cr are elevated and the urinalysis is positive for blood and protein.

ED Management

Consult a nephrologist and hematologist, as management is supportive and specific to the patient's presentation. Transfuse packed RBCs for patients with an Hgb <6 g/dL to a conservative goal of 9 g/dL. Transfuse slowly to avoid further fluid overload and subsequent cardiac compromise. Platelet transfusions are not routinely needed and are indicated for patients with significant bleeding or if a surgical procedure is required. Manage fluid and electrolyte disturbances as for AKI (pp. 671–673). See the specific sections for the treatment of hypertension (pp. 684–688) and seizures (pp. 531–535). Indications for intensive care unit admission and dialysis include life-threatening laboratory abnormalities (severe hyperkalemia or acidosis), and symptoms that are refractory to medical therapy, such as, cardiopulmonary compromise from fluid overload, symptomatic uremia, or oliguria >24 hours.

Indications for Admission

- Suspected HUS.

Bibliography

Greenbaum LA. Atypical hemolytic uremic syndrome. *Adv Pediatr.* 2014;**61**(1):335–356.

Loirat C, Fakhouri F, Ariceta G, et al. An international consensus approach to the management of atypical hemolytic uremic syndrome in children. *Pediatr Nephrol.* 2016;**31**(1):15–39.

Scheiring J, Rosales A, Zimmerhackl LB. Clinical practice: today's understanding of the haemolytic uraemic syndrome. *Eur J Pediatr.* 2010;**169**:7–13.

Sperati CJ, Moliterno AR. Thrombotic microangiopathy: focus on atypical hemolytic uremic syndrome. *Hematol Oncol Clin North Am.* 2015;**29**(3):541–559.

Trachtman H. HUS and TTP in children. *Pediatr Clin North Am.* 2013;**60**(6):1513–1526.

Henoch–Schönlein Purpura

HSP is an immune-mediated small vessel vasculitis associated with IgA deposition. Ninety percent of cases occur in children 3–17 years of age (peak incidence at 4–6 years of age). Patients present with one or more of the following: a purpuric rash on the extensor surfaces of the lower extremities and buttocks, abdominal pain, hematochezia, and arthritis/arthralgias of the large joints, although not all of these features may be present at the same time. There is often a history of a preceding URI. The most common etiologies are Group A *Streptococcus*, parvovirus, adenovirus, and *Mycoplasma*. Renal involvement may be the initial manifestation of HSP, or the nephritis can develop after other features of the disease have resolved.

Clinical Presentation

The clinical symptoms are a consequence of the small vessel damage occurring in the skin, GI tract, and kidneys. The rash may initially be urticarial. It then evolves into a palpable purpura that occurs in crops on the lower extremities, especially the buttocks and extensor surfaces. Colicky abdominal pain and hematochezia may also be present. The most common gastrointestinal (GI) complication of HSP is intussusception, most often ileoileal.

Arthralgias usually occur in the large joints of the lower extremities (knees, hips, ankles). There may be significant limited range of motion with swelling and tenderness. The joint involvement may precede the skin manifestations by a few days.

Renal involvement occurs in 25–50% of children within four weeks of presentation. It can range from isolated microscopic or gross hematuria with or without low-grade proteinuria to nephrotic syndrome.

Scrotal edema or pain may also occur, although testicular torsion is extremely rare.

Diagnosis

The rash as described above is characteristic. Before the classic purpuric rash evolves, the diagnosis may be confused with other diseases that present with the similar symptom complex of rash, edema, arthralgias, abdominal complaints, and renal findings.

In Wegener's granulomatosis the majority of patients present with upper airway complaints such as persistent rhinorrhea, purulent nasal discharge, or sinus pain. In SLE about one-third of patients present with the classic malar rash and hematologic abnormalities are common, including anemia or thrombocytopenia.

Acute hemorrhagic edema of infancy (AHEI) is a small vessel vasculitis that occurs in patients under two years of age. It can present with edema, including of the scalp, associated with palpable purpura in a distribution that differs from HSP (face, ears, limbs). There is no renal involvement.

Pay close attention to the blood pressure. Obtain a CBC, ESR, CRP, PT/PTT, IgA, complement levels, BUN and creatinine, and a throat culture. Complement levels, platelet count, and PT/PTT will be normal in HSP. Also obtain urine for RBC casts, and urinary protein-to-creatinine ratio (abnormal if >0.2).

ED Management

Fluid management and the treatment of hypertension are similar to that for AGN (pp. 671–673) and require consultation with a nephrologist. Treat scrotal pain and edema with elevation and cool compresses. See pp. 273–275 for the evaluation and management of a possible intussusception. Steroids are not routinely indicated for outpatient treatment, but are helpful if the patient has severe abdominal pain without intussusception or severe joint involvement limiting ambulation. Use methylprednisolone 1 mg/kg/day for two weeks, 60 mg/day maximum.

Follow-up

- Primary care every 2–3 days until the blood pressure is normal and arthralgias are resolving
- Refer to a nephrologist if the patient required treatment for hypertension

Indications for Admission

- GI hemorrhage or compromise, protein-losing enteropathy, decreased GFR, or nephrotic-range proteinuria with hypertension
- Severe arthralgias interfering with weight bearing or ambulation

Bibliography

Bluman J, Goldman RD. Henoch–Schönlein purpura in children: limited benefit of corticosteroids. *Can Fam Physician*. 2014;**60**(11):1007–1010.

Chen JY, Mao JH. Henoch–Schönlein purpura nephritis in children: incidence, pathogenesis and management. *World J Pediatr*. 2015;**11**(1):29–34.

Davin JC, Coppo R. Henoch–Schönlein purpura nephritis in children. *Nat Rev Nephrol*. 2014;**10**(10):563–573.

Reid-Adam, J. Henoch–Schönlein purpura. *Pediatr Rev*. 2014;**35**(10):447–449.

Trnka P. Henoch–Schönlein purpura in children. *J Paediatr Child Health*. 2013;**49**(12):995–1003.

Hypertension

Hypertension is estimated to occur in about 5% of children between the ages of 8 and 17 years of age. An identifiable cause of secondary hypertension (mostly renal) is more common in children younger than ten years of age, whereas in older patients primary hypertension is the leading cause.

Table 22.3 Classification of systolic and diastolic blood pressures

Normortensive	<90th percentile
Elevated blood pressure	≥90th to <95th percentiles, or >120/80 (whichever is lower)
Hypertension	≥95th percentile, or
	<95th percentile + 12 mmHg, or
	≥130/80 (whichever is lower)

The evaluation of blood pressure in children is dependent on the individual's age, gender, and height. Use age-specific blood pressure tables adjusted for height (e.g., the *Harriet Lane Handbook*) to confirm the normal ranges of blood pressure in children. The classification of blood pressure in children is summarized in Table 22.3.

In the ED, hypertension is often an incidental finding and the elevation is generally mild. The ED is not the clinical setting for diagnosing hypertension, unless it is the chief complaint or the cause of the patient's symptoms (e.g., headache), so defer diagnostic testing to a primary care setting.

Hypertensive crisis requires immediate intervention. Hypertensive crises can be divided into "urgent" or "emergent," depending on whether there is end-organ dysfunction (i.e., seizures) as determined by the history, physical examination, or laboratory tests, rather than the absolute increase in the blood pressure. Emergent hypertension in children is unusual. It is most often caused by renal parenchymal disorders, renal vascular lesions, pheochromocytoma, and drug (accidental/intentional) ingestions.

Clinical Presentation

The clinical presentation of hypertension varies from asymptomatic to hypertensive encephalopathy and evidence of end-organ dysfunction. A patient with emergent hypertension has symptoms (disorientation, seizures) that can be ascribed to the increase in blood pressure, the blood pressure exceeds the 99th percentile in both upper extremities on at least two manual readings over ten minutes, or the primary disease demands emergency treatment (increased intracranial pressure, renal failure).

Otherwise, patients may present with headache, dizziness, vomiting, visual changes, ataxia, or obtundation. Hypertensive infants may present with nonspecific symptoms such as crying, irritability, respiratory distress, or congestive heart failure.

Diagnosis

It is imperative to choose the correct blood pressure cuff size, as a cuff that is too narrow will result in a falsely high reading. The bladder width should be 40% of the circumference of the arm at midpoint between the acromion and the olecranon, and the bladder length should cover 80–100% of the circumference of the arm. When the choice of cuff size is between one that is too small versus one that is too large, select the larger size cuff. If using an automated blood pressure device, repeat by auscultation using a manual device when the blood pressure measurement is >90th percentile.

Obtain a hypertension-oriented history: neonatal history (prematurity, umbilical line catheterization), congenital anomalies, medication use (sympathomimetics, oral contraceptives), illicit drug (cocaine) or alcohol use, cardiac or renal disease (especially hematuria or repeated episodes of pyelonephritis), history of pregnancy, the nature of any previous hypertensive episodes (particularly if sporadic), and a family history of hypertension, renal, cardiovascular, or endocrine disease, as well as stroke.

Useful physical examination findings include height, weight, and differential blood pressure and pulses between upper and lower extremities (found with coarctation of the aorta). Look for evidence of neurologic dysfunction; AV nicking, hemorrhages or papilledema on fundoscopy; heart murmur or pulmonary findings (rales) of CHF; as well as abdominal mass/bruits, skin lesions (purpura in HSP), or virilization. When the heart rate as well as the blood pressure is elevated, consider hyperthyroidism, neuroblastoma, or pheochromocytoma.

If a secondary cause of the hypertension is suspected (young children, significantly elevated blood pressure, physical examination abnormalities, or contributory family history), obtain a urinalysis, serum electrolytes, glucose, BUN and creatinine, chest x-ray, ECG, and a renal ultrasound. If an adrenal cause is suspected (virilization, Cushingoid appearance), obtain a serum cortisol and 17-hydroxyprogesterone. If there are symptoms suggestive of a pheochromocytoma (headache, sweating, nausea, vomiting, pallor), obtain a serum metanephrine level and a 24-hour urine collection for catecholamine excretion.

In general, defer the diagnostic evaluation of asymptomatic mild to moderate hypertension to a primary care setting where further testing can be done if sustained hypertension is confirmed by repeated measurements.

ED Management

Hypertensive Emergencies

See Table 22.4. Immediate parenteral therapy is required for severe hypertension associated with end-organ damage (seizures, encephalopathy, pulmonary edema). The goal of acute antihypertensive therapy is a decrease in BP by 25% over the first hour, and then down to normal within eight hours. Lowering the BP too quickly can potentially result in ischemic target-organ damage (cerebral ischemia), although this is more common in adults with preexisting cardiovascular disease. A continuous IV infusion with meticulous monitoring is the safest way to lower the blood pressure. Alternatively, IV boluses may be used, although these may lead to BP fluctuations, which may worsen end-organ damage. Establish IV access, institute continuous cardiac monitoring, and measure urine output. Nicardipine (see Table 22.4) is an effective first-line drug for hypertensive emergencies, especially when the patient's medical history is unknown (e.g., asthma, diabetes).

Hypertensive Urgencies

A patient with BP >99th percentile who is asymptomatic and without history, physical examination, or laboratory evidence of end-organ damage requires a slower reduction in blood pressure with the use of oral antihypertensives; hospitalization may not be required. If a patient with known hypertension presents with severe hypertension, give an oral antihypertensive and monitor in the ED for 4–6 hours. The use of a long-acting antihypertensive is warranted, because short-acting drugs could lead to profound hypotension and

Table 22.4 Antihypertensive treatment for emergent hypertension (IV) and urgent hypertension (oral)

Drug	Class	Route/dose	Comments
IV infusions for emergent hypertension			
Labetalol	α- and β-blocker	0.4–1 mg/kg/h	Contraindicated in asthma, CHF, pulmonary edema
		3 mg/kg/h maximum	May start with 0.2–1 mg/kg bolus (20 mg maximum)
			Onset 2–5 minutes
Nicardipine	Ca^{++} channel blocker	0.5 mcg/kg/min	Useful when etiology or history unknown (asthma, diabetes mellitus)
		Titrate to 2 mcg/kg/min	Onset 2–5 minutes
			Can cause ↑→HR
		3 mcg/kg/min maximum	
IV bolus for emergent hypertension			
Enalaprilat	ACE inhibitor	0.05–0.1 mg/kg/dose up to 1.25 mg/dose	Can cause prolonged hypotension and acute kidney injury, particularly in neonates and infants
Hydralazine	Vasodilator	0.1–0.2 mg/kg q 4h	Can cause ↑ or extended hypotension
		20 mg/dose maximum	Onset 5–20 min
Oral for urgent hypertension			
Amlodipine	Ca^{++} channel blocker	0.1–0.3 mg/kg/dose	Long-acting
			May require dose adjustments every seven days
Atenolol	β-antagonist	0.25–0.5 mg/kg/dose daily or bid	Cardioselective
			Can cause bradycardia
Clonidine	Central α-agonist	2.5–5 mcg/kg/dose tid	May initially cause sedation
			Reflex hypertension with abrupt discontinuation
Enalapril	ACE inhibitor	0.2 mg/kg/dose daily or bid	May cause cough and hyperkalemia
			Check electrolytes after one week
			Contraindicated in pregnancy
			May cause laryngeal edema (very rare)

Table 22.4 (cont.)

Drug	Class	Route/dose	Comments
Hydrochloro-thiazide	Thiazide diuretic	0.5–1 mg/kg/ dose daily or bid	Monitor electrolytes and triglycerides
Isradipine	Ca^{++} channel blocker	0.05–0.1 mg/ kg/dose	Stable suspension can be compounded
Labetalol	α- and β-blocker	1–1.5 mg/kg/ dose bid	Weak alpha-blockade in oral formulation
Minoxidil	Vasodilator	0.1–0.2 mg/kg daily	Contraindicated in pheochromocytoma
		5 mg/dose maximum	Onset 30 minutes; long-acting Hypertrichosis common

cerebral or myocardial ischemia. The goal is reduction of the blood pressure to the targeted normal in three steps, with the first occurring within the first 4–6 hours. Adequate follow-up must be in place to ensure that the patient's blood pressure is reduced by another one-third in 24–36 hours, and the final third by 96 hours.

Follow-up

- Asymptomatic or mild to moderate hypertension: primary care follow-up in 1–2 weeks
- Hypertensive urgency after BP control attained and with assurance of good follow-up: pediatric nephrologist in 24–36 hours for BP check and further evaluation

Indications for Admission

- Hypertensive emergency (intensive care unit)
- Symptomatic or severe hypertension (sustained systolic and/or diastolic >99th percentile for age and sex)
- Hypertension of any degree associated with acute glomerulonephritis, chronic renal failure, or other urgent underlying condition

Bibliography

American Academy of Pediatrics. The fourth report on the diagnosis, evaluation, and treatment of high blood pressure in children and adolescents. *Pediatrics*. 2004;114:555–576.

Anyaegbu EI, Dharnidharka VR. Hypertension in the teenager. *Pediatr Clin North Am*. 2014;**61**(1):131–151.

Daniels SR. Diagnosis and management of hypertension in children and adolescents. *Pediatr Ann*. 2012;**41**(7):1–10.

Engorn B, Flerlage J. *Johns Hopkins: Harriet Lane Handbook* (20th ed). Philadelphia, PA: Elsevier Saunders, 2015; 129–137.

Nephrolithiasis

Nephrolithiasis can be caused by either metabolic diseases or structural abnormalities. The most common metabolic causes of stones are hypocitraturia and hypercalciuria (calcium excretion >4 mg/kg/day), which is frequently idiopathic and results in the formation of calcium oxalate stones. Urinary tract abnormalities and, rarely, infections, are other etiologies. Stones composed of calcium phosphate, uric acid, struvite, and cystine are less common.

Clinical Presentation

The typical adult presentation of colicky flank pain radiating to the ipsilateral groin and hematuria is less common in children, although adolescents may present similarly with intermittent severe pain, nausea, and vomiting. Younger children may have vomiting, urinary symptoms (dysuria, hematuria, or frequency), or colicky abdominal pain. Infants may be misdiagnosed as colic due to nonspecific symptoms. Up to 90% of children in all age groups will have microscopic or gross hematuria.

Diagnosis

Elicit a detailed history, including medical history (cystic fibrosis, metabolic disorders, recent immobilization), dietary intake (soda, high protein), and a family history of nephrolithiasis, renal, or metabolic abnormalities. Ask about the onset, duration, and location of the pain, oral intake, medication use (loop diuretics), and intake of calcium. Useful physical examination findings include abdominal tenderness or mass and costovertebral angle tenderness. The presence of hypertension or edema with hematuria suggests an alternate diagnosis, such as glomerular disease.

Obtain a urinalysis (hematuria) and urine culture. Microscopy may be particularly helpful if crystals or stones are visualized. Also send a spot urine for calcium/creatinine ratio, which is normally <0.2 in children older than two years of age, but may be up to three-fold higher in younger infants. Confirmation requires a 24-hour urine collection with calcium excretion of >4 mg/kg/day.

Calcium oxalate stones can be identified on plain radiographs, but other types of stones are generally not seen. A sonogram can identify most stones >5 mm, including those that are radiolucent on plain film. The finding of unilateral hydronephrosis on a sonogram may also suggest a stone. If the diagnosis is not confirmed on ultrasound or plain radiographs, obtain a *noncontrast* CT scan, which is the most sensitive imaging study and will identify very small stones (1 mm).

ED Management

Hydration and analgesia are the priorities, regardless of the etiology. Give morphine (0.1–0.2 mg/kg, 15 mg maximum) and/or ketorolac (0.5 mg/kg IV, 30 mg maximum), and hydrate the patient orally, or IV if there is nausea, vomiting, or severe pain. Consult a urologist for urinary obstruction or stones >5 mm to determine whether urologic stone removal is necessary, via shock wave lithotripsy, percutaneous nephrolithotomy, or ureteroscopy. Discontinue the ketorolac three days prior to a urologic procedure to minimize the risk of bleeding. Stones <5 mm often pass spontaneously. Instruct the patient and family to collect or strain the urine and arrange urology follow-up so that the stone can be analyzed. If the stone passes unnoticed, a 24-hour urine collection can reveal the underlying cause of stone formation.

Follow-Up

- Urology referral within 1–2 weeks. At that time a 24-hour urine collection will be helpful to evaluate for an underlying metabolic cause of stone formation if no anatomical abnormality can be identified.

Indications for Admission

- Inability to tolerate oral hydration or pain medications
- Severe pain recalcitrant to pain medications in the ED
- Urinary obstruction or infection
- Surgical stone removal required

Bibliography

Cambareri GM, Kovacevic L, Bayne AP, et al. National multi-institutional cooperative on urolithiasis in children: age is a significant predictor of urine abnormalities. *J Pediatr Urol.* 2015; **11**:218–233.

Copelovitch L. Urolithiasis in children: medical approach. *Pediatr Clin North Am.* 2012;**59** (4):881–896.

Hernandez JD, Ellison JS, Lendvay TS. Current trends, evaluation, and management of pediatric nephrolithiasis. *JAMA Pediatr.* 2015;**169**(10):964–970.

Tasian GE, Copelovitch L. Evaluation and medical management of kidney stones in children. *J Urol.* 2014;**192**(5):1329–1336.

Proteinuria

Normal urine can contain small amounts of protein (<100 mg/m^2), while proteinuria in excess of this is abnormal. Qualitative proteinuria is prevalent (5–15% of normal individuals), since the urine dipstick is very sensitive to albumin (but not to low molecular weight proteins) and detects protein concentrations as low as 10–15 mg/dL. Transient proteinuria can be found incidentally in an otherwise healthy child with stress, fever, urine that is highly concentrated (specific gravity >1.025) or alkaline (pH >8.0), or after vigorous exercise. Orthostatic proteinuria is also a common finding in children. In contrast, false-negative results on urine dipstick can occur with very dilute urine.

Significant proteinuria (>2+ on dipstick) is defined as a urinary protein-to-creatinine ratio >0.2 on an early-morning specimen. This occurs in only 1–2% of patients. When proteinuria is ≥1+ by dipstick on several occasions, further investigation is warranted.

Clinical Presentation

Although fever can induce transient proteinuria, most often, proteinuria is an unexpected finding in a child being examined for an intercurrent illness. Edema, hypoalbuminemia

(<3 g/dL), hypercholesterolemia, apparent hypocalcemia (secondary to the decreased albumin), and ascites are findings of nephrotic syndrome. These patients are at increased risk for spontaneous bacterial peritonitis, usually caused by *Streptococcus pneumoniae*. In patients with isolated proteinuria or nephrotic syndrome, the blood pressure and renal function are normal, although urine output may be decreased. With renal disease such as glomerulonephritis, there may be edema, hypertension, oliguria, or associated microscopic hematuria.

Orthostatic proteinuria can be found in a urine sample collected later in the day, after the patient has been in an upright position for a prolonged period of time. This is a variant of normal and is often found in children and adolescents.

Nephrotic Syndrome

The nephrotic syndrome is defined as edema, hypoalbuminemia (<3 g/dL), hyperlipidemia, and heavy proteinuria with a urinary protein/creatinine ratio >2. A glomerular protein leak is the primary disturbance in this syndrome. The edema, which can become generalized, usually begins in the periorbital region and may be the primary complaint. In contrast to AGN, the GFR is usually normal, although patients are at risk for electrolyte disturbances, infections (cellulitis, spontaneous bacterial peritonitis), pleural effusions, and thromboembolism (due to the loss of antithrombotic factors).

The nephrotic syndrome is classified as primary (no systemic disease) or secondary (associated with a systemic disease or another glomerular injury, such as post-infectious AGN, SLE). Although there are numerous causes of nephrotic syndrome, minimal change disease (MCD) causes 75% of cases in childhood, with a peak incidence at 2–5 years of age. Patients with MCD are normotensive, have normal complement levels, no hematuria, and (by definition) will respond to glucocorticoid therapy. Other primary causes are focal segmental glomerulosclerosis (often associated with hypertension), membranoproliferative glomerulonephritis, and membranous nephropathy, which occur at a later age.

Secondary causes include systemic disorders such as HSP, SLE and sickle cell disease, chronic infections (syphilis, HIV, hepatitis B), diabetes, and medications (penicillamine, nonsteroidal anti-inflammatory drugs).

Diagnosis

Since very few patients with dipstick-positive proteinuria truly have renal disease, in the absence of edema, hypertension, oliguria, or associated hematuria, merely arrange for the urinalysis to be repeated in 2–4 weeks. If the proteinuria persists, test the first voided morning specimen for protein-to-creatinine ratio. Instruct the patient to urinate prior to going to bed the night before. In orthostatic proteinuria the protein-to-creatinine ratio is normal (<0.2).

Consider causes other than MCD if the child is under one year old or older than 12, or if there are associated clinical findings, such as fever, rash, or arthralgias. A patient with associated microscopic hematuria is more likely to have glomerular disease, but up to 30% of children with MCD may have microscopic hematuria.

Although edema is a cardinal feature of the nephrotic syndrome, extrarenal causes of edema include cirrhosis, congestive heart failure, capillary leak syndrome, and protein-losing enteropathy. Significant proteinuria is absent in these conditions.

ED Management

A patient with edema, hypertension, oliguria, or associated gross hematuria requires an immediate and more complete evaluation, including serum electrolytes, BUN, calcium, creatinine and creatinine clearance, cholesterol, total protein and albumin, complement (C3, C4), ANA, VDRL, and serology for hepatitis B and C, and HIV testing (if clinically indicated).

Nephrotic Syndrome

Admit a patient with nephrotic syndrome who has moderate edema with hypertension or severe edema with inability to tolerate oral medications, or complications associated with nephrotic syndrome (peritonitis) and consult with a pediatric nephrologist to initiate therapy. For a patient who can be discharged, instruct the parents to restrict water intake and restrict salt intake by avoiding prepared foods and by reducing salt in home-cooked food.

Follow-up

- Patient with known nephrotic syndrome: nephrologist within one week
- Patient with newly diagnosed nephrotic syndrome: nephrologist within 1–2 days

Indications for Admission

- Proteinuria in association with signs or symptoms of renal disease (severe edema, hypertension, oliguria, electrolyte disturbances, infection, thromboembolism)
- Infant with nephrotic syndrome
- Suspected spontaneous bacterial peritonitis
- Significant gut edema that may interfere with enteral absorption of medication.

Bibliography

Andolino TP, Reid-Adam J. Nephrotic syndrome. *Pediatr Rev.* 2015;**36**(3):117–126

Greenbaum LA, Benndorf R, Smoyer WE. Childhood nephrotic syndrome: current and future therapies. *Nat Rev Nephrol.* 2012;**8**(8):445–458.

Hahn D, Hodson EM, Willis NS, Craig JC. Corticosteroid therapy for nephrotic syndrome in children. *Cochrane Database Syst Rev.* 2015;**3**:CD001533.

Samuel S, Bitzan M, Zappitelli M, et al. Canadian Society of Nephrology commentary on the 2012 KDIGO clinical practice guideline for glomerulonephritis: management of nephrotic syndrome in children. *Am J Kidney Dis.* 2014;**76**(3):354–362.

Sinha A, Bagga A. Nephrotic syndrome. *Indian J Pediatr.* 2012;**79**(8):1045–1055.

Urinary Tract Infections

Overall, urinary tract infections (UTIs) occur in approximately 2–3% of children annually. Uncircumcised boys under one year of age have a higher incidence of UTIs than girls, but in all other age groups, girls have a higher incidence. Uncircumcised boys under six months of age have a 10–12-fold relative risk of having a UTI compared to circumcised boys. The two most common types of infection are cystitis (infection confined to the bladder) and pyelonephritis (infection in the renal parenchyma). The most frequent etiology is *E. coli*; other causative organisms include *Klebsiella, Pseudomonas, Enterococcus, Staphylococcus saprophyticus*, and *S. epidermidis*, which are not contaminants if cultured repeatedly, particularly in adolescent girls. *Proteus* is an important pathogen in uncircumcised boys, but in girls it is less common and may be a contaminant. In addition, UTIs due to *group B Streptococci* can occur in neonates.

Clinical Presentation

The presentation in infancy is nonspecific and includes poor feeding, vomiting, diarrhea, irritability, jaundice, and seizures. From one month to two years, fever is more common, and some urologic symptoms (change in voiding pattern, foul-smelling urine) occur. Preschool- and school-aged children usually have specific urologic complaints, such as frequency, urgency, dysuria, suprapubic pain, hematuria, and enuresis. Less specific symptoms, such as abdominal pain and vomiting, may be seen in this age group as well. Higher fever (>38.5 °C; 101.3 °F), flank (CVA) tenderness, and systemic toxicity are consistent with pyelonephritis.

Diagnosis

Traditionally, the amount of bacterial growth required for the diagnosis of UTI is $>10^5$ CFU/mL in a midstream clean-catch urine. This definition is a statistical one, indicating an 80% chance of true infection, so that two consecutive positive cultures increase the likelihood of infection to 95%, In addition, a culture with a pure growth of $>10^3$ CFU/mL from a suprapubic specimen and $>10^4$ in a catheterized specimen in the context of symptoms associated with UTI may be indicative of infection. Prompt plating of the specimen is as important as meticulous cleaning of the perineum and urethral meatus for reducing the frequency of false-positive urine cultures. If the urine specimen cannot be plated immediately, refrigerate at 4 °C (39.2 °F) to prevent over-growth of contaminating bacteria. A bagged urine specimen is unreliable unless the culture demonstrates no growth.

Although the urinalysis is a useful screening test in the ED, abnormal findings are not sufficient for a definitive diagnosis. If a complete urinalysis is normal (including dipstick testing for leukocyte esterase and nitrite, and microscopic examination for bacteriuria), the likelihood that the patient *does not* have a UTI exceeds 95%. The presence of bacteriuria and pyuria (>10 WBC/hpf) has a positive predictive value over 84%, although in some culture-proven UTIs, pyuria may be absent. Alternatively, only 50% of patients with WBCs in the urine have a culture-proven UTI, as pyuria can occur with infections near but outside the urinary tract (appendicitis), glomerulonephritides, and viral infections of the urinary tract. With a UTI, proteinuria and hematuria are often present, and the leukocyte esterase is generally positive on dipstick testing.

The dipstick nitrite test has a low sensitivity in infants and young children who void frequently, as the urine must remain in the bladder for at least four hours for bacteria to produce nitrite. Also, Gram-positive organisms do not reduce nitrates to nitrites so the dipstick will be negative.

In the symptomatic child, the presence of any organisms on Gram's stain of an uncentrifuged urine correlates with a colony count $>10^5$/mL, and is presumptive evidence of a UTI, with higher sensitivity, specificity, and positive predictive value than urinalysis and dipstick. The urine culture, however, remains the definitive diagnostic test.

WBC casts (not clumps) are usually diagnostic of pyelonephritis. Other laboratory findings with pyelonephritis are leukocytosis (WBC >15,000/mm^3) and an elevated sedimentation rate (>30 mm/h) or CRP.

Symptoms of a UTI are not sufficient for a definitive diagnosis. Dysuria, frequency, and urgency among patients with suprapubic tenderness and gross hematuria without pyuria or bacteriuria suggest viral cystitis or idiopathic hypercalciuria. The same findings in a patient with pyuria but no hematuria are compatible with the dysuria–pyuria (acute urethral) syndrome. The symptoms of vaginitis and balanitis can mimic a UTI. Negative urine cultures are necessary to confirm these diagnoses.

The coexistence of another source for fever, such as a URI, does not exclude the possibility of a UTI. Consider UTI for all children under two years of age with fever, and girls of any age with fever without an identifiable source for more than 2–3 days.

ED Management

Inspect the external genitalia for signs of inflammation or infection (epididymitis, epididymo-orchitis, vaginitis), and measure the blood pressure. Examine the sacral region for abnormalities such as a dimple or pit, which may indicate a neurogenic bladder. Obtain a catheterized or suprapubic urine specimen for culture from a patient who lacks bladder control, has evidence of vaginitis, or is unable to provide an adequate midstream specimen. A bagged specimen can be used for a screening urinalysis if the clinical condition of the child does not warrant immediate antimicrobial therapy. If the urinalysis suggests an infection, obtain a suprapubic or catheterized urine specimen for culture. In an older child or adolescent, when a midstream specimen is used, collect samples from two separate voids to increase the likelihood of a noncontaminated culture. A large number of epithelial cells in the specimen suggests contamination. The finger-tap method is an alternative noninvasive method for obtaining midstream urine in infants.

After urine cultures are obtained, treat a nontoxic patient with signs or symptoms and microscopy results consistent with a urinary tract infection on an outpatient basis if the patient has adequate fluid intake, is not vomiting, and reliable follow-up can be assured. Give the first dose of antibiotics in the ED in order to assess the patient's ability to tolerate the medication. Base empiric treatment on the most likely uropathogen and the prevailing local resistance patterns. There are increasing rates of E. coli resistance to trimethoprim-sulfamethoxazole, amoxicillin, ampicillin, and first-generation cephalosporins (cephalexin). Therefore, start with amoxicillin-clavulanate (45 mg/kg/day div q 12h). Other empiric therapeutic agents include cefixime (16 mg/kg/day div q 12h on day 1, followed by 8 mg/kg/day div q 24h, 400 mg/day maximum) or cefdinir (14 mg/kg/day div q 12–24h, 600 mg/day maximum). Treat for a 7–10-day course.

Treat an afebrile, nonpregnant adolescent girl with an uncomplicated lower-tract infection (symptoms for fewer than three days) and a normal urinary tract, with ciprofloxacin 250 mg bid for three days. This therapy may be especially useful when compliance with a ten-day oral regimen is not assured. Three-day treatment is inadequate for infants, children, and febrile adolescent girls. Treat pregnant adolescents >12 years of age with nitrofurantoin (100 mg bid for seven days). Tailor subsequent antibiotic therapy according to culture and sensitivity results when available. Repeat urine cultures are not necessary when the patient has the expected response to the appropriate therapy.

Prescribe oral phenazopyridine (Pyridium) for short-term use (under two days) in children six years old onwards to treat symptoms of burning, urgency, and frequency. Give 4 mg/kg/dose tid with food. Inform the patient that the urine may become orange and the drug may discolor contact lenses.

Indications for admission and IV antibiotics include toxic appearance, inability to tolerate oral intake (including antibiotics), dehydration, immunocompromise, or adherence to treatment and/or follow-up seems unlikely. Also admit an infant under three months old, regardless of clinical appearance. Treat as follows.

<4 Weeks of Age

Perform a full evaluation for sepsis (pp. 391–392) and treat with ampicillin (<1 week of age: 100 mg/kg/day, div q 12h; >1 week of age: 200 mg/kg/day, div q 6h) *and* cefotaxime (<1 week: 100 mg/kg/day, div q 12h; 1–4 weeks: 150 mg/kg/day, div q 8h).

≥4 Weeks to Three Months of Age

Admit the patient and treat with ceftriaxone 100 mg/kg/day div q 12h. Obtain a CBC and blood culture, but complete a full sepsis work-up if the infant appears ill.

≥3 Months of Age

Indications for admission and treatment with ceftriaxone (50 mg/kg/day) include toxic appearance, inability to tolerate oral intake (including antibiotics), dehydration, immuno-compromise, risk for pyelonephritis (known high-grade reflux, abnormal GU anatomy), failed outpatient therapy (patient remains febrile after >72 hours of antibiotics), or unreliable adherence to treatment and/or follow-up. Otherwise outpatient management (as above) will suffice.

Radiologic Evaluation

It is important to determine if there is anatomic or functional uropathology, particularly vesicoureteral reflux (VUR). The presence of an abnormality may increase a child's risk for renal dysfunction and scarring. Radiographic evaluation is indicated for the following: all male patients with their first UTI; children under five years old with a febrile UTI; UTI in a girl below three years of age; after two or more episodes in a girl more than three years of age; a patient who does not respond appropriately to antibiotic therapy; and any patient after an episode of pyelonephritis or an atypical UTI with hypertension or a flank mass.

For children under three years of age, obtain an ultrasound to evaluate urinary tract anatomy and a voiding cystourethrogram (VCUG) under fluoroscopy to detect VUR. Although ultrasonography may be performed at any time after a UTI is diagnosed, a sterile urine culture must be obtained, or antibiotic prophylaxis provided, before the VCUG is performed. If the renal sonogram demonstrates hydronephrosis, assume that the patient has VUR and initiate prophylactic antibiotics. For children over three years of age, ultrasonography is sufficient. Obtain a VCUG if there are findings suggestive of reflux. Siblings of patients with VUR require urinary tract imaging, as this can be a heritable abnormality.

Follow-up

- Children with persistent symptoms on appropriate antibiotic therapy: within two days to repeat a urine culture
- For children requiring imaging studies for evaluation of the urinary tract: at the completion of antibiotic therapy to assess the need for prophylaxis

Indications for Admission

- UTI in patient <3 months of age.
- Any age: toxic-appearing, dehydrated, inability to tolerate oral intake, immunocompromised, at risk for nonadherence to treatment/follow-up
- Febrile UTI in a patient at risk for decreased renal function (decreased GFR, single kidney)

Bibliography

American Academy of Pediatrics Subcommittee on Urinary Tract Infection, Steering Committee on Quality Improvement and Management. Urinary tract infection: clinical practice guideline for the diagnosis and management of the initial UTI in febrile infants and children 2 to 24 months. *Pediatrics.* 2011;**128**:595–609.

Becknell B, Schober M, Korbel L, Spencer JD. The diagnosis, evaluation and treatment of acute and recurrent pediatric urinary tract infections. *Expert Rev Anti Infect Ther.* 2015;**13**(1):81–90.

Kowalsky RH, Shah NB. Update on urinary tract infections in the emergency department. *Curr Opin Pediatr.* 2013;**25**(3):317–322.

Paintsil E. Update on recent guidelines for the management of urinary tract infections in children: the shifting paradigm. *Curr Opin Pediatr.* 2013;**25**(1):88–94.

Schroeder A, Chang P, Shen M, Biondi E, Greenhow T. Diagnostic accuracy of the urinalysis for urinary tract infection in infants <3 months of age. *Pediatrics.* 2015;**135**:965–971.

Tran A, Fortier C, Giovannini-Chami L, Demonchy D, et al. Evaluation of the bladder stimulation technique to collect midstream urine in infants in a pediatric emergency department. *PLoS One.* 2016;**11**(3):e0152598.

Rheumatologic Emergencies

Joyce Hui-Yuen and Noé Romo

Acute Rheumatic Fever

Acute rheumatic fever (ARF) is a non-suppurative sequela of Group A *Streptococcus* (GAS) pharyngitis that can affect the heart, joints, subcutaneous tissue, and central nervous system. ARF occurs primarily between 5 and 15 years of age and is rare in children under three. The estimated incidence is 1–3% in patients who receive inadequate treatment for GAS pharyngitis and it is very uncommon when appropriate treatment is given.

Clinical Presentation and Diagnosis

ARF typically presents 2–4 weeks after an acute infection with GAS, which can sometimes be asymptomatic. There is no single test for the condition and the diagnosis is based on clinical features embodied in the Jones Criteria. Evidence of a recent GAS pharyngitis and the presence of two major, or one major and two minor, features are required for diagnosis. The criteria are described in Table 23.1.

Recent advances in echocardiography (ECHO) have made the detection of subclinical carditis (valvular damage detected only on ECHO) readily available. However, the use of ECHO for the diagnosis of ARF in a patient who has no clinically audible murmur is still controversial. Auscultatory findings remain the basis for the diagnosis of carditis.

Joint involvement is both a major and minor criterion. Migratory arthritis is defined as arthritis in an affected joint that resolves *before* another joint is affected. Since migratory polyarthritis (major criterion) often improves dramatically with the use of NSAIDS, corticosteroids, or aspirin, only arthralgia (minor criterion) may be evident. Therefore, delay symptomatic treatment if a definite diagnosis of ARF has not been established. In patients presenting with arthritis, other etiologies must be ruled out (see pp. 700–703), especially septic arthritis.

Post-streptococcal reactive arthritis (PSRA) occurs in patients who have arthritis and evidence of a preceding GAS infection, but do not fulfill the Jones Criteria. Symptoms can occur as early as ten days after GAS infection, but can last two months (longer than ARF). Although it is a known entity, it is not clear whether it is truly separate from ARF. In contrast to ARF, the arthritis typically does not respond dramatically to aspirin or NSAIDs, and patients do not present with carditis. Nonetheless, give ARF prophylaxis for one year after diagnosis of PSRA.

The World Health Organization's revised Jones Criteria include several exceptions to the criteria presented above for the following circumstances:

- Recurrent attack of rheumatic fever (RF): requires two minor features and evidence of recent GAS infection in a patient with established rheumatic heart disease.
- Rheumatic chorea or insidious onset of rheumatic carditis: evidence of GAS infection is not required.
- Chronic valvular lesions of rheumatic heart disease: no other criteria are required.

Table 23.1 Jones Criteria and the diagnosis of acute rheumatic fever

Evidence of GAS[1]

Throat culture and rapid strep test are positive in 25% of cases
Streptococcal Ab (ASLO, anti-DNase B, streptokinase, antihyaluronidase) is more sensitive

Major criteria[2]

(J)oints (polyarthritis)	Pain, erythema and swelling of large joints that "migrates" Persists for up to one week in each joint Pain is disproportional (↑↑ severe) to the physical findings
(O) Carditis	Endocarditis is most common; also peri-, epi-, and myocarditis Chest pain, friction rub, aortic and mitral regurgitation murmurs
(N)odules (subcutaneous)	Firm, symmetric, 1–2 cm, painless nodules Located over bony prominences or tendons, commonly the elbow
(E)rythema marginatum	Non-pruritic, evanescent, macular serpiginous rash with raised erythematous borders Central part of each lesion returns to normal as the rash spreads or resolves Typically on the trunk and inner thighs, upper arms
(S)yndenham chorea	Abrupt, purposeless, involuntary movements Associated with weakness and emotional lability

Minor criteria[3]

Arthralgia	Significant pain in a single joint with minimal findings of inflammation Cannot use as a minor criteria if polyarthritis used as a major
Fever	
Prolonged P–R interval	
Elevated acute phase reactants: ESR, CRP, WBC	

[1] Required for all criteria.
[2] Need two major alone, or one major and two minor.
[3] Need two minor along with one major.

ED Management

Since the diagnosis is based on the Jones Criteria, obtain a CBC, CRP, ESR, chest radiograph, ECG, throat culture, rapid *Streptococcus* swab, ASLO, and anti-DNAse B antibodies. The throat culture and rapid strep tests may be negative as the GAS pharyngitis can resolve, even

Table 23.2 Primary prevention of rheumatic fever

Antibiotic[1]	Dose
Penicillin G benzathine	≥27 kg: 1,200,000 units IM × 1 < 27 kg: 600,000 units IM × 1
Penicillin VK	250 mg tid or qid or 500 mg bid PO × 10 days
Amoxicillin	50 mg/kg daily PO × 10 days
First-generation cephalosporin	20 mg/kg/day PO × 10 days (dosing frequency varies)
Erythromycin ethylsuccinate	40 mg/kg/day PO div bid or tid × 10 days

[1] Trimethoprim, sulfonamides, and tetracyclines are not effective for eradicating GAS infections

Table 23.3 Secondary prophylaxis of rheumatic fever

Antibiotic	Dose
Penicillin G benzathine IM	1.2 million units IM q 4 weeks
Penicillin V	250 mg bid PO
Sulfadiazine or sulfisoxazole	<27 kg: 0.5 g/day PO ≥27 kg: 1 g/day PO
Penicillin-allergic	Erythromycin 250 mg bid PO

without antibiotic treatment. When the ASLO and anti-DNAse B are performed simultaneously, however, evidence of a preceding GAS infection can be found in >90% of patients.

Once the diagnosis is certain, treat migratory polyarthritis with aspirin 50–75 mg/kg/day div tid or qid or naproxen 15–20 mg/kg/day div bid for 2–4 weeks. Arthritis in ARF is exquisitely sensitive to NSAIDS and resolves shortly after institution of therapy.

Treat mild to moderate carditis with high-dose aspirin 80–100 mg/kg/day div qid for 4–8 weeks, depending on response, then gradually discontinue. Give prednisone (2 mg/kg/day) for severe carditis and congestive heart failure, but first consult a pediatric cardiologist.

Chorea resolves spontaneously over 2–3 weeks and most patients do not need to be medicated. Treat severe symptoms with haloperidol, but consult a pediatric neurologist prior to instituting therapy.

Once the diagnosis is established, the eradication of any existing streptococcal infection or carriage is necessary (Table 23.2). Secondary prophylaxis is critical for preventing disease recurrences (Table 23.3). Carditis is the single most important prognostic factor for ARF, but only valvulitis leads to permanent damage. Therefore, patient age and the presence of valvulitis determines the length of prophylaxis.

Follow-up

- Pediatric rheumatologist within one week
- Primary care monthly for antibiotic prophylaxis; other pediatric specialists (cardiologist, neurologist) based upon symptomatology

Indications for Admission
- Suspected acute rheumatic fever
- Recurrent episode of rheumatic fever

Bibliography

Gewitz MH, Baltimore RS, Tani LY, et al. Revision of the Jones Criteria for the diagnosis of acute rheumatic fever in the era of Doppler echocardiography: a scientific statement from the American Heart Association. *Circulation.* 2015;**131**(20):1806–1818.

Reyhan I, Goldberg BR, Gottlieb BS. Common presentations of pediatric rheumatologic diseases: a generalist's guide. *Curr Opin Pediatr.* 2013;**25**(3):388–396.

Uziel Y, Perl L, Barash J, Hashkes PJ. Post-streptococcal reactive arthritis in children: a distinct entity from acute rheumatic fever. *Pediatr Rheumatol Online J.* 2011;**9**(1):32.

Van Driel ML, De Sutter AI, Habraken H, Thorning S, Christiaens T. Different antibiotic treatments for group A streptococcal pharyngitis. *Cochrane Database Syst Rev.* 2016;**9**:CD004406.

Yanagawa B, Butany J, Verma S. Update on rheumatic heart disease. *Curr Opin Cardiol.* 2016;**31**:162–168.

Arthritis

Arthritis results from synovial inflammation due to infectious and noninfectious causes (Table 23.4). In contrast, arthralgia is pain or tenderness *without swelling.*

Clinical Presentation

The hallmarks of arthritis are joint swelling, pain, warmth, and limitation of motion, of which at least two must be present to diagnose arthritis. The patient may limp or refuse to use the affected extremity, which will have a decreased range of motion as the patient holds it in the position that maximizes the volume of the joint. The hip will be flexed, abducted, and slightly externally rotated; the knee and elbow flexed; and the ankle held in plantar flexion. Particularly worrisome symptoms include pain that consistently wakes the child from sleep, which raises the possibility of leukemia, and refusal to move the hot, swollen joint, which is consistent with a septic arthritis.

The most common etiology of arthritis that has been present for less than six weeks in an afebrile, well-appearing child is infection (viral, bacterial, or fungal). Post-infectious or reactive arthritis can occur within seven days of onset of infectious symptoms, and can take up to six weeks to resolve.

Juvenile idiopathic arthritis (JIA) is a chronic condition in which the arthritic symptoms have been constant and present for longer than six weeks. Children usually also complain of pain and stiffness in the morning and/or after long periods of rest, including naps for younger children. Patients will often exhibit adaptations to the pain in their daily activities, such as limping when walking, continuing to play sports with their best efforts, or typing instead of writing long essays.

In contrast, pain that can wake a child from sleep, and is described as localized over long bones, but is easily resolved with massage and reassurance is more likely associated with benign growing pains that do not require a work-up.

Table 23.4 Common etiologies of joint pain in children

Diagnosis	Differentiating features
Infection/infection-related	
Acute rheumatic fever	Pain is out of proportion to physical exam findings
	Classic migratory polyarthritis involves knees, ankles, elbows, and wrists
Gonococcal arthritis	Subacute onset
	Initially, pauciarticular and often migratory; can be monoarticular
	Adolescents may have tenosynovitis and papular or vesiculopustular rash
Lyme disease	Acute onset of swelling and tenderness without warmth or erythema, most often involving the knee
	Can be extremely painful
	Mostly monoarticular, sometimes migratory, rarely polyarticular
	Can persist for weeks to months and recur
Post-infectious	Subacute onset 2–3 weeks after an illness (URI or gastroenteritis) Duration <6 weeks
	Mono or asymmetric oligoarthritis commonly in knees and ankles
	Moderate pain, minimal swelling, no erythema, low-grade or no fever
Septic arthritis	Most common at 1–3 years of age in one large joint (knee, hip)
	Abrupt onset of painful, persistent and progressive arthritis
	Erythema, warmth, swelling, pain, and decreased range of motion (especially infants)
	Absence of joint effusion on ultrasound has a high negative predictive value for septic arthritis
Toxic synovitis	Occurs in as many as 3% of 2–10-year-olds
	Good response to NSAIDS
	Can last for 2 weeks, but resolves without complications
Inflammatory	
Dermatomyositis	Frequently involves the small joints of the hands
IBD	Acute onset of a persistent oligoarthritis involving large joints, including hips
JIA	Arthritis lasting >6 weeks in a child <16 years old
	Typically less painful than swelling suggests
	Worse in the morning, with associated stiffness
Kawasaki disease	Subacute onset polyarthritis involving the small joints of the hands and feet

Table 23.4 (cont.)

Diagnosis	Differentiating features
Serum sickness	Arthralgia/arthritis of the knees, ankles, shoulders, wrists, spine, and temporomandibular joint
	Associated with myalgias, urticaria, angioedema, and hematuria
SLE	Subacute onset of symmetric polyarthritis involving peripheral joints of the hands or feet
	Large joints may be involved during disease exacerbation
	Despite severe pain, arthritis is nondestructive and may be persistent or intermittent
Malignancy	
Leukemia/	Gradual onset of a persistent mono-, poly-, or migratory arthritis
bone tumors	Pain out of proportion to physical findings and may be worse at night, can awaken child from sleep
	Can be associated with fever, weight loss, and anemia
Non-inflammatory	
Benign growing	Pain is mild, generally localized to long bones
pains	Pain can wake child from sleep but easily resolved with massage and reassurance
RSD	Pain severely out of proportion with examination
	Affected joint/limb in preferred position of comfort
	Often the affected limb is cool to touch.
Trauma/overuse	
Fracture	Point tenderness, can be associated with some peri-articular swelling
Hypermobility	No objective arthritis, usually only arthralgias
	Can affect upper and/or lower extremities
Traumatic arthritis	Acute or chronic onset of intermittent pain that is worse with activity
	Typically one joint is involved (elbow, shoulder, knee, hip)
	May have an associated fracture, ligamentous injury, bursitis, or tenovitis

Adapted from Tse S, Laxer R. Approach to acute limb pain in childhood. *Pediatr Rev.* 2006;27:170–179.
IBD: inflammatory bowel disease; JIA: juvenile idiopathic arthritis; NSAIDS: nonsteroidal anti-inflammatory drugs; RSD: reflex sympathetic dystrophy; SLE: systemic lupus erythematosus; URI: upper respiratory infection.

Diagnosis

A detailed history helps to guide the initial approach to a child with arthritis. Inquire about antecedent or recurrent trauma, history of similar episodes in the past, fever, recent immunizations or illnesses, pharyngitis or gastroenteritis, medication use, travel, tick exposure, weight loss, or fatigue. Ascertain the location of the pain, the number of joints

Table 23.5 Rashes associated with arthritic diseases

Diagnosis	Skin manifestations
Acute rheumatic fever	Erythema marginatum
Systemic lupus erythematosus	Malar and discoid rashes
Systemic-onset juvenile idiopathic arthritis	Evanescent salmon-pink macular rash
Inflammatory bowel disease	Erythema nodosum
Dermatomyositis	Gottron papules, heliotrope rash, shawl sign
Lyme disease	Erythema migrans
Gonococcal arthritis	Erythematous, hemorrhagic, papular, or vesiculopustular lesions
Serum sickness	Angioedema, urticaria

involved, timing and severity of the pain, and any associated swelling, warmth, or limitation in range of motion. In the review of systems ask about ocular symptoms, oral ulcers, rashes (Table 23.5); a history of pulmonary disease, endocarditis, hematologic disorders, vasculitis, sexually transmitted infections, infectious or inflammatory gastroenteritis, hepatitis; and psychiatric and renal diseases.

On examination, document that arthritis is present, as opposed to arthralgias, myalgias, sprains, or bruises, and whether it is monoarticular or polyarticular. It is critical to distinguish joint pain from that originating from muscle, tendon, bursa, bone, soft tissue, or nerve. Compare the affected joint(s) to the contralateral side to confirm the presence of joint fluid. Finally, look for evidence of systemic illness, such as lymphadenopathy, hepatosplenomegaly, murmur or edema. Since most patients will have an infectious, post-infectious, or traumatic etiology for the arthritis, a limited evaluation is usually sufficient to make a presumptive diagnosis. In the ED it is prudent to involve the primary care physician, orthopedist, and/or rheumatologist if a more involved work-up seems necessary, so that proper follow-up can be arranged.

ED Management
Obtain a CBC with differential, ESR or CRP, complete metabolic panel, and infectious serologies as appropriate. Obtain radiographs of the affected joint(s) to look for trauma (fracture) and possible erosions, which suggest that the arthritis has been present for longer than six weeks. After the appropriate studies have been obtained, afebrile, well-appearing, weight-bearing patients with good follow-up may be discharged for further outpatient management. Give ibuprofen (10 mg/kg PO every six hours) for symptomatic relief.

Follow-up
- Afebrile patient with nonmigratory arthritis: primary care follow-up within one week
- Afebrile patient with nonmigratory arthritis for more than six weeks: rheumatology within 1–2 weeks

Indications for Admission
- Suspected septic arthritis, acute rheumatic fever, or malignancy
- Migratory polyarthritis
- Inability to bear weight

Bibliography
John J, Chandran L. Arthritis in children and adolescents. *Pediatr Rev.* 2011;**32**:470–479.

Reyhan I, Goldberg BR, Gottlieb BS. Common presentations of pediatric rheumatologic diseases: a generalist's guide. *Curr Opin Pediatr.* 2013;**25**(3):388–396.

Sen ES, Clarke SL, Ramanan AV. The child with joint pain in primary care. *Best Pract Res Clin Rheumatol.* 2014;**28**(6):888–906.

Monoarticular Arthritis
Monoarticular arthritis is arthritis affecting only one joint, usually a large joint in the lower extremity (knee, ankle). Consider monoarticular arthritis to be infectious until proven otherwise.

Clinical Presentation and Diagnosis
If the affected joint is hot, swollen, and extremely tender on attempted movement, septic arthritis must be ruled out, especially if the symptom onset was abrupt. Septic arthritis is an emergency requiring *immediate* orthopedic consultation, as bone destruction can occur in a short time.

Similarly, Lyme arthritis (pp. 417–420) commonly affects large joints, particularly the knee. It can be exquisitely painful, but a good range of motion is maintained. In addition, the joint is not erythematous. Lyme arthritis is typically a late, not early, manifestation of Lyme disease.

Consider toxic synovitis (pp. 581–583) in a well-appearing patient who can partially bear weight and responds to NSAIDS, and osteomyelitis (pp. 585–586) in a patient with apparent arthritis but a negative joint aspiration. Juvenile idiopathic arthritis can present with a monoarticular arthritis that persists for more than six weeks.

ED Management
Obtain a CBC with differential, ESR or CRP, and blood culture. Obtain a Lyme titer if the evaluation is highly suggestive (timing from exposure, joint is not erythematous, history of rash consistent with erythema migrans). Occasionally, a migratory or polyarticular arthritis may initially present with single joint involvement. Therefore, also keep two additional red-top tubes in the event that septic arthritis is ruled out.

Obtain an x-ray of the affected joint, and arrange for immediate arthrocentesis. The *only exceptions* to performing arthrocentesis are a traumatic effusion (unless indicated for pain relief), probable Lyme disease, an obvious case of Henoch–Schönlein purpura (see pp. 683–684), or a known autoimmune disorder. Culture of the joint fluid is critical; inoculate the specimen into a blood culture bottle. A Gram's stain and cell count of the joint fluid are also necessary, but crystal analysis is rarely helpful in children. The interpretation of joint fluid analysis is summarized in Table 23.6.

Table 23.6 Synovial fluid findings

Diagnosis	Color	Clarity	Viscosity	Mucin clot	WBC/mm^3	% polys
Normal	Straw	Transparent	High	Good	<200	<25
Chronic arthritis	Yellow	Cloudy	Low	Poor	15,000–20,000	75
Lyme arthritis	Purulent	Turbid	Low	Low	3000–100,000	>90
Rheumatic fever	Yellow	Slightly cloudy	Low	Fair	5000	10–50
Septic arthritis	Serosanguinous	Turbid or purulent	Low	Poor	50,000–300,000	>75
Traumatic arthritis	Straw to bloody to xanthochromic	Transparent to turbid	High	Fair to good	<2000	<25
			Few to many RBCs			
Tuberculosis arthritis	Yellow-white	Cloudy	Low	Poor	25,000	50–60

Adapted from Petty RE, Cassidy JT. Chronic arthritis in childhood. In Cassidy JT, Petty RE, Laxer RM, Lindsley CB (eds). *Textbook of Pediatric Rheumatology* (6th ed.). Philadelphia, PA: Saunders Elsevier, 2011; 228.

The Kocher criteria employs four features to assess the risk of septic arthritis of the hip (versus toxic synovitis and other conditions) in a patient with a painful limp: nonweight-bearing, fever, ESR >40 mm/h, and WBC >12,000/mm³. The probability of a septic hip is 99% if all criteria are present, 93% with three criteria, 40% with two, and 3% with one criterion. The criteria are less reliable in younger patients.

For septic arthritis, joint drainage is necessary to remove the organism's debris and enzymes, which can damage the articular cartilage and underlying bone. It is crucial to start intravenous antibiotics for treatment after arthrocentesis and blood and fluid cultures are performed. Use nafcillin (150 mg/kg/day div q 6h), cephalexin (100 mg/kg/day div q 6h), or clindamycin (40 mg/kg/day div q 6h), but add vancomycin (40 mg/kg/day div q 6h) if there is *any* concern about MRSA.

Admit the patient for further investigations which may include a technetium bone scan, MRI, and a bone or synovial biopsy to help identify conditions such as osteomyelitis, myositis, or tuberculosis.

Follow-up

- Lyme arthritis: primary care follow-up within one week
- Transient synovitis: 2–3 days, if symptoms have not resolved

Indications for Admission

- Suspected septic arthritis
- Inability to bear weight

Bibliography

Deanehan JK, Nigrovic PA, Milewski MD, et al. Synovial fluid findings in children with knee monoarthritis in Lyme disease endemic areas. *Pediatr Emer Care.* 2014;**30**:16–19.

Genes N, Chisolm-Straker M. Monoarticular arthritis update: current evidence for diagnosis and treatment in the emergency department. *Emerg Med Pract.* 2012;**14**(5):1–19.

John J, Chandran L. Arthritis in children and adolescents. *Pediatr Rev.* 2011;**32**:470–479.

Pääkkönen M, Peltola H. Management of a child with suspected acute septic arthritis. *Arch Dis Child.* 2012;**97**(3):287–292.

Polyarticular Arthritis

Polyarticular arthritis is arthritis affecting more than one joint, including the smaller joints in the hands and feet. It can be migratory, meaning an affected joint can have resolution of swelling and other symptoms before another is affected, or additive/nonmigratory, meaning another joint develops arthritis while previously affected joints remain with arthritis.

Clinical Presentation and Diagnosis

Migratory polyarthritis can be a sign of acute rheumatic fever (pp. 697–700). Suspect gonococcal arthritis in an adolescent with monoarticular or polyarticular arthritis associated with tenosynovitis, pustules, or necrotic lesions.

Other infections that can result in polyarticular arthritis, particularly in smaller joints of hands and feet, include parvovirus, Epstein–Barr virus, and *Mycoplasma*. Consider the diagnosis of juvenile idiopathic arthritis if an arthritis persist for over six weeks.

ED Management
Obtain a CBC with differential, ESR or CRP, LDH, and urinalysis, as well as confirmation of a group A streptococcal infection (rapid strep test, ASLO titer) and other serologies as appropriate (*Mycoplasma* IgM and IgG, Epstein–Barr virus IgM and IgG, parvovirus IgM and IgG). Do not obtain a "rheumatology panel" for a patient with a low probability of having a rheumatologic condition, as this will likely yield false-positive results and create undue stress for the patient and family. Therefore, order specialized tests (HLA-B27, anti-SM antibody, rheumatoid factor, etc.) only after consultation with a rheumatologist.

Obtain genital, rectal, and pharyngeal cultures for gonorrhea in addition to cultures already mentioned. If gonococcal infection is likely, use IV or IM ceftriaxone 50 mg/kg daily (1 g/day maximum) or cefotaxime (100 mg/kg/day IV div q 8h, 1 g/day maximum) for seven days, along with nafcillin, cephalexin, or clindamycin (as for monoarticular arthritis) until the diagnosis is confirmed.

For *Mycoplasma* infections with positive IgM serology, give a five-day course of azithromycin.

Follow-up
- Afebrile patient with nonmigratory arthritis: primary care follow-up within one week
- Afebrile patient with nonmigratory arthritis for more than six weeks: rheumatologist within 1–2 weeks
- Infectious cause of polyarthritis (e.g., gonococcal arthritis): follow-up with pediatrician at end of treatment course

Indications for Admission
- Inability to bear weight
- Suspected ARF

Bibliography
Balan S. Approach to joint pain in children. *Indian J Pediatr*. 2016;**83**(2):135–139.

John J, Chandran L. Arthritis in children and adolescents. *Pediatr Rev*. 2011;**32**:470–479.

Sen ES, Clarke SL, Ramanan AV. The child with joint pain in primary care. *Best Pract Res Clin Rheumatol*. 2014;**28**(6):888–906.

Spencer CH, Patwardhan A. Pediatric rheumatology for the primary care clinicians: recognizing patterns of disease. *Curr Probl Pediatr Adolesc Health Care*. 2015;**45**(7):185–206.

Webb K, Wedderburn LR. Advances in the treatment of polyarticular juvenile idiopathic arthritis. *Curr Opin Rheumatol*. 2015;**27**(5):505–510.

Juvenile Dermatomyositis
Juvenile dermatomyositis (JDM), also known as idiopathic inflammatory myopathy, is a rare autoimmune disease of unknown etiology affecting the skin and muscles.

Clinical Presentation

JDM is more common in girls with a peak age of 5–10 years. It has an insidious onset, with skin involvement of exposed areas being the typical initial complaint. Lesions are often photosensitive and severe pruritus may occur. The major cutaneous manifestations are:

- heliotrope rash: a violaceous, symmetrical eruption involving the upper eyelids with or without associated edema;
- Gottron's sign: violaceous papules and plaques found over bony prominences of the finger joints, elbows, knees, and/or feet;
- calcinosis cutis: cutaneous deposits of calcium crystals, commonly seen over the joints, while sparing the digits.

Muscle disease may precede or follow skin disease by weeks to years. Systemic manifestations also occur and include non-erosive/deforming arthritis, arthralgia, pulmonary fibrosis/pneumonitis, cardiac arrhythmias, dysphagia, and dysphonia. Approximately 25% of patients are ANA positive.

A visceral vasculopathy is an uncommon complication. It presents with diffuse abdominal pain, melena, hematemesis, and sometimes acute mesenteric infarction. Free intraperitoneal air can occur with hollow viscus perforation.

Diagnosis

The initial diagnosis requires a high clinical suspicion. Inquire about skin nodules, weakness, voice changes, joint pain, dyspnea, and dysphagia. Specific diagnostic criteria for JDM have been established:

- characteristic cutaneous changes;
- symmetric proximal muscle weakness;
- elevated muscle enzymes (CPK, LDH, aldolase, transaminases);
- biopsy is the gold standard (inflammatory myopathy with characteristic histopathology);
- inflammatory myopathy based on electromyographic findings.

The diagnosis of JDM can be made if the patient has a typical rash and three of the four other criteria. With the rash and two additional criteria present, the diagnosis is probable, and with the rash and just one criterion, it is possible. MRI has now been shown to be sensitive in evaluation for JDM but is not part of the diagnostic criteria.

ED Management

If JDM is suspected, obtain a CBC, comprehensive metabolic panel, CPK, LDH, aldolase, chest x-ray, and ECG. Consult a rheumatologist regarding further evaluation (EMG and MRI, muscle biopsy) and the initiation of treatment with corticosteroids.

Follow-up

- Rheumatology consult within 1–2 weeks

Indications for Admission

- Significant disability or severe systemic illness with esophageal, diaphragmatic, or cardiac involvement

Bibliography

Huber A, Feldman B. An update on inflammatory myositis in children. *Curr Opin Rheumatol.* 2013;**25**:630–635.

Nistala K, Wedderburn LR. Update in juvenile myositis. *Curr Opin Rheumatol.* 2013;**25**(6):742–746.

Quartier P, Gherardi RK. Juvenile dermatomyositis. *Handb Clin Neurol.* 2013;**113**:1457–1463.

Rennebohm R. Juvenile dermatomyositis. *Pediatr Ann.* 2002;**31**:426–433.

Systemic Lupus Erythematosus

Systemic lupus erythematosus is a chronic autoimmune inflammatory disorder that is characterized by multisystem involvement and a variable clinical course. The hallmark of the disease is the presence of antinuclear antibodies (ANA) and antibodies to double-stranded DNA (dsDNA).

Although the majority of patients are adults, up to 20% of cases involve children under 18 years of age. There is a female predominance, with African-American females at the highest risk of developing SLE.

Clinical Presentation

Patients with SLE may present to the ED with arthritis, edema or complications of renal disease, hypertensive crises, chest pain or shortness of breath, or infection with fever. There are a number of potential findings and complications in patients with SLE:

- Renal disease is present at diagnosis in up to 85% of pediatric patients, or develops within the first two years of disease onset. Hypertension, proteinuria, and red cell casts may be seen.
- Anemia may be normochromic/normocytic, as in anemia of chronic disease; microcytic/hypochromic suggestive of occult blood loss (gastritis, GI vasculitis); or hemolytic/autoimmune.
- Thrombocytopenia is most commonly a mild autoimmune process, although it can also be a sign of ensuing thrombotic thrombocytopenic purpura (TTP) with microangiopathic hemolytic anemia, rapidly declining renal function, and CNS dysfunction.
- Antiphospholipid antibody syndrome with arterial and venous thrombosis, livedo reticularis, and the presence of lupus anticoagulant.
- Pulmonary manifestations include pleurisy, pleural effusion, or hemorrhage. Suspect hemorrhage in patients with hemoptysis, declining hemoglobin, and shifting pulmonary infiltrates.
- Gastrointestinal (GI) manifestations include gastritis, sterile peritonitis, enteritis, or pancreatitis. GI bleeding may be secondary to medications (NSAIDS), gastritis, mesenteric vasculitis (small intestine), or thrombocytopenia.
- Cardiac complications include pericarditis, myocarditis, and valvulitis. Pericardial effusions can occur, but tamponade is rare.
- Raynaud's phenomenon is a triphasic change in color of the digits in response to cold or stress. Fingers or toes first turn pale then blue, then red upon rewarming. Recurrent

Table 23.7 1997 SLE classification criteria

(R)enal disorder: proteinuria, hematuria, cellular casts

(A)rthritis: usually non-erosive

(S)erositis: pleuritis, pericarditis

(H)ematologic disorder: hemolytic anemia, leukopenia, lymphopenia, thrombocytopenia

(O)ral and/or nasal mucocutaneous ulcers

(N)eurologic disorder: seizures, psychosis, stroke

(M)alar rash

(A)nti-nuclear antibody

(I)mmunologic findings: anti-double-stranded DNA, anti-Smith, antiphospholipid antibody positivity

(D)iscoid rash

(S)un sensitivity: photosensitive rashes

vasospasm predisposes to digital ulcers that can lead to superinfection or autoamputation of digits.
- Arthritis can be present, but it is usually non-erosive and can include ligamentous laxity (Jaccoud's arthropathy).

Diagnosis

Many of the features of SLE are not specific; therefore maintain a high index of suspicion to consider SLE in the differential diagnosis. Determine whether the patient has constitutional symptoms such as fever, weight loss, or fatigue. Ask about rashes, arthritis, renal manifestations (edema, hematuria, proteinuria), chest pain, and seizures. Explore any family history of SLE or other immune-mediated disorders. On physical examination look for evidence of systemic involvement, including edema, pleurisy, pericardial or pulmonary effusions, ascites, arthritis, and occult infections.

The diagnosis of SLE is made based on American College of Rheumatology classification criteria, revised in 1997 (Table 23.7). The patient must meet 4 of the 11 criteria, either simultaneously or at any time during follow-up. However, these are classification and not diagnostic criteria, so patients may have SLE and not fulfill the criteria, or conversely may meet the criteria but have another illness, including overlapping autoimmune diseases.

ED Management

The management of SLE depends on presenting symptoms and severity of the disease. When the initial diagnosis of SLE is suspected, consult a pediatric rheumatologist to guide further work-up and therapy. Other consultants may include a nephrologist and cardiologist, depending on the presentation. Obtain a CBC with differential, ESR, CRP (usually normal in an uninfected child with SLE), comprehensive metabolic panel, C3 and C4 (complement levels usually are low), ANA with an ENA panel, dsDNA, a urinalysis, and urine protein:creatinine ratio.

If a patient with known SLE is ill-appearing or neutropenic, obtain blood and urine cultures, a chest x-ray, and a lumbar puncture, if clinically appropriate. Initiate broad-spectrum antibiotics if a serious infection cannot be excluded. In particular, patients on immunosuppressive therapy are at increased risk of developing viral, fungal, or other opportunistic infections. If the patient is febrile and neutropenic, obtain blood and urine cultures and admit for intravenous antibiotics. Obtain a Coombs test, LDH, haptoglobin, and stool guaiac for patients with significant anemia. Patients with cardiac or pulmonary disease may need an ECG, echocardiogram, or CT of the chest. Management of a hypertensive crisis is discussed elsewhere (pp. 686–687).

There is no specific treatment algorithm for SLE. As outpatients, most patients with lupus receive maintenance hydroxychloroquine, which reduces lupus flares. Treat mild disease manifested by arthritis with NSAIDs (naproxen 15–20 mg/kg/day div bid). Severe systemic disease is an indication for hospitalization and IV methylprednisolone pulses (30 mg/kg/day, 1000 mg maximum) and other immunosuppressive therapy. Consult a rheumatologist.

Treat Raynaud's by avoidance of the cold, although severe Raynaud's may require nitroglycerin ointment to the webs of the fingers or volar surfaces of the wrists (do not apply for more than ten hours to prevent tachyphylaxis) and calcium channel blockers.

Follow-up
- Suspected new-onset SLE: pediatric rheumatologist and/or nephrologist within one week

Indications for Admission
- New-onset SLE
- Worsening renal disease in a known lupus patient
- CNS manifestations (seizures, psychosis, chorea)
- Severe systemic disease (pulmonary hemorrhage, pleuritis, pancreatitis, pericarditis)
- Serious infection

Bibliography

Borgia RE, Silverman ED. Childhood-onset systemic lupus erythematosus: an update. *Curr Opin Rheumatol.* 2015;27:483–492.

Reyhan I, Goldberg BR, Gottlieb BS. Common presentations of pediatric rheumatologic diseases: a generalist's guide. *Curr Opin Pediatr.* 2013;25(3):388–396.

Sawhney S. Childhood lupus: diagnosis and management. *Indian J Pediatr.* 2016;83(2):146–155.

Weiss JE. Pediatric systemic lupus erythematosus: more than a positive antinuclear antibody. *Pediatr Rev.* 2012;33:62–73.

Chapter 24

Sedation and Analgesia

Sandra J. Cunningham, Katherine J. Chou, and
Robert M. Kennedy

Overview

The recognition, assessment, and management of pain in children can be challenging, given the wide range of developmental stages, the difficulty in differentiating pain from anxiety, and the concern that relieving pain may obscure the diagnosis. Therefore, provision of analgesia to younger patients is often suboptimal. In fact, making the child more comfortable can facilitate the physical examination and required diagnostic testing. This includes patients with abdominal pain, headache, and trauma victims.

The goals of sedation are to provide optimal patient comfort during a procedure while maintaining patient safety. Adhere to strict protocols when administering procedural sedation in order to minimize adverse effects. Persons involved in the sedation process must be experienced in resuscitation in the case of an untoward event. Most importantly, ensure that the provider(s) administering the sedation and monitoring the status of the child are not the same person as the individual who is performing the procedure.

Several factors can affect the success of sedation, such as the patient's psychological development, pain threshold, and the pre-procedural anxiety level. Parental presence decreases both child and parent anxiety and does not negatively impact the procedure success rate. Adult behaviors that help to decrease pain or distress are distraction, direct commands to use a coping strategy, praise, and allowing the child to make some choices rather than giving overall control of the procedure to the child. Conversely, some adult behaviors may increase pain or distress and these are not always intuitive, e.g., reassurance and apology. Criticism of the child's behavior must be avoided.

Procedural Sedation and Analgesia

Procedural sedation and analgesia (PSA) employs sedatives or dissociative agents, which are administered at dosages and rates that allow the patient to maintain airway control, protective reflexes, and cardiorespiratory function. Be prepared, however, to intervene to support airway and ventilation, if necessary.

Acceptable candidates for PSA in the ED are patients who are American Society of Anesthesiology (ASA) Physical Status Classification Classes I or II (see Table 24.1). Perform the assessments and reassessments for PSA pre-sedation, intra-sedation, and post-sedation.

Pre-Sedation

When choosing a medication, take into account the physical and mental status of the patient, including age, vital signs, current medical condition, past medical and sedation

Table 24.1 American Society of Anesthesiologists (ASA) Physical Status Classification System

ASA Class	Patient description
I	Healthy, no underlying organic disease
II	Mild or moderate systemic disease that does not interfere with daily routines (e.g., well-controlled asthma, essential hypertension)
III	Organic disease with definite functional impairment (e.g., severe steroid-dependent asthma, insulin-dependent diabetes, uncorrected congenital heart disease)
IV	Severe disease that is life-threatening (e.g., head trauma with increased intracranial pressure)
V	Moribund patient, not expected to survive
E (suffix)	Physical status classification appended with an "E" connotes a procedure undertaken as an emergency (e.g., an otherwise healthy patient presenting for fracture reduction is classified as ASA physical status 1E)

Table 24.2 Pre-procedural fasting AAP/ASA guidelines

Age	Solids (includes milk)	Clears
<6 months	4–6 hours	2 hours
≥6–36 months	6 hours	2 hours
≥36 months	6–8 hours	2 hours

history, other medications given at home or in the ED, allergies, last oral intake of fluids or solids, and psychological state. Also consider the procedure being performed, including expected level of pain and likely duration.

The recent intake of solids or liquids is not an absolute contraindication for PSA. Determine the risks and benefits of immediately performing versus delaying the procedure. Data on aspiration risk have been extrapolated from anesthesia literature where the airway is being manipulated (e.g., endotracheal intubation). By definition, with appropriate PSA, the patient will maintain airway control and protective reflexes. See Table 24.2 for the American Academy of Pediatrics and the ASA preferred pre-procedural fasting guidelines.

Anticipate both common and uncommon complications. These include vomiting or aspiration, allergic reactions, paradoxical reactions, anaphylaxis, abnormal movements or seizures, airway compromise, respiratory depression and hypoxia, apnea, and cardiorespiratory arrest. Complications generally result from errors in medication dosing, inadequate monitoring, inadequate skill level of the provider, use of multiple agents (≥3), premature discharge of the patient, higher levels of ASA categorization, or young age. Patients are at the greatest risk of complications about five minutes after administration of PSA and after the procedure is completed, when the stimulus has been removed.

Table 24.3 PSA equipment

Blood pressure cuffs and sphygmomanometer	Bag-valve-mask apparatus
Cardiac monitor	Endotracheal tubes and stylets
Epinephrine (allergic reactions)	Large-bore suction device
Oral/nasal airways	Laryngoscope
Oxygen source	Pulse oximeter and $ETCO_2$
Resuscitation medications (atropine, epinephrine)	Specific antidotes

PSA Equipment

When administering medications with the potential for compromise of ventilation or circulation, continuously monitor the patient with a cardiorespiratory monitor, pulse oximeter, and end-tidal carbon dioxide monitor ($ETCO_2$). Equipment that must be immediately available at the patient's bedside include bag-mask apparatus with a proper-sized mask, suction with a large-diameter suction catheter, an oxygen source, and the correct size nonrebreather face mask (Table 24.3).

Other resuscitation equipment, such as laryngoscopes, endotracheal tubes, and resuscitation medications must be rapidly available, if needed.

Consent

Once the PSA medication has been chosen, explain to the parents the nature of the procedure and the expected effect of the drug, including possible side effects. Hospitals differ on whether a separate informed consent for PSA is required, although there is no evidence that a separate consent form enhances patient or parental satisfaction, and it is not required by the Joint Commission on Accreditation.

Intra-Sedation

During PSA, continually monitor airway, breathing, and circulation status, with written documentation at specified intervals (5–15 minutes). The provider performing the procedure *cannot also monitor the patient.*

Post-Sedation

Continue to monitor airway, breathing, and circulation status until the patient is awake and no longer at risk for cardiorespiratory compromise. Before discharge from the ED, the patient must return to a baseline level of alertness and motor ability. Give the parent appropriate discharge instructions, including a contact number for the ED.

Medication Administration

Medications can be given by a variety of routes, including intranasal (IN), inhalational, intramuscular (IM), intravenous (IV), oral (PO), and rectal (PR). The intravenous (IV) route provides the most reliable and predictable sedation. Many drugs can be titrated to accommodate the level of sedation needed and the length of the procedure. Rapid IV administration can lead to hypotension and cardiorespiratory compromise. Always infuse medications at an IV port close to the catheter hub to ensure that the drug reaches the vascular system immediately. When medications are given more distally in the IV tubing while fluids are running, there is a potential for a rapid bolus of the drug.

The intramuscular route can provide deep sedation without the need for an IV, but drugs cannot be titrated and this route lacks the precise control of the IV route. Oral, intranasal, inhalational, and rectal routes are generally appropriate for less painful procedures, procedures in which a local anesthetic will also be used, or as sedation for diagnostic procedures, such as a CT scan. The inhalation route (nitrous oxide) is appropriate for cooperative children of three years and older who are able to follow directions.

Before administration of the medication, use relaxation techniques such as guided imagery or hypnosis, and attempt to create a calm atmosphere (e.g., dim lighting, noise elimination). Insert an intravenous line, if needed, and place the child on a cardiorespiratory monitor, which includes continuous pulse oximetry. Pulse oximetry provides an early warning of desaturation, since visible cyanosis does not occur until 5 g/dL of hemoglobin are desaturated (generally at an oxygen saturation <70%). Although an oxygen source must be immediately available, the routine administration of oxygen during PSA will limit the provider's ability to detect hypoventilation when the pulse oximeter displays a decreasing oxygen saturation. Capnography measures $ETCO_2$, which is the highest value of carbon dioxide at the end of expiration of each breath and will detect early hypoventilation before oxygen desaturation. It is recommended for routine monitoring and specifically when using etomidate, ketamine, or propofol.

PSA Medications (See Table 24.4)

Opioids

Opioids are potent analgesics that elevate the pain threshold causing analgesia, euphoria, and respiratory depression. An advantage of opioids is that they are reversible with the pure antagonist, naloxone (Table 24.4). The serum half-life of naloxone is approximately 60 minutes, so be aware that the effects of the opioid may outlast the naloxone. For patients who require a prolonged course of naloxone, infuse a drip that delivers, per hour, two-thirds of the dose that was required to achieve the desired response initially.

Morphine

Morphine is the principal alkaloid of opium. It has minimal hemodynamic effects in the euvolemic patient when used in appropriate doses. Use morphine for procedures such as burn debridement and hydrotherapy, and abscess incision and drainage, and to control pain in patients with burns or sickle cell vaso-occlusive crisis.

Fentanyl

Fentanyl is a synthetic opioid that is 24–100 times more potent than morphine. Use fentanyl for painful procedures of short duration such as fracture reduction or incision and drainage of an abscess or pilonidal cyst.

Table 24.4 PSA medications

Drug	Route	Dose	Onset	Duration	Max Dose	Side Effects	Comments
Etomidate	IV	0.15–0.2 mg/kg	<1 min	<12 min	20 mg	Pain at injection site, vomiting $\downarrow$O2 sat, $\downarrow$BP Respiratory depression (with opioids) Myoclonus (not assoc. with EEG changes) Adrenal insufficiency (multiple doses)	Slow IV push over 1 minute May require a second dose
Propofol	IV	1.5 mg/kg	<1 min	<15 min	30 mg	Pain at injection site Apnea, $\downarrow$BP Lactic acidosis (continuous infusion)	Slow IVP over 1 min Additional dose: 0.5 mg/kg
Ketamine	IM IV IN	3–4 mg/kg 1.5 mg/kg 1 mg/kg in 0.5 mL 0.25 mL/nostril	4–5 min 1–2 min	20–30 min 10–15min	150 mg 75 mg	Vomiting, laryngospasm, $\downarrow$O2 sat Emergence reaction Post-procedure ataxia $\uparrow$ Oral and airway secretions $\uparrow$ Sympathomimetic activity $\uparrow$ Intraocular pressure	Slow IVP over 1 min Additional doses: 0.5 mg/kg
Propofol plus ketamine	IV	0.5–1 mg/kg/ 0.5–1 mg/kg					
Dexmedetomidine	IV Infuse	2 mcg/kg over 10 min 1 mcg/kg/h				$\uparrow$BP, nausea, vomiting	Can have slow onset and recovery

Drug	Route	Dose	Onset	Duration	Adverse effects	Comments
Nitrous oxide (see text)						
Morphine	IM IV SC	0.1–0.2 mg/kg	1–2 min	1–3 h	15 mg	Respiratory depression (especially when used with other agents) ↓ BP in if hypovolemic Nausea, vomiting Histamine release	Slow IVP over 1 min
Fentanyl	IV Infuse	1–5 mcg/kg 0.5 mcg/kg/min	1–2 min	30 min	100 mcg 25 mcg/min	Respiratory depression and hypoxia (can occur with appropriate dose and IV rate) Chest wall rigidity with rapid bolus ↓ Pulse, ↓BP Nausea, vomiting	Use in combination with midazolam Facial pruritus early sign of sedation Chest wall rigidity may require larger naloxone dose
Fentanyl (100 mcg/2 mL)	IN	1.5 mcg/kg Min 20 mcg	1–2 min		max 60 mcg		
Midazolam (5 mg/mL)	IV/IM PO PR IN	0.1 mg/kg 0.5–1 mg/kg 0.5 mg/kg 0.25–0.4 mg/kg	5–10 min 5–10 min	30–60 min 30–60 min	IV/IM: 5 mg PO: 20 mg IV: 5 mg	↓ Complications used as a single agent ↓ Respirations in combination with opioids	Administer before other agents Antidote: flumazenil (see below)
Methohexital	PR	25 mg/kg	<10 min	60–90 min	1 g	Minimal adverse effects at low doses ↓O2 sat, hiccups, cough, ↑salivation	Effects are dose-dependent and range from mild sedation to coma No analgesic effects

Table 24.4 (cont.)

Drug	Route	Dose	Onset	Duration	Max Dose	Side Effects	Comments
Pentobarbital	PO PR	2–6 mg/kg 2 mg/kg Min 30 mg	Up to 45 min	2–4 h	PO: 150 mg PR: 60 mg	Prolonged period to arousal Agitation	Most success in children <8 yrs Limited use due to onset and duration
Ketorolac	IM/IV	0.5 mg/kg	0.5–1 h	6 h	30 mg	Nausea, gastritis, drowsiness Interstitial nephritis	5 day course maximum Do not use in renal or hepatic failure Use for sickle cell pain and renal colic
Oxycodone	PO	0.05–0.15 mg/kg	0.5–1 h	6 h	5 mg	Nausea, vomiting, constipation, gastritis	Useful in sickle cell pain crisis
Codeine/ acetaminophen	PO	0.5–1.0 mg/kg as codeine	0.5–1 h	4–6 h	30 mg	Nausea, vomiting, constipation Abdominal pain	Useful in sickle cell pain crisis Various formulations available or dose codeine and acetaminophen separately
Acetaminophen	PO PR	15 mg/kg	0.5–1 h	4 h	650 mg		No anti-inflammatory effect
Ibuprofen	PO	10 mg/kg		6 hrs	800 mg	Gastritis, inhibits platelet aggregation	Has anti-inflammatory effects ↓ GI distress with food or milk Do not use with renal insufficiency

Antidotes

	Route	Dose	Onset	Duration	Max	Side effects	Notes
Naloxone (for opioids)	IV IM SC ETT	0.1 mg/kg	<1 min	60 min	2.0 mg first dose	Seizure risk if opioid dependent including newborns of drug-addicted mother	Have at bedside when using fentanyl Smaller doses (0.01 mg/kg/dose) may reverse respiratory depression but maintain analgesia Narcotic effects may outlast naloxone
Flumazenil	IV	0.02 mg/kg	1–3 min		1 mg	Crying, agitation	Administer via 0.2 mg increments over 15 sec Repeat dose in 60 sec, to 1 mg max Useful for iatrogenic/known overdose Not for reversal of known side effects Benzodiazepine may outlast flumazenil

Fentanyl combined with midazolam (see Benzodiazepines below) provides potent analgesia for short, painful procedures. Administer the midazolam first, followed by fentanyl. Generally, with this combination, the total dose of fentanyl can be decreased by about 50%.

Benzodiazepines

Benzodiazepines possess sedative-hypnotic, anxiolytic, and antegrade amnestic effects. When used as a single agent, they have a low risk of complications, although they are often combined with other drugs, such as opioids, for painful procedures. Untoward effects of benzodiazepines are reversible with the antagonist flumazenil (Table 24.4), which is appropriate for iatrogenic or known overdose of benzodiazepines. Do not use flumazenil routinely to reverse the known effects of benzodiazepines. Monitor the patient for resedation since the half-life of the benzodiazepine may outlast that of flumazenil.

Midazolam

Indications for use include anxiety-provoking or non-painful procedures such as CT scan or gynecologic examination, or procedures in which a local anesthetic will be used, e.g., laceration repair. Use midazolam in combination with an opioid to augment sedation for painful procedures.

Etomidate

Etomidate is a non-barbiturate sedative-hypnotic that has been used for several decades as an induction agent in the operating room. Initially in EDs it was used as a pre-intubation induction agent but has subsequently gained favor as a PSA medication. It has no analgesic properties, so patients undergoing a painful procedure will need additional medication, such as lidocaine or an opioid. Etomidate produces amnesia for the event in the majority of patients. Use etomidate for procedures of very short duration such as a CT scan of the head, reduction of a dislocation, foreign body removal, abscess incision and drainage, and lumbar puncture.

Propofol

Propofol is a potent sedative-hypnotic agent that has no analgesic or amnestic effects. Because of its potency, it can be used alone for painful procedures of short duration, such as fracture reduction and incision and drainage of an abscess or pilonidal cyst. It is contraindicated in patients with soy and egg allergies.

Nitrous Oxide

Nitrous oxide is a sedative-hypnotic that has no anesthetic qualities but causes a detached feeling in the patient. It is a two-tank system capable of delivering a mixture of up to 70% nitrous oxide and 30% oxygen. Attach a scavenger device from the nitrous oxide tank to wall suction to eliminate the potential for leakage of nitrous oxide into the atmosphere. Prepare an additional suction device in case the patient vomits, which is an indication for discontinuing the nitrous oxide. Administer 100% oxygen for 1–3 minutes before starting nitrous oxide, then initiate nitrous oxide at low levels (30–40%) for 2–3 minutes. Subsequently, increase nitrous oxide to 50–60% (steady state) and keep at this level for 2–3 minutes or throughout the procedure, if the desired level of comfort is met. During the most painful part of the procedure, 70% nitrous oxide can be used, with a return to the steady state percentage when complete. Dial down nitrous oxide in the same slow manner that it was raised. When nitrous oxide is discontinued, administer 100% oxygen for 3–5 minutes.

As a safety measure, the nitrous oxide delivery stops if the oxygen becomes diminished. Discontinue the nitrous oxide if there is no effect after 2–3 minutes; 10% of the population does not respond. Nitrous oxide is contraindicated in patients with head trauma or impaired mental status, abdominal distention or obstruction, pneumothorax, respiratory depression, and pregnancy.

Ketamine

Ketamine is a phencyclidine derivative that provides potent sedation and analgesia and dissociates the central nervous system (CNS) from outside stimuli such as pain, sight, and sound. Use ketamine for painful procedures of short or moderate duration such as fracture reduction, incision and drainage, or wound repair. It is not necessary to administer midazolam or an antisialagogue with ketamine.

Since there is no spectrum of dissociation (it is either present or absent), additional increments of the drug will not increase the level of dissociation. Titrate the drug to achieve the dissociated state over the length of the procedure.

Absolute contraindications of ketamine include age under three months and psychosis. Relative contraindications include procedures that stimulate the posterior pharynx (endoscopy), active respiratory disease, cardiovascular disease, history of airway problems (tracheal stenosis), CNS masses or hydrocephalus (ketamine is safe to use in head trauma), glaucoma or acute globe injury, hyperthyroidism, porphyria, or when there is a history of a previous adverse reaction. Perform meticulous oral suctioning if using for intraoral procedures to avoid pooling of secretions.

Propofol With Low-Dose Ketamine

This combination provides potent sedation with a good safety profile. Theoretically, propofol-related hypotension and respiratory depression are reduced by the increased norepinephrine induced by ketamine and the ketamine-related emesis is reduced by the antiemetic and anxiolytic properties of propofol.

Dexmedetomidine

Dexmedetomidine is a CNS α2-agonist that provides profound sedation with few cardiovascular and respiratory effects. Reported side effects include xerostomia, bradycardia, rash, orthostatic hypotension, and rebound hypertension. If necessary, the antidote atipamezole will reverse the sedative and cardiovascular effects.

Barbiturates

Barbiturates are sedative-hypnotics that can provide mild to deep sedation, depending on the dose. They have no analgesic qualities. Give barbiturates for anxiety-provoking procedures such as CT scan or procedures in which a local anesthetic will be used (e.g., laceration repair).

Methohexital

Methohexital is an ultra-short-acting barbiturate that is given rectally, avoiding the need for an IV catheter.

Pentobarbital

This is a short-acting barbiturate, although the onset of action may be delayed when given by the rectal or oral routes.

Bibliography

Bellolio MF, Puls HA, Anderson JL, et al. Incidence of adverse events in paediatric procedural sedation in the emergency department: a systematic review and meta-analysis. *BMJ Open*. 2016;6(6):e011384.

Godwin SA, Burton JH, Gerardo CJ, Hatten BW. Clinical policy: procedural sedation and analgesia in the emergency department. *Ann Emerg Med*. 2014;63(2):247–258.

Green SM, Roback MG, Kennedy RM. Clinical practice guidelines for emergency department ketamine dissociative sedation 2011 update. Ann Emerg Med. 2011;57:462–468.

Kannikeswaran N, Lai, ML, Malian, M, Wang B, Farooqi A, Roback MG. Optimal dosing of intravenous ketamine for procedural sedation in children in the ED: a randomized controlled trial. Am J Emerg Med. 2016;34:1347–1353.

Krieser D, Kochar A. Paediatric procedural sedation within the emergency department. *J Paediatr Child Health*. 2016;52(2):197–203.

Pacheco GS, Ferayorni A. Pediatric procedural sedation and analgesia. *Emerg Med Clin North Am*. 2013;31(3):831–852.

Local Anesthesia

Lidocaine

Lidocaine is a local anesthetic routinely used in the ED, most commonly for laceration repair. Lidocaine is available as either a 1% (10 mg/mL) or 2% (20 mg/mL) solution, with and without epinephrine. Epinephrine is contraindicated in areas with end-arteries (the fingers, toes, penis, nose, or ear).

Dose

With epinephrine: 7 mg/kg; without epinephrine: 4.5 mg/kg.

Administration

In order to decrease the pain of administration, administer slowly with a 27 gauge 1.5 inch needle, warm the solution to 40 °C (104 °F), and buffer with sodium bicarbonate in a 1:10 ratio, which will give the solution a pH of 7.2. For intact skin, infiltrate subcutaneously until a bleb is apparent. For open wounds, put a few drops directly into the wound, then infiltrate subcutaneously around the wound edge. In areas of large arteries, aspirate before infiltrating to check for blood return. Advance the needle slowly with constant infiltration of lidocaine. Withdraw and continue around the wound sequentially, placing the needle in the already anesthetized portion of the subdermis. Assure that the area is anesthetized by applying the needle to the skin out of view of the child. Anesthesia occurs in approximately five minutes.

Topical Anesthesia

LET

Lidocaine (4%), epinephrine (1%), and tetracaine (0.5%) is available in gel or liquid form and is indicated for laceration repair.

Dose

1–3 mL

Administration

Place half of the solution on the wound and half on a cotton pad. Do not use gauze as this will pull the LET away from the wound. Hold the cotton firmly in place for 30–45 minutes. Use an elastic bandage on suitable areas such as scalp or extremity lacerations. Otherwise, secure the cotton with firmly placed tape or have an adult hold it in place with pressure. Supplemental local lidocaine is generally required.

EMLA (Eutectic Mixture of Local Anesthesia)

EMLA contains 2.5% lidocaine and 2.5% prilocaine. Apply it on intact skin for IV placement, phlebotomy, and injections or minor procedures such as incision and drainage of a paronychia. It can be used on mucous membranes of the groin and on compromised skin (e.g., dermatitis). The major adverse event is the potential for methemoglobinemia, especially in infants with G-6-PD deficiency or children receiving other methemoglobinemia-inducing agents such as sulfa drugs.

Administration

Apply a thick layer to the area and cover with an occlusive dressing (Table 24.5), for a minimum of 60 minutes. The effects are maximal at 2–3 hours and may persist up to two hours after removal of the cream. The depth of anesthesia is 3 mm after one hour and 5 mm after two hours.

LMX4 (4% Liposomal Lidocaine)

Use LMX4 on intact skin (not mucous membranes) for procedures as listed above for EMLA. The onset of anesthesia is 30 minutes. Because it does not contain prilocaine, there is no risk of methemoglobinemia as with EMLA.

Table 24.5 Dose and application of EMLA

Age	Weight (kg)	Maximum dose (g)	Maximum duration (hours)	Maximum area (cm^2)
1–3 months	<5	1	1	10
4–12 month	5–10	2	4	20
1–6 years	>10	10	4	100
7–12 years	>20	20	4	200

Administration

Apply a thick layer to the area. An occlusive dressing will enhance absorption and keep the medication in place, but is not required.

Numby Stuff (Tetracaine 7%/Lidocaine 7% Patch)

The patch contains both analgesics as well as a warming element that enhances absorption and vasodilation. Apply the patch directly onto unbroken skin. Local analgesia is achieved in 20–30 minutes.

Ethyl Chloride

Ethyl chloride is a vapocoolant and not a local anesthetic. It transiently lowers the local temperature of the skin to –10 °C (14 °F) to –20 °C (–4 °F). The nerves are then desensitized for a brief period. Indications include IV placement, phlebotomy, injections, and incision and drainage of a paronychia or small abscess.

Procedure

Hold the can about six inches from the application site. Spray the desired area only until the skin appears white, which will be the point of maximal anesthesia. Perform the procedure immediately since the cooling effect is brief.

Hurricaine Spray (Benzocaine 20%)

Use Hurricaine Spray to anesthetize mucous membranes before draining a peritonsillar abscess or repairing intraoral lacerations. The onset of anesthesia is about one minute and the duration is 12–15 minutes. If swallowed, it may suppress the gag reflex. There is a potential risk of methemoglobinemia.

Procedure

Spray 1–2 inches from the intended site for one second.

Sucrose 12% Solution

The combination of sucrose and sucking can provide an analgesic effect in infants 0–3 months of age. Give 1.5–2.0 mL PO over two minutes through a nipple or on a gloved finger. Wait two minutes before starting the procedure. The effect lasts up to eight minutes.

Regional Anesthesia

In certain circumstances, use of local infiltration of anesthesia is undesirable. Examples include wounds in areas with little surrounding subcutaneous tissue where local infiltration will significantly distort the tissue architecture, large wounds where the amount of lidocaine needed to achieve anesthesia is excessive, and wounds in areas that are difficult and extremely painful to fully anesthetize, such as fingertips, toes, nailbeds, palms, soles, and the penis. Regional anesthesia provides effective anesthesia in these cases.

Equipment

- 1% lidocaine solution, without epinephrine;
- sodium bicarbonate (ratio of ten parts lidocaine to one part sodium bicarbonate);
- 25- or 27-gauge hypodermic needle, 0.5–1 inch in length;
- syringe (3–5 mL is usually sufficient);
- antiseptic solution for the skin;
- sterile gauze.

General Procedure

Assess for sensory deficits secondary to trauma before performing the nerve block. Cleanse the skin with antiseptic solution for percutaneous nerve blocks. No antiseptic is necessary with intraoral approaches. After inserting the needle, draw back on the syringe slightly before injecting lidocaine to ensure that the needle is not within a blood vessel. If insertion of the needle elicits paresthesias or a sharp jolt of pain in the nerve distribution, withdraw the needle slightly before injecting lidocaine to avoid infiltration directly into the nerve. Although anesthesia may be achieved within several minutes, 10–20 minutes may be needed for maximal effect to occur. Gently massage the area where the lidocaine is deposited to hasten the distribution of the anesthetic in the region of the nerve.

Supraorbital and Supratrochlear Nerve Blocks

Area of Effect
Forehead and frontal scalp.

Anatomy
The supraorbital nerve exits the supraorbital foramen at the orbital rim in the midpupillary line. The supratrochlear nerve exits the foramen just medial to the supraorbital nerve (Figure 24.1).

Technique
Locate the supraorbital foramen and insert the needle subcutaneously just lateral to the foramen. Direct the needle medially and advance it to the hub in a direction both parallel and adjacent to the superior orbital rim. Lay a track of 2–3 mL lidocaine along this line as the needle is slowly withdrawn.

Infraorbital Nerve Block

Area of Effect
Medial cheek to the nasal ala, upper lip, and lower eyelid.

Anatomy
The infraorbital nerve exits the infraorbital foramen approximately 1.5 cm below the inferior orbital rim, in the midpupillary line.

Technique
The intraoral approach is less painful and preferable to the percutaneous approach. Retract the upper lip. Using a cotton swab, apply a topical anesthetic (2% viscous lidocaine) for several

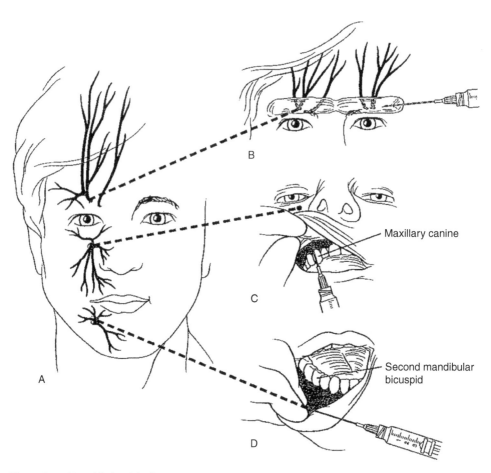

Figure 24.1 Nerve blocks of the face.
From: Trott AT. *Wounds and Lacerations* (3rd edn.). Philadelphia, PA: Elsevier Mosby, 2005, with permission.

minutes to the oral mucosa of the gingival-buccal sulcus at the level of the maxillary canine tooth or second bicuspid. Insert the needle at this location and direct it superiorly toward the infraorbital foramen. Advance the needle subcutaneously approximately 1–2 cm until the tip of the needle is at the level of the infraorbital foramen, then inject 1–2 mL of lidocaine.

Mental Nerve Block

Area of Effect
Lower lip and chin.

Anatomy
The mental nerve exits the mental foramen midway between the upper and lower borders of the mandible, in the midpupillary line, approximately 2–2.5 cm from the midline of the jaw.

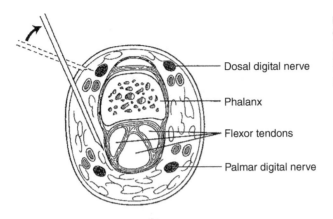

Figure 24.2 Dorsal and palmar digital nerves.
From: Trott AT. *Wounds and Lacerations* (3rd edn.). Philadelphia, PA: Elsevier Mosby, 2005, with permission.

Dosal digital nerve

Phalanx

Flexor tendons

Palmar digital nerve

Technique

The intraoral approach is less painful and preferable to the percutaneous approach. Pretreat the injection site with 2% viscous lidocaine (as above). Retract the lower lip. Insert the needle in the gingival-buccal sulcus at the second bicuspid, and advance the needle inferiorly toward the mental foramen. When the tip of the needle is at the level of the mental foramen, inject 1–2 mL of lidocaine.

Digital Nerve Block

Area of Effect

Finger or toe distal to the proximal phalanx.

Anatomy

Each digit is supplied by four nerves, two dorsal and two palmar. On a cross-section of the digit, the dorsal nerves are located at 2 o'clock and 10 o'clock; the palmar nerves are located at 4 o'clock and 8 o'clock. The nerves run adjacent to the phalanges. In addition, the great toe has nerve branches that come up the dorsal surface of the toe (Figure 24.2).

Technique

Insert the needle into the web space at the dorsolateral aspect of the proximal phalanx of the digit. Advance the needle until it touches the bone, then withdraw the needle slightly and inject 0.5–1 mL lidocaine. Redirect the needle toward the palmar nerve and advance adjacent to the bone. When the tip of the needle is at the level of the palmar nerve, inject 0.5–1.0 mL lidocaine. Repeat the entire process on the opposite side of the digit (Figure 24.3).

Alternatively, perform a transthecal block (tendon sheath block) by inserting the needle into the tendon sheath, resulting in complete finger anesthesia. Palpate the metacarpophalangeal joint and introduce the needle midline at a 45-degree angle just proximal to the joint. Advance the needle slowly toward the tendon sheath while maintaining slight constant pressure on the plunger of the needle. When the tendon sheath is entered, the anesthesia will

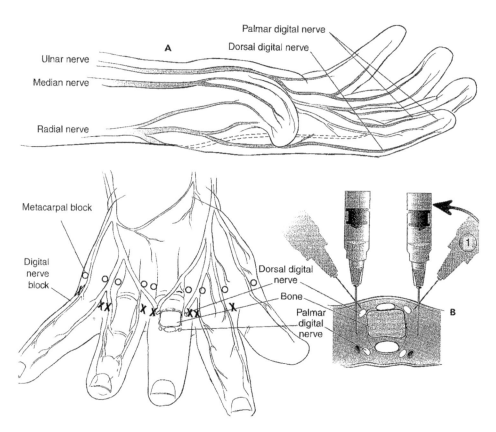

Figure 24.3 Digital nerve block.
From: King C, Henretig F (eds.) *Textbook of Pediatric Emergency Procedures* (2nd edn.). Philadelphia, PA: Lippincott Williams and Wilkins, 2008, with permission.

flow easily. Inject 1–2 mL lidocaine and withdraw the needle. If the anesthesia does not flow easily, the tendon may have been entered. Withdraw the needle slowly until the anesthesia flows freely.

To properly anesthetize the great toe, instill lidocaine circumferentially. After injecting lidocaine on either side of the great toe as described above, redirect the needle across the dorsal surface of the toe and advance the needle to the opposite side. Lay a track of lidocaine as the needle is slowly withdrawn. Repeat the process on the plantar surface of the toe (Figure 24.4).

Median Nerve Block

Area of Effect

The palmar surface of the thumb; second, third, and lateral aspect of the fourth fingers; and the dorsal surface of the tips of the thumb, second, third, and lateral aspect of the fourth fingers (Figure 24.5).

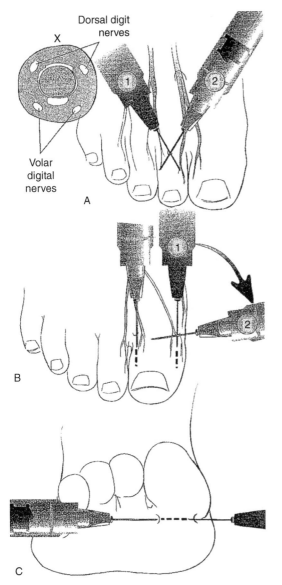

Dorsal digit nerves

X

Volar digital nerves

A

B

C

Figure 24.4 Digital nerve block of great toe. From: King C, Henretig F (eds.) *Textbook of Pediatric Emergency Procedures* (2nd edn.). Philadelphia, PA: Lippincott Williams and Wilkins, 2008, with permission.

Anatomy

The median nerve lies between and below the palmaris longus and flexor carpi radialis tendons. For patients who do not have a palmaris longus tendon (up to 20% of the population), the median nerve is just medial to the flexor carpi radialis (Figure 24.6).

(a)

(b)

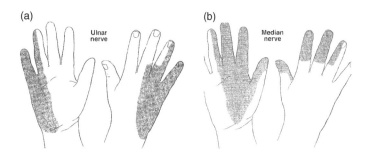

Ulnar nerve

Median nerve

Figure 24.5 Sensory distribution of median and ulnar nerves.
From: McCreight A, Stephan M. Local and regional anesthesia. In King C, Henretig F (eds.) *Textbook of Pediatric Emergency Procedures* (2nd edn.). Philadelphia, PA: Lippincott Williams and Wilkins, 2008, pp. 450–451.

Technique

Insert the needle between the palmaris longus and flexor carpi radialis tendons at the level of the proximal wrist crease. Insert the needle at the same level, just medial to the flexor carpi radialis for patients who do not have a palmaris longus tendon. Advance the needle approximately 1 cm. A "popping" sensation may be felt as the needle passes through the flexor retinaculum (Figure 24.6). If paresthesias are elicited, withdraw the needle slightly, and inject 2–3 mL of lidocaine. If no paresthesias are elicited, inject 3–5 mL of lidocaine as the needle is slowly withdrawn.

Ulnar Nerve Block

Area of Effect

Dorsal and palmar surfaces of the fourth and fifth fingers, medial aspect of the hand, and dorsal surface of the medial aspect of the third finger (Figure 24.5).

Anatomy

The ulnar nerve divides into the palmar and dorsal cutaneous branches several centimeters proximal to the wrist. The ulnar nerve lies beneath the flexor carpi ulnaris tendon at the level of the wrist, and runs adjacent to the ulnar artery. Both palmar and dorsal cutaneous branches must be blocked to achieve full anesthesia.

Technique

To block the palmar branch of the ulnar nerve, insert the needle just lateral to the flexor carpi ulnaris tendon at the level of the proximal wrist crease. Advance the needle approximately 1 cm. Check that the needle has not entered the ulnar artery by drawing back on the syringe, then inject 2–3 mL lidocaine. Block the dorsal branch of the ulnar artery by injecting 1–2 mL lidocaine subcutaneously at the dorsal aspect of the wrist just distal to the ulnar styloid.

Alternatively, insert the needle at the medial aspect of the wrist at the level of the proximal crease, just dorsal to the flexor carpi ulnaris tendon. Advance the needle laterally approximately 1 cm, then inject 2–3 mL lidocaine. Withdraw the needle and redirect it toward the distal end of the ulnar styloid. Inject 1–2 mL lidocaine

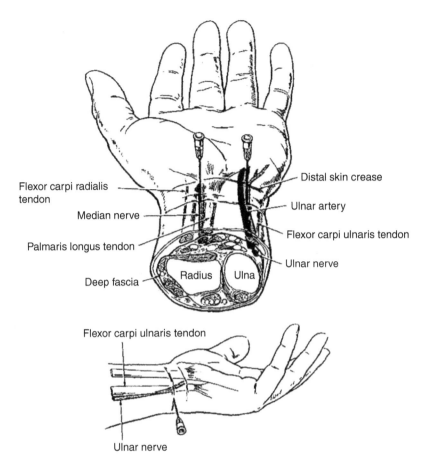

Flexor carpi radialis tendon

Median nerve

Palmaris longus tendon

Deep fascia

Distal skin crease

Ulnar artery

Flexor carpi ulnaris tendon

Ulnar nerve

Radius   Ulna

Flexor carpi ulnaris tendon

Ulnar nerve

Figure 24.6 Median and ulnar nerve blocks.
From: Roberts JR, Hedges JR (eds.) *Clinical Procedures in Emergency Medicine* (3rd edn.). Philadelphia, PA: W.B. Saunders Co., 1998, with permission.

superficially in this area. This approach will block both the dorsal and palmar branches of the ulnar nerve (Figure 24.6).

Radial Nerve Block

Area of Effect
Dorsal surface of the thumb, second, and third fingers, and lateral aspect of the hand (Figure 24.7).

Anatomy
A superficial cutaneous branch of the radial nerve divides from the main radial nerve several centimeters proximal to the wrist. At the wrist, this branch fans out subcutaneously around the distal radius and the dorsolateral aspect of the wrist and hand (Figure 24.7).

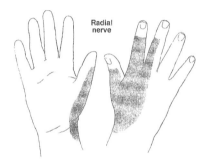

Figure 24.7 Sensory distribution of the radial nerve.
From: Roberts JR, Hedges JR (eds.) *Clinical Procedures in Emergency Medicine* (3rd edn.). Philadelphia, PA: W.B. Saunders Co., 1998, with permission.

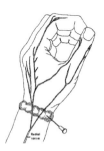

Figure 24.8 Radial nerve block.
From Roberts JR, Hedges JR (eds.) *Clinical Procedures in Emergency Medicine* (3rd edn.). Philadelphia, PA: W.B. Saunders Co., 1998, with permission.

Technique

Insert the needle at the dorsolateral aspect of the wrist at the level of the proximal wrist crease. Advance the needle 1–1.5 cm along the dorsum of the wrist toward the midline. Lay a track of 2–3 mL lidocaine while withdrawing the needle slowly. Before the needle is completely withdrawn, redirect it laterally toward the radial aspect of the wrist. Check that the needle is not inserted into the radial artery by drawing back on the syringe. Lay a track of 2–3 mL lidocaine along the lateral aspect of the wrist as the needle is slowly withdrawn (Figure 24.8).

Dorsal Penile Nerve Block

Area of Effect

Glans and shaft of the penis.

Anatomy

The right and left dorsal nerves of the penis are branches of the pudendal nerve, which arises from the second to fourth sacral nerve roots. On a cross-sectional view of the penis, the dorsal nerves are found at 2 o'clock and 10 o'clock (Figure 24.9a).

Technique

Insert the needle at the base of the penis at the 2 o'clock position. Advance the needle no more than 3–5 mm beneath the skin, just inside Buck's fascia. A "pop" may be felt as the needle passes through Buck's fascia. Inject 1–5 mL lidocaine, depending on the size of the child. Repeat the procedure at the 10 o'clock position (Figure 24.9b).

Alternatively, a single midline injection can also be used. Feel for the inferior edge of the symphysis pubis. Insert the needle perpendicular to the skin at the base of the penis in the midline. Advance the needle adjacent to the edge of the symphysis pubis to a depth of 3–5 mm beyond the symphysis pubis into Buck's fascia. A "pop" may be felt as the needle passes through Buck's fascia. Inject 1–5 mL lidocaine, which will anesthetize both dorsal nerves as the lidocaine diffuses through Buck's fascia.

A superficial ring block can be performed to augment the dorsal penile nerve block. Inject a subcutaneous ring of lidocaine circumferentially around the base of the penis. Two injection sites are generally sufficient, one on the ventral surface of the penis, and the other on the dorsal side. Direct and advance the needle both medially and laterally at each injection site. Inject the lidocaine subcutaneously as the needle is slowly withdrawn.

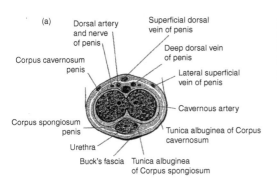

(a) Dorsal artery and nerve of penis — Superficial dorsal vein of penis — Deep dorsal vein of penis — Corpus cavernosum penis — Lateral superficial vein of penis — Cavernous artery — Corpus spongiosum penis — Tunica albuginea of Corpus cavernosum — Urethra — Buck's fascia — Tunica albuginea of Corpus spongiosum

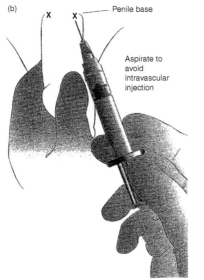

(b) Penile base — X X — Aspirate to avoid intravascular injection

Figure 24.9 Penile nerve block.
From: King C, Henretig F (eds.) *Textbook of Pediatric Emergency Procedures* (2nd edn.). Philadelphia, PA: Lippincott Williams and Wilkins, 2008, with permission.

Bibliography

Amsterdam JT, Kilgore KP. Regional anesthesia of the head and neck. In Roberts JR, Custalow CB, Thomsen TW, Hedges JR (eds.) *Roberts and Hedges' Clinical Procedures in Emergency Medicine* (6th edn.). Philadelphia, PA: Elsevier Saunders, 2014; 541–553.

McCreight A, Stephan M. Local and regional anesthesia. In King C, Henretig F (eds.) *Textbook of Pediatric Emergency Procedures* (2nd edn.). Philadelphia, PA: Lippincott Williams and Wilkins, 2008; 449–460.

Spektor M, Kelly JJ. Nerve blocks of the thorax and extremities. In Roberts JR, Custalow CB, Thomsen TW, Hedges JR (eds.) *Roberts and Hedges' Clinical Procedures in Emergency Medicine* (6th edn.). Philadelphia, PA: Elsevier Saunders, 2014; 554–557, 560–568, 571–574.

Trott AT. *Wounds and Lacerations: Emergency Care and Closure* (4th edn.). Philadelphia, PA: Elsevier Saunders, 2012; 41–72.

The Ouchless Emergency Department

Emergency department (ED) care is stressful and frightening for both children and their parents, as therapeutic procedures are often painful and seem beyond their control. Children fear separation from parents, loss of autonomy, frightening and painful procedures, and the unknown. Inadequately relieved procedure-related pain and anxiety can interfere with patient care and have negative physiological and psychological consequences for patients, parents, and healthcare providers. Parental presence, developmentally appropriate interactions, and effective pain management can help to moderate these issues.

Parental Presence

Children want their parent to be with them throughout their care, although the patient may, or may not, exhibit less upset behavior when the parent is present. Separating child and parent increases anxiety and interferes with coping skills of both. Parents believe they can help their child deal with the situation and they rarely interfere. In addition, parents are more satisfied with care when present for procedures. However, if parental distress is increased by being present during a procedure, the patient's anxiety is likely to increase. In such cases, use alternative strategies, such as ED staff assisting with distraction.

Use carefully considered language that does not frighten the child (Table 24.6) to inform parents of the plan of care and their role. Parents frequently know how best to distract their child, but may be overwhelmed by the situation. Specific recommendations help them understand how they can help. Table 24.7 provides some age- and development-oriented suggestions.

Developmentally Appropriate Approach to Establishing Trust

Toddlers (1–3 Years of Age)

Toddlers focus on the present, want autonomy, and are intensely curious about their environment. Use this to redirect their focus away from their injury by pointing out objects in the room, scenes in pictures, and tones on monitors, or allow them to hold your stethoscope. They need to feel as if they are doing things independently and like to engage

Table 24.6 Language and pediatric distress

	Neutral or reduces distress	Increases distress
Language	Pressure, tight squeeze, push, freezing Bother, uncomfortable Metal tube, squirter Sutures	Shot, sting, pinch, burning, hurt "I'm sorry" Needle, syringe Stitches
Behaviors	Redirecting attention Nonprocedural discussion (distraction) Talk before touch (avoid surprises) Firm, warm confidence Humor	Empathizing Apologizing Punishing Allow the child to delay Multiple adults talking

Adapted from Baxter AL. Common office procedures and analgesia considerations. *Pediatr Clin N Am.* 2013;60(5): 1163–1183.

Table 24.7 Developmentally directed distraction and comforting activities

All ages	Low, quiet, calm voice Maintain a calm, positive atmosphere
Infant	Position in comforting manner Sitting or upright in parent's lap/arms Secure to ensure minimal movement
Toddler	Position in comforting manner Hugging or maximum physical contact with parent Sitting or upright in parent's lap Use distractions, desensitization Secure to ensure minimal movement
Preschooler	Position in comforting manner Use distractions, desensitization Secure to ensure minimal movement
School-age	Use distractions, engage in conversation Secure to ensure minimal movement
Adolescent	Engage in conversation

Adapted from Khan KA, Weisman SJ. Nonpharmacologic pain management strategies in the pediatric emergency department. *Clin Ped Emerg Med.* 2007;8:240–247.

in making simple decisions, such as whether to sit in a parent's lap or on the bed alone, look at a book, or play a video game. Encourage the use of a favorite comfort object, such as a pacifier, blanket, stuffed animal. Call the patient by name and maintain eye contact. Avoid covering the child's face, and describe sensations during the procedure using non-frightening words. Provide hope, such as getting a Popsicle after the procedure (allow the child to choose which color). This small reward also signals completion of the procedure.

Redirect attention from the beginning. When first entering the treatment room, focus your interactions on the parents or older siblings while discretely observing the young patient. Shake hands with the parents as you introduce yourself. If applicable, chatting a bit and pointing out a humorous aspect of the situation may lead the parent to laugh. These interactions help the parent be more comfortable with you. The fearful toddler who is clinging to the parent, warily watching you, will sense you have established a rapport with their parent and may be more willing to trust you. As examples, you might humorously comment to the parent that the child's injury, e.g., a laceration or fracture, usually takes a "Y chromosome." Many parents laugh and acknowledge their child's tendency to play hard, whether it is a girl or boy. Alternatively, jokingly ask an older sibling whether he or she had anything to do with the injury. As the young patient begins to demonstrate less defensive posturing, try proffering your hand and ask the older toddler to "Give me five," then cause him to miss by quickly moving your hand. This often brings a smile from the patient and parents as they are surprised to see you playing.

For the young child who is still very fearful, try to focus their attention on something non-threatening by commenting on their shoes or their favorite comfort object if they are holding a blanket or doll. Speak in a calm, low voice, as if you have all day to do this. Try to desensitize the child to your touch by gently stroking an area of their body that is not painful. Generally, these techniques work better if you examine the fearful toddler or preschool child in their parent's lap or arms or with the parent sitting alongside on the stretcher.

Preschoolers (3–5 Years of Age)

Preschoolers have an emerging ability to engage in simple conversation, so try asking them about their siblings, pets, etc. They may act out emotions through temper tantrums, hyperactivity, shyness, or not speaking. They have a strong ability to fantasize and have magical thinking, so share limited information about a procedure *immediately* before performing it to prevent fantasies from becoming scary or overwhelming.

Give parents concrete information about the planned care so that they can be the child's primary source of explanation and comforting. Consider allowing the patient to explore equipment, if appropriate. For example, explain how the large syringe will be used to wash a wound and give the child a similar syringe to play with as you prepare equipment. Explain you will try to make the procedure not hurt, but ask the child to let you know if it does hurt. Use non-frightening language (Table 24.6) such as "pushing or squeezing too hard" as indicators of pain rather than "a stick and burn" or "bee sting" to describe injection of lidocaine. Distractions that work well involve active participation, such as playing a game on the parent's phone or computer tablet, singing a favorite song, picking out objects in a picture book, blowing bubbles, or deep breathing. Watching a movie or cartoons works best if the child already knows the story well and the screen is close (e.g., watching a favorite movie on a computer tablet). Use the screen to block direct visualization of the procedure as well.

School-Aged Children (6–12 Years of Age)

School-age patients fear death and disability associated with pain and they tend to display more overt distress than older children. Distress behaviors include crying, stalling, resisting, anger, fear, and withdrawal. While they may be developing a sense of competence, they may feel insecure in their ability to complete a task. To support their need to feel accomplishment, offer as many choices as possible. Be open about any pain/discomfort that may occur. Do *not* tell a child a procedure will *not* hurt if it is possible it may. A patient who is surprised by a painful stimulus tends to become more vigilant and less capable of engaging in distraction or relaxation exercises and may become more anxious and lose trust in providers.

It is very helpful to explain procedures beforehand, encourage cooperation, ask about preferences, give choices (if possible), and identify sensations. Try to use distraction and relaxation imagery, but alert the child to any sensations of pain they may feel. Enlist the parents to help provide support and comfort.

Adolescence (13–18 Years of Age)

Adolescents may try to "cover-up pain" or show bravado and may be more worried about the consequences of the injury. They often are ambivalent about parental presence as they try to assert independence. Give full explanations, encourage participation, allow questions, ensure privacy, allow control as appropriate, and use relaxation, imagery, and distraction. Reassure teens that their reactions are normal.

Altering Memory

The young child's memory of a distressful procedure may be altered to become less negative. Praising a young child after the procedure (e.g., complementing him on how brave he was, how much he helped by holding still, and how well he used his coping mechanisms) can reinforce the positive aspects of the experience. Lavish praise for desired behavior. Focusing on a reward such as a sticker or Popsicle can also help moderate the negative memories.

Language

Carefully choose words which avoid exacerbating distress (Table 24.6). For example, when preparing a preschooler for the discomfort of lidocaine injection, telling him "It will be like a little bee sting" guarantees a negative reaction. As an alternative, if buffered lidocaine is refrigerated, warn the child: "It may be cold and feel like freezing. Let me know if I'm pushing too hard and I will slow down." This gives the child a less frightening interpretation of the sensation.

Pain

Attention to pain early in treatment is critical. This may be pain of injury, illness, or impending procedures. A useful rule of thumb is that if the injury or procedure would be painful for you, the patient is, or soon will be, experiencing discomfort. If imminent care for the patient will cause pain – such as repositioning an injured area for radiographs – administer analgesia beforehand and allow time for effect.

In triage administer effective analgesia when a patient arrives with a possible fracture, burn, laceration, sickle cell pain, or other painful conditions. Splint potential fractures. Apply topical anesthetic cream over potential venous cannulation sites if an intravenous catheter or venipuncture is likely to be needed. These activities increase efficiency of care as well as patient and parent satisfaction.

Case-Based Recommendations

Lacerations

Apply topical anesthetic gel (lidocaine–epinephrine–tetracaine [LET]) directly into the wound at triage, then cover with a transparent nonabsorbent dressing to allow wound visualization. Thicken LET with methylcellulose to facilitate direct instillation into the wound; soaking liquid LET into cotton or gauze which is then placed in the wound reduces its effectiveness. As per institutional preferences and protocols, 30–60 minutes prior to wound cleansing and closure, administer an analgesic, such as oral oxycodone (0.2 mg/kg, 10 mg maximum), and/or a sedative such as intranasal midazolam (see Sedation and Analgesia, p. 717). If available, nitrous oxide administered via a continuous-flow facemask system is effective for the highly anxious child who cannot be calmed.

Parental support is crucial. Allow the infant and toddler to be held in the parent's lap. Instruct the parent about the plan, using careful language to avoid increasing the child's anxiety. Clarify what the parent is to do – e.g., give the child a gentle hug to control the child's movement, help with distraction, and provide comfort and reassurance. Parents usually know what works best for their child, but they will benefit from suggestions. Allow the child to become accustomed to your touch by gently stroking non-painful areas of their body, speaking in a calm, quiet voice, and engaging in distracting conversation. If available, use a computer tablet or parent's phone with games or video for distraction. Games that require patient interactions such as swiping or touching the screen are more effective. Try to use videos that are very familiar to the toddler or preschooler. Allow one person to attempt distraction, as multiple speakers increase anxiety.

Before cleansing the laceration, use a 30 gauge needle to slowly inject buffered lidocaine subcutaneously from within the wound to minimize pain of injection. Injecting all wound edges with buffered lidocaine after LET application ensures more reliable anesthesia, avoids painful surprises during suturing, and helps the patient become accustomed to your manipulating the wound. To reduce anxiety in young children, first show them the syringe without the needle, drip a few drops of lidocaine telling them that you are going to put more medicine into their cut to help it not hurt, then surreptitiously attach the 30 gauge needle for injection. Avoid allowing the child to see the needle by bringing the syringe from behind his head such that it is not in his field of vision. Inject very slowly to minimize pain. If the wound is not visibly contaminated, consider cleaning with wet gauze instead of irrigating. The spray from irrigation can frighten young children, especially if it gets into their eyes.

Avoid draping over the child's eyes for facial lacerations. Rather, place drape over the child's hair/forehead, beside the head, or below the chin to provide a sterile/clean surface over which to work. Use absorbable sutures when possible to negate the need for frightening suture removal. When using tissue adhesive to close the wound, anesthetize with LET before cleansing, since many adhesives release uncomfortable heat as they polymerize.

Many hand and finger lacerations do not need to be sutured if underlying tendons are not involved. If suturing of a finger laceration is necessary, direct injection of buffered lidocaine after LET application is less painful and therefore preferable to a digital block. If there is no evidence of a displaced fracture associated with the nailbed laceration, cyanoacrylate (tissue adhesive) is an acceptable alternative to suturing, but precise positioning of the involved nailbed is critical before application of the adhesive. Tissue adhesive allows a faster repair than suturing, with similar cosmetic and functional results.

Intravenous Catheter Insertion/Venipuncture

Needlesticks are frightening for children of all ages. Carefully consider whether the blood test or venous catheter is necessary. Allow the young child to sit in the parent's lap during venous catheter insertion or venipuncture to reduce distress.

Local Anesthesia for Venous Catheter Insertion or Venipuncture

Application of a topical local anesthetic at triage can improve efficiency, since most agents require 20–60 minutes to be effective. Relatively painless direct inoculation of buffered lidocaine using compressed gas or injection with a 30 gauge needle provides immediate and more effective anesthesia. Assure that the lidocaine is infused subcutaneously up to the wall of the vein for best effect. For the extremely anxious child, administer nitrous oxide (if available) in addition to local anesthesia to reduce anxiety, provide additional analgesia, and reduce stress-induced vasoconstriction.

Fracture Management

Early attention to reducing the pain of fractures helps reassure both children and their parents. At triage, splint the injured area and administer appropriate analgesia (oxycodone 0.2 mg/kg, 10 mg maximum). Repositioning the injured area for radiographs can be the most painful part of fracture care. Deep procedural sedation is usually necessary for fracture reduction.

Burn Debridement

When subsequent painful treatment procedures are likely, effective management of pain and anxiety during the initial procedure is especially important in order to decrease future distress related to care. For small burns that can be gently debrided, oral oxycodone 0.2 mg/kg or intranasal fentanyl (use 2 mcg/kg if the sole agent) may provide sufficient analgesia. Covering the burn with lukewarm wet gauze may soften the blisters sufficiently to allow blunt debridement by wiping with the gauze. For the especially anxious child, consider additional use of nitrous oxide, but the likelihood of emesis may be increased by the co-administration of opioid.

Lumbar Puncture (LP)

Injection of buffered lidocaine along the LP track using a 30 gauge needle provides effective local anesthesia and reduces the likelihood of a traumatic (bloody) tap. Topical anesthetic creams will reduce the pain of skin puncture, but do not provide deeper local anesthesia. For infants less than two months of age, a concentrated sucrose solution dripped onto their pacifier or into their mouth reduces distress. For older infants and children, administer midazolam to reduce anxiety. Nitrous oxide also reduces anxiety and provides additional analgesia.

Nasogastric (NG) Tube Placement

No techniques effectively reduce the pain and subsequent discomfort of NG tube insertion. Carefully consider whether this procedure is necessary. Prior to insertion administer oxymetazoline or phenylephrine nasal spray to shrink the nasal mucosa and reduce epistaxis. Administer intranasal 2% lidocaine at 4 mg/kg (0.2 mL/kg of 2%) as a gel or atomized spray to children at least five minutes prior to tube insertion.

Bibliography

Baxter AL. Common office procedures and analgesia considerations. *Pediatr Clin N Am.* 2013;**60** (5):1163–1183.

Cramton RE, Gruchala NE. Managing procedural pain in pediatric patients. *Curr Opin Pediatr.* 2012;**24**(4):530–538.

Krauss BS. Video: managing procedural anxiety in children. www.nejm.org/doi/full/10.1056/NEJMv cm1411127 (accessed May 17, 2017).

McNaughton C, Zhou C, Robert L, Storrow A, Kennedy RM. A randomized, crossover comparison of injected buffered lidocaine, lidocaine cream, and no analgesia for peripheral intravenous cannula insertion. *Ann Emerg Med.* 2009;**54**:214–220.

Zimmerman, R. When the doctor says this won't hurt a bit – and incredibly, it's true. http://com monhealth.legacy.wbur.org/2012/09/doctor-says-it-wont-hurt (accessed May 17, 2017).

Chapter 25

Trauma

Anthony J. Ciorciari

Cervical Spine Injuries

Among children in the United States, there are approximately 1300 new cases of spinal cord injury each year, with most occurring at the cervical level. Cervical spine injuries may accompany serious head trauma, such as severe deceleration injuries caused by high-speed motor vehicle crashes or falls from extreme heights. Sports injuries are another common mechanism. Less often, they may result from injuries to the top of the head or the back of the neck.

Clinical Presentation

Cervical spine injuries are most common in patients with severe head injuries. Therefore, cervical spine injury is always a possibility in a child who is unconscious or has an altered mental status after head trauma. This is especially true in younger children, whose horizontally aligned facet joints and more elastic intervertebral ligaments can predispose to subluxation without bony injury. This occurs when the angular momentum resulting from forceful impact levers the proportionately larger head on the fulcrum of the upper cervical spine. The result is a condition known as spinal cord injury without radiographic (including CT and MRI) abnormality (SCIWORA), which predisposes the victim to paraplegia and neurogenic shock or respiratory arrest. Approximately 20% of all pediatric spinal injuries are SCIWORA.

In the alert patient the most common finding is midline cervical tenderness. Less often, there is weakness, pain, or paresthesias along the affected nerve roots. In the unconscious patient with high-grade partial or complete cord transection, common findings include spinal shock (flaccidity and areflexia instead of spasticity, hyperreflexia, and Babinski's sign) and neurogenic ("warm") shock (hypotension that is poorly responsive to volume resuscitation but is paradoxically associated with bradycardia, "normal" urine output, and warm extremities).

Diagnosis

Assume that a cervical spine injury may have occurred in a patient who is unconscious or has an altered mental status after head trauma. Spinal cord injury is sometimes overlooked during the initial evaluation of a comatose patient with severe traumatic brain injury.

See pp. 749–758 for the general approach to the patient with multiple trauma and pp. 521–527 for the general approach to the patient with head trauma.

741

Often, an awake, alert patient arrives in the ED immobilized on a backboard, in a semirigid extrication collar. Ask about the presence of pain at the top of the head (C2–3) or back of the neck, and about paresthesias of the hands, arms, or legs. If none of these are present, without moving the patient, carefully remove the cervical restraint while maintaining in-line stabilization of the neck. Palpate the spinous processes for local tenderness-associated interspinous muscle spasm, or obvious deformity. The first spinous process that can be palpated is C2; C6 and C7 are the largest. Ask the patient to move the fingers and hands, feet and toes, and to raise the arms and legs. If there is no tenderness, hyperesthesia or paresthesias in the extremities, or evidence of trauma, and the patient moves all extremities easily, ask him or her to move the neck gently from side to side, then up and down. *Do not attempt to move the patient's neck yourself; insist that the patient stop immediately if any movement causes pain.*

Suspect a cervical spine injury in a patient with any of the following: unresponsiveness after head trauma; paresthesias or weakness; hyperesthesia; limitation of neck motion; inability to cooperate with the examination; pain on top of the head; neck trauma; or injury above the clavicles. Assume that there is a cervical spine injury until proven otherwise in a patient who is intoxicated or has a distracting injury that interferes with response to pain.

ED Management

Begin by performing an assessment of the ABCs, the initial component of the primary survey (see Resuscitation, pp. 1–4). Immediately stabilize the head and neck of every patient suspected of having a cervical spine injury, if temporary immobilization was not accomplished earlier in the field. The preferred method is with an appropriate-size semirigid extrication collar and head immobilizer. A thin layer of padding placed beneath the torso from shoulders to hips is required for a young child to assure maintenance of a neutral position, as the prominent occiput predisposes the neck to slight flexion unless this precaution is taken. A soft collar, sandbags, or large IV bags placed on both sides of the patient's head (despite being well-secured with tape across the forehead) do not provide adequate immobilization of the head and neck. Finally, because ventilation may be impaired by the very techniques required to achieve adequate immobilization, monitor the patient carefully for signs of respiratory compromise.

If intubation is necessary, apply bimanual in-line stabilization to the sides of the head and remove the extrication collar, if one is present. Have an assistant apply slight downward pressure over the larynx (the Sellick maneuver), if necessary, to bring the vocal cords into view. Avoid hyperextending or flexing the neck during the procedure. *Never delay intubation when indicated, because a cross-table lateral cervical spine x-ray has not been obtained or interpreted.*

Once the airway has been secured and the head and neck have been properly immobilized, order a cross-table lateral x-ray of the cervical spine. The base of the skull, all seven cervical vertebrae, and the top of the first thoracic vertebra must be visualized. Continuity of the normal lordotic curves of the cervical spine and important anatomic measurements (Table 25.1) must be confirmed by a physician experienced in interpretation of pediatric cervical spine radiographs. Be aware of certain anatomic features of young children that mimic vertebral injuries, including unfused epiphyses (particularly at the base of the dens), widening of the prevertebral soft tissue spaces on forced expiration (crying), and hypermobility of the upper cervical spine (resulting in the slight forward shifting of C2 on C3 and C3

Table 25.1 Normal cervical spine measurements

Measurement	<8 years	≥8 years
C2–3 override (flexion)	<4.5 mm	<3.5 mm
Predental space	4–5 mm	3 mm
Prevertebral space	½–⅔ thickness of C2	5–7 mm at level of C2
Spinal cord area	Varies with age	10–13 mm
Most commonly injured	C1–4	C5–7

on C4, known as pseudosubluxation). Suspect that the cervical spine is unstable in a child under eight years of age if >4.5 mm of subluxation is present at C2–3 or C3–4, or in an older patient if >3.5 mm of subluxation is noted at any level.

A lateral cervical spine radiograph alone can miss certain vertebral fractures. Thus, once this film is obtained and interpreted as normal, transport a patient with *stable vital signs* to the x-ray suite for AP and open-mouth views. An open-mouth view permits visualization of the odontoid process (dens) of the axis (C2) and the ring of the atlas (C1). Obtain a CT of the cervical spine when it is impossible to obtain a full radiographic series, there is a suggestion of fracture on radiograph without the actual fracture being seen (e.g., increased prevertebral soft tissue), or to look for additional fractures despite a fracture already having been identified on x-ray. Given that cervical injuries to children under eight years of age are more likely to be ligamentous than bony, do not use a CT scan as a screening tool in this population.

There is no immediate need to ascertain the integrity of the cervical spine in the comatose patient. Normal x-rays cannot definitely exclude spinal cord injury because of SCIWORA, while the patient's inability to relate symptoms compromises the reliability of the physical exam. Thus, it is safest to presume that spinal cord injury may be present, maintain full spinal immobilization, and defer comprehensive evaluation of the cervical spine to a later time. SCIWORA can be evaluated with an MRI. Findings include spinal cord transection or hemorrhage, or ligamentous or disk injury, although some MRIs may be normal.

When a cervical spine injury is diagnosed clinically or radiographically, immediately call the appropriate surgical specialist (neurosurgeon, orthopedist) to assist in further management (e.g., application of Gardner-Wells tongs). Admit any patient in whom cervical spine injury cannot be definitively ruled out in the ED.

Indications for Admission

- Cervical spine fracture
- Focal neurologic deficit
- Inability to exclude cervical spine injury

Bibliography

Adib O, Berthier E, Loisel D, Aubé C. Pediatric cervical spine in emergency: radiographic features of normal anatomy, variants and pitfalls. *Skeletal Radiol.* 2016;45(12):1607–1617.

Heini PF. Cervical spine injury in the young child. *Eur Spine J.* 2012 **21**:2205–2211.

Leonard JR, Jaffe DM, Kuppermann N, et al. Cervical spine injury patterns in children. *Pediatrics.* 2014;**133**(5):e1179–e1188.

Tat ST, Mejia MJ, Freishtat RJ. Imaging, clearance, and controversies in pediatric cervical spine trauma. *Pediatr Emerg Care.* 2014;**30**(12):911/–915

Tilt L, Babineau J, Fenster D, Ahmad F, Roskind CG. Blunt cervical spine injury in children. *Curr Opin Pediatr.* 2012;**24**:301–306.

Hand Injuries

The injured hand requires a thorough evaluation, as improper management may lead to permanent disability. A systematic approach is essential to avoid overlooking subtle injuries.

Clinical Presentation

Lacerations

Hand lacerations may affect the skin only or may be deep and involve underlying structures. Active extension of a digit is possible despite partial laceration of the extensor tendon. A dorsal hand laceration associated with pain on extension of the digit against resistance suggests a partial tendon injury.

Bites

Bites (pp. 763–766) are actually lacerations combined with crush injuries. Suspect that an irregular laceration over the metacarpophalangeal (MCP) joint is a human bite sustained by punching another person in the mouth. This is a serious injury, as oral flora can be inoculated into the MCP joint.

Fractures and Dislocations

Phalangeal Fractures

These fractures are common but not serious unless they are malrotated or the joint, volar plate, or collateral ligament is affected.

Wrist Fractures

Wrist fractures are less common in children than in adults. The most commonly fractured carpal bone is the scaphoid. Key findings include tenderness on deep palpation in the anatomic snuffbox area (between the extensor pollicis longus, extensor pollicis brevis, the prominent edge of the base of the first metacarpal and the styloid process of the radius); pain with longitudinal pressure placed on thumb; pain on pronation followed by ulnar deviation of the wrist; pain in the snuff box with resisted pronation or supination (ask the patient to "shake hands" with you while resisting your efforts to twist the wrist); and tenderness to palpation of the scaphoid tubercle (extend the child's wrist with one hand and apply pressure to the tuberosity at the proximal wrist crease with the opposite hand).

Metacarpophalangeal Joint Dislocations

MCP dislocations are rare. They usually involve the thumb and index and fifth fingers. Most of these dislocations can only be detected on lateral radiographs.

Proximal and Distal Interphalangeal (PIP and DIP) Joint Dislocations

PIP and DIP joint dislocations present with obvious deformity, unless already reduced at the scene by the patient or an onlooker.

Tendon Injuries

Gamekeeper's (Skier's) Thumb

Gamekeeper's thumb is caused by acute radial deviation of the thumb at the MCP joint that tears the ulnar collateral ligament. Typically the injury occurs when a patient falls with the thumb abducted. On examination, there is tenderness along the ulnar aspect of the first MCP joint, associated with >15 degrees of joint laxity on passive radial abduction (performed under local anesthesia) when compared to the unaffected thumb.

Mallet (Baseball) Finger

A mallet finger results from a direct blow to the tip of an extended digit, rupturing the DIP extensor tendon or avulsing it from the base of the distal phalanx (a Salter I, II, III or IV fracture). The finger is flexed at the DIP joint. Radiographs, which must contain a view of the PIP joint, may reveal an avulsed bone chip remaining attached to the extensor tendon.

Boutonnière (Buttonhole) Deformity

A boutonnière deformity follows violent flexion of the PIP joint. It presents with PIP flexion and DIP hyperextension. The lateral bands of the intrinsic muscles are pulled volar to the PIP axis, such that the lateral bands become PIP flexors while hyperextending the DIP. As a result, the PIP "buttonholes" through the torn extensor hood.

Jersey Finger

This is a partial or complete rupture of the flexor digitorum profundus at the point of attachment at the distal phalanx, caused by hyperextension at the DIP joint. The patient cannot flex the finger at the DIP joint.

Nail Bed Injuries

Blunt trauma to the nail can cause a subungual hematoma, bleeding between the nail and the nailbed. A very tender nail with blue-black subungual discoloration is seen.

Infections

Paronychia — A paronychia is an infection of the soft tissues around the fingernail. It usually begins as a hangnail and is more common in patients with a history of finger sucking or nail biting. There is exquisite tenderness to palpation of the nail as well as erythematous swelling along the nail margin. There may also be a purulent collection or discharge and/or an associated felon (see below).

Felon — A felon is a serious distal pulp space infection. Tense, tender, erythematous swelling of the volar surface of the distal phalanx is seen.

Purulent Tenosynovitis — This infection of the flexor tendon sheath is a true surgical emergency. There is usually a history of penetrating trauma. Kanavel's four cardinal signs of tenosynovitis are: (1) symmetric swelling; (2) slight flexion of the finger; (3) tenderness over the flexor tendon sheath; and (4) increased pain on passive finger extension (most likely to be present early in the disease). Tenosynovitis may progress to a palmer space infection.

Palmar Space Infection — A palmar space infection presents with tense, tender, erythematous swelling of the palmar surface with pain and decreased mobility of the third and fourth fingers (midpalmar space) or thumb (thenar space). In certain circumstances, the dorsum of the hand may be more swollen than the palmar surface. These infections can spread to the flexor tendon sheaths. Associated signs may include fever, lymphangitis, and lymphadenitis.

Ganglion

A ganglion is a benign, well-defined, smooth, cystic lesion of synovial origin. It is fixed to the deep tissues, typically tendon sheaths, or. less commonly, herniated joint lining. Usually less than 3 cm in diameter, it is most often found on the volar or dorsal surface of the wrist or on the palmar surface at the base of a digit.

Traumatic Amputations

Most traumatic amputations involve the distal fingertip only. Loss of the entire nail bed results in a more significant injury. Children have remarkable regenerative ability, so consider reimplantation of virtually any amputated part.

Diagnosis

The evaluation begins with a careful history, including hand dominance, tetanus immunization status, and description of any previous hand injuries. Inquire about the mechanism of injury, including the hand position at the time of injury, the time elapsed since injury, and whether the trauma occurred in a clean or dirty environment.

Expose and inspect the entire upper extremity. Note any discrepancy between active and passive mobility of upper-extremity joints. Inspect the hand and evaluate the vascular status. Look for an alteration in the usual resting cascade of the digits, suggestive of a tendon or nerve injury. Check the color and temperature of the injured digit, and assess capillary refill.

Before anesthetizing the hand in preparation for a surgical procedure, assess sensory function by evaluating two-point discrimination with two points of a paper clip. Apply both points to the radial side of each digit. Then move the points closer together until the patient can no longer distinguish between them. Use an uninjured digit as a control. Repeat the exam on the ulnar side. Then, evaluate the median (volar index fingertip), radial (dorsal web space between the thumb and index finger), and ulnar (volar fifth fingertip) sensory nerves. The "immersion test" can substitute when an adequate two-point discrimination test cannot be obtained. Failure of the skin to wrinkle after 5–10 minutes in water suggests sensory nerve injury.

Motor (nerve, muscle, and tendon) function must be evaluated in a systematic manner. First, test the extrinsic flexors: the IP joint of the thumb (flexor pollicis longus), the DIP joints of the fingers while the PIP joints are held in extension (flexor digitorum profundus), and then the PIP joints of each finger while the other fingers are held completely extended (flexor digitorum superficialis). Next, have the patient flex the wrist against resistance, and palpate the three tendons (flexor carpi ulnaris, palmaris longus, and flexor carpi radialis, from medial to lateral) at the base of the wrist. The palmaris longus is best seen by flexing the wrist against resistance with the thumb and fifth finger opposed; however, it is absent in approximately 15–20% of children.

Evaluate the thenar muscles and median motor function by opposing the pulp of the thumb with that of the other four fingers. Test thumb adduction (adductor pollicis) and ulnar nerve function by having the patient grasp a piece of paper between the thumb and radial surface of the proximal index finger. Weakness is indicated by Froment's paper sign, contraction of the flexor pollicis longus with flexion of the IP thumb joint. To check the hypothenar muscles, ask the patient to abduct the small finger. Evaluate the interosseous muscles (ulnar nerve) by having the patient spread the fingers apart. Test the lumbricals (median and ulnar nerves) by asking the patient to flex the digits at the MCP joints while keeping the PIP and DIP joints extended. Assess motor function of the radial nerve by having the patient extend the wrist against resistance.

ED Management

Manage profuse bleeding with elevation and pressure. *Never use clamps for hemostasis,* as the nerves traveling with the blood vessels can be damaged.

Palpate for localized bony tenderness or soft tissue swelling, and examine for obvious deformities, ecchymoses, and functional deficits. Obtain x-rays if any of these findings are present over the wrist or hand. Radiographs of the fingers are indicated for gross deformities, lacerations in association with crush injuries, or loss of IP joint mobility.

Instill local anesthesia for surgical procedures only after a satisfactory sensory examination has been completed. If a digital block is required, allow the skin to dry after preparing it with povidone-iodine. Use a 25 or 27 gauge needle to inject 2–4 mL of 2% lidocaine *without* epinephrine into both medial and lateral sides of the digit at the level of the metacarpal head. The maximum allowable dose of lidocaine is 4–5 mg/kg (without epinephrine). Before administration, be sure to inquire about personal or family history of previous reactions to local anesthetics.

Lacerations and Bites

Carefully debride and irrigate these wounds after administration of local anesthesia (see pp. 722–724). Close with 5-0 or 6-0 nylon, using simple sutures that are left in place for seven days. Avoid the use of deep sutures due to the risk of infection. A drain may be needed if the laceration is large. Carefully evaluate human bite wounds adjacent to MCP joints for evidence that the joint capsule has been violated. Open irrigation in the operating room is necessary if the wound has penetrated the capsule.

All deep lacerations and bite injuries of the hand require prophylactic antibiotics for seven days. Treat human and animal bite wounds with an IV dose of ampicillin/sulbactam (45 mg/kg). Follow this with amoxicillin/clavulanate alone (875/125 formulation, 45 mg/kg/day of amoxicillin div bid). Alternatively, give penicillin VK (50 mg/kg/day div qid) *plus* 40 mg/kg/day of either cephalexin (div qid) *or* cefadroxil (div bid) for five days. For other deep or potentially contaminated lacerations, discharge the patient with cephalexin or cefadroxil, as above. Administer tetanus toxoid for all tetanus-prone wounds unless it is certain that the patient received a booster within the last five years. Administer tetanus immune globulin if the patient's tetanus immunization status is incomplete or is unknown.

Fractures and Dislocations

Refer patients with fractures (except distal tuft), MCP dislocations, or non-radiographic suspicion of a scaphoid fracture to an appropriate surgical specialist (orthopedic, plastic, or hand surgeon). Treat distal tuft phalangeal fractures with a hairpin splint or bulky dressing.

A PIP dislocation can be reduced with traction and splinted after x-rays rule-out an associated avulsion fracture. To reduce a dorsal (most common) PIP joint dislocation, first anesthetize the finger with a digital block. Hold the finger proximal to the injury, then use a distracting force to hyperextend at the PIP joint to bring it back to its normal anatomic position. If successful, repeat the examination of active and passive range of motion and immobilize the joint for three weeks. If abnormal, or reduction was unsuccessful, consult with a hand specialist. A dorsal DIP joint dislocation can also be reduced using distracting force at the involved joint.

Tendon Injuries

Refer a patient with a gamekeeper's thumb, boutonnière deformity, or jersey finger to an appropriate surgical specialist. Treat a mallet finger with a short dorsal splint, ensuring mild DIP joint hyperextension with free PIP joint mobility, for 6–8 weeks. A paper clip or tongue blade wrapped in tape can serve as a temporary splint for a mallet finger.

Nail Bed Injuries

To drain a subungual hematoma, first soak the digit in warm water for 20 minutes. Then, "screw" through the nail with an 18-gauge needle. After several holes are made, soak the digit in warm water to permit blood to escape. Remove the nail only if there is disruption of the nail or nail margin. Repair lacerations of the nail bed with 6-0 absorbable sutures to prevent abnormal growth of the new nail. If the nail is present, suture or glue (Demabond) it in place to act as a dressing and splint. With crush injuries, however, it may be necessary to remove the nail in order to identify and repair occult lacerations to the nail bed. If the nail cannot be used as a splint, insert petrolatum gauze into the eponychial fold until the wound heals and the nail begins to grow.

Infections

Treat a paronychia without fluctuance with warm soaks q 2–3h, elevation, and 40 mg/kg/day of cephalexin (div qid), cefadroxil (div bid), or if MRSA is a concern, clindamycin (div q 6h), for 3–5 days. If fluctuance is present, soak the digit, then lift the edge of the eponychial fold with a No. 15 scalpel blade in order to remove pus from the eponychium. If is not clear whether all of the pus was removed, place a wick under the eponychium. Warm soaks and elevation are also necessary. If pus extends under the nail, partial nail removal is indicated.

Refer a patient with a felon to an appropriate surgical specialist (orthopedic, plastic, or hand surgeon) for immediate drainage. Admit patients with purulent tenosynovitis (culture for gonococcus) and palmar space infections for IV ampicillin/sulbactam (200 mg/kg div qid) or, if MRSA is prevalent in the community, either IV clindamycin (40 mg/kg/day div q 6h) or vancomycin (45 mg/kg/day div q 8h). Immediately consult with an appropriate surgical specialist.

Ganglion

Elective surgical removal is indicated if the lesion is painful or very disfiguring.

Traumatic Amputations

Rinse the amputated part gently in saline, wrap it in saline-soaked (but not dripping) gauze, and place it in a sealed plastic bag immersed in ice (do not allow direct contact with the ice). Distal fingertip amputations may require wrapping in petrolatum gauze. For more serious injuries, obtain a CBC and type and cross-match, start an IV line with maintenance fluids, treat pain with morphine sulfate (0.1–0.15 mg/kg IV or IM), and give IV ampicillin/sulbactam (200 mg/kg of ampicillin div qid). Gently cleanse the wound and cover it with petrolatum gauze or saline-soaked gauze until the patient can be taken to the operating room. Obtain an x-ray if there is suspicion of a crush injury to the distal phalanx.

Follow-up

- Bite wound or laceration being treated with prophylactic antibiotics: 2–3 days
- Drained subungual hematoma: two days
- Paronychia with wick in eponychial fold: 1–2 days; without wick: 3–5 days

Indications for Admission

- Felon, purulent tenosynovitis, or palmar space infection
- Any fracture requiring open reduction in the operating room
- Intra-articular fracture (>25% articular surface) or MCP dislocation
- Amputations other than distal fingertip
- Extensor tendon laceration that requires operative repair
- Flexor tendon laceration

Bibliography

Fufa DT, Goldfarb CA. Fractures of the thumb and finger metacarpals in athletes. *Hand Clin.* 2012;**28**(3):379–388

Liu EH, Alqahtani S, Alsaaran RN, et al. A prospective study of pediatric hand fractures and review of the literature. *Pediatr Emerg Care.* 2014;**30**(5):299–304.

Meals C, Meals R. Hand fractures: a review of current treatment strategies. *J Hand Surg Am.* 2013;**38**(5):1021–1031.

Patel L. Management of simple nail bed lacerations and subungual hematomas in the emergency department. *Pediatr Emerg Care.* 2014;**30**(10):742–745

Sendher R, Ladd AL. The scaphoid. *Orthop Clin North Am.* 2013;**44**(1):107–120.

Multiple Trauma

Trauma is the leading cause of death in children 1–14 years of age, exceeding all other causes combined. Each year, over 20,000 children and teenagers die from serious injury. Blunt injuries are most common at all ages, although the incidence of penetrating trauma increases in adolescence. The main factors contributing to early morbidity and mortality are upper airway compromise and respiratory failure or arrest due to central neuraxis injury (brain and cervical spinal cord). Intracranial and intra-abdominal hemorrhages are less common. Late deaths are caused chiefly by traumatic brain injury. Posttraumatic pulmonary insufficiency, respiratory distress syndrome, or "shock lung," and multiple organ system failure are not common.

Children are subject to unique mechanisms of injury that interact with their immature anatomic features and physiologic responses to produce distinct patterns of trauma. Children are struck by cars or fall from heights while playing, are propelled into the windshields or ejected through the windows of moving vehicles in which they ride as unrestrained passengers, and fall while bicycle riding, in-line skating, scooter riding, or skateboarding. Because the head is proportionately larger and heavier in the child than in the adult, it bears the brunt of the forces of injury, even if other body regions are involved. Thus, serious head injury is more common in multiple blunt trauma in childhood, while internal organ injury is less common. It is estimated that at least 80% of multiple injury cases involve the head.

As a result, pediatric trauma is far more often a disorder of airway and breathing than of bleeding and shock. Apnea, hypoventilation, and hypoxia occur five times more often than hypovolemia with hypotension in the seriously injured child. The mortality associated with neuroventilatory derangements (concomitant abnormalities in mental status and respiratory function) approaches 25%. The late finding of hypotensive (decompensated) shock is present in <10% of all cases of major pediatric trauma, but mortality in those cases exceeds 50%. Eight percent of all injuries in children involve the chest, and over two-thirds of children with chest injuries have multiple injuries.

Initial management of the injured child must be expeditious, in accordance with consensus protocols with which all participants in the resuscitative effort must be thoroughly familiar. This is best accomplished through the use of an aggressive team approach, with one member serving as team leader who takes responsibility for directing and coordinating the resuscitative effort. Although trauma resuscitation may be initiated in the ED, major trauma is a surgical illness that requires the immediate participation of experienced surgeons. The most common cause of preventable trauma death in children is inadequate initial resuscitation. Other preventable deaths are due to missed internal injuries, both intracranial and intra-abdominal. Surgical interventions are ultimately required in more than 50% of major pediatric trauma victims, despite the greater reliance on nonoperative management in children than adults.

Clinical Presentation

The presentation usually depends on the extent of central neuraxis injury, respiratory compromise, and blood loss. Head injuries are the most common anatomic findings, followed by axial skeletal injuries; internal organ injuries are least common. Abnormalities in level of consciousness and respiratory status are the most common physiologic findings. While hypotensive shock is uncommon in the pediatric trauma victim, particularly after blunt injury, a child may be in early shock with little or no external evidence (see Shock, pp. 28–35), leading to what may be called the "deceptive" presentation of shock in the child.

Diagnosis and ED Management

Primary Survey

The first priority is the primary survey, a rapid initial assessment that combines rapid cardiopulmonary assessment (the foundation of pediatric advanced life support) with rapid

Table 25.2 Management options for life-threatening conditions

Finding	Problem	Management
Asymmetric breath sounds and dull percussion note	Possible massive hemothorax	Chest x-ray Insert chest tube through separate incision in mid-axillary line at level of nipple
Asymmetric breath sounds and hyperresonant percussion note	Possible tension pneumothorax	Insert over-the-needle plastic catheter (second ICS in MCL) or chest tube
Difficulty breathing	Respiratory failure	Bag-valve-mask ventilation, intubation
External bleeding	External wound	Direct pressure
Hypotension	Decompensated shock Transient response to volume resuscitation	Transfusion: emergency: type O (Rh-neg for ♀); urgent: type-specific
Neck pain, spasm, tenderness Head injury	Possible C-spine fracture	Immobilize neck (semirigid extrication collar, tape, head immobilizer)
Noisy breathing, stridor	Upper airway obstruction	Jaw thrust/C-spine control, intubation
Orthostasis (pale, cool skin)	Compensated shock	Establish two large-bore IVs Give up to two 20 mL/kg boluses
Paradoxical chest wall movement	Flail chest	Positive pressure ventilation for respiratory failure
Penetrating chest wound with difficulty breathing	Possible sucking chest wound	Apply occlusive dressing Insert chest tube through separate incision in mid-axillary line at level of nipple
Penetrating chest wound with distended neck veins	Possible pericardial tamponade	Pericardiocentesis (subxiphoid or fourth ICS 1 cm lateral to muffled heart sounds or left sternal border)
Unconsciousness	Severe traumatic brain injury	Intubation, mild hyperventilation
Upper abdominal distension	Gastric dilation	Insert nasogastric tube (use orogastric tube if major hyperresonant percussion note orofacial trauma or an infant)

cranial-truncal examination, to *identify life-threatening problems that require immediate intervention* (Table 25.2). Note the patient's general condition, and take the following actions (*A, B, C, D, E*):

1. Assess the *Airway* for patency and maintainability. Confirm spontaneous air movement and listen for gurgling or stridor while protecting the cervical spine from flexion and extension. If needed, use a jaw-thrust maneuver with in-line spinal immobilization to open the airway. Placing a 2 cm thick layer of padding under the infant's or toddler's torso will preserve this alignment.
2. Check the adequacy of *Breathing* by simultaneously watching chest excursions, listening for breath sounds, and evaluating respiratory effort and rate. Palpate the trachea and ribs, and search for other signs of immediately life-threatening chest injuries.
3. Evaluate the *Circulation* for signs of shock by obtaining the pulse (tachycardia is the earliest measurable response to hypovolemia). In addition, examine the skin for pallor, cyanosis, mottling, and moisture. Check for the presence of active bleeding and delayed capillary refill (>2 seconds). Obtain a core temperature to assess for hypothermia.
4. Estimate the degree of *Disability* by noting the response to verbal and painful stimuli using the "AVPU" score (A = alert, V = responsive to verbal stimuli, P = responsive only to painful stimuli, U = unresponsive). Record pupillary size and reaction to light.
5. Fully *Expose* the patient, taking quick note of all external signs of injury (especially in penetrating trauma) before covering him or her to prevent heat loss.
6. Resuscitation. Trauma resuscitation is conducted concurrently with the primary survey. If life-threatening problems are identified, the team leader must immediately begin treatment, summon surgical assistance, and organize a sequence of therapy, corresponding to the alphabetical order listed below.

A: Airway/Cervical Spine. As described in the section on cardiopulmonary resuscitation (pp. 5–9), establish and maintain a patent airway. Noisy or stridulous breathing suggests airway obstruction, most often due to the tongue falling against the posterior pharyngeal wall. Perform a modified jaw thrust and combine with bimanual in-line stabilization of the cervical spine in a neutral position (as described above). Keep the plane of the midface parallel to the spine board in a neutral position. If the child is *A* (alert) or *V* (responsive to verbal stimuli) and is breathing spontaneously, administer humidified 100% oxygen. Use a nonrebreathing mask with a flow rate high enough to keep the nonrebreathing bag inflated throughout the respiratory cycle. If the child is *P* (responsive only to painful stimuli) or *U* (unresponsive), insert an oropharyngeal airway and ventilate with humidified 100% oxygen via a bag-valve-mask device. If these measures are unsuccessful in effectively maintaining or immediately restoring spontaneous ventilation and oxygenation, or if the child is comatose as determined by a GCS ≤8, perform orotracheal intubation while continuing to apply bimanual in-line stabilization to the head and neck.

Inability to ventilate with a bag-mask or failed attempts to intubate, are indications for placing a laryngeal mask airway (LMA) or needle cricothyroidotomy. The LMA comes in various sizes and choice is based upon the child's weight.

Perform needle cricothyroidotomy by inserting a large-bore (16–18 gauge) over-the-needle catheter through the cricoid membrane (located between the thyroid cartilage and the cricoid ring). Then attach oxygen tubing containing a side hole or a Y-connector to the hub of the catheter, and insufflate oxygen by intermittently occluding (one second) and releasing (four seconds) the open end of the side hole or Y-connector, thereby avoiding chest overexpansion. Alternatively attach the Luer-lock tip of a 3.0 mL syringe from which the plunger has been removed to the hub of the catheter. Administer oxygen by ventilating with a bag-valve device through a no. 7.5 endotracheal tube adaptor inserted into the open end of the barrel of the syringe.

Severe multiple trauma, significant head or neck trauma, neck pain and tenderness, cervical muscle spasm, or a history of a sudden deceleration suggests the possibility of cervical spine and spinal cord injury. Immobilize the neck once the airway has been secured with a semirigid cervical extrication collar and a head immobilizer (soft collar or sandbags or large IV bags and tape are inadequate) until AP, lateral, and open-mouth radiographic views of the cervical spine and a careful neurologic examination rule-out an injury (see Cervical Spine Injuries, pp. 741–743). For a child under three years of age, place a 2–3 cm thick layer of padding beneath the torso to preserve alignment of the spinal column. Note that a lateral cervical spine x-ray, by itself, is insufficient to rule-out cervical spine injury, due to possible SCIWORA. Therefore, it is neither necessary nor indicated as part of the initial management of the multiply injured child. Despite the importance of early cervical spine control, however, do not sacrifice the airway by efforts to maintain neck immobilization; never delay intubation because a radiologist or neurosurgeon has not reviewed the radiographs and confirmed that the film shows no fracture.

B: Breathing/Chest Injuries. Administer humidified 100% oxygen to all victims of major trauma without waiting for ABG results. Immediately intubate a patient who is unconscious, has decreased breath sounds, or has persistent evidence of respiratory failure after opening the airway.

The mobility of mediastinal structures makes a child more prone to a tension pneumothorax. Look for contralateral tracheal deviation, a hyperresonant percussion note, subcutaneous emphysema, distended neck veins, and continued respiratory distress after intubation (see Pneumothorax, pp. 760–761). If they are found, immediately decompress by inserting a large-bore (16–18 gauge) over-the-needle catheter into the second intercostal space, above the third rib, in the midclavicular line on the affected side, without waiting for x-ray confirmation and follow with immediate thoracostomy.

Asymmetric breath sounds associated with a hyperresonant percussion note and subcutaneous emphysema but without tracheal deviation or distended neck veins suggest a simple pneumothorax. Asymmetric breath sounds associated with a dull percussion note suggest a simple hemothorax. Tube thoracostomy is indicated for both, after the airway, breathing, and circulation have been adequately addressed.

Hypotension after a penetrating chest wound suggests the possibility of pericardial tamponade. Tachycardia is the most common finding. Distant heart sounds, distended neck veins, and pulsus paradoxus are variable. Emergency thoracotomy is required, but pericardiocentesis (see Pericardial Tamponade, pp. 758–759) is indicated if emergency thoracotomy is not initiated in the ED.

Also examine the patient for rib fractures, subcutaneous emphysema, and signs of penetrating chest trauma. A flail chest, though rare in children, can cause paradoxical chest wall movement after blunt chest trauma. Positive pressure ventilation is required if large flail segments are impairing ventilation. Small flail segments are associated with enough muscle spasm that they rarely impair ventilation. They require supportive treatment only, primarily for the underlying pulmonary contusion that is invariably present. Once the patient is stable, give analgesics as necessary.

Penetrating chest trauma can cause an open pneumothorax (sucking chest wound). Cover penetrating chest wounds completely with petrolatum gauze, and perform tube thoracostomy to prevent the subsequent development of tension pneumothorax.

After securing the airway, obtain a chest radiograph if any of the above abnormalities are found on examination of the chest (except tension pneumothorax, which must be treated immediately). Review the film carefully for intrapleural air (simple or tension pneumothorax), intrapleural fluid (hemothorax), rib fractures, lung densities (pulmonary contusion), mediastinal emphysema, and widened mediastinum and loss of aortic contour (traumatic dissection of the aorta). Do not rely on normal chest radiographs when there is a suspicion of traumatic dissection of the aorta; obtain a CT of the chest.

Obtain an ECG to assess for the possibility of cardiac contusion, although no single finding is pathognomonic. Nonspecific changes, including sinus tachycardia, are present in up to 80% of the ECGs obtained in patients with suspected blunt cardiac injury. Assume that a child has a possible cardiac contusion and consult with a pediatric cardiologist if there are ECG changes such as relative tachycardia, relative bradycardia, conduction delays, or atrial or ventricular dysrhythmias.

C: Circulation/Bleeding and Shock. Cardiopulmonary arrest in a pediatric trauma victim may be an indication for emergency thoracotomy with pericardiotomy in the ED for relief of pericardial tamponade, cross-clamping of the descending aorta, or both, if personnel experienced in these techniques are available. ED thoracotomy is not indicated for victims of blunt trauma, including those with pulseless myocardial electrical activity, but it is occasionally successful in victims of penetrating trauma, particularly those who have pericardial tamponade or develop profound hypotension during the course of the resuscitative effort. ED thoracotomy is also indicated for victims of penetrating trauma who have lost pulses en route to the hospital. A patient with penetrating parasternal chest wounds or pericardial tamponade who is not in hypotensive shock should immediately be transported to the operating room for urgent thoracotomy. Summon the surgical team immediately upon the arrival of any such patient, and notify the operating room that the need for surgery may be imminent.

Control external bleeding with direct digital or manual pressure, pressure dressings, or pneumatic splints. Additionally, commercial tourniquets are an emerging treatment modality for presurgical management of limb-threatening hemorrhage. Secure two large-bore (16–18 gauge) peripheral IV lines using over-the-needle catheters. Substitute a tibial intraosseous line, provided the extremity is uninjured, if two attempts at antecubital IV access have failed or if venous access is impossible secondary to circulatory collapse. The distal femur (3 cm above the external condyle) can be used if the tibia is fractured. Give 20 mL/kg of warmed isotonic crystalloid (normal saline or Ringer's lactate) as a rapid IV bolus after obtaining blood for type and cross-match and a CBC. Monitor the blood pressure carefully, and repeat the bolus every 5–10 minutes, as needed. If 40 mL/kg does not raise the blood pressure, give another 20 mL/kg bolus and prepare for a transfusion of 10 mL/kg of packed RBCs. In an emergency, when there is evidence of hypotensive shock, use type O blood, which is available immediately: O-positive for males, O-negative for females; transfusion reactions are extremely rare. Type-specific blood that is not cross-matched can be available in ten minutes; it can be used in urgent but not emergency circumstances. An emerging trend is that patients with traumatic injuries, particularly to the thoracoabdominal region, may have better outcomes when crystalloid is restricted, permitting lower systolic blood pressure (BP) until the bleeding is controlled. The exception would be the patient with multitrauma who also has traumatic brain injury (TBI). For such a patient, the targeted blood pressure must be higher in order to preserve adequate cerebral perfusion pressure and prevent secondary brain injury.

Base ongoing volume resuscitation on the response to the initial fluid challenge. Remember that fewer than 10% of children present in hypotensive shock after major trauma. Many hospitals have rapid transfusion protocols for patients with profound hemorrhage and ongoing blood loss, with a targeted ratio of 1:1:1 of packed RBCs, fresh frozen plasma, and platelets. Consult with the local trauma service to determine whether to initiate this protocol.

Attempt to identify sources of potential or ongoing blood loss. Following a careful physical examination, obtain a chest radiograph to rule-out hemothorax and obtain a pelvic x-ray, since a pelvic fracture is a common cause of retroperitoneal hemorrhage. Obtain urine for urinalysis. Hematuria (>50 cells/hpf) may indicate urinary tract injury (see Genitourinary Trauma, pp. 299–302) or injury to other intra-abdominal organs, as 80% of blunt renal injuries are associated with damage to adjacent organs. Although isolated hematuria is rarely a life-threatening problem, expeditious imaging of the urinary tract is indicated.

If the patient remains in shock or has a falling hematocrit, reassess for occult blood loss in the pleural cavities, abdomen, retroperitoneum, and pelvis; repeat diagnostic tests, if indicated, and transport the patient to the operating room.

Diagnostic peritoneal lavage is not routinely employed for injured children with suspected intra-abdominal bleeding to determine the need for urgent laparotomy. Conservative, nonoperative management of solid organ (liver, spleen, kidney) injury is standard, so a positive result (>100 RBC/mm^3) does not constitute an automatic indication for surgery. Abdominal CT with IV contrast enhancement is the diagnostic procedure of choice for identifying injuries and bleeding sites in a hemodynamically stable patient. For an unstable patient, use a focused assessment sonography in trauma (FAST). It is noninvasive and does not interfere with resuscitation. It is accurate for the identification of free abdominal fluid as well as pericardial fluid (see Bedside Ultrasound, p. 659). Reserve abdominal paracentesis for a patient with unstable vital signs in whom the source of the bleeding is unknown or the FAST examination is suboptimal, and/or the child with stable vital signs who is going immediately to the operating room for treatment of intracranial or musculoskeletal injuries. If necessary, the paracentesis can be performed in the operating room.

D: Disability (Neurologic). Once vital signs have been stabilized, direct resuscitative efforts toward the diagnosis and treatment of central neuraxis injuries (see Head Trauma, pp. 521–527 and Cervical Spine Injuries, pp. 741–743). Priorities in the neurologic evaluation are accurate determination of the level of consciousness, pupillary size and reactivity, eye movements, and motor, sensory, and reflex responses. Asymmetry in pupillary size and reactivity or in motor, sensory, or reflex responses suggests the possibility of serious intracranial or spinal cord injury.

Request neurosurgical assistance and arrange immediate CT of the brain for a patient under two years of age with a Glasgow Coma Scale ≤14, a palpable skull fracture, alteration of mental status (agitation, somnolence), occipital, parietal, or temporal scalp hematoma, history of a loss of consciousness for five or more seconds, not acting normally as per parent, or a severe mechanism of injury. For a patient two years of age or older, indications for CT scan include a GCS ≤14, signs of basilar skull fracture (hemotympanum, raccoon eyes, Battle's sign), and alteration of an alert mental status. Relative indications also include history of a loss of consciousness, vomiting, severe headache, or severe mechanism of injury.

Monitor the patient fully (ECG, vital signs, pulse oximetry) throughout the study, and ensure that someone (emergency physician, trauma surgeon, physician-anesthesiologist, nurse-anesthetist) capable of emergency management of the pediatric airway is present. The leading cause of the increased intracranial pressure commonly observed after pediatric closed head injury is not intracranial hematoma, as in adults, but cerebral swelling due to the secondary brain injury that is caused by cerebral hypoxia. For this reason, and because the outcome of traumatic brain injury in children is far better than it is in adults, children with traumatic brain injury who present in coma require aggressive resuscitative efforts.

A number of factors contribute to the development of cerebral hypoxia in the child with severe closed head injury. Normal cerebral blood flow increases to nearly twice that of adult levels by the age of 5, and then decreases. Unconsciousness produces hypotonia in the muscles supporting the soft tissues of the larynx and oropharynx, resulting in passive closure of the upper airway. Both primary brain injury (direct trauma) and secondary brain injury (cerebral hypoxia) can cause temporary paralysis of cerebrovascular autoregulation, resulting in cerebral vasodilation and cerebral hyperemia, leading to progressive increases in intracranial pressure. These, in turn, decrease cerebral perfusion pressure and disrupt medullary control of breathing, thereby worsening cerebral hypoxia and leading to further increases in intracranial pressure.

Immediate intubation and mild hyperventilation, if instituted promptly, may interrupt this vicious cycle, which otherwise leads to uncal herniation and brain death. Intubation reopens the airway, permitting oxygen to reach the circulation and facilitating hyperventilation. Hyperventilation induces alkalosis, normalizing cerebral blood flow and allowing blood to perfuse the brain. Immediately intubate any child who presents with a GCS ≤8 and initiate mild hyperventilation with tidal volumes of 10 mL/kg, at a rate that lowers the pCO_2 to approximately 35 mm Hg. Mild hyperventilation is preferred due to the potential risk of cerebral ischemia associated with aggressive hyperventilation.

Rapid-sequence intubation is indicated for the head-injured child who presents in coma, and it must be performed only by personnel experienced in emergency intubation of the pediatric patient and familiar with the use of neuromuscular blockers. It is technically more difficult in the trauma patient whose neck must remain in a neutral position throughout the procedure because of the possibility of spinal cord injury. A number of therapeutic regimens are in common use (see Airway Management, pp. 5–9).

Treat ongoing seizures with lorazepam (0.1 mg/kg) or diazepam (0.15–0.2 mg/kg) slowly over two minutes, followed by fosphenytoin (20 phenytoin equivalents (PE)/kg, IV over 10–15 min), phenytoin (20 mg/kg, IV at a rate of 1 mg/kg/min), or levetiracetam (30–60 mg/kg, 4500 mg maximum, IV over one hour).

Corticosteroids have no established role in the acute management of head injuries. Avoid the use of diuretic agents such as IV mannitol (0.5–1 g/kg) or furosemide (1 mg/kg) unless there is evidence of uncal herniation (unilateral dilated pupil or other lateralizing signs). Carefully document key neurologic findings before rapid-sequence intubation or other treatments that alter neurologic status, but never delay treatment of life-threatening neurotrauma while awaiting arrival of neurologic or neurosurgical consultants.

E: Expose (Examine). Expose the patient completely, and perform a rapid but thorough physical exam (including the back, buttocks, and all skin creases), looking for associated injuries. Palpate all bones, including the pelvic and facial bones, and palpate and percuss the teeth. Check the extraocular movements and corneal clarity, and recheck pupillary reactivity and symmetry. Look for signs of depressed (scalp hematoma or laceration with underlying deformity or crepitance) and basilar (hemotympanum, clear rhino- or otorrhea, infraorbital and retroauricular ecchymoses) skull fractures. Once the exam is completed, cover the patient with a blanket to prevent hypothermia. The diagnosis and management of other traumas is detailed elsewhere: ocular (pp. 548–553), dental (pp. 87–92), orthopedic (pp. 565–573), genitourinary (pp. 299–302), and soft tissue (pp. 762–784).

F: Foley Catheter. Insert a catheter into the bladder to monitor the urine output closely in all multiple-trauma patients. The sole exception is a patient with suspected urethral disruption, suggested by blood at the urethral meatus, and males with scrotal hematoma or a "high-riding" or "boggy" prostate. These injuries are usually associated with a pelvic fracture, straddle injury, or penetrating wound. Call a urologist immediately to obtain a retrograde urethrogram; urine output can be monitored with a suprapubic catheter if needed. The desired urine output is at least 2 mL/kg/h in an infant, 1 mL/kg/h in a child, and 0.5 mL/kg/h in an adolescent. Gross or significant microscopic (>50 RBC/hpf) hematuria requires radiologic evaluation to rule-out renal injury.

G: Gastric Decompression. Insert a nasogastric tube and attach to intermittent (Levin tube) or continuous (sump tube) suction to prevent aspiration and improve ventilation by reducing gastric dilation. Use an orogastric tube instead if there is evidence of significant orofacial trauma.

Secondary Survey

Once the primary survey has been completed and the resuscitation phase is underway, proceed with the secondary survey: a careful, complete head-to-toe examination of the trauma patient to determine the full extent of tissue injury. Be sure to perform a rectal exam to exclude GI bleeding and evaluate anal sphincter tone. If life-threatening problems are not identified during the primary survey, but the mechanism of injury indicates that the patient is potentially at risk for life-threatening problems, secure a large-bore IV, obtain frequent vital signs, arrange for initial blood and x-ray studies, order a urinalysis as a screen for occult intra-abdominal injury, and admit for observation.

Obtain a CBC and type and cross-match for any patient admitted for observation to a critical care unit. In addition, obtain serum lipase (looking for pancreatic injury) and hepatic transaminases for a patient admitted for evaluation of abdominal trauma. CPK and urine myoglobin are indicated for the child with suspected crush injury, as well as electrolytes, BUN, and creatinine. The last three, as well as serum glucose, are useful as baseline studies in children with severe traumatic brain injury.

Most multiple-trauma victims require x-rays of the chest and pelvis. A lateral cervical spine x-ray is also commonly obtained, although as discussed previously, it cannot reliably rule-out spinal cord injury. Therefore, maintain full spinal immobilization of any patient in whom spinal cord injury has not been or cannot be properly ruled out. If the vital signs are stable but intra-abdominal injury is suspected (based on physical signs of internal hemorrhage, such as abdominal tenderness, distention, bruising, or gross hematuria), prepare the patient for a CT scan of the abdomen with IV and oral contrast (to follow CT scan of the head when obtained). For oral contrast, the dose of Gastrografin for a child older than ten years is 15 mL in 485 mL of water. Give 8–10 mL in 350 mL water to a patient 8–10 years old and 5 mL in 245 mL water to a child 1–5 years of age. Oral contrast is not helpful in children unless the full dose can be given (usually requires a nasogastric tube). If this is not possible, obtain the CT scan with IV contrast, only. Plain x-rays may then be ordered as necessary. Victims of minor trauma with stable vital signs who are awake, alert, and able to ambulate normally require x-rays only if indicated by historical and physical findings.

Indications for Admission

- Serious head or neck injury
- Respiratory distress or compromise
- Hypotension or orthostatic vital sign changes
- Suspected intrathoracic or intra-abdominal injury
- Serious fracture or soft tissue injury
- Minor injuries caused by major trauma
- Gunshot or stab wound unless surgical evaluation determines it to be superficial

Bibliography

Drexel S, Azarow K, Jafri MA. Abdominal trauma evaluation for the pediatric surgeon. *Surg Clin North Am.* 2017;**97**(1):59–74.

Miele V, Piccolo CL, Trinci M, Galluzzo M, Ianniello S, Brunese L. Diagnostic imaging of blunt abdominal trauma in pediatric patients. *Radiol Med.* 2016;**121**(5):409–430.

Naik-Mathuria B, Akinkuotu A, Wesson D. Role of the surgeon in non-accidental trauma. *Pediatr Surg Int.* 2015;**31**(7):605–610.

Pandya NK, Upasani VV, Kulkarni VA. The pediatric polytrauma patient: current concepts. *J Am Acad Orthop Surg.* 2013;**21**(3):170–179.

Rossaint R, Bouillon B, Cerny V, et al. The European guideline on management of major bleeding and coagulopathy following trauma. *Crit Care.* 2016;**20**(1):100.

Tovar JA, Vazquez JJ. Management of chest trauma in children. *Paediatr Respir Rev.* 2013;**14**(2):86–91.

Pericardial Tamponade

Pericardial tamponade is a life-threatening emergency requiring immediate intervention. The most common cause is penetrating thoracic trauma, when blood accumulates in the pericardial sac and interferes with cardiac filling. Tamponade is rare after blunt thoracic trauma.

Clinical Presentation

Suspect pericardial tamponade if there are failing vital signs or pulseless electrical activity after penetrating chest trauma, especially following a poor response to tube thoracostomy. Shock associated with tachypnea, clear lungs with equal breath sounds bilaterally, and neck vein distention (if the patient is not hypovolemic) suggests the diagnosis. The pulse pressure may be narrowed, and pulsus paradoxus (a >10 mm Hg drop in the systolic blood pressure on inspiration) may be present but is not necessary to establish the diagnosis. Deterioration can lead to pulseless electrical activity and death.

Diagnosis

See pp. 749–758 for the approach to the multiple-trauma patient. The clinical presentation of pericardial tamponade may resemble that of other life-threatening chest injuries; often, they occur simultaneously. Distended neck veins and pulsus paradoxus can both be seen in a patient with non-traumatic disorders such as congestive heart failure. Pulsus paradoxus may also be noted in a patient with severe asthma (wheezing, poor air movement). Tachypnea and tachycardia are frequent in patients with pneumothorax or hemothorax.

In acute pericardial tamponade, the chest x-ray frequently reveals a normal heart or a waterbag cardiac shadow, but the pericardial effusion is usually evident on the FAST examination.

Insert a right atrial catheter or central venous pressure (CVP) line if the diagnosis is uncertain. The CVP is usually elevated (>15 cm H_2O), unless the patient is hypovolemic from other injuries. The ECG in pericardial tamponade may reveal low voltage and non-specific ST–T-wave changes. Electrical alternans (alternating variations in the height of the QRS complex, due to shifts in the QRS axis from beat to beat as the heart swings to and fro in the pericardial sac) is diagnostic of a pericardial effusion. Also, generalized low voltage (R-waves height <1 cm in all leads) may be observed.

ED Management

Once the diagnosis is made, immediately consult a surgeon to perform a thoracotomy or pericardiotomy in the operating room. If an experienced surgeon is not available, pericardiocentesis is indicated. Monitor the patient's vital signs and ECG before, during, and after the procedure. Use a large-bore (16–18 gauge) over-the-needle catheter, attached by three-way stopcock to a 30 mL syringe and by alligator clip (placed just beyond the hub of the needle) to the chest lead (V_1) of an ECG machine. Puncture the skin inferior to the xiphoid process, directing the needle toward the tip of the left scapula, at a 45° angle to the skin. Free flow of nonclotted, nonpulsatile blood suggests that the pericardium has been entered. If the needle touches the epicardial surface, a "current of injury pattern" (ST segment elevation) will be seen on the ECG; withdraw the needle slightly. An improvement in vital signs may follow removal of as little as 10–20 mL of blood. After aspiration is complete, withdraw the needle but leave the catheter in with the stopcock closed in case fluid reaccumulates. A negative tap does not rule-out tamponade, since blood in the pericardial sac clots rapidly.

Indications for Admission

- Pericardial tamponade
- Pericardial effusion

Bibliography

Guttman J, Nelson BP. Diagnostic emergency ultrasound: assessment techniques in the pediatric patient. *Pediatr Emerg Med Pract.* 2016;**13**(1):1–27.

Pearson EG, Fitzgerald CA, Santore MT. Pediatric thoracic trauma: current trends. *Semin Pediatr Surg.* 2017;**26**(1):36–42.

Smith AT, Watnick C, Ferre RM. Cardiac tamponade diagnosed by point-of-care ultrasound. *Pediatr Emerg Care.* 2017;**33**(2):132–134.

Tovar JA, Vazquez JJ. Management of chest trauma in children. *Paediatr Respir Rev.* 2013;**14**(2):86–91.

Pneumothorax

Pneumothorax can result from blunt or penetrating thoracic trauma. It can also occur in asthmatics, patients with cystic fibrosis, newborns (pneumothorax occurs most commonly among neonates), and in association with smoking "crack" cocaine or marijuana. Occasionally, a pneumothorax occurs without trauma in an otherwise healthy adolescent.

Clinical Presentation

Pneumothorax presents with signs of respiratory distress, including tachypnea, nasal flaring, accessory muscle use, and anxiety or altered mental status. Breath sounds may be decreased or absent on the affected (ipsilateral) side. The percussion note can be tympanitic. Pulsus paradoxus (>10 mm Hg drop in the systolic blood pressure on inspiration) may be noted.

Signs of a tension pneumothorax may include all of the above, along with deviation of the trachea away from the affected side and, if severe, may include cyanosis, jugular vein distention (if the patient is not hypovolemic), and deterioration of the vital signs, leading to pulseless electrical activity and death. Pneumomediastinum can occur with or without pneumothorax. Although a pneumomediastinum requires no immediate treatment, its presence suggests the possibility of barotrauma and an associated pneumothorax.

Diagnosis

See pp. 749–758 for the general approach to the patient with multiple trauma. Always be suspicious of the possibility of pneumothorax in a trauma victim. Air can leak from the lung, the tracheobronchial tree, or the esophagus or through a sucking wound in the chest wall. Trauma can produce pneumothorax directly in penetrating injury, or indirectly in blunt injury (by fracturing ribs); however, a pneumothorax can occur in the absence of either.

Tension pneumothorax may be confused with other immediately life-threatening chest injuries (Table 25.3). In massive hemothorax, breath sounds are decreased on the affected side, as in tension pneumothorax, but the percussion note is dull and the neck veins are flat. In pericardial tamponade, the neck veins may be distended (if the patient is not hypovolemic), but breath sounds are adequate, and ECG monitoring may reveal low voltage. In hypovolemic shock, vital signs will have deteriorated, but breath and heart sounds are usually equal on both sides and the neck veins are flat.

Table 25.3 Diagnosis of immediately life-threatening chest injuries

	Tension pneumothorax	Massive hemothorax	Cardiac tamponade
Physical sign			
Breath sounds	Ipsilateral decrease	Ipsilateral decrease	Normal
Neck veins	Distended	Flat	Distended
Percussion note	Hyperresonant	Dull	Normal
Tracheal location	Contralateral shift	Midline	Midline

The diagnosis of tension pneumothorax is made on clinical grounds alone. *Treat immediately if it is suspected*, without waiting for a confirmatory chest x-ray; however, a chest x-ray is indicated to confirm the diagnosis of simple pneumothorax. A pleural effusion in the asthmatic with pneumonia can mimic hemopneumothorax.

ED Management

Immediately give humidified 100% oxygen with a flow rate high enough to keep the nonrebreathing bag inflated throughout the respiratory cycle and secure a large-bore (16–18 gauge) IV line, unless the patient has severe respiratory distress.

Tension Pneumothorax

Decompress immediately, without waiting for x-ray confirmation. Insert a large-bore over-the-needle plastic catheter into the chest above the top of the third rib, in the midclavicular line of the affected side. A rush of air and improvement in the patient's ventilatory status confirm both the diagnosis and the adequacy of the therapy. Remove the needle and leave the catheter in place. Then insert a chest tube in the fifth intercostal space above the sixth rib in the anterior to mid-axillary line, attach it to an underwater seal device once the tube has been properly secured, and remove the over-the-needle catheter used for decompression.

Simple Pneumothorax

If the patient is alert, with an oxygen saturation >90% and stable vital signs, provide 100% oxygen via nonrebreather mask and consult with a pediatric surgeon regarding the possible placement of a chest tube or pigtail catheter. If the clinical condition deteriorates, immediately place a chest tube.

Indications for Admission

• Any pneumothorax or hemothorax

Bibliography

Goodwin SJ, Flanagan SG, McDonald K. Imaging of chest and abdominal trauma in children. *Curr Pediatr Rev.* 2015;**11**(4):251–261.

Gutierrez IM, Ben-Ishay O, Mooney DP. Pediatric thoracic and abdominal trauma. *Minerva Chir.* 2013;**68**(3):263–274.

Guttman J, Nelson BP. Diagnostic emergency ultrasound: assessment techniques in the pediatric patient. *Pediatr Emerg Med Pract.* 2016;**12**(12):1–28.

Pauzé DR, Pauzé DK. Emergency management of blunt chest trauma in children: an evidence-based approach. *Pediatr Emerg Med Pract.* 2013;**10**(11):1–22.

van As AB, Manganyi R, Brooks A. Treatment of thoracic trauma in children: literature review, Red Cross War Memorial Children's Hospital data analysis, and guidelines for management. *Eur J Pediatr Surg.* 2013;**23**(6):434–443.

Chapter 26

Wound Care and Minor Trauma

Anthony J. Ciorciari

Abscesses

A cutaneous abscess is a localized collection of pus, usually secondary to disruption of skin integrity. The organisms most often involved are methicillin-sensitive *Staphylococcus aureus* (MSSA), methicillin-resistant *Staphylococcus aureus* (MRSA), and *Streptococcus pyogenes* (GAS).

Clinical Presentation and Diagnosis

An abscess presents as a discrete, well-circumscribed swelling with central fluctuance. It is tender and is usually associated with erythema and warmth of the overlying skin. There may be an area of cellulitis adjacent to or surrounding the abscess. Lymphangitis and lymphadenitis are complications that can herald hematogenous dissemination and sepsis.

A patient with a significant abscess may exhibit signs of systemic disease such as temperature >38 °C, tachycardia, or tachypnea, and possibly an abnormal white blood count (>12,000/mm^3 or < 4000/mm^3).

ED Management

The definitive treatment of an abscess is incision and drainage, which can usually be performed in the ED. When the abscess is in immediate proximity to neurovascular structures, first perform either a needle aspiration to confirm purulence or obtain an ultrasound to avoid incising a vascular aneurysm. This precaution applies to abscesses in the neck, supraclavicular fossa, antecubital fossa, popliteal fossa, and inguinal and axillary areas.

Maintain strict aseptic technique to prevent the spread of the infection; prepare the skin with a povidone-iodine solution. Although total anesthesia may be difficult to achieve, use a combination of a regional field block (a ring of 1% lidocaine outside the perimeter of the abscess and erythema) and a linear injection of 1% lidocaine into the roof of the abscess along the planned incision line. The maximum dose of lidocaine is 4–5 mg/kg without epinephrine and 7 mg/kg with epinephrine. If this technique is unsuccessful, provide sedation and analgesia (pp. 715–722).

Make the incision along the natural dynamic skin tension lines to prevent excessive scarring. In view of the increasing incidence of MRSA, after the incision, obtain a specimen for culture in case the patient subsequently requires antibiotic therapy. Explore the abscess cavity with a blunt instrument or sterile gloved finger to break up any loculated pockets of purulence. Copiously irrigate the cavity with NS under moderate pressure, pack it loosely with iodoform gauze to promote drainage and ensure hemostasis, and apply a sterile dressing.

Oral antibiotics are of no additional benefit after incision and drainage of uncomplicated abscesses <5 cm in otherwise healthy children. Antibiotics are indicated when the abscess is >5 cm or there is an area of surrounding cellulitis. Use cephalexin (40 mg/kg/day div qid) or cefadroxil (40 mg/kg/day div bid), but if MRSA is prevalent in the community, treat with clindamycin (20 mg/kg/day div qid) alone *or* add trimethoprim-sulfamethoxazole (which does not reliably cover group A *Streptococcus*) to one of the above regimens (8 mg/kg/day of trimethoprim div bid). Treat for 5–7 days. Arrange for follow-up in 24–48 hours to evaluate for complications, remove the packing, and repeat the irrigation. Loosely repack the cavity only if pus is found again. Usually, by 48 hours, the incision remains open without packing while the cavity heals from below. Instruct the family to irrigate the cavity under running warm water or to apply warm wet soaks three times daily at home for five days.

Refer breast, perirectal, fingertip (pulp), hand, and deep abscesses of the neck to an experienced surgeon.

Follow-up
- After abscess drainage: daily for 2–3 days

Indications for Admission
- Abscess associated with lymphangitic streaking, fever >38.9 °C (102 °F), or signs of toxicity
- Abscess in an immunocompromised patient
- Severe injuries and soft tissue infections
- Infections that interfere with oral intake, urination, defecation

Bibliography
Gupta AK, Lyons DC, Rosen T. New and emerging concepts in managing and preventing community-associated methicillin-resistant *Staphylococcus aureus* infections. *Int J Dermatol*. 2015;**54**(11):1226–1232.

Korownyk C, Allan GM. Evidence-based approach to abscess management. *Can Fam Physician*. 2007;**53**:1680–1684.

Mistry RD. Skin and soft tissue infections. *Pediatr Clin North Am*. 2013;**60**(5):1063–1082.

Montravers P, Snauwaert A, Welsch C. Current guidelines and recommendations for the management of skin and soft tissue infections. *Curr Opin Infect Dis*. 2016;**29**(2):131–138.

Schmitz GR. How do you treat an abscess in the era of increased community-associated methicillin-resistant *Staphylococcus aureus* (MRSA)? *J Emerg Med*. 2011;**41**(3):276–281.

Stevens DL, Bisno AL, Chambers HF, et al. Practice guidelines for the diagnosis and management of skin and soft tissue infections: 2014 update by the Infectious Diseases Society of America. *Clin Infect Dis*. 2014;**59**:e10.

Bite Wounds
About 1% of all ED visits are for bites, the majority of which are caused by dogs. More than one-half of bite victims are children, most of them toddlers. While a patient may seek

medical attention because of cosmetic concerns, bleeding, or fear of rabies, the most common complication is infection. An increased risk of infection occurs with puncture wounds, hand wounds, or when there has been a delay (>24 hours) in seeking medical attention.

Clinical Presentation and Diagnosis

Usually, the history of an animal bite is readily obtained, so the diagnosis is evident. The three major types of bite wounds are puncture wounds, lacerations, and closed-first injuries (CFIs). Puncture wounds are of particular concern, as the small break in the skin belies the significant risk of infection. Suspect that a laceration over the metacarpophalangeal joint of an adolescent represents a CFI, sustained when the patient punched another person in the mouth.

ED Management

General Measures

Thoroughly clean every bite wound with soap and water. Moderate-pressure irrigation in the ED is indicated for lacerations and CFIs, but it is probably ineffective for punctures. Use an 18 or 20 gauge IV catheter attached to a 1 L bag of NS, around which a blood transfusion cuff is inflated to 300 mm Hg. If the irrigation is not tolerated, anesthetize the intact skin margins of the wound with 1% lidocaine and then irrigate. Debride devitalized tissue, which is an excellent culture medium. This is particularly important with dog bites, which are, in part, crush injuries.

Suturing

Dog Bites

Do not suture puncture wounds; hand, forearm, or foot lacerations; wounds more than eight hours old (except the face in children over one year old); wounds over a joint; crush wounds that cannot be debrided; or if the patient is immunosuppressed. In these circumstances, if the wound appears clean and cosmesis is a concern, close the wound in approximately four days (delayed primary closure). Alternatively, allow the wound to granulate (secondary closure). Low-risk dog bite wounds can be sutured, but avoid deep closure to minimize the possibility of infection.

Cat Bites

Because the infection rate is high, leave cat bite wounds open. Exceptions are easily cleaned wounds that are not on the hand, forearm, or foot. Once again, avoid deep closure to minimize the possibility of infection.

Human Bites

Do not close wounds on the distal extremities, but suture facial bites less than eight hours old that can be cleaned adequately.

Other Bites

Consult with a pediatric infectious disease expert to determine the risk of infection.

Antibiotics

Dog and Cat Bites

Organisms causing infections include *Pasteurella multocida, Staphylococcus aureus*, and *Streptococcus* species. Give antibiotics for puncture wounds, hand and forearm wounds, injuries that are considered deep or have penetrated the joint capsule, and lacerations that are sutured. Also give antibiotics to a patient who is immunocompromised, asplenic, or has moderate to severe injuries to the hand and/or face. Use amoxicillin-clavulanate (875/125 formulation; 45 mg/kg/day of amoxicillin div bid). If MRSA is a concern, use either clindamycin (20 mg/kg/day div qid) alone *or* add trimethoprim-sulfamethoxazole (which does not reliably cover group A *Streptococcus*) as described for an abscess (p. 763).

Human Bites

Etiologies of infections include *Eikenella corrodens, Staphylococcus aureus, Streptococcus* spp., *Haemophilus* spp., *Fusobacterium* spp., *Veillonella* spp., and *Pervotella* spp. Use the same guidelines as for dog and cat bites (above).

Other Bites

Consult a pediatric infectious diseases expert (as above).

Tetanus

Clostridia can be present in the mouths of coprophagic animals. Give tetanus toxoid unless it is certain that a booster was received in the previous five years. For patients under seven years of age, use 0.5 mL of DTaP, unless pertussis vaccination is contraindicated, in which case use DT. For patients 7–10 years old, use 0.5 mL of dT. If the patient is ≥11 years old, use 0.5 mL of Tdap.

Rabies

Decisions regarding rabies treatment depend on the prevalence of the disease in the species in the area where the animal lives. See pp. 771–772 for the indications for prophylaxis. Give post-exposure prophylaxis (PEP) for any patient with a bite, scratch, or mucous membrane exposure to a bat, unless the bat is available for testing and is negative for evidence of rabies. Also give PEP when direct contact between a child and a bat has occurred, unless the exposed person can be certain that there was no bite, scratch, or mucous membrane exposure. If a bat is found indoors and there is no history of bat–human contact, the likely effectiveness of PEP must be balanced against the low risk of such an exposure. PEP may also be indicated for a patient who was in the same room as a bat and might be unaware that a bite or direct contact had occurred (e.g., a sleeping person awakens to find a bat in the room or an adult witnesses a bat in the room with a previously unattended child, mentally disabled person, or intoxicated person) and rabies cannot be ruled out by testing the bat.

Follow-up

- Bite wound: daily for 2–3 days; initiate antibiotic therapy if the patient develops fever, increasing pain or erythema, or a purulent discharge

Indications for Admission

- Bite wound infections unresponsive to oral antibiotics
- Infected bite wounds in patients who initially seek attention >24 hours after the bite
- Bite wounds in immunocompromised patients

Bibliography

Aziz H, Rhee P, Pandit V, et al. The current concepts in management of animal (dog, cat, snake, scorpion) and human bite wounds. *J Trauma Acute Care Surg.* 2015;**78**(3):641–648.

Ellis R, Ellis C. Dog and cat bites. *Am Fam Physician.* 2014;**90**(4):239–243.

Lohiya GS, Tan-Figueroa L, Lohiya S, Lohiya S. Human bites: bloodborne pathogen risk and postexposure follow-up algorithm. *J Natl Med Assoc.* 2013;**105**(1):92–95.

Rothe K, Tsokos M, Handrick W. Animal and human bite wounds. *Dtsch Arztebl Int.* 2015;**112**(25):433–442.

Foreign Body Removal

Small fragments of wood or pieces of glass are the most common foreign bodies embedded in the skin.

Clinical Presentation

A fresh wound is usually tender, and the foreign body is often seen or palpated just below the skin surface. Delayed presentations are associated with induration and tenderness, often with purulent or serosanguinous drainage.

Fishhooks embedded in the skin merit special consideration, as there may be more than one barb. The barb may completely penetrate a finger or earlobe, emerging from the other side, leaving the hook shaft still embedded.

Diagnosis

Radiographs can be helpful in identifying and locating foreign bodies. Use a radiopaque marker, such as a bent paperclip taped to the overlying skin, as a reference point for estimating the exact location of the object. A radiograph is also indicated when the presence of a foreign body cannot be ruled out, as when an old wound does not heal, continues to drain serosanguinous or purulent material, or remains tender. Virtually all glass is radiopaque, and wooden splinters can occasionally be seen if they are covered with dirt particles. Obtain an ultrasound to locate a nonradiopaque foreign body such as a thorn or piece of plastic.

ED Management

Attempt to remove a foreign body in the ED only if it is close enough to the surface to be seen or palpated. Cleanse the skin with povidone-iodine, and anesthetize the area by local infiltration, field block, or regional nerve block. Using the paperclip marker and x-rays for reference, make a stab incision with a No. 11 blade directed at the foreign body. Carefully explore the wound with a small hemostat to find and remove the object. Then gently palpate over the wound with a gloved finger to identify any remaining fragments.

When removal attempts are prolonged or unsuccessful, consult with a surgeon to plan for a definitive operative procedure under fluoroscopic or sonographic guidance. Foreign bodies in the plantar surface of the foot are especially difficult to remove in the ED. Refer patients with foreign bodies in the face or hand to a surgeon, and consult with a surgeon before attempting to remove a foreign body from the neck, unless it is clearly superficial.

When the foreign body is small or cannot be palpated, probing the wound is usually fruitless. If the wound is tender and crusted over, however, unroof it with the point of an 18 gauge needle to facilitate the drainage of any pus; the object may emerge over the next several days. Continue with warm soaks at home, and reevaluate the wound in 48 hours.

To remove a fishhook, advance the barbed end until the skin is tented and anesthetize that area with 1% lidocaine. Then advance the point until the barb leaves the skin, sever the barbed point with wire cutters, and pull the shaft of the hook back out through the original entrance wound. Small-barb hooks may be removed in a retrograde fashion through the original wound site. If the fishhook has several barbs, separate them with wire cutters and remove each one individually. If the barb is already through the skin, cut it off and pull the shaft out without using any anesthetic.

Give tetanus toxoid unless it is certain that a booster was received in the previous five years. For patients under seven years of age, use 0.5 mL of DTaP, unless pertussis vaccination is contraindicated, in which case use DT. For patients 7–10 years old, use 0.5 mL of dT. If the patient is ≥11 years old, use 0.5 mL of Tdap.

Follow-up
- Small or nonpalpable foreign body: 48 hours

Bibliography

Davis J, Czerniski B, Au A, et al. Diagnostic accuracy of ultrasonography in retained soft tissue foreign bodies: a systematic review and meta-analysis. *Acad Emerg Med.* 2015;22(7):777–787.

Sidharthan S, Mbako AN. Pitfalls in diagnosis and problems in extraction of retained wooden foreign bodies in the foot. *Foot Ankle Surg.* 2010;16(2):e18–e20.

Varshney T, Kwan CW, Fischer JW, Abo A. Emergency point-of-care ultrasound diagnosis of retained soft tissue foreign bodies in the pediatric emergency department. *Pediatr Emerg Care.* 2017;3 (6):434–436.

Insect Bites and Stings

Insect bites and stings usually cause a local reaction. Systemic anaphylactic reactions occur after 1–3% of Hymenoptera stings (honeybees, wasps, hornets, yellow jackets, harvester and fire ants) in susceptible patients.

Clinical Presentation

Reactions can be classified as immediate (within two hours) or, rarely, delayed (after two hours). Immediate reactions may be local or systemic.

Immediate Local Reactions

These include local pain, erythema, swelling, tingling, warmth, and pruritus at the sting site. Local reactions usually last 24–48 hours; they can be extensive, although all affected skin is contiguous with the sting site.

Delayed Reactions

These can occur after a 1–2-week interval. They present as large local reactions, serum sickness (fever, arthralgia, urticaria, lymphadenopathy), and rarely, peripheral neuritis, vasculitis, nephritis, or encephalitis.

Immediate Systemic Reactions

The hallmark of a systemic reaction is swelling that occurs at locations not contiguous with the sting site. The reaction may be mild, with itching and urticaria. More severe anaphylactic reactions can occur with hypotension, wheezing, laryngeal edema, and shock. Eighty-five percent of sensitive patients manifest symptoms within five minutes; all have symptoms within 1–2 hours.

Diagnosis

The diagnosis is suggested by the history of a sting or by the typical appearance of a local reaction in the warm-weather months. Stings, as opposed to insect bites, are always painful. Cellulitis may look similar, but a bacterial infection usually does not develop abruptly. A cellulitis may be associated with fever, lymphangitic streaking, and local lymphadenopathy.

Consider other causes of systemic allergic reactions, such as drugs (penicillins, sulfonamides, contrast dyes) and foods (shellfish, eggs). Try to ascertain whether the insect was a member of the Hymenoptera order, and inquire about a history of allergies and any previous systemic reactions to insect stings.

ED Management

Local Reactions

Among the Hymenoptera, only honeybees lose their stingers, which may remain at the sting site. Remove the stinger (if it is still in place) by grasping as close to the puncture site as possible with a small forceps. Cleanse the site, apply ice or cool compresses to the area, and give oral diphenhydramine (5 mg/kg/day div qid, 50 mg/dose maximum) or hydroxyzine (2 mg/kg/day div tid, 50 mg/dose maximum). If the erythema continues to spread during the 24 hours after the bite or sting, consider the wound to be infected. Treat with 40 mg/kg/day of cephalexin (div qid) or cefadroxil (div bid), warm compresses every two hours, and elevation. If MRSA is a concern, use either clindamycin (20 mg/kg/day div qid) alone *or* add trimethoprim-sulfamethoxazole (which does not reliably cover group A *Streptococcus*), to one of the above regimens (8 mg/kg/day of trimethoprim div bid).

Systemic Reactions

Treat mild reactions (itching, urticaria) with oral diphenhydramine or hydroxyzine. The management of severe systemic reactions is the same as for anaphylaxis (see pp. 38–40). Prescribe an EpiPen and refer the patient to an allergist for evaluation and possible immunotherapy.

Follow-up

- Local reaction: 24 hours, if the erythema is spreading
- Systemic reaction (not anaphylaxis): 2–3 days

Indications for Admission

- Systemic anaphylactic reaction

Bibliography

Golden DB. Large local reactions to insect stings. *J Allergy Clin Immunol Pract.* 2015;3(3):331–334.

Lee H, Halverson S, Mackey R. Insect allergy. *Prim Care.* 2016;43(3):417–431.

Niedoszytko M, Bonadonna P, Oude Elberink JN, Golden DB. Epidemiology, diagnosis, and treatment of Hymenoptera venom allergy in mastocytosis patients. *Immunol Allergy Clin North Am.* 2014;34(2):365–381.

Tan JW, Campbell DE. Insect allergy in children. *J Paediatr Child Health.* 2013;49(9):E381–E387.

Marine Stings and Envenomations

Marine stings and envenomations can be caused by either invertebrates or vertebrates. Invertebrates such as the jellyfish, Portuguese man-of-war, sea anemones, and corals can contain thousands of stinging cells (nematocysts); others contain toxin that can be transmitted by contact (certain sponges, sea urchins).

Envenomation from vertebrates results from contact with toxin on the dorsal spines of the *Scorpaenidae* family (scorpionfish, stonefish, and lionfish) or the spines on the tail of a stingray.

Clinical Presentation and Diagnosis

Invertebrates

The presentation can vary substantially depending upon the species, the number of nematocysts coming into contact with the skin, the amount and duration of the contact, and the patient's body weight. Signs and symptoms can vary from mild dermatitis with pain, burning, swelling, and erythema at the site of the sting to anaphylactic reactions.

The Portuguese man-of-war produces a single long strap dermatitis, along which are small blisters. There may also be generalized muscular cramps, vomiting, and cardiovascular collapse.

Sponges deposit silica spicules, causing pruritic or irritant dermatitis that can lead to epidermal desquamation.

The barbs of sea urchins can become deeply embedded with venom injection. Local reactions, as well as muscle spasms, shortness of breath, and cardiovascular collapse can ensue.

Vertebrates

Contact with the dorsal spines of scorpionfish, stonefish, and lionfish causes excruciating pain (especially the stonefish), associated with erythema, swelling, and paresthesias of the affected extremity, which is sometimes followed by vesicle formation. The pain will peak in about an hour and can last for 12 hours if not treated, although milder pain can persist for weeks. Examination usually reveals one or more puncture wounds. The patient may also have GI and respiratory symptoms. Serious envenomations can lead to dyspnea and shock.

The tail of a stingray can cause a severe laceration, without venom release. If venom is released from the tail spines, local pain and burning ensue, followed by muscular cramping, vomiting, diarrhea, diaphoresis, fasciculations, weakness, and on occasion, cardiac arrhythmias and seizures.

ED Management

As a rule, the venoms are heat labile. Soaking the affected area in hot water (43.3–45.0 °C; 110–113 °F) for 30–90 minutes may greatly reduce the pain. Additional therapy consists of local wound care, analgesia, tetanus prophylaxis (if indicated), antihistamines (hydroxyzine 2 mg/ kg/day div tid, 50 mg/dose maximum or diphenhydramine 5 mg/kg/day div qid, 50 mg/dose maximum) for itching, and antibiotics (40 mg/kg/day of cephalexin div qid or cefadroxil div bid) for lacerations.

Invertebrates

Immobilize the limb and inactivate the nematocysts by applying vinegar or acetic acid for 10–15 minutes. Do not apply alcohol or fresh water, which may cause nematocyst discharge. Lift away the tentacles, then shave the area (shaving cream can be used) to remove any remaining nematocysts.

Treat the dermatitis from sponges by removing the stingers and soaking the contact area in dilute acetic acid, vinegar, or isopropyl alcohol.

Remove sea urchin spines carefully, as they are easily broken. If the sea urchin possesses pedicellariae, apply shaving cream and shave the area.

Vertebrates

Immerse the area in hot water for at least one hour. Provide local wound care and systemic support as necessary. Surgically remove spines that are in proximity to nerves, vessels, or joints. Radiographs and/or ultrasonography may assist in the identification of retained spines.

Stonefish antivenin is available via the regional poison control center for your area.

Indications for Admission

- All marine animal envenomations associated with signs or symptoms of systemic toxicity

Bibliography

Berling I, Isbister G. Marine envenomations. *Aust Fam Physician*. 2015;44(1–2):28–32.

Diaz JH. Marine Scorpaenidae envenomation in travelers: epidemiology, management, and prevention. *J Travel Med*. 2015;22(4):251–258.

Hornbeak KB, Auerbach PS. Marine envenomation. *Emerg Med Clin North Am*. 2017;35(2):321–337.

Lakkis NA, Maalouf GJ, Mahmassani DM. Jellyfish stings: a practical approach. *Wilderness Environ Med*. 2015;26(3):422–429.

Rabies

Most rabies viruses are transmitted by the bite of infected mammals. While the issue of rabies PEP is considered most often after domestic animal (dog and cat) bites, wildlife (skunks, raccoons, bats, foxes, ferrets, opossums, weasels, wolves, woodchucks) now constitute the major reservoir of rabies in the United States. Rodents (squirrels, hamsters, rats, mice) and rabbits can be infected, but they do not secrete the virus in their saliva, so they rarely transmit the disease.

Clinical Presentation

The most common scenario in which rabies is considered is when a patient comes to the ED after an unprovoked bite (such as while attempting to feed an animal). On occasion, abnormal behavior (abnormally aggressive, reserved, or withdrawn) on the part of the animal is noted. Exposure can be by bite (any penetration of the skin by the animal's teeth) or by scratch, abrasion, or saliva. Petting alone, contact with blood, urine, or feces, or contact with saliva on truly intact skin does not constitute exposure.

The incubation period of rabies ranges from four days to one year, with an average of 20–90 days. Clinical rabies presents with a nonspecific 1–10 day prodrome of fatigue, anxiety, fever, headache, and abdominal pain that may be associated with pain, paresthesias, and fasciculations at the bite site. This is followed by the neurologic stage which can last 2–7 days. There will be increasing agitation, incoordination, ascending paralysis, hyperactivity, hallucinations, seizures, pharyngeal spasm, and hydrophobia (the patient will not drink water). Rabies is virtually universally fatal once the virus becomes established in the CNS.

Diagnosis

The definitive diagnosis is made from examination of the animal's brain. Since the specimen is not always available, management decisions must be based on the likelihood of rabies in that species in the particular locale. The best information will come from the local health authorities. Post-exposure prophylaxis for any bat contact is recommended, even if there is no evidence of soft tissue injury, although the risk of rabies varies with the type of exposure (see Table 26.1).

Clinical rabies can be confused with a variety of neurologic conditions, including poliomyelitis, Guillain-Barré, herpes simplex, brain abscess, vaccine reaction, sepsis, and psychosis.

ED Management

Recommend confinement and observation of healthy domestic animals for ten days. If any signs of rabies develop, the animal must be sacrificed and the head sent to an appropriate laboratory. Contact the local veterinary public health service to arrange for transportation of stray domestic animals to the ASPCA.

Regardless of the nature of the attack, thoroughly clean all wounds. Infiltrate high-risk wounds with 1% lidocaine, then thoroughly irrigate to the depth of the wound. Give prophylactic antibiotics, if indicated (see Bite Wounds, pp. 763–766).

The indications for PEP are summarized in Table 26.2. Use human rabies immune globulin (HRIG) and human diploid cell vaccine (HDCV) at the initial time of presentation. Give a single dose of 20 units/kg of HRIG. Infiltrate as much of the dose as is anatomically possible in and around the wound, and inject the remainder in a site that is distant from the wound. Give

Table 26.1 Rabies risk from bats

Exposure unlikely	Exposure reasonably possible
Bat droppings found in sleeping quarters	Bat found in same room of someone sleeping, mentally disturbed, intoxicated, or an unattended child
Patient touches bat, but is certain there is no scratch	Young child touches bat, but may be unaware or unable to communicate about the bite
Bat swoops by patient who does not feel it touch, or there is no contact with bare skin	Bat flies into patient, touching bare skin and unable to determine what contact occurred
Patient has contact with carcass of bat	Patient with bare feet steps on a live bat
Bats are heard or seen in the attic or walls	Patient puts hand in firewood or brush, feels pain, then sees a live bat

Table 26.2 Rabies post-exposure prophylaxis guide

Animal species	Condition at time of attack	Treatment
Dogs, cats, ferrets	Healthy (observed for ten days)	None[1]
	Rabid or suspected rabid	HRIG and HDCV
	Unknown (escaped)	Consult local public health officials[2]
Bats, foxes, skunks, raccoons, woodchucks, and most other carnivores	Regard as rabid unless area is free of rabies or laboratory tests prove otherwise	HRIG and HDCV
Livestock, rodents, lagomorphs (rabbits, hares)	Consider individually	Consult local public health officials

Bites of squirrels, hamsters, guinea pigs, gerbils, chipmunks, rats, mice and other rodents, rabbits, and hares almost never require antirabies prophylaxis.
HRIG = human rabies immune globulin; HDCV = human diploid cell vaccine.
[1] During the holding period, immediately begin prophylaxis if the dog or cat develops any signs of rabies. Sacrifice the animal and test its brain.
[2] The incidence of rabies in the community determines the need for prophylaxis.
Adapted from: Kimberlin D, Brady M, Jackson M, Long S (eds.). *Red Book: 2015 Report of the Committee on Infectious Diseases*. Elk Grove Village, IL: American Academy of Pediatrics, 2015; 661.

1 mL IM of HDCV, with subsequent doses 3, 7, and 14 days after the first. Use the deltoid area for adolescents and older children; the anterolateral aspect of the thigh may be used in younger children. Do not give the vaccine at the same site as HRIG (may cause prophylaxis failure).

Follow-up

- Rabies prophylaxis initiated: three days

Indications for Admission

• Clinical rabies

Bibliography

Jackson AC. Human rabies: a 2016 update. *Curr Infect Dis Rep.* 2016;**18**(11):38.

Kimberlin D, Brady M, Jackson M, Long S (eds.). *Red Book: 2015 Report of the Committee on Infectious Diseases.* Elk Grove Village, IL: American Academy of Pediatrics, 2015; 658–666.

National Association of State Public Health Veterinarians, Inc. Compendium of animal rabies prevention and control, 2011. *MMWR Recomm Rep.* 2011;**60**(RR-6):1–17.

Willoughby RE Jr. Rabies: rare human infection – common questions. *Infect Dis Clin North Am.* 2015;**29**(4):637–650.

Zhu S, Guo C. Rabies control and treatment: from prophylaxis to strategies with curative potential. *Viruses.* 2016;**8**(11). doi: 10.3390/v8110279.

Scorpion Stings

There are 650 species of scorpions worldwide, although only one species in the United States, *Centruroides exilixauda,* produces serious toxicity. This scorpion, also known as the "bark scorpion" because it lives in the bark of trees, is found in Arizona and to a lesser extent in other southwestern states. Scorpions are nocturnal and will frequently enter houses to feed on cockroaches.

The scorpion has two claws anteriorly and a tail which ends in a telson, which contains poisonous glands and a stinger. The venom contains a neurotoxin that can cause autonomic and neuromuscular dysfunction.

Clinical Presentation

In children, immediate systemic symptoms are common. These may include fever, respiratory distress, sympathetic (tachycardia, hypertension, diaphoresis, altered mental status), parasympathetic (hypotension, bradycardia, salivation, bronchorrhea, urination), and neuromuscular (extremity jerking, cranial nerve dysfunction, fasciculations, opisthotonos) findings.

Diagnosis

In most cases, there is a definite history of a scorpion sting. When the history is lacking, consider a scorpion bite when local pain and numbness are accompanied by autonomic symptoms.

ED Management

As soon as the patient arrives in the ED, apply an ice bag to the area of the sting. Immobilize the affected area in a functional position below the level of the heart. If there is mild to moderate pain without neurotoxicity, give ibuprofen (10 mg/kg). If the pain is severe, use fentanyl (1–5 mcg/kg IV or 1.5 mcg/kg intranasal). Treat anxiety with midazolam (0.1 mg/kg IV/IM), hypertension with labetalol (0.1 mg/kg IV) or diazoxide (1 mg/kg minibolus IV push), and the parasympathetic effects with atropine (0.01 mg/kg IV). Monitor IV fluids carefully as these patients are at risk for pulmonary edema and hypertension. Although commercially prepared antivenin is produced in other parts of the world for endemic scorpions, in the United States commercially prepared scorpion antivenin is available only in Arizona.

Indications for Admission

- *Centruroides* bite, if the patient is symptomatic after four hours of ED observation

Bibliography

Rodrigo C, Gnanathasan A. Management of scorpion envenoming: a systematic review and meta-analysis of controlled clinical trials. *Syst Rev.* 2017;6(1):74.

Skolnik AB, Ewald MB. Pediatric scorpion envenomation in the United States: morbidity, mortality, and therapeutic innovations. *Pediatr Emerg Care.* 2013;29(1):98–103.

Tuuri RE, Reynolds S. Scorpion envenomation and antivenom therapy. *Pediatr Emerg Care.* 2011;27(7):667–672

Snakebites

Although most snakes in the United States are not venomous, snakebites cause approximately 5–15 deaths annually. Poisonous snakes indigenous to the United States include the Crotalidae (rattlesnakes, water moccasins, copperheads) and the Elapidae (coral snake). Crotalids account for 99% of venomous snakebites occurring in the wild, and can be found in virtually any state in the continental United States. The poisonous coral snake (which is the only elapid found in the United States) is found in southeastern and Gulf Coast states, as well as Arizona. On occasion, victims are bitten by exotic snakes that are kept as pets.

Clinical Presentation

Crotalid Envenomation

The pain usually starts within one minute of the bite, although a deep bite or one not on an extremity can cause more rapid symptoms. Crotalid envenomation can affect the following organ systems:

- Skin and soft tissue: local necrosis.
- Cardiovascular: increased capillary permeability leading to progressive edema and local hemorrhage. In the most severe cases, pulmonary edema, hemorrhage and hypotension may occur.
- Hematologic: thrombocytopenia and defibrination may occur. Hemorrhage, hemolysis, and DIC may also develop.
- Renal: acute tubular or cortical necrosis can occur, especially in the presence of marked hemolysis and shock.
- Immune: anaphylactic-like symptoms.
- Neurologic: symptoms are uncommon, although the Mojave rattlesnake may cause neuromuscular blockade. Cranial nerve palsies are often seen as the first manifestation.

Elapid Envenomation

- Skin and soft tissue: small amount of local erythema and swelling. There is also a possibility that the snake will chew the skin, leading to a large laceration.

- Neurologic: paresthesias, nausea, emesis, muscle fasciculations, tremors, and bulbar paralysis can occur. Severe cases can lead to respiratory and muscular paralysis.

Diagnosis

The diagnosis of a snakebite is generally clear from the history. The key diagnostic issue is determining the type of snake. The crotalids can be identified by their large triangular heads and heat-sensing pits located above the nostrils. Elapids have red and yellow bands adjacent to each other.

ED Management

Nonvenomous

Clean the wound, give tetanus prophylaxis if necessary (pp. 783–784), and appropriate pain medication. Prescribe a five-day course of oral antibiotics, using either amoxicillin/clavulanic acid (875/125 formulation; 45 mg/kg/day of amoxicillin div bid) or the combination of penicillin VK (50 mg/kg/day div qid) and cephalexin (40 mg/kg/day div qid). If there is any uncertainty about the identity of the snake, contact the regional poison control center, and observe for venomous symptoms for at least 3–4 hours.

Venomous

In the field, the priority is expedient transfer to a medical facility. Splint the affected extremity and remove jewelry that could cause a tourniquet effect. Do not apply cold packs or tourniquets. Although up to 20% of bites from venomous snakes are "dry" bites and are therefore asymptomatic, emergency medical treatment is needed to clean the wound and evaluate the need for antivenin.

Once the patient arrives in the ED, the decision to use antivenin is based on the type of snake and the duration and progression of symptoms. Contact the regional poison control center to consult with someone experienced in managing snakebites. For all patients, start an IV in the contralateral side and keep the affected extremity at heart-level. Give antibiotics and pain medication as for nonvenomous snakebites, but do not give aspirin or NSAIDs. Obtain blood for CBC, electrolytes, BUN, creatinine, PT, PTT, fibrinogen level, and blood type. Also obtain a urinalysis to look for hematuria and proteinuria.

CroFab is indicated for the management of a patient with a minimal or moderate North American crotalid bite. Early use of CroFab (within six hours) can prevent clinical deterioration and the occurrence of systemic coagulation abnormalities. The initial dose is 4–6 vials. Carefully observe the patient for up to one hour to determine if initial control of the envenomation has been achieved, as defined by the complete arrest of local manifestations, reversal of the systemic signs, and the return of coagulation tests to normal. If this is not accomplished with the first dose, give additional doses of 4–6 vials until control of the envenomation syndrome has been achieved. After initial control has been established, administer additional two-vial doses every six hours for up to 18 hours. It is not necessary to adjust the dosage for age.

Debridement is often necessary after the first 48 hours, but fasciotomy is rarely required for treatment of compartment syndrome. Warn the patient that serum sickness may occur 10–14 days after treatment. This presents with a pruritic urticarial rash, which can be

776 | Chapter 26: Wound Care and Minor Trauma

associated with fever, nausea, headache, arthralgias, and adenopathy. Admit all sympto-matic patients for at least 24 hours, regardless of whether antivenin was given.

Indications for Admission

- Snakebite with signs of envenomation or requiring antivenin treatment

Bibliography

Daley BJ, Torres J. Venomous snakebites. *JEMS*. 2014;**39**(6):58–62.

Del Brutto OH, Del Brutto VJ. Neurological complications of venomous snake bites: a review. *Acta Neurol Scand*. 2012;**125**(6):363–372.

Kularatne SA, Senanayake N. Venomous snake bites, scorpions, and spiders. *Handb Clin Neurol*. 2014;**120**:987–1001.

Spider Bites

There are 50 species of North American spiders with fangs capable of penetrating human skin, although only two species (black widow and brown recluse) can cause fatalities.

The black widow (*Latrodectus*) is distinguished by a red hourglass marking on the abdomen. The spiders are found throughout North America, except in Alaska. The female can grow up to 4 cm (including leg span), with a male being about one-quarter to one-half smaller.

The brown recluse (*Loxosceles*) is the most common cause of serious spider bites in the United States. They can be up to 3 cm in length and are distinguished by a dark-orange violin-shaped marking on the cephalothorax. It generally lives in dark, dry environments such as abandoned houses or vacation homes, and is most active at night.

Clinical Presentation

Black Widow

The bite causes a pinprick sensation with slight local erythema, pain, and swelling. Within 10–90 minutes there are systemic symptoms, including muscle cramps, especially in the abdomen and back after bites of the lower extremities. Agitation and irritability may also be part of the initial presentation. There may be spasms with intense pain, paresthesias (particularly intense in the soles of the feet), headache, dysphagia, dizziness, nausea and vomiting, facial edema, tachycardia, and hypertension (which can be life-threatening). A venom dose that may cause only pain in an adult may lead to respiratory and cardiac arrest in a child.

Brown Recluse

The bite of this spider is generally trivial. Within ten minutes to several hours there is sharp, stinging, or burning type of pain at the bite site, followed by an aching pain and pruritus. The lesion becomes an irregular violaceous blister surrounded by an erythe-matous halo. In about 50% of cases, over 2–3 days the blister becomes an eschar that later sloughs, leaving an ulcer that is very slow to heal. The larger South American *Loxosceles* genus gives a more pronounced cutaneous picture, with intense pain and accompanying facial edema.

Systemic involvement is rare but can occur in any *Loxosceles* envenomation. The manifestations include fever, chills, nausea, vomiting, malaise, and a confluent scarlatiniform rash. There may be an associated hemolytic anemia presenting as hemoglobinuria, as well as thrombocytopenia and renal failure. The systemic response is usually not seen until 24 hours after the bite, making the diagnosis difficult.

ED Management

Assess the ABCs and treat as necessary (see Shock, pp. 28–36). Insert an IV on the contralateral side and infuse D_5 ½ NS (use NS if the patient has signs of shock), and obtain a CBC, electrolytes, CPK, calcium, PT, and PTT. Apply ice to the bite site to reduce toxin absorption and decrease the pain.

Black Widow

Give diazepam (0.05–0.2 mg/kg IV) and morphine (0.05–0.2 mg/kg) for analgesia, anxiety, and muscle relaxation. For most cases this will be the only treatment needed. Give labetalol (0.1 mg/kg IV) if hypertension is present despite the benzodiazepine and morphine.

For severe envenomations an antivenin is available. Dilute one vial in 100 mL of normal saline and give over 30–60 minutes. Immediate and delayed hypersensitivity reactions may occur.

Brown Recluse

Apply repeated ice compresses for 2–3 days; these will reduce pain and the local cutaneous inflammation. There is no demonstrable benefit for any specific treatment for brown recluse bites other than routine wound care. Persistent ulceration may require skin grafting. If hemolysis occurs, ensure a good urine output (at least twice normal).

Follow-up

- Black widow: daily until the patient is asymptomatic
- Brown recluse: daily, until the wound is healing well

Indications for Admission

- Systemic symptoms

Bibliography

Juckett G. Arthropod bites. *Am Fam Physician.* 2013;88(12):841–847.

Kang JK, Bhate C, Schwartz RA. Spiders in dermatology. *Semin Cutan Med Surg.* 2014;33(3):123–127.

Monte AA. Black widow spider (*Latrodectus mactans*) antivenom in clinical practice. *Curr Pharm Biotechnol.* 2012;13(10):1935–1939.

Peterson ME. Black widow spider envenomation. *Clin Tech Small Anim Pract* 2006;21:187–190.

Shackleford R, Veillon D, Maxwell N, et al. The black widow spider bite: differential diagnosis, clinical manifestations, and treatment options. *J La State Med Soc.* 2015;167(2):74–78.

Wound Management

Most lacerations can be treated in the ED using basic principles of aseptic technique and wound closure. Plastic surgical consultation may occasionally be required for complex wounds, cosmetic concerns, functional deficits, or loss of subcutaneous tissue.

Clinical Presentation and ED Management

History

Determine the elapsed time since the injury. Most wounds <8–12 hours old may be closed primarily without an increased risk of infection; scalp and face wounds can be sutured up to at least 12–24 hours after injury. Delayed closure of face, head, and neck wounds does not cause an increased rate of wound infection. Knowing the mechanism of injury is helpful in predicting the likelihood of infectious complications: wounds resulting from compressive forces (blunt scalp trauma) often cause stellate lacerations which may be more susceptible to infection than linear lacerations due to shearing forces (razor). Assess the general health of the patient, and ask about any possible immunocompromise that may increase the risk of an infection, such as underlying chronic illnesses (diabetes, vasculitis), steroid use, or chemotherapy.

Examination

Determine the extent of the injury, and evaluate sensation, general strength, vascular supply, motor function, and range of motion with and without resistance (looking for tendon injuries). This is difficult in an uncooperative young child, but if an extremity is involved, observe that the patient is able to move it normally through a full range of motion before closing the wound. During the assessment, keep the wound edges moist by applying gauze pads moistened with NS.

Radiology

Radiographs are indicated when the mechanism of injury or physical examination suggests a bony injury or a retained foreign body. Metal fragments and glass can be seen on plain films, and wood fragments are visible if coated with radiopaque particles of dirt. If a foreign body is still suspected despite negative radiographs, arrange for an ultrasound. Obtain radiographs of a crush injury to rule-out a compound fracture. When possible, irrigate the wound before radiographs or ultrasound are performed to remove superficial debris.

Shaving

Shaving has the potential to increase the risk of infection. Therefore, clip the hair around a wound with scissors only if it interferes with wound closure. Never shave eyebrows, since there is no guarantee that they will grow back.

Anesthesia

Local anesthesia may be required to perform adequate irrigation and debridement. Apply a solution of either LET or LMX4 (see Topical Analgesia, pp. 723–724) prior to administering the local anesthetic. Topical anesthesia is especially useful for lacerations of the face and scalp. To prepare the wound for local anesthesia, apply povidone-iodine solution twice to the skin surrounding the wound, allowing it to dry for four minutes between applications. Lidocaine is the usual anesthetic agent. To minimize the possibility of a toxic reaction, use the 1% strength in children, although 2% can be used when only a limited volume of anesthetic is to be injected (small child's finger). Use lidocaine with epinephrine for vascular areas (scalp, face), but epinephrine is contraindicated in areas with end-arteries (digits, pinna, nose). Do not exceed a total dose of 5 mg/kg of lidocaine (7 mg/kg when used with epinephrine). Procaine is the alternative in the patient allergic to lidocaine (extremely rare).

In unquestionably clean wounds, inject the lidocaine through the open wound (less painful), but in wounds likely to be dirty, administer it through the surrounding skin to avoid injecting debris into the deeper tissues.

Debridement and Irrigation

After anesthesia has been achieved, debride any devitalized tissue, including fat. Irrigate the wound using a large (35 mL) Luer-lock syringe attached to a splash shield, which will produce 5–8 psi, an adequate pressure for wound irrigation. The solution of choice for irrigation is NS; use copious amounts (at least 100 mL, but often >1 L, depending on the wound size). Tap water may be an effective alternative, especially for preliminary cleansing before radiographs are obtained.

Exploration

Examine every wound for foreign substances and any associated trauma to blood vessels, ligaments, tendons, and bone. Remove fragments of hair, pieces of clothing, other debris, and blood clots, which may camouflage other injuries and be a source of infection. For scalp wounds, examine with a sterile gloved finger to determine any disruption of the galea and the outer table of the skull.

Suturing

For skin closure, nonabsorbable suture material is indicated, the least reactive of which is monofilament nylon. For typical outpatient wounds, deep sutures must be absorbable. Synthetics (Dexon) are less reactive than naturally occurring substances (gut). The appropriate suture size for different areas is given in Table 26.3. For areas where there is an increase in tension, such as over joints, choose the next heavier size.

Hemostasis may be accomplished with a simple ligature, a loop of absorbable suture either around the bleeder or tied in a small figure-eight (Figure 26.1). Never use a hemostat to clamp blindly, as a tendon, tendon sheath, or nerve may be clamped and destroyed.

Close deep wounds in two layers to obliterate dead space (Figure 26.2). When using deep sutures, bury the knot (Figure 26.3), except where it will cause friction (fascia, tendon sheaths), and cut the ends fairly short.

Most wounds can be closed with simple interrupted sutures (Figure 26.4). The skin edges must be everted and touching. Inverted edges result in poor healing but can be avoided by ensuring that the suture is at equal depth on both sides of the wound, that the depth is greater than the width (B > C), and that the width at the bottom of the suture (C) is greater than at the top (A). Evenly space the sutures so that the tension is distributed equally.

A vertical mattress (Figure 26.5) is a good method of closing a wound when there are problems with wound edge eversion or tension on the wound edge or when a wound is deep but does not require a two-layer closure. It is also useful in areas of skin laxity – for example, the back of the hand. The area inside the suture has all the tension, leaving the edges with

Table 26.3 Suggested suture size

Site	Suture Size
Scalp (consider wounds at the hairline to be facial)	3-0, 4-0
Face, orbit	5-0, 6-0
Neck	
Ventral	5-0, 6-0
Dorsal	4-0, 5-0
Arms, legs, trunk	4-0, 5-0
Hands and fingers	5-0, 6-0
Feet	
Dorsum	4-0, 5-0
Plantar	3-0, 4-0
Toes	5-0, 6-0
Deep (absorbable)	
Hemostasis	4-0, 5-0
Deep closure	3-0, 4-0, 5-0*

* The more superficial the subcutaneous suture, the smaller the size of suture material.

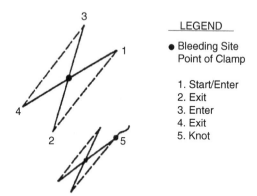

LEGEND

● Bleeding Site
Point of Clamp

1. Start/Enter
2. Exit
3. Enter
4. Exit
5. Knot

Figure 26.1 Figure-eight suture.

none. The suture must be of equal depth on the two sides of the wound, to prevent a stepping scar.

Employ a horizontal mattress (Figure 26.6) when there are problems with wound edge eversion; do not use it where there will be any tension or to eliminate a two-layer closure. Note that each horizontal mattress takes the space of two sutures, so this is a fast way to close a wound.

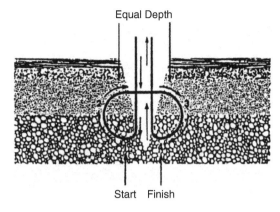

Figure 26.2 Suture for a deep wound.

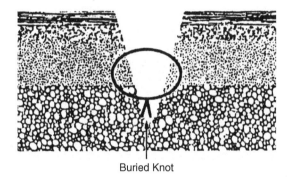

Figure 26.3 Suture for a deep wound burying the knots.

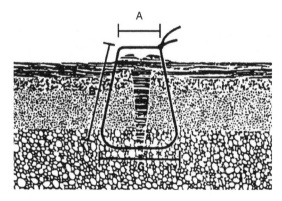

Figure 26.4 Interrupted suture.

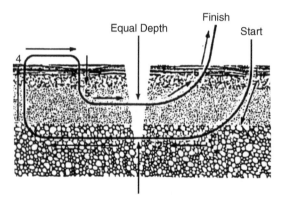

Figure 26.5 Vertical mattress suture.

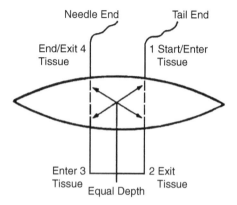

Figure 26.6 Horizontal mattress suture.

The half-horizontal mattress is the best way to handle any sharp corner (Figure 26.7a,b) and can be used for a "v," "y," "t," "z," or stellate type of wound (Figure 26.7c–f).

In wounds of the lip, the first suture must bring together the edges of the vermilion border; otherwise, a noticeable scar results.

Wound Adhesives

Cyanoacylates, such as Dermabond, can be used for minor facial lacerations that are small (<5 cm), clean, under minimal tension, with sharp edges. Anesthesia may not be necessary and wound closure time can be decreased by as much as 50%. The adhesive polymerizes in about one second; hold the wound margins together with forceps or the wooden ends of swabs placed about 3–5 mm from the edges. Do not use Dermabond if there is evidence of active infection or on mucosal surface wounds, skin exposed to body fluid regularly, or areas with dense hair.

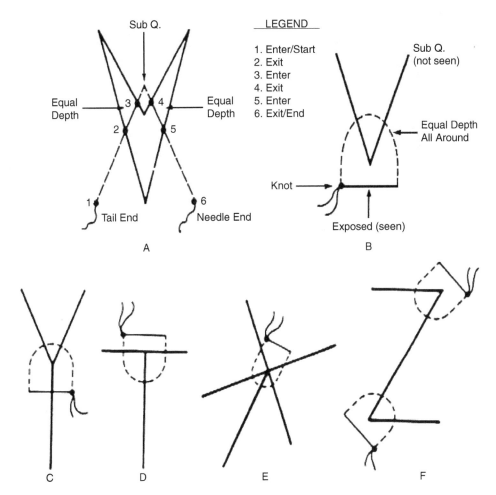

Figure 26.7 Half-buried horizontal mattress suture.

Referral

Refer complex wounds, in which underlying structural injury is a possibility, to a surgeon. Among these are deep lacerations of the wrist or hand, chest, abdomen, perineum, or anterior neck. Also refer ear and eyelid wounds.

Tetanus

Clean minor wounds require tetanus prophylaxis only if the patient has not had at least three documented previous tetanus toxoid doses or if a previously immunized patient has not had a tetanus dose in at least ten years. Serious wounds at greater risk for tetanus include contaminated (dirt, feces, saliva) and puncture wounds and wounds with devitalized tissue. With these wounds, give tetanus toxoid to a patient who has had three previous doses but more than five years has elapsed since the last dose. For patients with fewer than three previous doses, use toxoid and tetanus immune globulin

Table 26.4 Approximate timetable for removing sutures*

Location	Days to suture removal
Scalp	8 ± 2
Face	4 ± 1
Orbit	4 ± 1
Neck	
Dorsal	6 ± 1
Ventral	5 ± 1
Chest, arms, legs	7 ± 1
Back	11 ± 1
Hands	7 ± 1
Fingertips	9 ± 1
Feet	
Dorsal, toes	9 ± 1
Plantar	10 ± 2
Skin over joints	12 ± 2

* Remove any packing in 24 hours and reevaluate the wound.

(250–500 units IM). When tetanus toxoid is indicated for a patient under seven years of age, use 0.5 mL of DTaP, unless pertussis vaccination is contraindicated, in which case use DT. For a child 7–10 years old, use 0.5 mL of dT. If the patient is ≥11 years old, use 0.5 mL of Tdap.

Other Measures

Splint wounds in areas of great mobility (across joints, on the hand) using a thick wrapping of gauze for two days, until healing is underway. Advise the patient to avoid getting the wound wet for the first 24 hours; after that, it can be cleaned gently and allowed to air-dry. Give the parents dry bandages to apply in case the original dressing becomes wet.

No antibiotics are necessary for small, uncomplicated wounds that are not a result of an animal or human bite. Give antibiotics for facial wounds >24 hours old; other wounds >12 hours old; contaminated wounds; and wounds in immunosuppressed patients. Use amoxicillin-clavulanate (875/125 formulation; 45 mg/kg/day of amoxicillin div bid). For penicillin-allergic patients, give clindamycin (20 mg/kg/day div tid) or erythromycin (40 mg/kg/day div qid).

Suture Removal

Remove sutures according to Table 26.4. When sutures are removed, cut them just below the knot with suture scissors or a curved blade and pull them out. This prevents pulling contaminated material through the tissue. After sutures are removed, apply Steri-Strips to give additional strength for a few days without the risk of infection or foreign body reaction.

Follow-up

- Immediately for signs of infection (fever, erythema, proximal streaking, induration, purulence). Otherwise, return for suture removal.

Bibliography

Black KD, Cico SJ, Caglar D. Wound management. *Pediatr Rev.* 2015;36(5):207–215.

Childs DR, Murthy AS. Overview of wound healing and management. *Surg Clin North Am.* 2017;97(1):189–207.

Tayeb BO, Eidelman A, Eidelman CL, et al. Topical anaesthetics for pain control during repair of dermal laceration. *Cochrane Database Syst Rev.* 2017;2:CD005364.

Chapter 27

Special Considerations in Pediatric Emergency Care

Joshua Vova, Kirsten Roberts, Daniel Rogers, Frank A. Maffei, and David P. Sole

Children With Special Healthcare Needs (CSHCN)

Only 13–18% of children have special healthcare needs, but they are responsible for approximately 80% of pediatric healthcare costs. The complexity of their care often results in emergency department (ED) visits, and they are much more likely to be hospitalized as children without disabilities. In addition, approximately 1 in 1000 CSHCN requires technology-assistive care, and complications from these devices are often the reasons for ED visits. The family may also use the ED as the medial home, especially if there is no established relationship with a primary healthcare provider.

The ED physician must determine whether the chief complaint is a manifestation of the underlining diagnosis or a new acute problem. The patient may also have difficulty cooperating and communicating, adding to the challenge of making a diagnosis. In addition, there are over 800 congenital syndromes responsible for childhood disability, so no physician can be familiar with every aspect of a given disease. Moreover, obvious inexperience with a CSHCN may make a parent less trusting. It is important to understand the child's functional status and abilities prior to the incident that brought them into the ED. Incorrect assumptions about the patient's capabilities may obscure the physician's clinical assessment.

Some CSHCN may also present with behavioral challenges that can cause examination, imaging, or simple diagnostic testing to be more challenging. The patient may be nonverbal, have a decreased ability to communicate, or be unable to cooperate. Therefore, attempt to communicate in a manner that is familiar to the patient, including the use of augmentative communication devices or sign language when relevant. Also, take steps to ease the stress for the child and family, such as reducing stimulation, using objects from home that may provide some comfort, and minimizing the number of staff that are interacting with the patient. If available, a child life specialist may be helpful. When behavioral modifications are not effective, the ED physician may have to use pharmacological methods in order to perform procedures safely.

Enterostomy Tubes

Many CSHCN require an enterostomy tube because of oral motor problems, dysphagia, inadequate calorie intake, unpalatable medications, or severe aspiration. Tubes are classified as gastrostomy (GT), gastrojejunostomy (JT) or jejunostomy, depending upon the location of the distal end. Advise the parents to keep a detailed record of their child's current tube size and type in order to facilitate any future replacements.

Dislodgement

Dislodgement is the most common reason for an ED visit concerning a GT or JT. This may occur due to trauma, tension on the tube (intentional or unintentional), rupture of the balloon, or unintentional balloon deflation. A feeding tube may also malfunction due to deterioration over time or obstruction.

Early Dislodgement

Dislodgement in the first four weeks after insertion is the most common complication of feeding tubes. A tract for the tube will begin to mature within 7–10 days, although it may not be complete for up to three months. However, if a tube dislodges within the first 2–4 weeks, there is a risk that the stomach may separate from the anterior abdominal wall, so that blindly reinserting a new feeding tube may result in placing it within the peritoneal cavity. Using aseptic technique, stent the site with a replacement tube, then consult the service that originally placed the tube, as there is considerable institutional variation as to when a tract is considered to be mature. Do not use the feeding tube at this point. Instead, place an NG tube while awaiting consultation.

Later Dislodgement

If the dislodged tube was from an older stoma, immediately replace it with either a Foley catheter or an appropriate-sized replacement tube. Lubricate the distal end with petroleum jelly using aseptic technique. Reinsert the tube carefully to avoid placing it into the peritoneal cavity through a false tract. Always inflate the balloon with sterile water (not saline). Abdominal pain upon balloon inflation is an indication of improper position; remove the tube and retry.

If excessive time has elapsed prior to the family seeking medical attention, the stoma may have constricted. To avoid this, do not delay replacement while seeking the correct size replacement tube. If the proper-size feeding tube is unavailable, insert a Foley catheter to stent the stoma until a replacement can be obtained. If the stoma has partially closed and the original size gastrostomy tube or Foley does not fit, use a smaller tube, but do not use excessive force when attempting reinsertion.

After a GT has been reinserted, check for proper placement. To confirm, aspirate gastric fluid and test the pH (should be <5) and/or inject 10–15 mL of air while listening over the stomach for borborygmi. Otherwise, obtain an abdominal film after injecting 5–10 mL of water-soluble radiocontrast material to confirm the location of the tube. Apply an abdominal binder or a loose-fitting ace bandage wrap to secure the enterostomy tube flush against the stomach and reduce the risk of recurrent dislodgement.

A dislodged JT must be replaced by either interventional radiology or surgery, as there is a risk of subsequent ischemia and bowel necrosis.

Removing a GT

Generally, there is no reason to remove a GT in the ED. However, if it is necessary, use a 20 mL syringe to deflate the balloon prior to removing the tube. Alternatively, some tubes have an internal bumper. In order to determine whether there is an internal bumper or a balloon, inspect the outer ports. If the port is meant for inflating a balloon it is typically white and labeled with the volume of fluid needed to maintain the balloon. If the situation remains uncertain, use a syringe and aspirate the contents of the port.

Redness and Bleeding

Skin Irritation

Frequent complaints are redness or bleeding around the tube site due to leakage, tape sensitivity, infection, or granulation tissue. If the tube is not properly secured against the skin, the stoma may become widened over time and gastric contents can leak around the tube. It is important to determine whether leakage is caused from a defect in the tube itself, or from gastric contents refluxing around the tube. Shield the skin from leaking gastric contents with a plastic barrier (e.g., Tegaderm), or a barrier agent, such as sucralfate, hydrocolloid agents, or zinc oxide. Add an antacid to the feeding regimen to increase the pH of the leaking gastric contents, and refer the patient to the primary physician for further care.

Granulation Tissue

Granulation formation around the tube is a common complaint. While these areas are usually painless and only rarely become infected or cause obstruction of the stoma, on occasion they may bleed. Apply warm saline compresses and cauterize with silver nitrate. Then apply a topical antibiotic cream and dress with sterile gauze. Alternatively, use a topical steroid ointment (e.g., triamcinolone), which may help reduce the redness and size of the granuloma.

Local Infection

Approximately 20% of patients will experience a local infection after placement of an enterostomy tube. Although most infections are minor, there is a small risk of progression to a necrotizing fasciitis. See Cellulitis (pp. 108–109) for the treatment of a local infection in a nontoxic-appearing patient.

Vomiting

Vomiting is common in a child with an enterostomy tube, although it is most often related to gastroesophageal reflux disease or dysphagia. However, there are several possible tube-related causes: tube occlusion, tube migration, and intestinal obstruction due to adhesions.

Occlusion

Gastrostomy tube occlusion may occur in up to 45% of patients, secondary to kinking or obstruction of the lumen by the accumulation of formula or medications. The usual complaint is an inability to flush the tube or infuse liquid into it. Attempt to flush the tube with sterile water using a 30 mL or larger syringe to avoid excessive pressure. Use 20–30 mL of warm water to unclog PEG tubes. If conservative measures fail, replace the gastrostomy tube or use a Foley catheter of equal size. However, newly placed gastrostomy tubes, as well as jejunostomy tubes, and nasoenteric tubes may be difficult to replace. In these cases, consult the appropriate subspecialist and do not remove the tube.

Migration

Although rare, it is possible for a GT to migrate. A traditional GT or JT (not a button) will have about 4–6 cm of tube outside the stoma, although this may vary based on the size of the patient. Compare the centimeter markings on the outside of the tube with what the parent has typically observed. If there is a discrepancy, gently pulling back on the tube until the balloon is against the abdominal wall may relieve an obstruction.

Buried Bumper

Buried bumper syndrome occurs when the internal bumper erodes through the stomach wall with subsequent re-epithelialization which covers or buries the bumper. Often this is a result of excess traction on the enterostomy tube. It usually presents as resistance to flow or vomiting and/or abdominal pain during feedings. Suspect a buried bumper if the tube cannot be freely rotated. Consult a surgeon or gastroenterologist to plan removal and replacement of the tube.

Tracheostomy

Tracheostomy tubes are sized according to three dimensions: the inner diameter, the outer diameter, and the length. Regardless of the brand, the inner diameter is consistent among manufacturers and is always imprinted on the flange. In contrast, outer diameters and lengths are not consistent and may or may not be printed on the tube. Discrepancy in the outer diameter may cause a replacement tube to not fit into the stoma, so it may be necessary to select a smaller-size tube. Therefore, before replacing a tracheostomy, always have a smaller-size back-up available in case the original size cannot be reinserted.

The proper tube diameter optimizes airway resistance and limits the risk of aspiration, without irritating the mucosa or damaging the airway wall. Typically, the outer diameter is less than two-thirds of the tracheal diameter and the end of the tube is >2 cm beyond the stoma, but no closer than 1–2 cm from the carina. To prevent esophageal obstruction, trachea-esophageal fistula, or a tracheo-innominate artery fistula, use a curved tube to ensure that the distal end is concentric and parallel to the trachea. The standard pediatric tracheostomy tube has a 15 mm connector at the proximal end that allows for a connection to a bag-mask or a ventilator. However, a metal tube will not have this adapter.

A tracheostomy tube may be cuffed or uncuffed. The limited indications for a cuffed tube include a patient with chronic aspiration or one who requires high positive pressure for ventilation. The patient cannot speak with the cuff inflated.

The tracheal lumen may be fenestrated or non-fenestrated. A fenestrated tracheostomy tube is usually reserved for a patient who is able to speak, but may require intermittent mechanical ventilation.

Hypoxia

The most common causes of hypoxia are infection related, either tracheitis or pneumonia. However, dislodgment or obstruction also occur frequently and must be identified. A false tract is also a possibility, especially in tracheostomy tubes less than a week old or that have been recently changed by an inexperienced caregiver.

Bleeding

Any significant bleeding from the tracheostomy site requires an endoscopic evaluation of the airway. If the tip of the tracheostomy tube rests against the tracheal wall it may cause irritation, inflammation, and ulceration with bleeding. This tends to be more common in a patient receiving mechanical ventilation. If the erosion occurs on the anterior tracheal wall it has the potential to cause a hemorrhage of the innominate artery, which typically lies 9–12 rings below the cricoid cartilage. This is a potentially life-threatening event and a surgical emergency which presents with a pulsating tracheostomy tube, bleeding around the tracheostomy site, or massive hemoptysis. If an innominate artery hemorrhage is suspected, do not remove the tracheostomy, as it may be the only way to ensure an adequate airway. If the patient does have a cuffed tracheostomy, overinflating the cuff may help to tamponade the bleeding.

Infection

A patient with a tracheostomy, especially one requiring ventilatory support, is at high risk for infection involving the stoma and lower respiratory tract. A child with a neuromuscular disease is at particularly high risk. A tracheostomy is usually colonized with potential pathogens, including *Pseudomonas aeruginosa, Streptococcus* spp., *Staphylococcus aureus, Haemophilus influenza*, and *Candida albicans*. Signs of an acute infection include a change from the baseline respiratory status, fever, tachypnea, increased oxygen requirement, and changes in tracheal secretions, cough, or accessory muscle use. Minor bleeding may also be a sign of infection if accompanied by other symptoms.

Tracheoesophageal Fistula

A tracheoesophageal fistula can occur when the posterior wall of the trachea is exposed to chronic pressure from the tip of the tracheostomy. This is potentially life-threatening because of bacterial contamination of the tracheobronchial airway. Symptoms include more copious secretions, new or increased aspiration of food contents, dyspnea, cuff leak, or gastric distention. The diagnosis can be made with a CT scan or barium esophagography. Treatment is usually surgical.

Granuloma Formation

This is the most frequent complication of a tracheostomy and can be caused by frictional trauma from the tube, inflammation from stasis of secretions, infection, poor tube position, or traumatic suction technique. Granulomas are most common just superior to the internal stoma site on the anterior tracheal wall, but may also be seen along the posterior tracheal wall. Up to 80% of pediatric tracheostomies develop suprastomal granulation tissue, but in the majority of cases they are small and asymptomatic and require no intervention. Large granulomas may cause bleeding and may delay decannulation or pose an obstruction for recannulation after accidental decannulation. Treat granulation tissue along the external stoma with silver nitrate.

Stenosis

Stenotic lesions are classified according to the anatomical site, including suprastomal, stomal, cuff, and at the tip of the cannula. Most patients with tracheal stenosis remain

Table 27.1 Pressure Ulcer Staging System

Grade	Finding
I	Non-blanchable erythema of intact skin
II	Partial-thickness skin loss with exposed dermis
III	Full-thickness skin loss
IV	Full-thickness skin and tissue loss
Unstageable	Obscured full-thickness skin and tissue loss
Deep tissue injury	Persistent non-blanchable deep red, maroon, or purple discoloration

Adapted from: National Pressure Ulcer Advisory Panel. NPUAP pressure injury stages. www.npuap.org/resources/educational-and-clinical-resources/npuap-pressure-injury-stages (accessed June 26, 2017).

asymptomatic until the original tracheal lumen diameter is reduced by 50–75% or the actual diameter is <5 mm. Symptoms include cough, inability to clear secretions, and dyspnea.

Skin Breakdown and Pressure Injuries

Pressure injuries are common in a patient who is immobilized, wheelchair-dependent, or has insensate skin. Other predisposing factors are fecal or urinary incontinence, chronic steroid use, muscle atrophy, elevated tissue temperatures, chronic malnutrition, and improper transfer techniques. In addition, many CSHCN are malnourished due to oral motor control issues, predisposing them to pressure ulcers. The most frequently affected sites are bony prominences, such as the sacrum, greater trochanter, and ischial tuberosity, as well as the occipital region in a younger child. Ulcers can be further complicated by osteomyelitis and sepsis. Use the National Pressure Ulcer Advisory Panel Pressure Ulcer Staging System to assess skin breakdown (Table 27.1).

When evaluating skin breakdown, document the anatomical location, pressure injury stage, length, width, depth, type of tissue present at the wound base and its color, presence of exudate (none, minimum, moderate, large amount), and odor. Note whether there is undermining (destruction beneath intact tissue) or tunneling at the wound base, which can create dead space and lead to abscess formation. Several factors may interfere with an accurate assessment, including the presence of either an eschar or copious necrotic material, although necrosis may begin deeper within the tissue at the bony prominence. Also, multiple ulcers within a limited area may be indicative of interconnecting fistula tracts. Areas of deep tissue and pressure injury may present as a dark purple/maroon discoloration, particularly over a bony prominence, and can be mistaken for a bruise. These are potentially serious injuries.

Clean the wound to remove the necrotic, devitalized tissue and exudate while minimizing trauma to the wound bed. First, irrigate with a 30–35 mL syringe attached to an 18 or 19 gauge needle (delivers 8 lb per square inch). Use normal saline, but do not add an antiseptic solution, which may be cytotoxic. Debridement is then necessary if there is a fibrinous

Table 27.2 Wound dressings

Dressing type	Properties	Brand names
Calcium alginates	Fibers absorb exudates and convert into a gel, providing moisture for healing	Kaltostat
	Absorbs moderate to heavy drainage	Aquacel Ag
	Controls minor bleeding	(antimicrobial)
	Provides a moist healing environment	
	Use under a dressing (ABD pad, gauze or transparent film)	
Enzymatic debriding agents	Will chemically lyse necrotic tissue	Medihoney
	Must use within moist environment	Santyl
	Will chemically lyse necrotic tissue	
Film dressing	Use on skin tears	Bio Occlusive
	Use on wounds with little or no drainage	Tegaderm
	Allows water and oxygen into wound, keeps bacteria out	Op-site
	If too much exudate in wound it will interfere with evaporation and oxygen diffusion and cause maceration	
Foam dressing	Absorbs moderate to heavy exudates	Mepilex Border
	Nonadherent	Mepilex Lite
Hydrocolloid	Forms occlusive gel by interacting with wound barrier	Duoderm
	Provides barrier to external contaminates	
	Use with low to moderate exudates	
	Provides autolytic debridement	
	Do not use with infected wounds	
Hydrogel	Use with minimal to moderate exudates	Saf-gel
	Promotes autolytic debridement of devitalized tissue/eschar	
	Maintains moist environment	
	May ease pain and inflammation	

exudate. Use autolytic debridement, which involves keeping the wound moist to allow the body to debride on its own (may use Medihoney), or enzymatic debridement with a topical medication containing collagenase (e.g., Santyl). Use calcium alginate, foam (Mepilex) or hydrogel dressing (Aquacel Ag or Kaltostat) (Table 27.2) for exudative wounds.

Wound cultures are not useful, as most wounds above Stage I are colonized with bacteria. Arrange for daily cleansing and dressing changes to help control colonization as wound healing will not occur if the bacterial count is excessive. Give antibiotics only if there is a cellulitis (erythema and warmth) or the patient has signs of a systemic infection (fever, chills, toxicity). If a wound infection is suspected, consult a burn specialist or dermatologist to perform a wound biopsy or obtain fluid via needle aspiration. A bacterial count $>10^5$/gram of tissue indicates an infection. Prescribe topical mupirocin, bacitracin, or polymixin, all of which are effective against Gram-negative and Gram-positive organisms.

Dressing Selection

Wounds heal better in a moist environment, which enhances cell migration, granulation tissue formation, and white blood cell (WBC) effectiveness. Select a dressing (Table 27.2) which provides an appropriate environment while managing the amount of exudate that the wound is producing. Use these guidelines as a framework to provide temporary care measures until the patient can be evaluated by a wound management expert. All pressure injuries require close follow-up, as superficial-appearing wounds may reflect a deeper injury.

For Stage I and II injuries, use transparent film, hydrocolloid, or foam. For Stage III and IV wounds, use calcium alginate, foam, or hydrogel, but obtain surgical consultation to determine whether inpatient management is needed. When applying a dressing leave at least a 1–1½ inch margin around the wound. In addition, removing the weight load/ pressure to the injured area is a priority. Limit the use of an orthotic device that may be causing pressure and refer the patient to the orthotist to modify or fabricate a new orthosis.

If the injury is in an area of continued pressure, use a hydrocolloid dressing (e.g., Duoderm) or foam dressing (Mepilex) to protect the skin. Review with the parents the proper techniques for preventing wounds, including recognizing potential skin hazards such as radiators, car heaters, hair dryers, and hot plates on laps that can cause burns. In the summer, warn parents about hot sidewalks, metal storm drains, and hot sand. Teach proper positioning, including weight shifts every 15–20 minutes for 30 seconds while sitting, and bed turns every two hours. Encourage the patient to participate in wound checks and arrange for follow-up with either the primary care provider or a local skin specialist (i.e., physiatrist, plastic surgeon) the next day.

Special Considerations in Patients With Spinal Cord-Related Conditions

Autonomic Dysreflexia

Autonomic dysreflexia is a life-threatening syndrome characterized by excessive uncontrolled sympathetic output below the level of a spinal cord injury, particularly in a patient whose injury level is above T6. A noxious stimulus causes an afferent impulse along an intact spinal reflex mechanism below the level of injury, leading to hypertension. Above the level of lesion there is an excess of parasympathetic output that results in peripheral vasodilation and the symptoms that characterize this condition. The most common causes of autonomic dysreflexia include bladder distention, fecal impaction, pressure sores, infection (most commonly urinary tract infection [UTI]), ingrown toenails, fractures, hemorrhoids, heterotopic ossification, and hip dislocation. Less common triggers include menstruation, appendicitis, gallstones, urinary stones, delivery, syringomyelia, testicular torsion, deep vein thrombosis, and pulmonary emboli. Medications such as nasal decongestions, methylphen-idate, or illicit drugs such as cocaine may also produce these symptoms.

Clinical Presentation

The presenting symptoms include hypertension, pounding headache, sweating above the level of injury, bradycardia or tachycardia, piloerection, blurred vision, and anxiety. In the infant or young child there may be sleepiness or irritability. If unrecognized, the hypertensive episodes can lead to retinal hemorrhage, stroke, subarachnoid hemorrhages, seizures, and cardiac arrhythmias (including atrial fibrillation).

When evaluating a child or young adult with a spinal cord injury, it is important to recognize that resting blood pressure is lower due to decreased tone below the level of the injury. The median systolic blood pressure for a patient with a spinal cord injury is (90 + [age in years × 2]). A systolic blood pressure of 150 mmHg or 20–40 mmHg above baseline is consistent with autonomic dysreflexia.

ED Management

Obtain IV access and place the patient on a cardiac monitor. Sitting the patient upright, with the legs dangling off the stretcher, will cause an orthostatic decrease in blood pressure. Loosen the patient's clothing and remove any anti-embolism stockings or abdominal binder, if present. Catheterize the bladder, but first apply lidocaine jelly. If there is an indwelling catheter, check for obstruction and either irrigate it or replace it. If the blood pressure is labile, apply 2% nitropaste (nitroglycerin) ½–1 inch above the level of the injury. If the above measures do not decrease the blood pressure, add nifedipine (0.25–0.5 mg/kg, maximum 10 mg), using the bite and swallow method rather than sublingually, which can cause rebound hypotension. If symptoms persist, manually disimpact the bowel, but use lidocaine jelly first. Consult with a neurologist and admit the patient if symptoms persist and no precipitant is found that can be successfully addressed in the ED.

Neurogenic Bladder

A patient with a spinal cord injury or spina bifida with resultant neurogenic bladder is at increased risk of developing a UTI due to incomplete voiding, elevated intravesical pressure, and catheter use. An indwelling catheter is the most important risk factor, while repeated antibiotic exposure increases the likelihood of resistant organisms.

For a patient with a neurogenic bladder, significant bacteriuria is defined as >10^2 CFU/mL for catheter specimens from a child with intermittent catheterization; >10^4 CFU/mL for clean void specimens from a catheter-free male using condom catheter devices; or any detectable growth from a patient with an indwelling catheter or from a suprapubic aspirate. The patient may reuse catheters, which may become colonized with bacteria and then yield confusing results. Therefore, use a clean catheter to obtain a culture specimen. If the patient has an indwelling catheter, replace it before collecting a specimen. Since chronic catheterization may cause pyuria in the absence of a UTI, use 50 WBC/hpf in an unspun urine to suggest a UTI.

Signs and symptoms suggestive of a UTI (pp. 692–693) include fever, pain over the bladder or kidney, urinary incontinence, increase in spasticity, cloudy urine with increased odor, malaise, lethargy, feelings of anxiety, or autonomic dysreflexia (see pp. 793–794).

Bibliography

Behar S, Cooper J. Best practices in the emergency department management of children with special needs. *Pediatr Emerg Med Pract.* 2015;**12**(6):1–25.

Bernabe KQ. Pressure ulcers in the pediatric patient. *Curr Opin Pediatr.* 2012;**24**(3):352–356.

Mitchell RB, Hussey HM, Setzen G, et al. Clinical consensus statement: tracheostomy care. *Otolaryngol Head Neck Surg.* 2013;**148**(1):6–20.

Powell A, Davidson L. Pediatric spinal cord injury: a review by organ system. *Phys Med Rehabil Clin N Am.* 2015;**26**(1):109–132.

Soscia J, Friedman JN. A guide to the management of common gastrostomy and gastrojejunostomy tube problems. *Paediatr Child Health.* 2011;**16**(5):281–287.

Royal Children's Hospital Melbourne. Gastrostomy acute replacement of displaced tubes. www.rch .org.au/clinicalguide/guideline_index/Gastrostomy_Acute_replacement_of_displaced_tubes (accessed June 26, 2017).

Failure to Thrive

Failure to thrive (FTT) represents an inability to maintain appropriate growth for age. It is essentially a sign of undernutrition, and not a diagnosis *per se*. By definition, a patient under two years of age is found to have a weight that is below the third percentile for age (or <80% of the ideal weight for age) or has a history of crossing two major percentiles (90th, 75th, 50th, 25th, 10th, and 5th) downward on a standardized growth chart. While weight is the usual concern, in severe cases height and head circumference can also be affected. The possible etiologies of FTT can be divided into three major categories (Table 27.3), although a patient may have more than one problem contributing to growth failure.

Clinical Presentation

Inadequate Caloric Intake

Lack of Appetite

This usually occurs in the toddler age group. The parents report a refusal of foods and frustration with their inability to get their child to eat. Psychosocial stressors, including lack of food/resources, domestic violence, and parental mental illness can play an important role. Anemia, lead poisoning, and chronic infections (recurrent otitis media) may also contribute to poor appetite.

Difficulty Ingesting

Infants with congenital anomalies, such as cleft palate or choanal atresia, as well as toddlers with poor dentition or severe tonsillar hypertrophy, may have difficulty ingesting adequate calories. Dyspnea due to congestive heart failure or bronchopulmonary dysplasia can interfere with oral intake. The parents may report that the patient seems to be exhausted during feeds and needs to rest frequently. Neuro-developmental problems such as cerebral palsy and oral motor dysfunction are some of the most common causes of FTT. In such a case, growth may be adequate in the first 6–8 months, then FTT develops after solid foods are introduced. The child often has difficulty with textures, and finds solid foods aversive,

Table 27.3 Differential diagnosis of failure to thrive

Diagnosis	Possible etiologies
Inadequate caloric intake	
Difficulty ingesting calories	Central nervous system disorder (cerebral palsy, mental retardation)
	Craniofacial anomaly
	Oral motor dysfunction
	Tracheoesophageal fistula
Lack of appetite	Anemia
	Chronic infection
	Psychosocial
Unavailability of calories	Inappropriate feeding
	Insufficient food
	Withholding of food
Vomiting	Central nervous system pathology
	Gastrointestinal obstruction
	Gastroesophageal reflux
Inadequate calorie absorption	
Diarrhea	Infection
Malabsorption	Celiac disease
	Food allergies
Increased calorie requirements	
Increased metabolism	Cardiopulmonary disease
	Chronic infection
	Endocrine disease
	Malignancy
	Toxins (lead)
Inefficient use of calories	
	Diabetes mellitus
	Inborn error of metabolism
	Renal tubular acidosis

thereby making eating an unpleasant experience. The parents report prolonged mealtimes and a preference for liquids. The patient commonly also presents with speech and language delays. An infant who was critically ill and therefore not given oral feeds during the first months of life may have difficulty acquiring oral feeding skills.

Recurrent Vomiting

Gastroesophageal reflux with subsequent esophagitis can lead to refusal to eat because of pain upon swallowing. The parents may report irritability and grimacing with feeds, but there may not be a history of frank vomiting. Increased ICP of any etiology can cause recurrent vomiting leading to inadequate intake. Gastrointestinal obstruction in an infant (pyloric stenosis, malrotation) can present as poor weight gain and recurrent vomiting. The infant typically appears very hungry since appetite is unaffected.

Lack of Available Calories

Inadequate availability of calories is a common cause of FTT, and may be due to economic problems, stresses within the family, mental health problems (maternal depression leading to neglect), and intentional abuse. Improper breastfeeding technique or mixing of formula, and feeding primarily foods that are nutritionally empty ("junk food") can result in inadequate calorie intake.

Inadequate Calorie Absorption

Once ingested, foods may be inadequately digested, malabsorbed, or eliminated too rapidly. Malabsorption generally presents with a history of failure to grow accompanied by chronic diarrhea. Enzyme deficiencies, severe food allergies, and celiac disease are possible etiologies. The parents may be able to correlate onset of symptoms with introduction of specific foods. Cystic fibrosis can cause malabsorption, usually in association with other manifestations of the disease, but FTT may be the initial presentation. Inflammatory bowel disease can also lead to chronic malnutrition through malabsorption. Diarrhea due to bacterial or parasitic infection can interfere with nutritional uptake by shortening transit time, as well as consumption of nutrients by the parasites. Hepatic dysfunction secondary to biliary atresia, cirrhosis, or hepatitis can also result in malabsorption of nutrients.

Increased Calorie Requirements

Conditions that cause increased metabolic rate or inefficient use of calories resulting in FTT typically are secondary to a disorder that is not difficult to diagnose. Chronic infection with tuberculosis (TB) or human immunodeficiency virus, malignancy, hyperthyroidism, chronic cardiac or pulmonary disease, metabolic diseases, renal tubular acidosis, and diabetes mellitus can all cause defective or inefficient use of calories and subsequent FTT.

Diagnosis

Obtain a complete, detailed history, including feeding history: adequacy of breastfeeding, formula preparation, amounts consumed, feeding techniques, patient's feeding behavior, what types of food the child can and cannot tolerate, timing of solid foods introduction, and any parentally imposed dietary restrictions such as no sugar, no fat, or vegan diet. Ask about the perinatal and developmental history (prematurity, delayed oral feeds, intrauterine growth restriction [IUGR], congenital infections, developmental milestones, child's temperament), psychosocial history (ability to buy food, household stresses such as illness or domestic violence, history of abuse or neglect, environmental exposure to lead or other toxins, and travel to areas with high rates of intestinal parasites, TB, or hepatitis). Ask about the details of the FTT, including the age of onset and rate of growth deceleration, history of diarrhea or constipation, vomiting, food intolerance, and recurrent infections.

On physical examination, observe a feeding to assess the quality of child and caregiver interaction, the quality of suck/swallow, abnormal use of tongue and lips, aversion to oral stimulation, and any evidence of pain during or after feeding. Plot the weight, height, and head circumference on an appropriate, gender-specific growth chart. Whenever possible, include previous measurements to assess changes in growth velocity. Examine an infant for dysmorphic features and congenital facial anomalies. Check the oral cavity of a toddler, looking for dental caries and tonsillar hypertrophy. Other priorities on physical examination are the cardiopulmonary (tachypnea, cyanosis, murmur, rales, hepatosplenomegaly), gastrointestinal (hepatomegaly, jaundice), neurologic (micro- or macrocephaly, asymmetry) examinations as well as signs of abuse or neglect (unexplained bruises or burns, poor hygiene, inappropriate behavior). Assess for developmental delay.

In less than 1% of patients, laboratory testing will establish a diagnosis in the absence of specific abnormalities noted on history or physical examination. If no likely diagnosis is suggested, obtain a limited battery of routine laboratory tests (CBC, urinalysis, urine culture, serum electrolytes) to ensure that there is no immediate life-threatening pathology. Further tests, such as a sweat test, chest radiograph, or stool analysis are indicated only if history or physical examination suggests a particular diagnosis.

The majority of cases of FTT in infants and toddlers represent "undernutrition" secondary to inadequate provision (quantity or quality of food) or inadequate intake (improper feeding or eating). The best diagnostic test is the response to proper nutrition. This requires very close follow-up as an outpatient or sometimes as an inpatient, with feeding supervised or performed by the nursing staff.

ED Management

The goal of ED management is to rule-out the presence of an immediate life-threatening condition, assess the severity of the malnutrition, and ensure that adequate outpatient services (medical subspecialist, speech or occupational therapist, nutritionist, family support services) and follow-up with a primary provider are arranged. As noted above, the results of a thorough history and physical usually indicate the diagnostic and therapeutic course to follow.

Follow-up

• Primary care or subspecialty follow-up in 3–5 days

Indications for Admission

• Infant <4 months with FTT
• Severe malnutrition or ill appearance
• Underlying disease which requires hospitalization
• Suspicion of abuse or neglect in a child with moderate or severe malnutrition
• Poor response to outpatient evaluation and therapy

Bibliography

American Academy of Family Practitioners. Failure to thrive: an update. www.aafp.org/afp/2011/04 01/p829.html (accessed May 31, 2017).

Cole SZ, Lanham JS. Failure to thrive: an update. *Am Fam Physician*. 2011;**83**(7):829–834.

Jaffe AC. Failure to thrive: current clinical concepts. *Pediatr Rev*. 2011;**32**:100–107.

Larson-Nath C, Biank VF. Clinical review of failure to thrive in pediatric patients. *Pediatr Ann.* 2016;45(2):e46–e49.

Rabago J, Marra K, Allmendinger N, Shur N. The clinical geneticist and the evaluation of failure to thrive versus failure to feed. *Am J Med Genet C Semin Med Genet.* 2015;169(4):337–348.

The Critically Ill Infant

Infants may develop signs of severe illness due to a congenital disorder that was not initially apparent or become ill due to environmental forces or infectious agents that produce severe disease. Establishing the correct diagnosis can be difficult owing to the variety of pathologic processes that can cause rapid deterioration in the young infant. Additionally, the initial stabilization can be difficult and requires expertise in airway, respiratory, circulatory, and neurological support. The approach to the critically ill-appearing infant demands a high index of suspicion for acute illness along with the simultaneous initiation of diagnostic and therapeutic measures.

Clinical Presentation

The clinical presentation of the critically ill infant ranges from subtle findings, including poor feeding, irritability, and minor behavioral changes, to profound derangements in respiratory, cardiovascular, and/or neurological function. A meticulous and ordered examination can help to quickly narrow the diagnostic possibilities and facilitate the timely initiation of specific therapies. Physical examination findings are summarized in Table 27.4.

Table 27.4 Physical examination findings in the critically ill-appearing infant

Examination finding	Diagnoses
General appearance	
Cyanosis	Congenital heart disease, respiratory failure, methemoglobinemia, sepsis
Dehydration/emesis	Congenital adrenal hyperplasia, gastroenteritis, insufficient intake, volvulus
Hypotonia	Botulism, sepsis
Skin	
Purpura	Sepsis, inflicted trauma
Vesicles	Herpes simplex
HEENT	
Bulging fontanelle	Abusive head trauma, increased intracranial pressure, inborn error of metabolism, meningitis
Miosis	Toxic ingestion
Ptosis/mydriasis	Botulism
Retinal hemorrhages	Abusive head trauma

Table 27.4 (cont.)

Examination finding	Diagnoses
Respiratory	
Apnea	Bronchiolitis, increased intracranial pressure, sepsis
Wheeze/rales	Bronchiolitis, congenital heart disease, myocarditis
Cardiovascular	
Bradycardia	Increased intracranial pressure (abusive head trauma, meningitis), sepsis, toxic ingestion
Poor perfusion	Congenital heart disease, hypovolemia, myocarditis, sepsis, tachyarrhythmia
Tachycardia	Hypovolemia, myocarditis, sepsis, supraventricular tachycardia, toxic ingestion
Gastrointestinal	
Distention/tenderness	Hirschsprung's enterocolitis, necrotizing enterocolitis volvulus
Hepatomegaly	Congenital heart disease, inborn error of metabolism, myocarditis
Mass	Intussusception, pyloric stenosis
Neurologic	
Bulbar findings	Botulism
Irritability/lethargy	Abusive head trauma, inborn error of metabolism, head trauma

Diagnosis and ED Management

A basic tenet when dealing with a critically ill infant is to assume sepsis (pp. 391–394) and administer antibiotics quickly. The mnemonic "THE MISFITS" for altered mental status in a neonate also serves as a useful guide to the approach to the critically ill infant. Although the mnemonic focuses on neonates with altered mental status, the broad differential outlined makes it a useful guide in the approach to any critically ill neonate or infant.

T Trauma
H Heart disease and hypovolemia
E Endocrine (e.g., congenital adrenal hyperplasia [CAH], thyroid, etc.)
M Metabolic (e.g., electrolyte disturbance, hepatic dysfunction, hyperbilirubinemia, etc.)
I Inborn error of metabolism
S Sepsis (e.g., pneumonia, UTI, meningitis, bacteremia)
F Formula mishaps (e.g., concentration errors)
I Intestinal catastrophies (e.g., intussusception, pyloric stenosis, volvulus, necrotizing enterocolitis [NEC])
T Toxins
S Seizures

Obtain the following studies:

- blood and urine cultures – preferably before antibiotics are given;
- lumbar puncture – defer until the patient is stabilized (but initiate antibiotics);
- basic laboratory tests – CBC, electrolytes, liver function tests, coagulation profile, and urinalysis;
- viral studies, if a severe viral infection suspected (e.g., RSV, HSV, enterovirus) – cultures, rapid antigen testing, and PCR (if available).

Other diagnostic studies to consider based on clinical suspicion include:

- capillary or venous blood gas (acid–base and ventilatory status), but obtain an arterial blood gas if the clinical work-up requires precise measurement of PaO_2;
- methemoglobin level (unexplained cyanosis);
- metabolic studies (inborn errors of metabolism): serum lactate, pyruvate, ammonia, and amino acids, as well as urine for organic acids;
- cortisol and 17-hydroxyprogesterone (adrenal insufficiency);
- blood and urine for toxicological testing (accidental or intentional ingestion);
- imaging studies (as indicated by the clinical presentation): chest and/or abdominal radiographs (intestinal catastrophes), head CT, skeletal survey, echocardiogram;
- EEG (seizure).

Proceed with stabilization in a systematic manner (see Resuscitation, pp. 1–28). Following an expanded "ABCDs" format will aid in stabilization and early initiation of life-saving therapies, but keep in mind several unique attributes of young infants, as discussed below.

Airway

Small neonates and infants have proportionately larger tongues, increased soft tissue, a more cephalad and anterior larynx, and a smaller, more compliant subglottic airway than an older child or adult. As a result, they are at greater risk for upper airway obstruction. Additionally, neonates tend to have a larger occiput, which results in exaggerated neck flexion and further airway compromise. When intubating a neonate or infant, also be aware that the narrowest point of the infant airway is at the cricoid cartilage. Consequently, it may be challenging to place an ETT despite easy passage through the vocal cords.

Breathing

If there is evidence of respiratory failure or insufficiency, begin bag-mask ventilation with 100% oxygen and prepare for endotracheal intubation (see Respiratory Failure, pp. 653–655). If there is coexisting hemodynamic compromise, provide volume expansion while preparing for intubation, as positive pressure ventilation may impede venous return.

Circulation

To help differentiate a primary pulmonary process versus congenital heart disease with restriction of pulmonary blood flow, perform a hyperoxia test with 100% O_2 for ten minutes (see Cyanosis, pp. 70–71). With a pulmonary process the SaO_2 and PaO_2 (by ABG) will increase by >10% and >30 mmHg respectively, while in congenital heart disease there will be minimal improvement in SaO_2 and PaO_2. Consider a left-sided heart lesion with ductal-dependent systemic blood flow (i.e., coarctation of the aorta, critical aortic stenosis, hypoplastic left heart syndrome) in an infant with poor to absent distal pulses, a gallop rhythm, enlarged liver, abnormal chest radiograph, and acidosis. In contrast, right-sided lesions with ductal-dependent pulmonary blood flow (i.e., pulmonary stenosis/atresia, tricuspid atresia) often present shortly after birth with cyanosis as the primary abnormality. Start a prostaglandin E_1 infusion (0.05–0.1 mcg/kg/min) as soon as possible and consult with a pediatric cardiologist. Continuous cardiopulmonary monitoring is essential during prostaglandin infusion as apnea is a known side effect.

A rapid (>220 bpm), regular, narrow complex tachycardia is suggestive of supraventricular tachycardia (pp. 49–54). The P-waves may be normal, inverted, or absent. In a hemodynamically stable infant, attempt vagal maneuvers.

Recognize the signs of poor perfusion, including delayed capillary refill, central and peripheral pulse discrepancy, urine output <1 mL/kg/h, altered mental status, and lactate elevation. Administer intravenous, isotonic crystalloid fluid boluses of 20 mL/kg over five minutes until perfusion is reestablished. The need to administer up to 60 mL/kg of crystalloid fluid is not unusual, and some patients may require more based on clinical picture and hemodynamics.

Disability

An infant with meningitis, intracranial injury (abusive head trauma), or certain metabolic disorders (Reye's syndrome, inborn error producing hyperammonemia) may have progressively increasing intracranial pressure. Perform a rapid neurologic assessment, looking for associated signs (i.e., altered mental status, hypertension, bradycardia, bulging fontanelle). See pp. 528–529 for the treatment.

Dextrose

Obtain a rapid glucose determination promptly in *every* critically ill infant. Treat hypoglycemia (pp. 196–197) with 0.5–1 g/kg of dextrose (2–4 mL/kg of D_{25} or 5–10 mL/kg of D_{10}). Inadequate intake, limited glycogen stores, and an increase in glucose utilization during stress states (gastroenteritis, pneumonia, sepsis) can lead to clinically significant hypoglycemia. A primary endocrine or metabolic abnormality (congenital adrenal hyperplasia, fatty acid oxidation disorders) may also lead to hypoglycemia.

Drugs

Inquire about medications given to the infant and those taken by a breastfeeding mother. Also, consider specific medications needed for further stabilization (i.e., antibiotics, intubation medications, prostaglandin, inotropes and/or pressors).

Environment/Equipment

Due to a relatively large surface area, reduced subcutaneous fat stores, and immature thermoregulatory mechanisms, a young infant is at risk for significant heat loss. Hypothermia (pp. 224–226) leads to increased oxygen consumption and pulmonary and systemic vasoconstriction, and it impedes effective resuscitation. If necessary, perform rewarming slowly. Avoid active rewarming in the post-cardiac arrest situation and in cases where severe neurological injury exists, as this may promote tissue reperfusion injury. In such cases, allowing the infant to remain hypothermic while permitting passive rewarming may be beneficial.

Check equipment for proper functioning. An acute decompensation during stabilization may be secondary to equipment failure, rather than a true physiologic change. Assume that any decompensation after endotracheal intubation is the result of endotracheal tube displacement or obstruction until proven otherwise.

Foley

A bladder catheter is necessary to assess urinary output during volume resuscitation.

Gastric tube

If the airway is secured, insert a gastric tube and decompress the stomach. This is especially important if prolonged bag-mask ventilation was employed prior to intubation. A gastric tube also plays a role in gastric decompression in the setting of small bowel obstruction secondary to acute abdominal processes (e.g., volvulus, intussusception, NEC). Gastric decompression may have an added benefit of improving respiratory mechanics and ventilation, by relieving abdominal pressure that may impede lung expansion.

Hematology/Hydrocortisone

Consider the need for packed red blood cell infusion in infants with ongoing blood loss or the need for surgery. Check for the possibility of congenital or acquired coagulopathy and treat with fresh frozen plasma if needed. Consider the need for steroid replacement in an infant with suspected adrenal insufficiency (i.e., congenital adrenal hyperplasia, hypopituitarism, adrenal hemorrhage from overwhelming infection).

Specific Diagnostic Considerations

Sepsis

Early recognition and management of sepsis is essential. Clinical signs such as altered mental status, tachycardia/bradycardia, hypothermia/hyperthermia, delayed capillary refill (>2 seconds), urine output <1 mL/kg/h, inconsistency between central and peripheral pulses, and an elevated serum lactate require aggressive resuscitation measures and administration of broad-spectrum antibiotics.

Neonatal Sepsis (Sepsis Neonatorum)

Group B Streptococcal Disease (GBS)

GBS is a major cause of systemic and focal infections in infants and accounts for 70% of all early-onset sepsis, although the incidence has fallen dramatically since the initiation of prophylaxis protocols. Early-onset disease usually occurs within the first 24 hours of life (range 0–6 days). There is often a history of maternal perinatal complications, such as prolonged rupture of membranes, premature birth, or chorioamnionitis. It may present as fulminant sepsis, pneumonia, and occasionally, meningitis. Pulmonary disease often mimics respiratory distress syndrome and may be further complicated by severe pulmonary hypertension.

In contrast, an infant with late-onset disease (range 7–28 days) often presents with fever, sometimes associated with bacteremia. Meningitis occurs in 25% of cases, and focal infections, such as septic arthritis, osteomyelitis, and adenitis, may occur. In contrast to early-onset disease, these infants do not usually have multisystem involvement.

Herpes Simplex Virus (HSV)

Most infants are infected at the time of delivery and become symptomatic at 7–16 days of life, although with *in utero* transmission the patient is symptomatic at birth. In addition, infection can be horizontally acquired, from close contact with fever blisters, whitlow, or other skin infections. Neonatal herpes presents in three forms: disseminated disease, localized CNS disease, and disease localized to skin, eyes, and mucosa (pp. 124–126).

Consider the diagnosis of HSV infection in any septic-appearing infant under four weeks of age, regardless of the presence or absence of cutaneous lesions. Infection can be confirmed by isolation of virus in tissue culture from lesions, mucosa, and cerebrospinal fluid or antigen identification techniques, such as ELISA and DFA. Polymerase chain reaction allows rapid detection of HSV in cerebrospinal fluid.

Cardiac Disease

There are two important milestones during the transition from neonatal to postnatal circulation that may "unmask" congenital heart disease: the closure of the ductus arteriosus (two days to three weeks of age) and the progressive decline in pulmonary vascular resistance (first 18 weeks of life). Infants with congenital heart disease may present with subtle symptoms such as poor feeding, failure to thrive, or irritability. Alternatively, severe congenital heart disease may present with obvious cyanosis (right-sided lesions with right-to-left shunting), circulatory shock (left-sided lesions with obstruction), and signs of congestive heart failure (lesions producing large left-to-right shunting).

Cyanotic Infant

Lesions where pulmonary blood flow is ductal-dependent (see Cyanosis, pp. 70–71) often present in the first few hours after birth. Clinically, these lesions are characterized by minimal respiratory distress, fair-to-good distal perfusion, variable presence of a murmur, a failed hyperoxia test, an abnormal chest x-ray (decreased pulmonary vascular markings, abnormal cardiac contour), and minimal metabolic acidosis. While definitive treatment is surgical, preoperative management includes restoration of pulmonary blood flow via the ductus arteriosus with the institution of prostaglandin E_1. Due to prostaglandin's propensity to induce apnea and its potent vasoactive affects, pay careful attention to respiratory mechanics, gas exchange, and hemodynamics.

Cardiogenic Shock

Lesions which obstruct systemic blood flow increase in severity and become apparent with closure of the ductus arteriosus. Clinically, obstructive left-sided lesions often present after newborn discharge with signs of cardiogenic shock, including poor distal perfusion, ashen to mildly cyanotic color, respiratory distress, severe metabolic acidosis, variable hepatomegaly, variable murmur, and a chest x-ray with pulmonary venous congestion and cardiomegaly. The diagnosis requires a high index of suspicion in infants under four months of age, as sepsis, myocarditis, and abusive head trauma can also produce profound circulatory changes. The early use of PGE_1 to reestablish systemic blood flow may be life-saving, while an inotrope infusion is often required for myocardial support.

Congestive Heart Failure

Lesions in which the natural fall in pulmonary vascular resistance lead to pulmonary overcirculation (pulmonary edema) may present in a delayed and/or indolent fashion.

Clinically, infants with significant left-to-right shunts may present with subtle complaints (failure to thrive, poor feeding, diaphoresis), moderate respiratory distress, hyperdynamic precordium usually with murmur, hepatomegaly, as well as cardiomegaly and increased pulmonary vascular markings on chest radiograph and right ventricular hypertrophy on ECG. See pp. 68–69 for the treatment of CHF.

Metabolic and Endocrine Disorders

Metabolic Disorders

A metabolic crisis secondary to an inborn error of metabolism (IEM) is a rare but serious cause of critical illness. It is typically a consequence of dysfunction, depletion, or absence of particular enzymes necessary for specific metabolic pathways. Suspect an IEM in every patient presenting without an obvious etiology, especially if there is a positive family history of an IEM, sudden infant death, or consanguinity. The infant with an IEM may present with a history of poor feeding, vomiting, failure to thrive, tachypnea or hyperpnea without obvious pulmonary pathology, temperature instability, cardiomyopathy, or what seems to be a primary neurological disorder (lethargy, encephalopathy, seizures, hypo/hypertonia) or sepsis. Because of the diversity, complexity, and nonspecific clinical presentation, the classification and thus diagnostic approach to IEM remains challenging.

   If an IEM is suspected, consult with a pediatric metabolic specialist and obtain blood for a CBC, glucose, electrolytes (anion gap), liver enzymes, simultaneous pyruvate and lactate (lactate:pyruvate > 20:1 suggests mitochondrial disorder), ammonia (urea cycle disorder), serum amino acids (amino acidopathy), and a venous or capillary blood gas. Also send urine: ketones (fatty acid oxidation disorders have small or absent ketones), reducing substances, and urine organic acids.

   Regardless of the ultimate diagnosis, the initial management of an infant with a suspected IEM consists of correction of metabolic derangements (hypoglycemia, acidosis, electrolyte abnormalities) and prevention of further catabolism by providing adequate glucose and immediately discontinuing protein intake.

Neurologic Conditions

Infantile Botulism

Infantile botulism (pp. 379–380) usually occurs in infants under six months of age. The initial symptom is often constipation, followed by signs of a descending paralysis beginning with the cranial nerves. Bulbar findings include a weak cry, poor suck, and bilateral ptosis. Loss of airway reflexes coupled with progressive muscular hypotonia often leads to respiratory failure. Treatment remains mainly supportive, although human-derived botulism immune globulin is effective when started early in the course. Avoid giving drugs known to impede neuromuscular transmission (e.g., aminoglycosides).

Abusive Head Trauma

Physical abuse (pp. 604–608) is the leading cause of serious head injury in infants. The classic triad seen includes retinal hemorrhages, subdural hematomas and few, if any, signs of external trauma. Although an infant who has been shaken can present with subtle symptoms, such as irritability and vomiting, the abused infant often presents with profound neurological dysfunction due to rising intracranial pressure. Respiratory failure and hemodynamic compromise are usually concomitant in such cases. If abusive head injury is suspected, obtain a complete skeletal survey and arrange for a dilated fundoscopic examination by a pediatric ophthalmologist, although these can be deferred until the patient is stable. In addition, on the first day, obtain photographs of any external injury, for use in any future legal proceedings, and notify social services.

Indications for Admission
- Critically ill infant, generally to a pediatric intensive care unit unless the primary process was easily identified and stabilized in the emergency department

Bibliography

Dellinger RP, Levy MM, Rhodes A, et al. Surviving sepsis campaign: international guidelines for management of severe sepsis and septic shock – 2012. *Crit Care Med.* 2013;**41**:580–637.

Opiyo N, English M. What clinical signs best identify severe illness in young infants aged 0–59 days in developing countries? A systematic review. *Arch Dis Child.* 2011;**96**(11):1052–1059.

Piteau SJ, Ward MG, Barrowman NJ, Plint AC. Clinical and radiographic characteristics associated with abusive and nonabusive head trauma: a systematic review. *Pediatrics.* 2012;**130**(2):315–323.

Rice GM, Steiner RD. Inborn errors of metabolism (metabolic disorders). *Pediatr Rev.* 2016;**37**:3–15.

Strobel AM, Lu le N. The critically ill infant with congenital heart disease. *Emerg Med Clin North Am.* 2015;**33**(3):501–518.

Zawistowski CA. The management of sepsis. *Curr Probl Pediatr Adolesc Health Care.* 2013;**43**:285–291.

The Crying Infant

On average, an infant can be expected to cry approximately two hours per day. The crying often has two peaks of occurrence during the day, with the first being in the late afternoon and the second later in the evening. Not surprisingly, after unsuccessful attempts to sooth a crying infant, parents may become distressed and seek medical evaluation. Persistent crying has been associated with maternal depression, exposure to tobacco smoke, and infant abuse and neglect.

Clinical Presentation

While the majority of afebrile, crying infants will have no apparent serious illness, there are several diagnoses that must be considered. These include colic, viral illness, corneal abrasion, hair tourniquet, gastroesophageal reflux, urinary tract infection, and constipation.

Colic

No single definition exists for colic (pp. 249–251), although the "rule of threes" is helpful: infants from three weeks to approximately three months of age with periods of crying lasting three hours a day on at least three days per week.

Viral Illness

The incompletely or unvaccinated infant presenting for evaluation of febrile crying poses challenges. Many institutions have policies requiring a full evaluation for bacterial sepsis in febrile infants (pp. 391–394). A thorough investigation is necessary to identify the source of fever.

Corneal Abrasion

Suspect a corneal abrasion (pp. 549–552) if a crying infant has scratches around the eyes. However, a history of eye trauma may be lacking and obvious physical findings may not be present.

Hair Tourniquet

Less commonly, crying may be caused by the strangulation of a digit, the penis, or clitoris by a strand of hair or a piece of thread or fiber, the so-called hair tourniquet. Use a magnification device, such as an ocular loop or ophthalmoscope, during the examination of the digits and genitalia.

Other potential etiologies include gastroesophageal reflux (pp. 291–292), anal fissures (p. 266), urinary tract infection (pp. 692–695), osteomyelitis (pp. 585–586), otitis media (pp. 143–145), thrush, (p. 93), meningitis, (pp. 422–425), intussusception (pp. 273–275), incarcerated hernia (pp. 304–306), testicular torsion (pp. 303–306), and inflicted injuries (pp. 604–608).

Diagnosis

Begin the emergency department (ED) evaluation by assuming that a crying infant has a true medical problem. Colic is a diagnosis of exclusion.

Obtain a comprehensive history, including feeding and sleeping patterns, medication changes (including those of a breastfeeding mother), and recent vaccination(s), and consider the possibility of neonatal withdrawal syndrome. Review the infant's medical record, looking for a pattern of encounters that may suggest infant neglect or abuse. While taking the history, pay particular attention to the interaction between the parents and the infant.

Perform a thorough physical examination. Document a complete set of vital signs, including weight, and inspect the undressed infant from head to toe. Priorities in the examination include the skin (rashes, abrasions, healing wounds), anterior fontanelle (fullness), cardiac auscultation and palpation of distal pulses (unrecognized congenital heart disease), abdomen (hard stool), external genitalia (diaper rash, inguinal hernia, penile hair tourniquet), and extremities (decreased range of motion secondary to trauma, hair tourniquet). If the infant has facial scratches or no other etiology is found, perform fluorescein staining of the cornea, looking for an abrasion.

In general, no routine laboratory testing or imaging studies are indicated. If the infant appears ill or if there is a concern for a serious cause of crying, obtain a CBC and additional studies based on clinical suspicion. A lumbar puncture may be required in a persistently crying febrile infant in whom no obvious etiology is identified on examination.

ED Management

The priority in the ED is to rule-out a life-threatening condition. Once that is assured, tailor the management to the specific diagnosis (refer to the specific sections elsewhere in this text). If the examination and work-up are unremarkable and a period of observation is reassuring, the infant can be discharged with close follow-up. Include in the documentation a review of the medical decision-making and discussion of caretaker counseling points.

Review the discharge instructions with the caretakers and answer their questions. Arrange for primary care follow-up within 24–48 hours. If the family seems overwhelmed with the infant's crying, respite admission may be necessary.

Follow-up
- Primary care in 24–48 hours

Indications for Admission
- Surgical emergencies (incarcerated hernia, testicular torsion, intussusception)
- Infectious disease emergencies (sepsis, meningitis, UTI, osteomyelitis)
- Cardiac emergencies (supraventricular tachycardia, anomalous coronary artery)
- Suspected child abuse
- Parents no longer able to cope with crying infant

Bibliography

Akhnikh S, Engelberts AC, van Sleuwen BE, L'Hoir MP, Benninga MA. The excessively crying infant: etiology and treatment. *Pediatr Ann.* 2014;**43**:e69–e75.

Douglas PS, Hill PS. The crying baby: what approach? *Curr Opin Pediatr.* 2011;**23**(5):523–529.

Freedman SB, Al-Harthy N, Thull-Freedman J. The crying infant: diagnostic testing and frequency of serious underlying disease. *Pediatrics.* 2009;**123**:841–848.

National Center on Shaken Baby Syndrome. The period of PURPLE crying. www.dontshake.org/pu rple-crying (accessed May 31, 2017).

Shope TR, Rieg TS, Kathiria NN. Corneal abrasions in young infants. *Pediatrics.* 2010;**125**:e565–e569.

Index